T0315340

Biomechanics of Injury

THIRD EDITION

Ronald F. Zernicke, PhD, DSc
University of Michigan

Steven P. Broglio, PhD
University of Michigan

William C. Whiting, PhD
California State University, Northridge

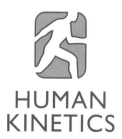

HUMAN
KINETICS

Library of Congress Cataloging-in-Publication Data

Names: Whiting, William Charles, author. | Broglio, Steven P., 1975-
author. | Zernicke, Ronald F., author.
Title: Biomechanics of injury / Ronald F. Zernicke, Steven P. Broglio,
William C. Whiting.
Other titles: Biomechanics of musculoskeletal injury
Description: Third edition. | Champaign, IL : Human Kinetics, [2024] |
William Charles Whiting's name is listed first on previous edition. |
Includes bibliographical references and index.
Identifiers: LCCN 2022023631 (print) | LCCN 2022023632 (ebook) | ISBN
9781718201590 (paperback) | ISBN 9781718201606 (epub) | ISBN
9781718201613 (PDF)
Subjects: MESH: Musculoskeletal System--injuries | Biomechanical Phenomena
Classification: LCC RD680 (print) | LCC RD680 (ebook) | NLM WE 140 | DDC
617.4/7044--dc23/eng/20221110
LC record available at https://lccn.loc.gov/2022023631
LC ebook record available at https://lccn.loc.gov/2022023632

ISBN: 978-1-7182-0159-0 (print)

Copyright © 2024 by Human Kinetics, Inc.
Copyright © 2008, 1998 by William C. Whiting and Ronald F. Zernicke

Human Kinetics supports copyright. Copyright fuels scientific and artistic endeavor, encourages authors to create new works, and promotes free speech. Thank you for buying an authorized edition of this work and for complying with copyright laws by not reproducing, scanning, or distributing any part of it in any form without written permission from the publisher. You are supporting authors and allowing Human Kinetics to continue to publish works that increase the knowledge, enhance the performance, and improve the lives of people all over the world.

To report suspected copyright infringement of content published by Human Kinetics, contact us at **permissions@hkusa.com**. To request permission to legally reuse content published by Human Kinetics, please refer to the information at **https://US.HumanKinetics .com/pages/permissions-information**.

This book is a revised edition of *Biomechanics of Musculoskeletal Injury, Second Edition*, published in 2008 by William C. Whiting and Ronald F. Zernicke.

The web addresses cited in this text were current as of July 2022, unless otherwise noted.

Acquisitions Editor: Jolynn Gower
Developmental Editor: Judy Park
Managing Editors: Anne Mrozek, Hannah Werner, and Melissa J. Zavala
Copyeditor: Heather Gauen Hutches
Proofreader: Lisa Himes
Indexer: Rebecca McCorkle
Permissions Manager: Laurel Mitchell
Senior Graphic Designer: Nancy Rasmus
Cover Designer: Keri Evans
Art Director: Joanne Brummett
Cover Design Specialist: Susan Rothermel Allen
Photograph (cover): SCIEPRO/Science Photo Library/Getty Images
Photographs (interior): © Human Kinetics, unless otherwise noted
Photo Asset Manager: Laura Fitch
Photo Production Manager: Jason Allen
Senior Art Manager: Kelly Hendren
Illustrations: © Human Kinetics, unless otherwise noted
Printer: Walsworth

Printed in the United States of America   10   9   8   7   6   5   4   3   2   1

The paper in this book was manufactured using responsible forestry methods.

Human Kinetics
1607 N. Market Street
Champaign, IL 61820
USA

United States and International
Website: **US.HumanKinetics.com**
Email: info@hkusa.com
Phone: 1-800-747-4457

Canada
Website: **Canada.HumanKinetics.com**
Email: info@hkcanada.com

E8250

In loving memory of my parents, Martha and
Clarence; and to Kathy, Kristin, and Eric.
—*Ronald F. Zernicke*

For Lily.
—*Steven P. Broglio*

In loving memory of my parents, Richard and
Charlotte; and to Marji, Trevor, Emmi, and Tad.
—*William C. Whiting*

Contents

Preface   vii

Acknowledgments   ix

PART I   Introduction and Foundations

1   Overview and Perspectives on Injury   3

Definition of Injury   4

Perspectives on Injury   5

2   Classification, Structure, and Function of Biological Tissues   19

Embryology   19

Tissue Types   21

Arthrology   45

3   Basic Biomechanics   51

Kinematics   53

Kinetics   55

Fluid Mechanics   69

Joint Mechanics   71

Material Mechanics   76

Biomechanical Modeling and Simulation   89

PART II   Tissue Mechanics and Injury

4   Tissue Biomechanics and Adaptation   99

Biomechanics of Bone   100

Adaptation of Bone   105

Biomechanics and Adaptation of Other Connective Tissues   111

Biomechanics of Skeletal Muscle   116

Adaptation of Skeletal Muscle   117

(5) Concepts of Injury and Healing 121

Overview of Injury Mechanisms 122

Principles of Injury 122

Inflammation and Entrapment Conditions 127

Bone Injuries 130

Injuries to Other Connective Tissues 135

Skeletal Muscle 140

Joint Injuries 144

Nonmusculoskeletal Injuries 145

PART III Regional Injuries

(6) Lower-Extremity Injuries 153

Hip Injuries 153

Thigh Injuries 161

Knee Injuries 166

Lower-Leg Injuries 185

Ankle and Foot Injuries 193

(7) Upper-Extremity Injuries 207

Shoulder Injuries 207

Upper-Arm Injuries 225

Elbow Injuries 227

Forearm Injuries 235

Wrist and Hand Injuries 240

(8) Head, Neck, and Trunk Injuries 245

Anatomy 245

Head Injuries 248

Neck Injuries 262

Trunk Injuries 271

Glossary 285

References 303

Subject Index 335

Name Index 345

About the Authors 349

The purpose of the first and second editions of *Biomechanics of Musculoskeletal Injury* was to explore the mechanical bases of musculoskeletal injury to better understand the mechanisms involved in causing injury, the effect of injury on musculoskeletal tissues, and, ultimately, how injury might be prevented. That fundamental purpose remains unchanged in this third edition as injury continues to be a pervasive and inevitable part of our lives. However, the title of this third edition has been updated to *Biomechanics of Injury* to reflect the expanded discussion of injury beyond those of the musculoskeletal system.

Biomechanics of Injury was written primarily for undergraduate students in the fields of exercise science, kinesiology, human movement studies, physical education, biomechanics, physical therapy, occupational therapy, and athletic training. The book may also serve as a supplemental reference for practitioners in the fields of orthopedics, sports medicine, sport performance sciences, rheumatology, physical medicine and rehabilitation, physical therapy, occupational therapy, chiropractic medicine, ergonomics, public health, and health and safety sciences.

In this third edition, the format of the inaugural two volumes is fundamentally preserved as the subject matter is enhanced by new research and updated statistics, greater emphasis on lifestyle issues and a life-span approach, new topics and technologies, updated figures, and more photographs.

We are very fortunate to have Dr. Steven Broglio collaborate with us in generating this third edition of the book. His expertise and professional experience significantly expanded key content in chapter 5 (Concepts of Injury and Healing) and chapter 8 (Head, Neck, and Trunk Injuries). At the University of Michigan, Dr. Broglio is a professor of athletic training and the director of the Michigan Concussion Center and the NeuroTrauma Research Laboratory, where he oversees clinical care, educational outreach, and multidisciplinary research aimed at answering fundamental questions about concussion prevention, identification, diagnosis, management, and outcomes.

How This Book Is Organized

In this expanded third edition, we begin chapter 1 with an introduction to the interdisciplinary study of biomechanics and explore the mechanical aspects of injury, briefly assessing the prevalence of injury in our society and the physical, monetary, and emotional costs that result.

Chapter 2 establishes the structural foundation to both appreciate the normal functions of the human musculoskeletal and neuromotor systems and understand how injury may affect these functions. The key roles of embryology and tissue development in determining the morphology and mechanical behavior of the mature human structure are explained, and we highlight the details of tissues that are most often involved in injuries (e.g., bone, cartilage, tendon, ligament, and neural structures). Because many functionally disabling injuries affect joints, chapter 2 concludes with an examination of arthrology, or joint mechanics.

Chapter 3 presents biomechanical concepts essential for understanding injury. These mechanical parameters, such as force, stress and strain, stiffness, and elasticity are explained in the context of tissue injuries. This third edition is expanded to include more in-depth discussions on the application of mechanical principles to tissue mechanics and injury. Although mathematics is inextricably intertwined with biomechanics, we keep mathematical calculations to a minimum, instead emphasizing mechanical concepts.

Chapter 4 includes an introduction to the principle of overload and how this principle applies to tissue adaptation. The chapter builds on information from earlier chapters to explain how tissues respond to mechanical loading in both normal and abnormal environments and how these tissues are tested experimentally to quantify their mechanical behavior. Because a multitude of factors affect the musculoskeletal and neural systems' responses to various forces, we discuss several of these factors, such as age, gender, nutrition, and exercise, with an emphasis on how a person's lifestyle choices might lessen the chance or severity of injury.

With a foundation in the scientific bases of tissue structure and function in place, we progress, in chapter 5, to the exploration of injury mechanisms. This third edition expands the link between basic mechanical properties of tissues and their clinical application and explores in greater depth applied topics such as ergonomics, osteoporosis, and nervous tissue injuries.

The final three chapters delve into the essentials of regional injuries. We begin with the lower extremity in chapter 6, looking in detail at injuries such as ankle sprains, stress fractures, compartment syndromes, and meniscal tears. Chapter 7 examines injuries of the upper extremity, including rotator cuff tears, impingement syndrome, and carpal tunnel syndrome. Finally, chapter 8 discusses injuries of the head, neck, and trunk, including concussion and intervertebral disc injury. With each of these three chapters, our goal is provide a deeper understanding of the mechanisms responsible for specific regional injuries in order to assist with more effective diagnosis, treatment, and prevention.

Special Features of This Book

This text includes the following features to help you understand and retain the information:

- *Objectives* at the start of each chapter highlight the main concepts.
- *Key terms* appear in **bold** in the text and are defined in the glossary.
- *Sidebars* cover special topics of interest, ranging from famous cases to closer examination of specific injuries.
- *Key Points* at the end of each chapter summarize central concepts.
- *Questions to Consider* appear at the end of each chapter to test your understanding and your ability to synthesize and apply the information presented.
- Updated *Suggested Readings* are included at the end of each chapter for students who wish to dive deeper into selected topics.

In each of the final three chapters we present a detailed exploration of a select injury in *A Closer Look*. These include new or expanded sections highlighting topics of current concern such as anterior cruciate ligament (ACL) injury, rotator cuff pathologies, and concussion.

Instructor Resources

In addition to these textbook features, we also provide ancillary products via HK*Propel*.

- *Presentation package.* The presentation package includes more than 300 slides based on the material in the book that you may use directly or modify for your lecture outlines.
- *Image bank.* The image bank includes most of the figures and tables from the book, separated by chapter, which you may use for lecture materials.
- *Test package.* The test package includes more than 190 questions in various formats: multiple-choice, true-false, fill-in-the-blank, and short answer or essay.
- *Instructor guide.* The instructor guide provides instructors with a sample syllabus and a sample course outline for organizing lectures and chapters. It also includes supplemental lecture aids, notes, and guidance. The instructor guide also presents outlines for suggested student answers to the review questions found at the end of each chapter.

Closing Thoughts

Knowledge of the biological responses of tissues to mechanical loading improves our understanding of injury and its consequences and will enable you, as a health professional, to reduce the likelihood that your clients, patients, or athletes will experience painful and debilitating physical injury.

Acknowledgments

A project of this scope involves the unique contributions of many more people than the three listed on the book's cover. We extend our appreciation to those friends and colleagues. We thank Rainer Martens and the staff at Human Kinetics, in particular the devoted efforts of Loarn Robertson, Elaine Mustain, Melissa Zavala, Jolynn Gower, and Judy Park for sharing our belief in the importance of this project. We acknowledge the hundreds of colleagues and thousands of students who shaped our philosophies, guided our progress, and provided inspiration for our professional work for more than 35 years. In particular, Ron Zernicke acknowledges and thanks two University of Michigan students (undergraduate Ishan Bhalgat and postdoctoral fellow Geoffrey Burns, PhD), who uniquely and creatively provided their perspectives and feedback on chapters 2 and 4. Most importantly, we thank our families for their support, patience, and love while we completed this project. Without them, our work and lives would have little meaning.

Introduction and Foundations

Overview and Perspectives on Injury

We must have perseverance and above all confidence in ourselves. We must believe that we are gifted for something and that this thing must be attained.

Marie Curie (1867-1934; Nobel Laureate 1903 and 1911)

OBJECTIVES

- To define and explain injury, mechanisms of injury, and biomechanics
- To explain the multidisciplinary nature of injury analysis
- To describe perspectives on injury, including historical, epidemiological, health professional, economic, psychosocial, safety professional, and scientific

Injury pervades everyday life. Although people may sustain injuries of varying severity, and some are injured more frequently than others, virtually no one is spared the pain, distraction, and incapacity caused by injury. Along with injury come inevitable physical, emotional, and economic costs, as well as loss of time and normal function.

The worldwide impact of these costs and losses is staggering. The World Health Organization (WHO 2014) reports more than 14,000 fatal injuries *daily*, which projects to more than 5 million injury-related deaths worldwide each year. As tragic as fatal injuries are, they account for only a small percentage of overall injury totals (figure 1.1).

Injury-related deaths are not evenly distributed across the socioeconomic spectrum. Accounting for population size, injury death rates are higher in lower-income countries than in higher-income countries (WHO 2014)—an estimated 90% of fatal

injuries occur in low- and middle-income countries. In reporting a systematic analysis of the "global burden" of 369 diseases and injuries in 204 countries and territories, Vos et al. (2020) also pointed to regional differences in health challenges worldwide. Haagsma et al. (2016) concluded that "injuries continue to be an important cause of morbidity and mortality in the developed and developing world. The decline in rates for almost all injuries is so prominent that it warrants a general statement that the world is becoming a safer place to live in. However, the patterns vary widely by cause, age, sex, region and time and there are still large improvements that need to be made" (p. 3).

U.S. National Safety Council (2022) estimates indicate that every 10 minutes, three people from the United States are killed as a result of injury. In the United States, unintentional injury ranks only behind heart disease, cancer, and as of 2020,

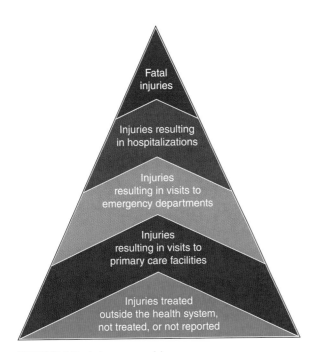

FIGURE 1.1 Injury pyramid.

Reprinted by permission from *Injuries and Violence: The Facts*, (Geneva, Switzerland: World Health Organization, 2014), 6.

COVID-19 as a leading cause of death. Prior to 2016, injury-related deaths also ranked behind cerebrovascular disease (stroke) and chronic obstructive pulmonary disease, but vaulted up the rankings based on Centers for Disease Control and Prevention (CDC) estimates from those years.

Such fatality statistics paint only a partial picture of the impact of injury. Nonfatal accident statistics are even more astounding. Disabling injuries affect more than 20 million people each year in the United States. Every 10 minutes, 885 people in the United States suffer an injury severe enough to require professional medical attention, adding up to an estimated 40 million injury-related emergency room visits in the United States in 2017 (National Center for Health Statistics 2017). (More extensive injury statistics are available on the CDC's Web-based Injury Statistics Query and Reporting System, or WISQARS.)

From the perspective of potential life span remaining and years of potential life lost, the impact of injury-related death is more significant than the impact of death from other causes. Using years of potential life lost as a measure of impact, in 2013 the NCIPC identified unintentional injuries as the leading cause of death, accounting for more than 2 million years lost, outpacing both cancer and heart disease.

Despite historically high rates of injury and significant negative consequences, all is not dark news. On a positive note, a study by Kegler et al. (2017) concluded that, "Increases in life expectancy of the magnitude considered in this report are arguably attainable based on long-term historical reduction in the US injury death rate, as well as significant continuing reductions seen in other developed countries. Contemporary evidence-based interventions can play an important role in reducing injury-related deaths" (p. 1).

Definition of Injury

As will become clear in the following chapters, many injuries have a mechanical cause. Forces and force-related factors can lead to injury and influence the severity of injury. Before delving into the multiple facets of injury, however, we will establish a working definition: **Injury** is the damage sustained by tissues of the body in response to physical trauma. This definition is less encompassing than other generally accepted notions of injury (which may include thermal, chemical, electrical, or radiation causes), but is useful in the context of the biomechanics of injury.

The term *injury* usually is associated with negative outcomes. In some situations, however, injury may be involved in events with positive consequences. In the bone remodeling process, for example, bone must first be "injured" to prepare it for subsequent positive adaptive changes.

Biomechanics is the area of science related to the application of mechanical principles to biological organisms and systems. The number of potential areas of study in biomechanics is immense. Topics as diverse as blood flow dynamics, human and animal locomotion, artificial limbs and prosthetic design, sports, and biomaterials fall under the rubric of biomechanics. The mechanical causes and effects of forces applied to the human musculoskeletal and nervous systems are the primary focal points of our text, within the broader area of biomechanics.

As we explore injury biomechanics, key terms will recur, so we define them at the outset. The first, **mechanics**, is the branch of science that deals with the effects of forces and energy on bodies, materials, and structures. Second, a **mechanism** is defined as the fundamental physical process responsible for a given action, reaction, or result. Chapters 6 through 8 examine in detail the mechanisms of many musculoskeletal and neural injuries.

Perspectives on Injury

The problem of musculoskeletal injuries cannot be addressed effectively by any single discipline examining injury in isolation. Exploration of the biomechanics of injury is an interdisciplinary endeavor that includes anatomy, physiology, mechanics, kinesiology, medicine, engineering, and psychology. In 1996, Caine et al. stated that extensive research on injury supported the notion that "we know many facts—but we lack integrated answers" (p. 1). Although progress has been made in recent decades, further meaningful progress in addressing the problems of injury biomechanics will require an interdisciplinary approach.

Those with an interest in studying injury include physicians, physical therapists, kinesiologists, prosthetists, orthotists, nurses, occupational therapists, chiropractors, osteopaths, ergonomists, safety engineers, strength trainers, athletic trainers, coaches, and athletes, each with their own perspective on injury.

Historical Perspective

As we know from lesions in vertebrate fossils and pathologies in prehistoric bones, injury is as old as life. Skeletal remains of the earliest humans reveal arthritis and fractures, suggesting that at no time have we been invulnerable to injury. The nature of injuries can provide insight into the history of an era. Some ancient Egyptian skeletons, for example, show a fracture of the left ulna, perhaps a result of self-defense from an overhead blow by a club. Today, these types of fractures are sometimes called *nightstick fractures*. Evidence of musculoskeletal disorders is commonly seen in the art of ancient civilizations (figure 1.2).

Attempts to treat the injured are nearly as old as injury itself. Archeologists have uncovered evidence of splints and primitive surgical implements (e.g., obsidian knives). Indian surgeons circa 1000 to 600 B.C., predating Hippocrates by several centuries, used instruments such as forceps, scissors, and knives. The Indian surgeon Sushruta documented diseases and drug treatments, as well as 300 or so surgical procedures and treatments for various injuries.

In Western cultures the evolution of medicine into a specialized profession with rational tenets of practice is generally acknowledged to have begun with Hippocrates. Although their knowledge of anatomy was scant and their procedures were often

What's in a Word: Accident or Injury?

Hear the word **accident** and most people envision an event that is unexpected, by chance, unintentional, or—as insurance companies like to say—an "act of God." *Accident* sometimes is used synonymously with *injury* in practical situations. However, this can be an ambiguous and misleading descriptor. *Accident* implies a degree of human error or involvement, but that is not always the case— not all accidents involve injuries and not all injuries are accidental in nature.

Robertson (2018) proffered an interesting take on the issue. He wrote:

"Accidents" refer to a very large and fuzzily defined set of events, only a small proportion of which are injurious. Any unintended, incidental event that interferes in one's daily pursuits is an accident. In writing these few paragraphs, I had several accidents in typing, but hopefully they will be corrected enough so as not to irritate the reader, and thus become irrelevant to my exposure to risk of injury. (p. 14)

Some years ago, Suchman (1961) provided a list of still-relevant indicators that increase the likelihood that an event is accidental. These indicators are the degree of expectedness, avoidability, and intention. If an event is unexpected, unavoidable, and unintentional, it likely is accidental.

No single definition of *accident* will satisfy everyone. So what should be done? Some organizations no longer officially include the word *accident* in their professional vocabularies at all. In some scientific circles, the word *accident* has been replaced with more specific terminology: What were formerly accidental injuries are now referred to as *unintentional injuries*, and car accidents are now commonly termed *motor vehicle crashes*.

In any case, as Eeyore mused in A.A. Milne's *The House at Pooh Corner*, "They're funny things, Accidents. You never have them till you're having them."

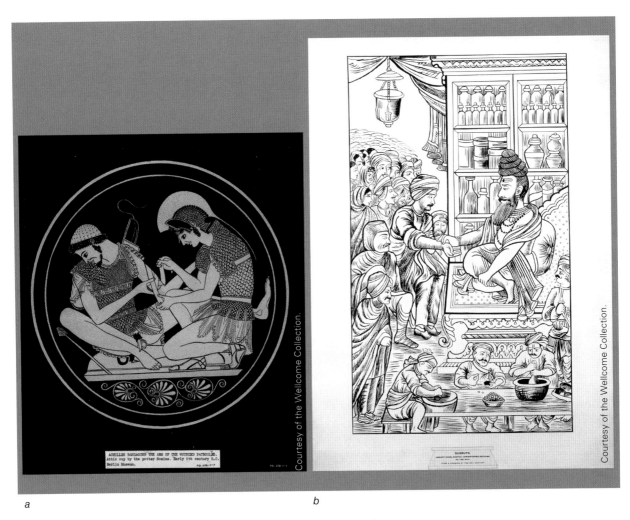

Courtesy of the Wellcome Collection.

Courtesy of the Wellcome Collection.

a   b

FIGURE 1.2   Ancient *(a)* Greek and *(b)* Indian depictions of injury and treatment.

crude by modern standards, Hippocrates and other Greek physicians established the foundations that form the basis for the study and treatment of injury today. Similar advances are documented in Eastern cultures. In China, for example, the *Huangdi Nei-jing*, a two-text set (*Suwen* and *Lingshu*), covered the theoretical bases of Chinese medicine, diagnostic methods, and acupuncture therapies.

Besides the physicians of the day who studied and treated injury, some of history's great names, often heralded for other pursuits and accomplishments, highlighted injury in some form and accorded it recognition in their work. The Greek poet Homer, in his classic *Iliad*, wrote often of trauma and treatment, describing more than 100 specific wounds and injuries (Apostolakis et al. 2010; Kayhanian and Machado 2020; Koutserimpas et al. 2017; Galanakos et al. 2015; Hutchison and Hirthler 2013; Mylonas et al. 2008; Swinney 2016).

With the decline and eventual fall (146 BC) of the Greek Empire, much of the accumulated Greek knowledge shifted to Byzantium (Asia Minor), Alexandria, and then Rome. Notable among practitioners of this era was Galen (AD 129-199). Galen's work has been credited with defining, for better or worse, the direction of medical treatment for the next 1,500 years. Among his contributions were an appreciation of the nature of muscle contraction; a fundamental understanding of anatomy (although human dissection was still centuries away); the treatment of spinal deformities such as kyphosis, scoliosis, and lordosis; and the use of pressure bandages to control limb hemorrhage (Rang 2000). Soon after Galen's death the Roman Empire declined, and with its abrupt fall in AD 476, western civilization entered the Dark Ages, virtually halting progress in medical science.

The entire world, however, did not suffer the ravages of Europe's Dark Ages. In China during the

Tang dynasty (AD 619-901), for example, surgery (e.g., orthopedic treatment of fractures and dislocations) was recognized as a special branch of medicine (LeVay 1990). During the Islamic Golden Age, Inb Sina (known in the West as Avicenna [AD 980-1037]) wrote extensively across many disciplines, including psychology, logic, theology, mathematics, physics, and medicine. His most notable works, *The Canon of Medicine* (1025) and *The Book of Healing* (1027), were used as the foundation of science and medicine in many medieval civilizations and universities for centuries.

Later, as Europe emerged from the Dark Ages, renewed creative energies were applied to medical problems. Anatomical investigation flourished, most notably by Vesalius (1514-1564), whose anatomical drawings still inspire wonder (figure 1.3). As knowledge of human anatomy advanced, so too did understanding of how the body functions.

Leonardo da Vinci (1452-1519), perhaps the best-known figure of the Renaissance, was intrigued by the nature of pain and trauma. In his art we find exquisite depictions of physical pain and agony. In his scientific writing we also find many references to trauma, especially that caused by what he termed *percussion* (impact). From his deep interest in human anatomy, da Vinci was aware that joints in the body serve as shock absorbers. Noticing that the pain produced by landing from a jump on the heels is much greater than when landing on the toes, he deduced "that which gives more resistance to a blow suffers most damage."

da Vinci had an abiding fascination with the body's senses and in particular with the sense of pain. Although he knew that pain served an important protective function, Leonardo also saw it as the "chief evil" in life, concluding that "the best thing is

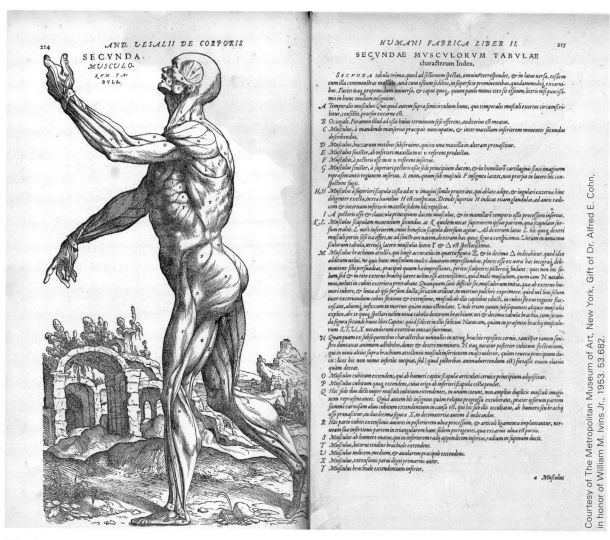

Courtesy of The Metropolitan Museum of Art, New York, Gift of Dr. Alfred E. Cohn, in honor of William M. Ivins Jr., 1953. 53.682.

FIGURE 1.3 A "muscle man" from Vesalius's *Fabrica*.

the wisdom of the soul; the worst thing is pain of the body" (Keele 1983, p. 237). The insights of da Vinci and other great thinkers of the Renaissance era may seem elementary, even naive, compared with current levels of understanding, but compared with the knowledge that was available and accepted for many centuries, their breakthroughs were extraordinary.

With the advent of the Industrial Revolution in the 19th century, medical progress accelerated. Although many new problems arose—notably injuries caused by machinery—the period brought a welcomed prospect for rapid developments in medicine. With the discovery of anesthesia and antiseptics, surgical success improved dramatically. Florence Nightingale (figure 1.4), recognized as the founder of modern nursing, also played a prominent role in introducing hygiene standards and reducing infections during the Crimean War (1853-1856). Furthermore, advances such as clinical arthroscopy, pioneered by Eugen Bircher in the early 1900s, showed the promise of rapidly developing technologies.

Progress continues today, and advancements in the diagnosis and treatment of injury show no sign of slowing. Even a few decades ago the suggestions of routine joint replacement, laser surgery, advanced imaging techniques, microsurgery, and computer- or robot-assisted surgery were viewed as futuristic specu-lation. Continuing advancements in materials science, computer technology, nanotechnology, robotics, tissue engineering, and genetic engineering promise even more spectacular advances to come. Although technological progress holds great promise, we must not forget that technology can be a double-edged sword. The technological saber swung in one direction has the potential to prevent injury and aid in its diagnosis and treatment, but wielded in the opposite direction has potential to create or exacerbate injury as well. As long as injury remains an unfortunate fact of everyday life, challenges will undoubtedly change but not vanish.

Epidemiological Perspective

Questions about injuries, such as how many, how often, what kind, and to whom, are central to epidemiology. Epidemiology is the study of the distribution and determinants of disease and injury frequency within a given human population. In most cases, the distinction between disease (e.g., measles) and injury (e.g., torn ligament) is clear. In other cases the picture is less clear, and deciding whether a malady is a disease or an injury may not be as obvious. Although we focus on musculoskeletal and neurological injuries, disease can be a contributing factor, because certain diseases may predispose an individual to injury (e.g., osteoporosis can lead to bone fractures).

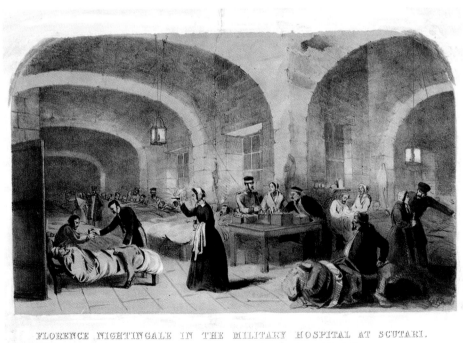

Courtesy of the Council of the National Army Museum, London.

FLORENCE NIGHTINGALE IN THE MILITARY HOSPITAL AT SCUTARI.

FIGURE 1.4 Florence Nightingale in the Military Hospital at Scutari, 1855.

Hippocrates and Injury

Hippocrates (460–377 BC), generally acknowledged as the "father of medicine," treated numerous injuries in his role as a physician and described in detail many of the orthopedic conditions he encountered. Although some of his descriptions were flawed in light of our current understanding, he successfully treated injuries on a regular basis and related his techniques and results in documentary form. Hippocrates' descriptions of treating shoulder dislocations, for example, gave numerous artists the material to depict the procedures. Hippocrates, with biomechanical insight, noted that even an old dislocated shoulder could be reduced (i.e., bones brought back to their normal position), "for what could not correct leverage move?" (LeVay 1990, p. 24).

Among the many injuries Hippocrates described were acromioclavicular dislocation ("I know many otherwise excellent practitioners who have done much damage in attempting to reduce shoulders of this kind"), spinal deformities (with vertebrae "drawn into a hump by diseases"), and leg fractures ("All bones unite more slowly if not placed in their natural position and immobilized in the same position, and the callus is weaker") (LeVay 1990, pp. 26–37).

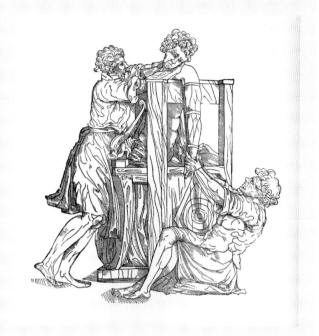

Depiction of historical technique of reducing a shoulder dislocation using a large wooden beam.
Reprinted from "Hippocrates," Wikipedia, accessed June 28, 2022, en .wikipedia.org/wiki/Hippocrates#/media/File:GreekReduction.jpg.

Hippocrates exhibited great insight in this summary observation:

> All parts of the body which have a function, if used in moderation and exercised in labours to which each is accustomed, thereby become healthy and well-developed: but if unused and left idle, they become liable to disease, defective in growth, and age quickly. This is especially the case with joints and ligaments, if one does not use them. (LeVay 1990, p. 30)

Epidemiological studies are typically either descriptive or analytical in nature. The first of these, **descriptive epidemiology,** is the most common form of epidemiological research. Types of descriptive epidemiological designs include case reports or case series, cross-sectional surveys, and correlational studies. The purpose of such approaches is to quantify the distribution of disease or injury and address questions pertaining to occurrence (how many injuries occur?), person (who is getting injured?), place (where are the injuries occurring?), and time (when are the injuries happening?).

On the surface, this process should be straightforward, and in most cases it is. However, identification and classification of a specific injury can be problematic, either because clinical manifestations may be similar although the underlying pathology differs, or because there may be multiple injuries resulting from a single incident, which makes classification difficult. Care is essential in classifying injuries so that the resulting categories are mutually exclusive (is an injury suffered in a delivery truck crash a vehicular injury or a work-related injury?), exhaustive (is there a category for every injury?), and useful (does the classification system have practical and meaningful application?).

Clear terminology is essential when we examine the biomechanics of injury. With respect to descriptive epidemiology of injury, results are most commonly reported as either incidence or prevalence rates. Many people use the terms *incidence* and *prevalence* interchangeably. However, incidence and prevalence are in fact distinctly different terms and, when one is analyzing injuries, provide very different estimates.

- **Prevalence** describes the number of cases (e.g., injuries), both new and old, that exist in a given population at a specific point in time. For example, the World Health Organization (WHO) reports that more than 200 million people suffer from osteoporosis worldwide (Kanis 2007). This equates to an overall prevalence rate of about 270 in 100,000 persons. However, the prevalence rate is much higher in older populations.

- **Incidence** describes the number of *new* cases that occur within a given population at risk over a specified time period. For example, there are about 340,000 hip fractures in the United States annually (IOF 2020), which equates to an incidence rate of about 103 in 100,000 persons, with higher incidence rates in older groups.

Analytical epidemiology involves complex research strategies to reveal the determinants or underlying causes of disease and injury. Questions such as *how* and *why* injuries happen are addressed by identifying and analyzing factors that may contribute to the occurrence of injury. These contributing factors are known as **risk factors** and are classified as either *intrinsic* or *extrinsic*. Intrinsic risk factors are characteristics of a biological or psychological nature that may predispose an individual to injury. Examples of intrinsic risk factors include physical characteristics such as gender, age, family history of injury or disease, and somatotype or body composition; performance characteristics such as muscular strength, balance, flexibility, or endurance; and cognitive characteristics such as level of anxiety, self-esteem, and self-efficacy.

In contrast, extrinsic risk factors are external or environmental characteristics that influence a person's injury risk, such as the safety conditions, programs, or the use or misuse of protective equipment within a workplace. With respect to sporting events, these factors might include the level of competition, training schedule, or weather conditions during the event. Difficulties arise in the identification of risk factors because in most situations, factors act in concert to result in injury or disease. Before a **causal association** between a risk factor and an injury outcome can be established, the factor under investigation must be examined through a multifactorial model of causation. Intrinsic risk factors are thought to predispose an individual to injury, and once a person is susceptible, extrinsic or "enabling" factors may interact with predisposing factors to increase the likelihood of injury (Meeuwisse et al. 2007) (figure 1.5). Investigators must exercise caution in assigning causal relations to injury by ruling out the possibility of mere correlation or coincidence. Much of the epidemiological information about the biomechanics of injury cannot be used directly because it is described according to circumstance (e.g., injury

Public Health Approach to Injury Prevention and Control

One valuable use of descriptive epidemiology in the community is public health surveillance. Surveillance is a systematic and ongoing collection, analysis, interpretation, and dissemination of public health information to assess public health status, define priorities, and evaluate programs set in place to improve the health of a community. Surveillance is carried out by health agencies for a number of reasons, such as estimating the magnitude of a problem, detecting epidemics, generating hypotheses, stimulating further research, evaluating present levels of health care, determining the geographic distribution of a disease, and facilitating planning and resource allocation. *Who*, *what*, *where*, and *when* are addressed, resulting in valuable information that is applicable and accessible to the public.

There are four steps to gathering this information, termed the **public health approach**:

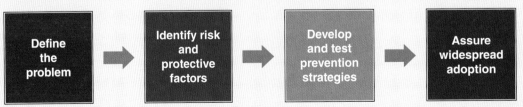

Reprinted from "Injury Prevention and Control: Our Approach," Centers for Disease Control and Prevention, accessed June 28, 2022, www.https://www.cdc.gov/injury/about/

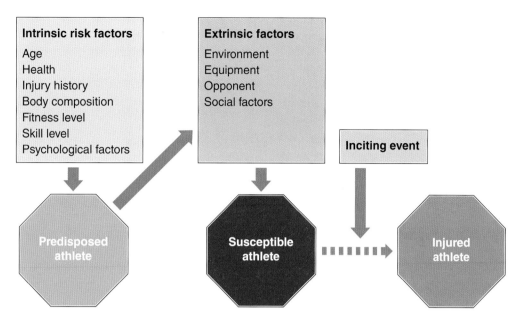

FIGURE 1.5   Sport injury risk assessment and causation: A multifactorial issue.

Adapted from Meeuwisse et al. (2007).

attributable to automobile collision) rather than by a specific causal agent or mechanism.

Recently, complex systems modeling has been used to improve our understanding of the relation between risk factors and injury causation patterns (Bittencourt et al. 2016; Fonseca et al. 2020; Hulme et al. 2019). These models seek to explore the interactions of what Philippe and Mansi (1998) termed the "web of determinants," rather than trying to evaluate singular risk factors.

Relative risk is an epidemiological measure used to quantify the likelihood of injury occurrence in one group versus another group. Relative risk is calculated as the injury incidence in group A divided by the injury incidence in group B. For example, you could calculate the relative risk of stress fractures for female long-distance runners as compared to same-age sedentary women with data for these two groups—but not their relative risk compared to other groups (e.g., male runners, sprinters, and older women). When using any statistical measure, investigators must ensure that injury rates are calculated from reliable data and that conclusions based on rates are valid. Caution, care, and clear thinking are warranted before using or accepting any statistical measures, including those for rates of injury.

These statistical data can be found from a variety of sources. The World Health Organization (WHO) reports a variety of international injury data, such as its

2014 publication *Injuries and Violence: The Facts*, as well as national reports such as *The High Burden of Injuries in South Africa* (2007). The International Labour Organization, a specialized agency of the United Nations, is another source of data through their efforts to promote safe work environments. Other global-region organizations, such as the European Injury Database (EU-IDB) and the Latin American Association of Safety and Hygiene at Work (ALASEHT), also provide a wide array of injury information.

Many countries have national organizations that gather and report injury-related data. In the United States, the National Safety Council, the Occupational Safety and Health Administration (OSHA), insurance companies, and traffic safety boards routinely collect and publish accident and injury data. Health Canada collects similar data annually for Canada, as does Safe Work Australia, the Japan Industrial Safety and Health Association, the Chinese Center for Disease Control and Prevention, and many others.

For two primary reasons, much of the available injury data are for injury-related deaths. First, the catastrophic nature of fatalities makes them prominent and definitive, and second, death statistics are easy to compile. Less attention is paid to the documentation of nonfatal injuries, especially those of a minor nature that may never be reported at all. This raises a question: What percentage of all injuries are actually reported? The answer to that question is unknown.

Certainly many injuries are never officially recorded, and therefore any published statistics undoubtedly underestimate the true injury toll.

In the United States in 2019, unintentional, preventable injury deaths totaled an estimated 173,040 (nearly two-thirds of them men), which translates to a rate of 51.1 injury deaths per 100,000 (National Safety Council 2022). In 2014, the World Health Organization estimated that on average, 9% of all mortality occurring in its member countries was attributable to unintentional injury. That percentage, however, varied substantially between high-income and low- and middle-income countries. Variation in injury-related death rates around the world is attributed to the influence of many economic, social, and cultural factors.

Deaths attributable to injury are also disproportionately higher in the young. According to the U.S. National Safety Council (2020), injury is the number one cause of death among individuals aged 1 to 44. Statistics for nonfatal injuries are equally daunting. In the United States, for example, the National Center for Health Statistics (NCHS 2022) estimated nearly 40 million injury-related emergency department visits in the United States in 2017. Virtually all nonfatal injury statistics are approximations based on hospital or commission records or extrapolations from interview surveys.

Health Professional Perspective

Many health professionals and organizations are involved in strategies to reduce the incidence and severity of injuries. In the United States, groups such as the National Safety Council, the Centers for Disease Control and Prevention, and the Consumer Product Safety Commission perform injury prevention analyses. Both Canada and New Zealand have injury prevention strategy organizations that function in much the same way. In Europe, Asia, Africa, and South America, the World Health Organization (WHO) is actively involved in similar analyses. At an individual level, safety engineers, ergonomists, safety consultants, job supervisors, health professionals, parents, teachers, coaches, and many others are in positions to stress safety and injury prevention.

Severe injuries often require immediate medical attention. Emergency medical personnel, such as paramedics, emergency room physicians, and support staff, provide life-saving emergency diagnosis and treatment. Less severe injuries may require nonemergency treatment. Physicians, athletic trainers, and other allied health professionals perform these less urgent diagnostic and treatment tasks. Many injuries, especially those requiring surgical treatment, require postsurgical rehabilitation to ensure a return to preinjury performance levels. Rehabilitation personnel (e.g., physical and occupational therapists) perform these essential services.

Economic Perspective

In addition to the physical and emotional costs, the financial costs of injury are enormous. Because public policy decisions are often based on fiscal considerations, the economic perspective of injury requires comment.

In comparison to long-recognized public health hazards such as cardiovascular disease and cancer, only in the last several decades has injury been recognized as a true public health hazard. A watershed study, *Injury in America* (Committee on Trauma Research 1985), helped bring injury into the public health spotlight and prompted the U.S. Congress to commission a study on the economic and noneconomic impact of injury. Results of that study showed that injury had a tremendous effect on both individuals and society as a whole (Rice and Max 1996).

The National Safety Council estimated the total cost of unintentional injuries for 2019 at more than $1 trillion (USD). On average, that breaks down to $118 million per hour! This includes estimates of such economic losses as employer costs, vehicle damage, fire losses, wage and productivity losses, medical expenses, and administrative expenses. If to that $1 trillion we add a similar estimated amount for lost quality of life from those injuries, the resulting comprehensive cost of injury for 2019 alone is well more than $2 trillion.

Soon after the landmark 1985 *Injury in America* study, Runge (1993) issued a challenge to health professionals to become more involved as advocates for injury prevention and control, thereby contributing to efforts to limit the present cost of injury. Because we all pay the price that injury exacts, his challenge remains germane today.

Psychosocial Perspective

The most obvious consequence of injury is the direct, physical damage to bodily tissues. However, often overlooked are the psychological and social factors that may be involved before, during, and after an injury. Collectively, consideration of all these areas has been termed a *biopsychosocial approach* to injury (Brewer and Redmond 2017). These factors can influence the likelihood and severity of injury and the course of healing and rehabilitation. Aspects of injury in which psychological factors may be integrally involved include risk behaviors and predisposition to injury, human error and accidents, theories of causation, risk evaluation, and emotional response to injury.

Ivarsson et al. (2017) performed a meta-analysis of psychosocial factors and sport injuries and concluded that psychosocial variables, along with psychological-based interventions, can influence injury risk in athletes. They specifically found that high levels of negative stress and strong stress responsivity were strongly associated with injury risk, and that psychological-based interventions reduced the rate of injuries (compared to control groups).

The likelihood of being injured depends largely on the task in which a person is engaged, the environment in which the injury occurs, and the person's psychological state. Some activities such as playing football or occupations such as oil drilling are inherently riskier than others. Certain environments, such as rugged outdoor terrain or construction sites, are more risk laden than an office environment. In addition, certain psychological states, such as inattention, distraction, fatigue, or stress, may predispose a person to injury.

Key points from a discussion of the role of human error, accident causation, and risk evaluation in injury prevention and control by Sanders and McCormick (1993) highlight the importance of including psychological factors in the overall context of injury analysis:

• Human error (defined as an inappropriate or undesirable human decision or behavior that reduces or has the potential to reduce effectiveness, safety, or system performance) is responsible for many events leading to injury. Human error leading to injury typically results from the direct action of the injured person but also may be an indirect human error, such as a poor decision made by an engineer in designing a particular product or device. Human error may be reduced by (1) selection of people with appropriate skills and capabilities to perform a particular task, (2) proper training, and (3) effective design of equipment, procedures, and environments. With regard to the third point, direct human error may be incorrectly identified as the cause of injury when the real culprit is indirect human error involved in poorly designed equipment or faulty construction.

• Many psychological theories have been proposed to explain accident causation (with due deference to our earlier comments on use of the word *accident*), including the following:

• *Accident-proneness theory* (some people are more prone to accidents than others)

• *Accident-liability theory* (people are prone to accidents in given situations and this tendency is not permanent)

• *Capability–demand theory* (accidents increase when job demands exceed the capability of workers)

• *Adjustment-to-stress theory* (accidents increase in situations with stress levels that exceed an individual's coping capabilities)

• *Arousal–alertness theory* (accidents are more likely when arousal is too low or too high)

• *Goals–freedom–alertness theory* (freedom of workers to set their own goals results in high-quality performance, which reduces accidents).

No single theory adequately explains all accidents and their resulting injuries; a more likely scenario is that a unique combination of factors is involved in each injury.

• **Risk** refers to the likelihood of injury or death associated with a particular object, task, or environment. The perception and evaluation of risk are important for determining whether an injury will occur and, if it does, the severity of the injury. Interestingly, studies indicate that although most people are quite capable of discerning the relative risk between various activities (e.g., using a computer is less risky than riding a bicycle), their ability to estimate the absolute risk is not nearly as accurate. Perception of risk may be distorted by overestimating the value of one's own expertise and experience, overemphasizing situations receiving media attention, and adopting a philosophy that "it can't happen to me."

Psychological factors are important influences before, during, and immediately following the injury and in the postinjury period, which may last for weeks, months, or even years. Although the psychological factors summarized by Heil (1993) are specific to athletes, many of the factors are applicable to general injury situations as well (table 1.1). Other factors that could be added to the list include family support structures, need to work, and malingering.

TABLE 1.1   Psychological Factors in Injury

Factors preceding injury	Factors associated with injury	Factors following injury
Medical history	Emotional distress	Culpability
Psychological history	Injury site	Compliance with treatment
Somatization	Pain	Perceived effectiveness
Life stress and change	Timeliness	Treatment complications
Sport stress and change	Unexpectedness	Pain
Approach of major competition		Medication use
Marginal player status		Social support
Overtraining		Personality conflicts
Sport-related health risk factors		Fans and the media
		Litigation

Adapted by permission from J. Heil, *Psychology of Sport Injury* (Champaign, IL: Human Kinetics, 1993), 75.

Many injuries, and certainly those that draw the most media attention, occur among athletes. The psychological profiles of highly competitive, elite athletes are in some ways different from those of the general population. These differences can be both beneficial and deleterious when dealing with injury and the recovery process. As noted by Heil (1993), the positive psychological attributes found in many athletes are high levels of motivation, pain tolerance, goal orientation, and good physical training habits. On the negative side, athletes may experience a higher sense of loss, greater threat to their self-image, unrealistic expectations, and desire for a quick recovery, and they may have higher, sport-specific demands to meet than do those in the general population.

Nixon (1992) described a "culture of risk" associated with high-level competitive athletes in which they have been socialized to accept and endure injury and pain as normal components of athletic participation, ignore pain and continue to play while hurt, and conceal their injuries. Nixon (1992) argued that "the willingness of athletes to risk pain and injuries is affected by structural features of their sports networks (called 'sportsnets'), by relations with individual sportsnet members, and by 'the culture of risk' that is deeply embedded in serious athletic subcultures (p. 127).

Whether among athletes or the general public, there is little doubt that psychological factors play an influential role in a comprehensive assessment of injury, and should be neither underestimated nor ignored.

Safety Professional Perspective

The prevention and control of injuries, although not the primary focus of this text, are integral to a broad discussion of injury, and we would be remiss not to mention the role of safety professionals, such as safety consultants, ergonomists, safety engineers, and health and safety educators, in dealing with injury and its prevention.

Injury prevention programs are typically of two types: *injury control programs* and *health and safety education programs*. Collectively, injury prevention programs apply three strategies:

1. Safety education programs seek to persuade (educate) those at risk of injury to alter their behavior to increase self-protection (e.g., to use helmets while cycling or to use seat belts while driving cars or flying in planes)

2. Injury control programs require changes in individual behavior by law or rules (e.g., enforce laws for mandatory seat belt use in cars, penalize football players who spear-tackle an opponent with the top of the helmet, and require protective eyewear while working with chemicals)

3. Injury control programs provide automatic protection by product or environmental design (e.g., airbags, passive restraints in cars, multi-directional release mechanisms for ski bindings, padding for fixed goalposts, and shock-absorbing heel materials for running shoes).

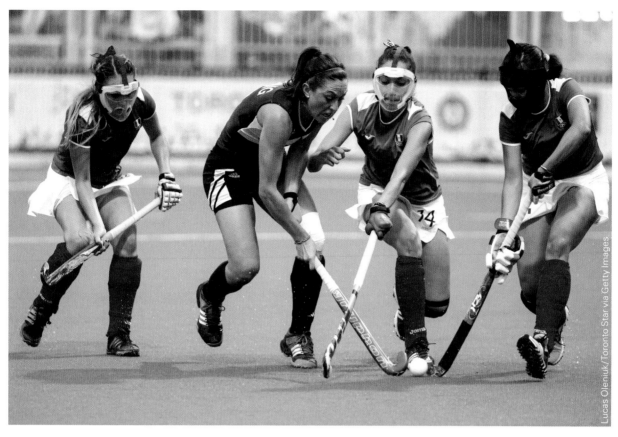

What injury prevention strategy is likely being applied in the scenario depicted here?

Of these three injury prevention strategies, automatic protection is the most effective, followed by requiring behavioral change. Persuading is the least effective of the three. Although education about injuries is important, many injuries result less from a lack of knowledge than from failure to apply what is known. Most people will acknowledge that it is safer to wear a mask as a baseball catcher or hockey goalie, but sometimes a mask is not available or the player chooses not to wear one. Health behavior research has shown that as the amount of individual effort required to adopt a safer behavior increases, the proportion of the population that will respond by adopting the behavior decreases. For example, the more difficult or cumbersome the protective equipment is to put on, the less likely players are to use it.

Education alone rarely has proven to be an adequate preventive strategy (Committee on Trauma Research 1985). The most successful attempts at changing individual behavior to prevent injuries have involved behaviors that were easily observable and required by law. For example, when laws required helmet use for motorcyclists, almost all

complied. In Thailand, for example, after enforcement of a helmet law, the number of helmet wearers increased five-fold (Ichikawa et al. 2003).

Over the past century, safety researchers have developed a wide variety of accident causation models that have sought to clarify the cause, process, and injury consequences of accidents. In a recent comprehensive review of accident causation models, Fu et al. (2020) proposed a classification method specifying linear and nonlinear models, which they divided into human-based, statistics-based, energy-based, and system-based accident models.

A final strategy for preventing musculoskeletal injury worthy of mention in this section is maintenance of personal strength, flexibility, and good physical condition. Whether in the home, in the workplace, or in sports, people with better physical conditioning and flexibility are less likely to be injured, suffer fewer severe injuries, and recover from injury faster than those who are in poor physical condition. Indeed, one of the most important benefits of regular stretching and flexibility training may be the prevention of musculoskeletal injury. Proper

WARNING: Hazardous to Your Health

Warning signs, it seems, are everywhere. Their purpose is to inform product users or people in a certain environment of potential dangers posed by the product or place. For any warning to be effective, it must be designed to include the following elements:

1. A clear statement of the danger
2. A pictogram or signal word (e.g., WARNING)
3. A signal to ensure that the person at risk senses the warning (e.g., bright colors or flashing lights) and receives and understands the message (e.g., the message must be short, simple, and unambiguous)
4. A statement of the potential consequences
5. Instructions on what to do to avoid the danger

Effective warnings can go a long way toward reducing the incidence of injury and death in both work and recreational situations.

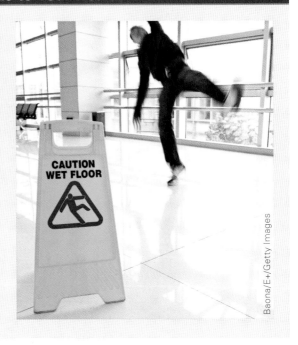

Baona/E+/Getty Images

flexibility training and pre-exercise stretching can reduce joint stiffness, muscle and tendon tightness, and exercise-related muscle soreness.

Considering the enormous numbers and types of injuries that occur, many challenges remain for safety professionals worldwide. The obstacles cross educational, legal, scientific, political, and economic disciplines, suggesting that the most effective solutions will likely be interdisciplinary or multidisciplinary in scope.

Scientific Perspective

Among all the perspectives on injury, the one that predominates in the following chapters is a scientific perspective. As stated earlier, many scientific disciplines have a role to play in a comprehensive understanding of injury. Anatomists, for example, study which structures and tissues are actually injured, physiologists examine the biological processes involved in tissue health and repair, psychologists are interested in the behavioral aspects of injury, and engineers design equipment and structures to minimize or prevent injury.

Of all the scientific disciplines, physics and its subdiscipline mechanics are arguably most central to the study of injury. The common denominator of this area of science is energy. Indeed, energy is called the agent of injury. Although thermal, electri-

cal, magnetic, and chemical energy can cause injuries, most injuries involve mechanical energy. The fundamental relation between mechanical energy and injury highlights biomechanics as the logical discipline to study the causes and effects of human musculoskeletal injury.

In *Injury in America,* the Committee on Trauma Research (1985) reinforced the important role of biomechanics research in the prevention of injury with the following conclusions, which remain highly relevant more than three decades later:

- High priority should be given to research that can provide a clearer understanding of injury mechanisms.
- Quantification of the injury-related responses of critical body areas (such as the nervous system, thoracic and abdominal viscera, joints, and muscles) to mechanical forces is needed.
- High priority should be given to defining limits of human tolerance to injury, particularly with regard to segments of the population for whom data are extremely limited, including children, women, and older adults.
- Improvement in injury assessment technology is needed, including the development of methods to assess important debilitating injuries and causes of fatality, improvement

of anthropomorphic dummies, and development of valid computer simulation models to predict injury in complex crash conditions.

- Organizations at all levels are needed to conduct research on injury mechanisms and injury biomechanics and ensure a supply of scientists trained in injury biomechanics.

Chapter Review

Key Points

- Statistics emphasize that injury is a serious public health problem that deserves our full attention, should be given greater priority, and should be addressed with combined approaches to prevention and control. Injury is a multifaceted problem, requiring a multidisciplinary approach to find and implement effective solutions.

- An accurate and comprehensive awareness of injury can be developed only by examining it from numerous perspectives. The historical perspective highlights the achievements of many individuals who advanced our knowledge in anatomy, physiology, injury, and trauma, and our current level of knowledge would not exist without the keen investigation, curiosity, and observations of these historical figures.

- An epidemiological perspective offers a chance to answer health questions both observationally (e.g., who, what, where, and when, with respect to injury) and analytically (how and why). Incidence, prevalence, and risk factors are key measures to consider from an epidemiological perspective.

- Health and safety professionals are involved with injury prevention and treatment. Injury control and safety education programs can reduce the incidence and severity of injury to some degree. Nonetheless, injuries will still occur, and thus health professionals, whether emergency medical personnel, physicians, or athletic trainers, are needed to perform essential services critical to injury diagnosis and treatment.

- The cost of injury is enormous: One must consider not only the direct costs of injury, such as medical expenses and lost wages, but also the indirect costs, such as lost quality of life. Estimated costs of injury exceed trillions of dollars per year worldwide.

- Often overlooked, but nonetheless extremely important to both prevention and recovery from injury, are the psychological factors that may affect a person before, during, or after injury. Many theories have been proposed identifying psychological state as a predisposing risk factor to injury. Additionally, psychological state after injury greatly affects rehabilitation and recovery.

- Many scientific disciplines collaborate to address etiology, affected tissues, and the biological processes underlying injury. Arguably, the scientific discipline of physics, and more specifically the subdiscipline of mechanics, is most pertinent to understanding musculoskeletal and neurological injuries and their prevention.

Questions to Consider

1. Explain why effective consideration of musculoskeletal injury requires a multidisciplinary approach.

2. Our understanding of injury mechanisms, diagnosis, and treatment has increased rapidly in recent decades. Looking into the future, if you were to write a chapter on the history of injury research from the present until the year 2040, what would you cover?

3. What are the limitations of examining injury from a single perspective (e.g., only from a biomechanical viewpoint)?

4. As an injury epidemiologist, you have been hired by a manufacturing company to investigate a recent increase in the rate of work-related injuries. What steps would you take to conduct a comprehensive assessment of the problem?

5. Consider a sport psychologist working with an Olympic-level athlete who has recently suffered a potentially career-ending injury. What factors should the psychologist keep in mind while assisting this athlete?

6. What do you see as the most important future areas of injury-related research?

Suggested Readings

Ahmad, C.S., and A.A. Romeo, eds. 2019. *Baseball Sports Medicine*. Philadelphia: Wolters Kluwer.

Caine, D.J., P.A. Harmer, and M.A. Schiff, eds. 2010. *Epidemiology of Injury in Olympic Sports*. Hoboken, NJ: Wiley-Blackwell.

Injury Prevention. Available: https://injuryprevention.bmj.com

National Center for Health Statistics. Injuries. Available: www.cdc.gov/nchs/fastats/injury.htm

National Institute for Occupational Safety and Health (NIOSH). Available: www.cdc.gov/niosh

National Safety Council. Available: https://injuryfacts.nsc.org

Robertson, L.S. 2018. *Injury Epidemiology* (4th ed.). Morrisville, NC: Lulu Books.

Schmitt, K-U., P.F. Niederer, D.S. Cronin, M.H. Muser, and F. Walz. 2014. *Trauma Biomechanics: An Introduction to Injury Biomechanics* (4th ed.). Berlin: Springer-Verlag.

U.S. Centers for Disease Control and Prevention. Injury prevention and control. Available: www.cdc.gov.injury

U.S. National Highway Traffic Safety Administration. Available: www.nhtsa.gov

Yoganandan, N., A.M. Nahum, and J.W. Melvin, eds. 2015. *Accidental Injury: Biomechanics and Prevention* (3rd ed.). New York: Springer-Verlag.

Classification, Structure, and Function of Biological Tissues

Form follows function.

Louis Henri Sullivan (1856-1924)

- To learn the embryonic origins of the body's tissues, focusing on the connective tissues that form the key elements of the musculoskeletal system
- To understand the common and unique constituents and features of musculoskeletal tissues, including bone, cartilage, tendons, ligaments, skeletal muscle, and joints
- To be able to describe the unique roles that connective tissues and skeletal muscles play during normal function and after injury
- To understand and appreciate how the anatomical structures of joints influence the ranges and planes of motion of the human musculoskeletal system

For centuries, load-bearing connective tissues, such as bone, ligament, tendon, and articular cartilage, were considered nonreactive structures, which reacted uniformly to mechanical stress. In reality, these tissues are dynamic and respond to varying physiological and mechanical stimuli—including injury. This chapter provides background on the formation, structure, and adaptability of musculoskeletal tissues (e.g., bone, cartilage, tendons, ligaments, skeletal muscle, and joints) so we can better understand the underlying mechanisms of their unique responses.

Embryology

To understand normal musculoskeletal system function and injury outcomes, we need to understand the formation and organization of body tissues. Just as woven threads form a fabric, cells, fibers, and other matrix components combine to form tissues. A tissue is an aggregation of cells and interstitia that interact to perform specialized functions.

Each tissue in the body has a unique function and a distinctive organization. To better understand how tissues are organized and how they function, it is important to understand where they come from and how they differentiate and form during **gastrulation**— the embryonic process during which a single layer of cells transforms into a gastrula containing multiple cell layers. The following overview of tissue **embryology** highlights common elements of tissues and lays the groundwork for later discussions about the role of cells in the repair and healing processes of tissues of the musculoskeletal and nervous systems.

The following descriptions are arranged in developmental, chronological order following the fusion of sperm and egg nuclei. The **embryonic stage** of human development refers to the time from fertilization to week 8, and the **fetal stage** is the time from week 9 until birth.

Fertilization of the egg (*oocyte*) by a sperm cell (*spermatozoa*) produces a **zygote** following the fusion of haploid nuclei. The zygote begins to mitotically divide in the fallopian tube 1 day after fertilization, and that division continues as the zygote travels toward the uterus (figure 2.1). Between days 1 and 4, the zygote undergoes rapid cell division by a process called embryonic cleavage (i.e., cells "cleave" in half, resulting in no growth in size) to produce a solid ball called the **morula**. This ball hollows out, fills with fluid, and "hatches" from the zona pellucida—the original membrane surrounding the oocyte. By day 5, the morula, now called the

embryo, consists of a mass of about 64 cells attached to the wall of a hollow ball shape, and this structure is the **blastocyst**. The previously mentioned "wall," or outer sphere, consists of trophoblast cells, and the dividing embryo cell cluster is referred to as the inner cell mass.

By day 8, the blastocyst is partially implanted in the uterine wall, and by day 10 two cavities have developed within the cell mass. The primitive amniotic cavity (sac) is associated with a layer of cells called the **ectoderm**, whereas the second cavity, the primitive yolk sac, is associated with a layer of cells called the **endoderm**. The embryo is where the endoderm and ectoderm are in contact (i.e., interface of ectoderm cells and endoderm cells in figure 2.2). These contiguous layers of cells form the **bilaminar embryonic disc**, which is the fundamental cellular mass that develops into the fetus.

The first traces of a primitive spinal cord (notochord) are apparent by day 16 of embryonic development. Further specialization and differentiation of cells in the embryo occur during the second and early third weeks of development. At this time, a third layer of cells, called the intra-embryonic mesodermal layer, is produced. The developing mesodermal cells invaginate and spread between the endodermal and ectodermal layers. This transformation of the bilaminar embryonic disc into a three-

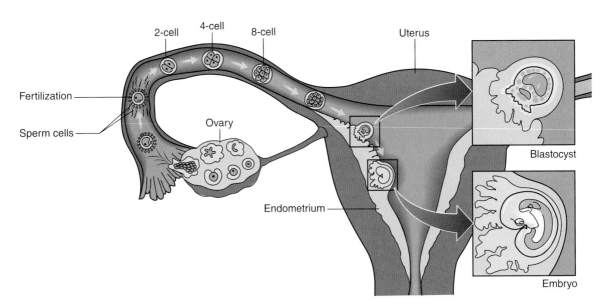

FIGURE 2.1 The zygote begins to divide about 24 hours after fertilization and continues the rapid mitotic divisions of cleavage as it travels down the fallopian tube. Three to four days after ovulation, the pre-embryo reaches the uterus and floats freely for 2 to 3 days, nourished by secretions of the endometrial glands. At the late blastocyst stage, the embryo is implanting into the endometrium; this begins at about day 7 after ovulation.

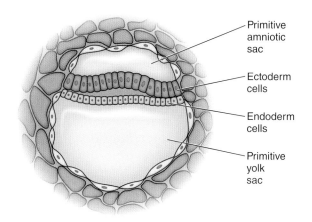

Primitive
amniotic
sac

Ectoderm
cells

Endoderm
cells

Primitive
yolk
sac

FIGURE 2.2 The bilaminar germ cell layers are shown (i.e., juxtaposed ectoderm cells and endoderm cells), as well as the primitive amniotic sac (associated with the ectoderm) and the primitive yolk sac (associated with the endoderm).

layered disc containing the three primary germ layers—ectoderm, **mesoderm**, and endoderm—is called *gastrulation*. By day 20 there is evidence of the formation of distinct neural structures (i.e., plate, groove, and folds).

The **somites** are cuboidal bodies that form distinct surface ridges and influence the external contours of the embryo. By the beginning of week 4 following fertilization, the ventral and medial walls of the somites show highly proliferative activity, become polymorphous in shape, congregate, and migrate toward the notochord. Collectively, the cluster of migrating cells is known as the **sclerotome**. After the sclerotome has condensed near the notochord, the remaining wall of the somite (i.e., dorsal aspect) gives rise to a new layer of cells called the **dermatome**. Cells arising from the dermatome form a tissue known as the **myotome**, which gives rise to the musculature. The chronology of key embryological events is presented in table 2.1.

The undifferentiated cells of the sclerotome form a loose tissue known as **mesenchyme** (primitive connective tissue). Mesenchyme is the precursor tissue of numerous adult connective tissues, such as cartilage, ligaments, fascia, tendons, blood cells, blood vessels, skin, bone, and muscle. One of the primary attributes of mesenchymal cells (**stem cells**) is their ability to differentiate into a variety of specialized cells among connective tissue types; thus, they are called **pluripotent**. They may become fibroblasts (associated with the formation of elastic or collagen fibers), chondroblasts (involved in the formation of cartilage matrix), or osteoblasts (associated with bone extracellular matrix).

Tissue Types

Tissue is classified as one of four types: epithelial, nervous, connective, or muscle (figure 2.3). These types of tissue and their structures and functions will be discussed in the following sections.

Epithelial Tissue

Epithelial tissue is a covering (lining) tissue that can be specialized to absorb, secrete, transport, excrete, or protect the underlying organ or tissue. Most of the epithelial tissues of the body are derived from the endoderm and the ectoderm. Epithelial membranes consist entirely of cells and have no capillaries, but they are nourished by secretions from nearby capillaries of connective tissues. These membranes are not strong and are typically bound firmly to connective tissue separated by a thin layer of material called a **basement membrane**, composed of a basal and reticular lamina.

Epithelial tissue is subject to wear, and its cells are constantly being lost and regenerated. Structurally, the number of cell layers and the arrangement of the cellular shapes provide the generic names of epithelial tissues. For example, a single layer of cells is described as *simple*. Tissue with two or more layers of cells is *stratified*. For cell shape, the usual categories include squamous, cuboidal, and columnar. For

TABLE 2.1 Chronology of Key Events in Early Embryology

Days after fertilization	Event
5	Cells arranged into blastocyst
8	Blastocyst partially implanted into uterine wall
10	Two cavities form within cell mass
16	Notochord forms
20	Evidence of distinct neural structures and somites

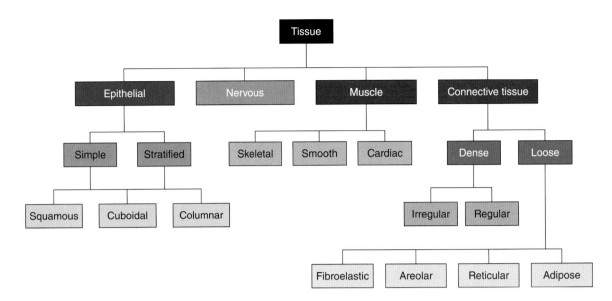

FIGURE 2.3 Organizational relations of tissue types.

example, an epithelial tissue could be classified as simple cuboidal or stratified squamous. Figure 2.4 illustrates four types of epithelial cells.

The layered or columnar arrangement of epithelial cells is mechanically weak. Epithelial tissues, however, play a prominent role in the diffusion of tissue fluid and heat and in bioelectric conduction.

Nervous Tissue

Nervous tissue, a second type of tissue, develops from the ectoderm. It comprises the main parts of the nervous system, including the brain, spinal cord, peripheral nerves, and sensory organs. The basic unit of nervous tissue is the **neuron**, or nerve cell. Communication, a vital feature of nervous tissue, is achieved through the movement of ions or other chemical messengers, thus allowing **irritability** (capacity to react to chemical or physical agents) and **conductivity** (ability to transmit impulses from one location to another). Nerve impulses are received by **dendrites** (fingerlike projections near the proximal end of the neuron), conducted toward the cell body and summed, and—if an action potential is generated—carried away from the cell body by the axon (the longer distal portion of the neuron). Nerve tissue can be injured by excessive tension (stretching) or compression because its prime physiological function is not load-bearing.

Connective Tissue

Connective tissues are aggregate materials consisting of cells, fibers, and other macromolecules embedded in a matrix that can also contain tissue fluid. The principal fibers in connective tissues are **collagenous**, **reticular**, and **elastic fibers**, although collagenous and reticular fibers are basically different forms of the collagen protein—types I and III, respectively (Nezwek and Varacallo 2019). Connective tissue is derived from the mesoderm but differs from the other three types of tissue primarily in the amount of extracellular substance. Connective tissue cells are soft, easily deformable structures that are mostly vascular (other than cartilage, tendons, and ligaments). Alone, they would be unable to transmit substantial loads, but the **extracellular matrix** that holds the connective tissues together gives them form and allows the tissues to transmit load. The ratio of cells to extracellular matrix and the composition of the matrix establish the physical characteristics of the connective tissue. The composition of the matrix can range from a relatively soft, gel-like substance (e.g., skin or ligament) to rigid (e.g., bone). A primary role of the cells in bone, cartilage, tendons, and ligaments is to produce and maintain the extracellular matrix. The arrangement and packing density of fibers distinguish these dense connective tissues, detailed in later sections of this chapter, from loose connective tissues.

Loose connective tissues are more prevalent than dense connective tissues and have four basic types: fibroelastic, areolar, reticular, and adipose tissues. All of these tissues contain some elastic fibers that provide flexibility to the tissues. Collagen fibers

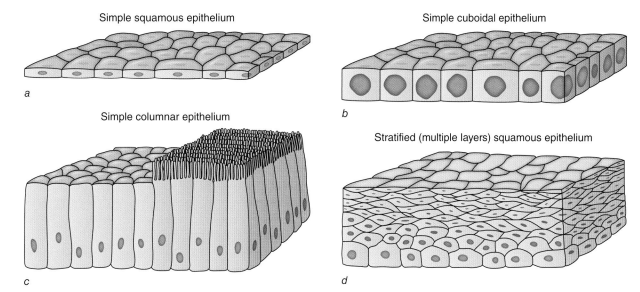

FIGURE 2.4 Examples of cellular shapes and arrangements of various types of epithelial tissue. *(a)* Simple squamous epithelium contains platelike cells organized in a single layer that adhere closely to each other by their edges to allow simple diffusion (i.e., alveoli in the lungs). *(b)* Simple cuboidal epithelium and *(c)* simple columnar epithelium may appear similar on the surface. From the side (e.g., *b* compared to *c*), however, the heights of these cell types are substantially different—one being essentially a cube arrangement and the other being a much taller column, which may or may not have hairlike cilia attached. *(d)* Stratified squamous epithelium consists of multiple layers—should some slough off when in contact with the environment (i.e., the mouth)—ranging from deep cuboidal or columnar cells to irregularly shaped polyhedral cells to superficial layers consisting of thin squamous cells.

are also evident in the tissues, along with a liquid extracellular matrix that bathes and nourishes the cells and fibers.

Fibroelastic tissue is a loose, woven network of fibers that covers most organs. The degree of flexibility of loose connective tissue is related to the organization of the collagen fibers. The tissue as a whole can be stretched without initially deforming the fibers. Because the collagen in loose connective tissue is configured as a mesh, the mesh is first deformed (slack), then the fibers are aligned before the individual collagen fibers are stretched elastically. This contrasts with dense fibrous connective tissues, such as tendon, in which the collagen is arranged in parallel rows. Because the tendon collagen is already more aligned with the tensile load, the fibers more quickly resist the applied tensile load. After a load deforms fibroelastic tissue, elastic fibers help return the stretched connective tissue back to its original position when the load is released.

Areolar tissue permeates almost every area of the body to bind different tissue types together (i.e., skin to muscle and the space between organs) for slight insulation and protection. The tissue is called *areolar* because this area is characterized by spaces or holes where only fluid extracellular matrices exist

(i.e., interstitial fluid between organs). Fibroblasts and macrophages are abundant and collagenous, and some elastic and reticular fibers give limited structural strength to areolar tissue. Nonetheless, areolar tissue is a weak connective tissue and can be easily pulled apart. Reticular network fibers act as a boundary between areolar connective tissues and other structures.

Reticular tissue contains reticular fibers and some primitive cells and thus resembles early mesenchymal tissues. The primitive cells within reticular tissue can differentiate into fibroblasts, macrophages, and even some plasma cells. Reticular tissue is found near lymph nodes and in bone marrow and the liver and spleen. Reticular fibrils are also found in many other areas of the body, such as around nerves, muscles, and blood vessels, as well as the **stroma** of organs.

Adipose tissue is the fourth type of loose connective tissue. Microscopically, this tissue appears as a collection of fat cells surrounded by areolar tissue. Each adipose cell has a fat droplet. Any loose connective tissue can accumulate fat, and when it predominates, the term *adipose tissue* is used. Reticular fibers enclose each fat cell, and capillaries are found between the cells. The rich vascularity is consistent with the elevated metabolism of adipose tissue. It can be mobilized for use in the body when carbohydrates are not immediately available and is readily stored when not needed. Adipose tissue is commonly found around the organs in the abdominal cavity, under the skin, and in bone marrow. When present under the skin, it may prevent heat dissipation and act as a cushion for the skeleton during external impacts. In adults, adipose tissue is primarily white and serves primarily for triglyceride storage. However, in young children, adipose tissue tends to appear brown due to an elevated mitochondrial density. The higher rates of adenosine triphosphate (ATP) production associated with brown adipose tissue is associated with greater heat production, allowing greater temperature control in young children.

Constituents of Connective Tissues

Cells, extracellular matrix (including fibers and matrix glycoproteins), and tissue fluid are the structural elements of connective tissues. The specific constituents of bone, cartilage, tendon, and ligament are discussed later in this chapter; here we present only the generic components of these tissues.

Cells Several cell types exist within connective tissues. They are classified as either **resident cells** (fixed) or **migratory cells** (wandering) (Fawcett and Raviola 1994). Resident cells are relatively stable within a tissue, and their role is to produce and maintain the extracellular matrix.

Undifferentiated mesenchymal stem cells are resident cells that can differentiate into a variety of connective tissue cells, including fat cells (**adipocytes**). An important characteristic of mesenchymal cells is that they can differentiate into fibroblasts, chondroblasts, or osteoblasts. Subsequently, chondroblasts and osteoblasts mature into chondrocytes

and osteocytes. Fibroblasts are the principal cells in many fibrous connective tissues. Their function includes the formation of fibers as well as other components of the extracellular matrix.

The migratory cells that enter connective tissue (e.g., macrophages, monocytes, basophils, neutrophils, eosinophils, mast cells, lymphocytes, and plasma cells) travel via the bloodstream. These cells are usually associated with the tissue's reaction to injury through the initiation and regulation of an immune response and inflammation. The numbers of these cells in connective tissues are quite variable, but two types of cells warrant further mention.

The first type, **macrophages**, contain vacuoles (empty reservoirs) and lysosomes that can accumulate and break down foreign material, old red blood cells, and bacteria. Because of this ability, the macrophage is part of a larger phagocytic ("cell-eating") system, the reticuloendothelial system, a major defense system in the body. The second type, **mast cells**, are relatively large cells that contain substantial amount of cytoplasm. The many granules in their cytoplasm are thought to contain **heparin**, which acts as a blood anticoagulant. **Histamine** (a vasodilator) and **serotonin** (a vasoconstrictor) may also be present in mast cells.

Extracellular Matrix The extracellular matrix in connective tissues is a blend of components, including protein fibers (**collagen and elastin**), simple and complex matrix glycoproteins, and tissue fluid, all of which interact and contribute to the mechanical properties (e.g., stiffness and strength) of connective tissues. The extracellular matrix can be attached or linked with cells via transmembrane **integrin** proteins, and those interactions may be involved in **mechanotransduction** (i.e., conversion of mechanical stimuli into biological responses).

Fibroblast Versus Fibrocyte

Mesenchymal cells are the undifferentiated progenitors of connective tissue cells. Fawcett and Raviola (1994) explained that the suffix—blast (derived from the Greek *blastos*, meaning *germ*) is frequently used to refer to the immature stages of some cell types. The term *fibroblast* has been used to describe the undifferentiated stage of a fibrocyte. In turn, the term fibrocyte is used to indicate the relatively quiescent and mature phase of the cell's development. That is a misnomer, however. Fibroblast already means a "fiber-forming" cell. Because the mature fibroblast is the principal site of collagen and elastin biosynthesis, it is not necessary to change the name to fibrocyte when the cell becomes mature. Although there is some difference of opinion, generally it is agreed that the terms *fibroblast* and *fibrocyte* are interchangeable; fibroblast is the preferred term, but fibrocyte is permissible. In the remainder of this text, we use only the term **fibroblast** to refer to this mature cell.

Collagen is the most abundant protein in the animal world and constitutes more than 30% of the total protein in the human body (Eyre 2004; Parry and Squire 2005). The fundamental unit of collagen is the tropocollagen molecule. The molecule is made from three spiraled polypeptide chains of about 1,000 amino acids that are intertwined to form a triple helix. Parallel rows of tropocollagen form microfibrils, and these microfibrils aggregate in a parallel fashion into fibrils (figure 2.5). Collagen fibrils are aligned into bundles to form collagen fibers. The stability of the collagen fibers can be enhanced with the formation of collagen crosslinks both within and between the collagen molecules (although excessive cross-linking makes the collagen overly stiff and inextensible). These fibers are present in varying amounts in all types of connective tissue. The organization of collagen fibers is tissue specific and can range from a relatively random arrangement of fibers in loose connective tissue to a very organized and parallel arrangement in dense regular connective tissues. All of the key cells of connective tissue (fibroblasts, chondroblasts, chondrocytes, osteoblasts, and osteocytes) are able to produce collagen.

Collagen is an umbrella term; at least 28 types of collagen have been reported (Ricard-Blum 2011). Collagen is classified according to its molecular organization as type I, type II, type III, and so forth. Type I collagen, which comprises 90% of collagen in humans, is found in skin, bone, tendon, ligament, and cornea. Type II collagen is primarily found in cartilage, and type III is most abundant in loose connective tissue, the dermis of the skin, and blood vessel walls.

Elastic fibers are comprised of elastin protein and microfibrils, which are aggregated into small bundles and embedded within a relatively amorphous elastin. They are more slender and extensible than collagen fibers, and can be stretched to about 150% of their original length before the fiber ruptures (Fawcett and Raviola 1994). The chemical composition of elastin has some components that are similar to collagen.

Besides the collagen and elastic fibers, another major protein fraction of the extracellular matrix is complex glycoproteins. Glycoproteins occupy the spaces between fibers and constitute the so-called *ground substance* of connective tissues. These complex matrix glycoproteins are negatively charged and hydrophilic (attract water molecules), attributes that have significant effects on the mechanical behaviors of connective tissue. One type of glycoprotein is a proteoglycan, a protein to which one or more specialized carbohydrate side chains (glycosaminoglycans) are attached (Lo et al. 2003; Silver and Bradica 2002).

In addition to proteoglycans, other specialized glycoproteins can also be found in the connective tissue matrix. These are called cell-associated glycoproteins, because they are important for the aggregation of cells. One type, fibronectin, plays an important role in cell migration. Cells involved with tissue repair can also use fibronectin as a stable attachment site during the repair process. Other types of cell-associated glycoproteins include chondronectin, which helps to stabilize the chondrocyte in its matrix (Lo et al. 2003).

Tissue Fluid   Tissue fluid is a filtrate of the blood and resides in the intercellular (interstitial) spaces. It aids in the transport of materials (e.g., nutrients,

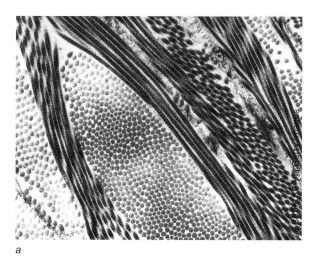

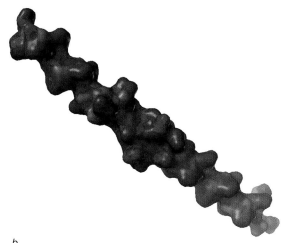

a   *b*

FIGURE 2.5   *(a)* Transverse collagen sections, ×26,000 magnification. *(b)* Structure of collagen.

trophic factors, and wastes) between the capillaries and cells in the extracellular matrix. The tissue fluid carries nutrients and oxygen to the cells by diffusing through the arterial end of the capillary (filtration). Moving in the opposite direction, the fluid either returns wastes to the venous end of the capillary for removal by the blood (reabsorption), or wastes are disposed of by the lymphatic system. The latter provides channels and filtering points (lymph nodes and spleen) to cleanse the tissue fluid before it is returned to the bloodstream. If blockage occurs in the lymphatics, the tissue fluid is trapped in the intercellular spaces, and edema (tissue swelling) results.

Tissue fluid is retained in the interstitial spaces of the intertwined proteoglycans and glycosaminoglycans. The interaction of the fluid with these macromolecules gives the extracellular matrix its gel characteristics and contributes to the mechanical behavior of the tissue.

Bone

Bone is one of the hardest and strongest specialized connective tissues in the body. The skeleton of humans and other vertebrates protects vital organs, serves as a mineral (calcium) storehouse, houses bone marrow hematopoietic cells (for formation of red blood cells), and provides levers that contribute to muscular generation and control of force production and movements. Bone is a dynamic structure that perpetually remodels and responds to alterations in mechanical loading, circulating hormone levels, and serum (blood plasma without clotting factors) calcium levels. Each of these factors is synergistically interrelated, and the anatomy of a bone reflects the interaction of these factors. One key feature of bone (and other connective tissues) is the altered response of the tissue to varying types of mechanical loading. For example, a bone subjected to tension (stretching) will react differently and fracture under a smaller load than a bone subjected to compression (compacting).

Bone can be studied as an organ, as a tissue, or at the cellular level, because it is a functional unit at each of these organizational levels. As an organ, bone accounts for a substantial percentage of the total body mass and is involved with metabolic processes such as **hematopoiesis** (formation of blood cells) and triglyceride storage. Bone tissue can be classified either as **cortical bone** (also called **compact bone**) or **trabecular bone** (also called **cancellous bone** or **spongy bone**). Although cortical bone and trabecular bone have the same cells, their mechanical behavior and adaptive responses are different. Cortical bone is the hard exterior, and trabecular bone provides internal structure and resists compressive loads. Persons with lower bone mineral density or osteopenia have lesser amounts of trabecular bone, leading to more fractures. Many types of cells are found in bone tissue, and these cells function interactively to maintain bone as a tissue and an organ.

Bone Development   Skeletal development begins when mesenchymal cells from the mesodermal germ layer condense. In certain bones (cranium and facial bones and, in part, ribs, clavicle, and mandible), the cellular condensations form fibrous matrices that subsequently ossify (form bone tissue) directly (**intramembranous ossification**). Figure 2.6 illustrates elements of ossification, which starts with the differentiation of mesenchymal cells into osteoblasts, which then secrete bone matrix (e.g., type I collagen). When the bone extracellular matrix

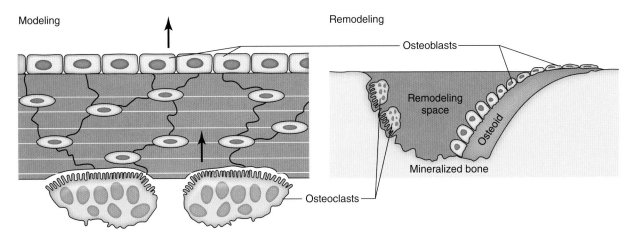

FIGURE 2.6   Intramembranous ossification.

calcifies, distinct **canaliculi** (channels) are left intact to permit communication between osteocytes.

In most limb and axial bones (e.g., cranium, vertebral column, and sacrum), mesenchymal condensations form a cartilaginous model (**anlage**) of the bones rather than proceeding directly to calcification and ossification. **Endochondral ossification** (figure 2.7) proceeds from the center of the bone towards the epiphyses (ends) during long-bone development through a cartilaginous **growth plate** (**physis**). Long bones typically have two physes (one at each end), although some bones (e.g., metacarpals) may only have one functional physis. Should the bone have two physes, there may be a dominant physis of the two, resulting in unequal growth rates (e.g., distal femoral physis and proximal humeral physis).

Longitudinal growth occurs when tissue is added to the **metaphyseal** side of the physis and also occurs through activity of the chondrocytes within three functionally distinct regions of the growth plate: the proliferation and growth region, maturation region, and transformation region.

Proliferation and Growth Region

- *Zone 1.* The region of proliferation and growth contains two types of chondrocytes. In zone 1, resting cells lie closest to the epiphyses and secondary ossification center. These cells are associated with the small arterioles and capillaries from the epiphyseal vessels, which are important in transporting undifferentiated cells to add to the pool of resting cells.

- *Zone 2.* Away from the resting cells is an area of active cell division. In this area, the cells are organized in longitudinal columns along the axis of the bone, and during a period of rapid growth the columns may account for more than half the height of the growth plate (Ogden et al. 1987).

Maturation Region

- *Zone 3.* Moving away from the epiphyses, the region of maturation is associated with hypertrophic (growing) chondrocytes that actively synthesize and secrete cartilaginous extracellular matrix for load bearing. Cells adjacent to the region of growth and ossification are large and actively produce matrix components, whereas the cells nearest the ossification front become trapped in the rapidly calcifying cartilage and, therefore, cannot be as active in matrix production.

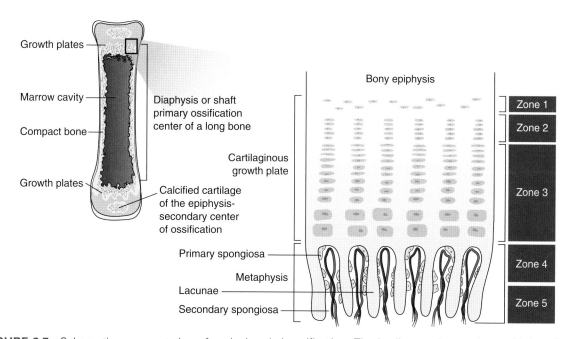

FIGURE 2.7 Schematic representation of endochondral ossification. The hyaline cartilage anlage with its primary ossification center is shown on the left. The transitional zones (1-5), ranging from a site of cell proliferation, through hypertrophy, to cell death and ossification. The active growth region is the primary site of bone accretion and, thus, is the primary site for long-bone growth.

Transformation Region

- *Zone 4.* The transformation region is where the cartilage matrix becomes increasingly calcified. The calcification of the matrix leads to the death of the chondrocytes (cartilage-forming cells).

- *Zone 5.* Here, only large empty spaces (lacunae) remain where the chondrocytes once resided. That lattice of calcified cartilage is known as the primary spongiosa. Blood vessels invade that lattice, perfuse the lacunae, and deliver cells of monocytic origin (septoclasts and osteoclasts) that degrade the calcified cartilage, as well as cells that secrete bone matrix (osteoblasts) to replace the degraded calcified cartilage. At that time, metaphyseal trabeculae are referred to as secondary spongiosa. Eventually, all of the cartilaginous trabeculae are replaced by bone. Simultaneously, bone grows in circumference as the perichondrium surrounding zone 5 thickens and lays down a thin layer of osteoid (bone) tissue that subsequently mineralizes, forming a bony collar (periosteal collar) at the midshaft level. Vascular channels penetrate the central region and bony collar, ultimately forming the **primary ossification center**. Ossification proceeds quickly toward the ends to form the bone diaphysis and metaphysis.

An important anatomical region within the developing long bone is the **zone of Ranvier**, found at the cortical margins of the growth plate toward the primary ossification center (Ogden and Grogan 1987). This complex zone is where the increase in metaphyseal diameter occurs during growth. Therefore, if trauma damages the zone of Ranvier, the normal circumferential growth of the long-bone metaphysis can be disrupted.

In the epiphyseal regions, the vascular channels directly invade the cartilage, which subsequently ossifies and forms **secondary ossification centers**. Vascular perfusion is an integral step in the formation of the primary and secondary ossific centers, because the blood supply ensures the arrival and subsequent differentiation of osteogenic precursor cells (Zelzer et al. 2004).

Between the bone formed by the primary and secondary ossification centers, the cartilage anlage persists as a physis between the shaft and ends of the long bone. As growth proceeds, the physes typically change from a relatively flat plate dividing the epiphysis and metaphysis to a complex series of curves and interdigitating epiphyseal and metaphyseal ridges and valleys. That change in geometry has significant implications for resistance to fracture. Cartilage can withstand large compressive loads but cannot withstand large shear and tensile loads. Because of that, physeal injuries in which the epiphysis "shears" off the metaphysis (e.g., slipped capital femoral epiphysis) are common in young children. The interdigitations in the physes that come about with growth may help prevent those shearing injuries by locking the epiphysis and metaphysis together, like two puzzle pieces that become harder to separate once connected.

Eventually, over many years, chondrocyte differentiation and proliferation slow in the regions of growth and maturation, allowing the bone mineralization (from the plate shaft edge) to catch up. This unites the bone formed by the primary and secondary centers, epiphyseal and metaphyseal vascularity, and marks the culmination of long-bone growth. That process is known as epiphyseal plate **closure**, culminating in the end of longitudinal growth. Physeal closure typically occurs 2 to 3 years earlier in girls than it does in boys, which can contribute to the shorter stature of women relative to men.

It is worth noting that both intramembranous and endochondral ossification can occur in the same bone. For example, the shaft of the clavicle is formed by intramembranous ossification, but a secondary ossification center develops within a cartilaginous epiphysis to form the sternal end of the bone. A primary ossification center is present in most bones at birth, but the secondary ossification center of the distal femur is the only secondary center present at birth and is often used to identify a full-term fetus. Both the endochondral and intramembranous ossification processes persist postnatally and are similar to those during fracture repair (endochondral) and periosteal bone deposition (intramembranous).

Movement and its related forces during skeletal development are among the stimuli that can influence the final skeletal form. Carter and colleagues (2004) proposed that the regulation of skeletal biology by mechanical forces is accomplished by the transfer of strain (deformation) energy that changes the length of the bone. To that end, they suggested that repeated shear (transverse) stresses generated during movement accelerate the rate of chondrocytic death and ossification, whereas compressive stresses tend to slow the same sequence. Carter and colleagues proposed that some of the energy imparted to the skeletal structures during movement is stored within the tissue and later released during unloading, as characteristic with most tissues. The remaining energy is transferred to the tissue in the form of heat or a change in internal energy. This latter form of energy transfer may be an important factor in a bone's ability to recognize and respond to mechanical stresses.

Extrinsic factors, such as hormones, influence the rate and extent of long-bone growth. Thyroxine, growth hormone, and testosterone can all stimulate cartilage cell differentiation in the growth plate. Estrogen exerts a greater stimulatory influence on the bony tissue while suppressing cartilage growth. The differential influences of testosterone and estrogen may account for the differences in the timing of epiphyseal plate closure between boys and girls.

Normal skeletal growth can also be interrupted by trauma or fracture. Physeal injuries account for approximately 15% of all fractures in children. Girls are more prone to physeal injury from 9 to 12 years of age, whereas boys are more prone between the ages of 12 and 15 years (Ogden 2000a). The periods of increased incidence of fracture correspond to the times of rapid growth, during which hormone-mediated changes in the growth plate cartilage may alter the response of the cartilage to mechanical stress (Sands et al. 2003). Most pediatric fractures are classified according to a system developed by Salter (Ogden 2000b). The system considers the location of the fracture, whether the fracture disrupts the growth plate, and the extent of the growth plate damage. Growth disturbances may result if the fracture and subsequent callus formation stimulate the premature closure of the growth plate, thereby preventing the normal longitudinal growth of the bone. Angular deformities may result if only one portion of the growth plate sustains damage while normal growth occurs in the remaining portion of the growth plate, leading to "curved" bone growth. An example of an angular deformity of the proximal radius is demonstrated in the X-ray in figure 2.8.

Bone Tissue Components The four primary bone cells are osteoblasts, osteocytes, bone-lining cells, and osteoclasts. **Osteoblasts**, mononuclear cells of mesenchymal origin, are located on the bony surface and are the primary bone-forming cells. Once osteoblasts have produced a sufficient amount of unmineralized matrix (**osteoid**) and become relatively inactive, one of three things can happen. Osteoblasts can (1) undergo cell death, (2) persist on the bone surface (i.e., become bone-lining cells), or (3) become trapped and surrounded by osteoid that mineralizes shortly after deposition, at which point they have become osteocytes.

Osteocytes encompass the entire bone cortex (25,000 cells/mm³ of tissue). When the active osteoblast begins the transition to osteocyte, cell volume decreases by 30% initially, and as the metabolic

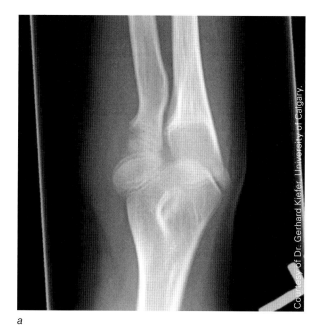

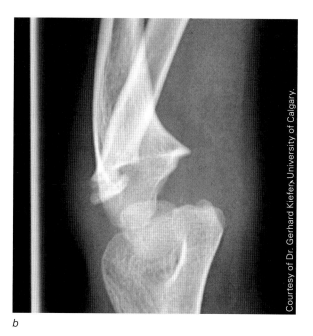

a   *b*

FIGURE 2.8 An X-ray of a bone deformity resulting from a damaged growth plate. (*a, b*) Orthogonal views of the deformed proximal radius.

activity of the osteocyte gradually decreases, cell volume also continues to decrease. The osteocyte slowly fills in its surrounding lacuna with matrix, and thus both cell and lacunar size decrease.

Osteocytes communicate with one another, and the deeper osteocytes communicate with the surface-covering osteoblasts by a network of interconnecting processes (gap junctions) housed in canaliculi within the extracellular matrix. The connections between adjacent processes between bone cells suggest that osteoblasts, osteocytes, and bone-lining cells form a functional syncytium that may play an integral role in many physiological functions, including the conversion of mechanical signals into remodeling activity and mineral movement into and out of the bone (Currey 2002).

Osteoclasts are multinuclear cells of hematogenous (from blood) origin that are located on the bony surface and are the primary bone-resorbing cells. The most distinguishing feature of the osteoclast is the extensive in-folding of the cell plasma membrane that gives rise to a ruffled border. That border is functionally significant because it greatly increases the surface area along which the cell can interact with the surrounding bony matrix (Rosier et al. 2000). Osteoclasts break down bone by anchoring to the bone surface and secreting hydrogen (H^+) ions and proteolytic enzymes across their plasma membrane. The enzymes are released into the extracellular matrix by lysosomes and digest the organic components of the matrix. Osteoclasts move along the bone surface and leave behind a trail of resorbed bone that has the appearance of an etched surface.

The **extracellular bone matrix** has inorganic (mineral), organic, and fluid components. Minerals, primarily in the form of calcium **hydroxyapatite** crystals ($Ca_{10}(PO_4)_6(OH)_2$), contribute about 50% of the total bone volume. Organic components constitute 39% of the volume (95% type I collagen and 5% proteoglycans), whereas fluid-filled vascular channels and cellular spaces constitute the remaining volume. Bone mechanical behavior reflects the properties of both mineral and organic phases, with minerals contributing stiffness and the organic matrix adding strength to bone.

Mineral content distinguishes bone from other connective tissues and provides bone with its characteristic rigidity; bone serves as a mineral storehouse (mainly calcium). The mechanism responsible for calcification of the extracellular matrix of bone (and not of other connective tissues) is not completely understood, but the ability of type I col-

lagen to bind mineral crystallites (hydroxyapatite) is unique among the collagen varieties. More than 200 noncollagenous proteins are also found within bone's extracellular matrix. In terms of concentration, however, collagen occupies the greatest portion of the matrix. Because collagen provides major structural support in connective tissues, abnormalities in collagen production can have far-reaching consequences in the ability of the skeleton to resist mechanical stresses. For example, should an arginine residue be replaced by a cysteine residue during collagen synthesis, the ensuing missense mutation is associated with Ehlers-Danlos Syndrome, producing a condition known as osteogenesis imperfecta, leading to fragile bones with higher likelihood of fracture (Cabral et al. 2007).

Bone, including the marrow, periosteum, **metaphysis**, **diaphysis**, and **epiphysis**, is richly supplied with blood vessels (figure 2.9). Studies report that approximately 7% of the cardiac output is sent to the skeleton (Shim et al. 1967; Tothill and MacPherson 1986). Blood reaches each area of the bone via extensive arterial interconnections (**anastomoses**).

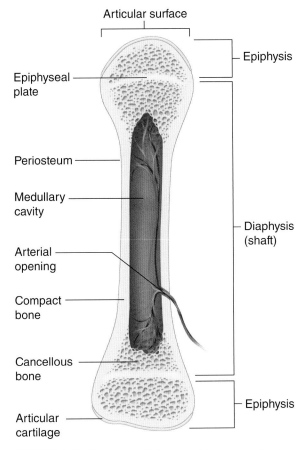

FIGURE 2.9 Diagram of the arterial supply of a long bone.

Those feed into a network of sinusoids (dilated venous channels), which, in turn, empty into central venous channels deep within the **medullary canal** in long bones or a central canal in flat bones. The primary nutrient artery enters the medullary canal via an oblique (slanted) nutrient foramen. Once within the marrow cavity, the artery divides into two longitudinal branches, one toward each of the epiphyses. Each branch gives rise to many parallel branches that can pierce through the cortex and anastomose with periosteal vessels that supply the outer third of the cortex. Within compact bone, primary arteries and veins travel relatively parallel to the osteonal longitudinal axes within structures called **Haversian canals**. Transversely oriented vessels are contained within structures called perforating or **Volkmann canals** (figure 2.10).

The terminal ends of the nutrient artery branches join with branches from the metaphyseal system. Preceding closure of the physes, the physes can be seen as a boundary largely separating the epiphyseal and metaphyseal systems; only a few metaphyseal

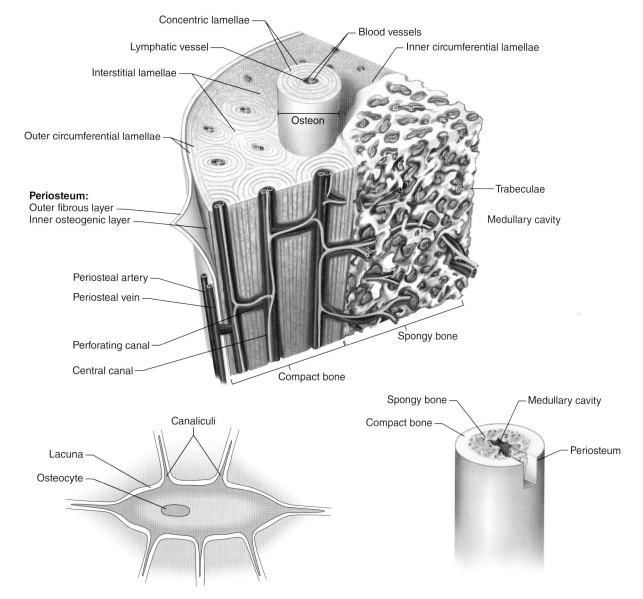

FIGURE 2.10 Ultrastructure of cortical bone, emphasizing the organization of intracortical Haversian (central) and Volkmann (perforating) canals containing blood vessels, as well as the canalicular connections within osteons and between osteocytes.

Reprinted by permission from W.C. Whiting, *Dynamic Human Anatomy,* 2nd ed. (Champaign, IL: Human Kinetics, 2019).

branches perforate the physes and anastomose with epiphyseal branches. After closure of the physes, the metaphyseal and epiphyseal branches are richly interconnected. Epiphyseal vessels branch into extensive networks that supply the bony ends.

Bone Macrostructure Despite differences in size and mechanical properties, bone tissue is basically similar in all bones. As described earlier, bone can be divided at a gross structural level into cortical (compact) and trabecular (cancellous or spongy) bone. At a tissue level, bone may be divided into three broad categories: woven, primary, and secondary bone. These categories are described in table 2.2.

Woven bone is laid down as a disorganized arrangement of collagen fibers and osteocytes. Although the mineral content of woven bone can be higher than that of primary and secondary bone, the disorganized pattern and generally lower proportions of noncollagenous proteins decrease the mechanical strength of woven bone compared with primary or secondary bone. Developmentally, woven bone is unique, because it can be deposited de novo (without a preexisting membrane, bone, or cartilaginous model; Martin et al. 1998). The cell-to-bone volume ratio is high in woven bone, confirming its role in providing temporary, rapid mechanical support, such as following traumatic injury.

In the adult skeleton, woven bone is not usually present but can be found in a fracture callus, in areas undergoing active endochondral ossification, and in some skeletal pathologies. During maturation, primary bone systematically replaces woven bone, providing the mature skeleton with the appropriate functional stiffness.

Primary bone comprises several types of bone, each with unique morphology and function. A common factor among the types of primary bone, however, is that unlike woven bone, primary bone must replace a preexisting structure, either a cartilaginous model (anlage) or previously deposited woven bone. Primary bone is composed of multiple thin layers (lamellae) of bone matrix and cells organized in parallel with the bone surface. This is referred to as **lamellar bone** and can exist within cortical and trabecular bone. Vascular channels are sparse in primary bone, and therefore it can be very dense. Where vascular channels are present, they are associated with several lamellae surrounding the vascular channels. The outermost lamella has a smooth surface. The units of vascular channels and lamellae are referred to as **primary osteons** or principal structures of compact bone.

Primary bone is also found in cancellous bone. For example, the trabeculae (small rods) found in the vertebral bodies and in long-bone epiphyses are mostly primary bone in adolescents. In this case, although vascular channels are not enclosed within the lamellar structure, the individual trabeculae of the cancellous bone are in intimate contact with a rich vascular supply. Because of that close proximity, cancellous bone has a very important role in mineral homeostasis, because calcium stores (hydroxyapatite) can be mobilized quickly via deep osteoclasts in response to decreased serum calcium via secretion of parathyroid hormone (Shaker and Deftos 2018).

Secondary bone is deposited only during remodeling and replaces preexisting primary cortical or trabecular bone. Remodeling can create osteons, but unlike primary osteons, the outermost lamellae of secondary bone have an indented surface. Differences between the developmental process of primary and secondary bone imply that a different controlling mechanism may be responsible for the endosteal or periosteal deposition of primary bone versus the intracortical deposition of secondary bone during remodeling.

TABLE 2.2 Bone Macrostructure

Type of bone tissue	Formation	Examples
Woven bone	Does not need preexisting membrane, bone, or cartilage model	Initial cortical bone development, fracture callus
Primary bone • Lamellar • Osteonal	Needs cartilage foundation, membrane, or woven bone	Embryonic bone development, trabecular bone
Secondary bone	Replacement of preexisting bone during remodeling	Human cortical bone

Adapted by permission from R.B. Martin and D.B. Burr, *Structure, Function, and Adaptation of Compact Bone* (New York, NY: Raven Press, 1989), 19.

Cartilage

Cartilage contains the basic elements of a connective tissue, namely cells and extracellular matrix composed of tissue fluid and macromolecules. The relative amounts and types of matrix constituents distinguish the three forms of anatomical cartilage: hyaline (articular), elastic, and fibrocartilage. Hyaline cartilage is the most abundant form. Cartilage does not have intrinsic blood vessels, nerves, or lymph vessels. The absence of vascular structures makes it imperative for cartilage cells (chondrocytes) to receive nutrients and remove metabolic waste by simple diffusion.

All cartilage develops from mesenchyme (primitive connective tissue). Mesenchymal cells produce the extracellular matrix (including collagenous fibrils) and differentiate into chondroblasts, which are the precursors of chondrocytes. After chondrocytes are formed, they are encapsulated in caves (lacunae) within the cartilage matrix. The functional unit of a chondrocyte and lacunae is termed a **chondron**. A connective tissue membrane (**perichondrium**) surrounds the new cartilage and gives it shape. Within the perichondrium are capillaries and lymph vessels and nerves, from which nutrients diffuse to enrich the chondrons within. The perichondrium also contains fibroblasts, collagen fibers, and elastic fibers.

Cartilaginous structures can grow by two mechanisms. **Interstitial growth** occurs in newly deposited cartilage as preexisting chondrocytes divide within the lacunae, forming cell nests. Because younger cartilage is more flexible than mature cartilage, the matrix can accommodate the interstitial expansion. **Appositional growth** proceeds in the cartilage layers immediately beneath the perichondrium. The mesenchymal cells in this superficial zone develop into new cartilage cells, which, in turn, are laid between the older cells and perichondrium, and new cartilage cells produce new matrix components.

Figure 2.11 shows the distribution of cells in articular cartilage from the surface of the perichondrium, through the chondrogenic layer immediately beneath the perichondrium (where appositional growth occurs), and on to the middle region where interstitial growth occurs within the chondrocytes. In the superficial tangential zone (perichondrium), the collagen fibers are arranged parallel to the joint surface to help resist shear forces. In the middle 40% to 60% of the cartilage, the collagen fibers appear more randomly organized. In the deepest layer of the articular cartilage, the collagen fibers are oriented perpendicular to the joint surface and penetrate

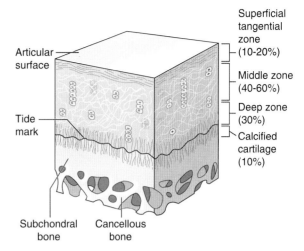

FIGURE 2.11 Cellular organization of hyaline cartilage. In the superficial tangential zone, cells are flattened, chondrogenic, and adjacent to the perichondrium. Progressing into the middle zone, there is a continuation of the perichondrium level as cartilage cells produce extracellular matrix to distance themselves from their neighboring cells. In the deep zone, columns of cartilage cells are seen in lacunae. In the orientation represented in the figure, the joint surface is at the top, and the deepest part of the cartilage is at the bottom near the attachment to bone. In addition to the cellular elements in the various depths of the hyaline cartilage, collagen fibers also have distinct regions and orientations. The superficial tangential zone is closest to the joint surface, and the collagen fibers are aligned parallel to the articular surface. In the middle zone, the collagen fibers are relatively random in orientation, and in the deep zone the collagen fibers are in a radial direction (with respect to the surface of the joint)—where collagen fibers penetrate through the **tide mark** (the transition zone between calcified and noncalcified articular cartilage) and into the calcified cartilage overlying the subchondral bone.

into the underlying calcified cartilage to maintain a solid adhesion to the underlying bone. This helps the bone resist both tension and compression forces.

Hyaline Cartilage   Hyaline cartilage gets its name from its glossy appearance. The fetal skeletal anlage is composed of hyaline cartilage before being replaced by bone later in life. The surfaces of most joints, the anterior portions of the ribs, and areas of the respiratory system (e.g., trachea, nose, and bronchi) are composed of hyaline cartilage throughout life. Hyaline cartilage within joints is known as **articular cartilage** and provides a suitable and relatively frictionless surface for joint lubrication. Degradation of articular hyaline cartilage is characteristic of the osteoarthritis pathology. Normally, the hyaline matrix appears blue and homogeneous in its fresh state, is firm and resilient in texture, and contains collagen fibers, 90% of which are type II collagen. The collagen fibers give cartilage its tensile strength, and the mechanical stiffness throughout the cartilage depth varies with the changes in collagen fiber orientation (Lo et al. 2003; Morel et al. 2005; Oinas et al. 2018; Silver and Bradica 2002). The perichondrium provides the nutrients for the cartilage and surrounds all hyaline cartilage except articular cartilage, which receives nutrients by diffusion via the joint synovial fluid.

Cells constitute less than 10% of total hyaline cartilage volume, with the principal components being macromolecules (about 20% of volume) and tissue fluid (about 70% of volume; Lo et al. 2003). The main structural macromolecule (besides type II collagen) in hyaline cartilage is a glycoconjugate known as a *proteoglycan*. The integrated structure–function relations among the collagen fibers, proteoglycans, and fluid contribute to the unique mechanical behavior of articular cartilage.

Hydrophilic proteoglycans tend to draw water into the matrix, and negatively charged sulfate groups located on attached glycosaminoglycans tend to repel each other. Articular cartilage wants to swell, but this expansion is resisted by the tensile restraint provided by the collagen fibrils. A dynamic interaction occurs between these matrix constituents during the loading of normal articular cartilage. Figure 2.12 illustrates the basics of this

dynamic interaction. Figure 2.12*a* illustrates articular cartilage without any external load applied. The cartilage is normally swollen with water that has been attracted by the proteoglycans, and the negative charges of the sulfate groups repel each other while the collagen fibers provide the restraining tensile forces to maintain the structure. In figure 2.12*b*, an external compressive load has been applied. Now the fluid exudes from the articular cartilage, and the proteoglycan monomers and **aggrecan** are forced closer together. If a constant load is applied, the cartilage will exhibit a **creep response** (slowly deform) until a new resting length has been established.

In adults, chondrocytes slowly continue to produce and renew proteoglycan macromolecules. With aging, however, the turnover rate of proteoglycan diminishes, and some of the proteoglycan monomers or individual glycosaminoglycans can become disconnected, which diminishes the resilience of the articular cartilage to external loads. Mutations associated with the glycoproteins that make up proteoglycan aggregates can lead to a variety of chondrodysplasia pathologies, including arthritis (Vynios 2014).

Other Types of Cartilage Elastic cartilage is found in the external ear, the epiglottis, portions of the larynx, and the Eustachian tube. Consistent with

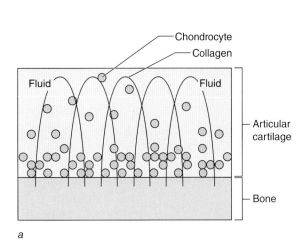

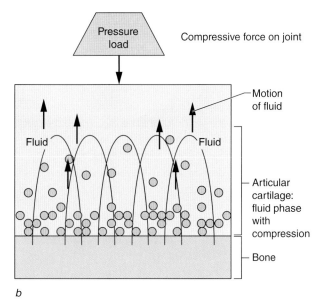

FIGURE 2.12 Unloaded and loaded extracellular matrix of articular cartilage. *(a)* Collagen provides the tensile restraint to the swelling pressures generated by the influx of tissue fluid (assisted by the hydrophilic, negatively charged proteoglycans). In resting articular cartilage, there is a normal swelling pressure. *(b)* An external load has been applied to the surface of the articular cartilage, and the matrix is being compressed. Tissue fluid exudes from the cartilage matrix, and the negatively charged proteoglycan monomers and aggrecan are being pushed closer together. For a given (constant) load, eventually a new equilibrium will be reached with the matrix in a compressed state.

its name, elastic cartilage possesses a great deal of flexibility. The extracellular matrix contains elastic fibers as well as collagen fibers and appears more yellow because of the higher percentage of elastic fibers. It is not translucent like hyaline cartilage. Elastic cartilage is able to develop both interstitially and through appositional growth.

• **Fibrocartilage** is strong and flexible because of its endogenous collagen fibers and is resilient because of its extracellular matrix. Fibrocartilage is found in many areas of the body, especially at stress points where friction could be problematic. It is distinct from hyaline and elastic cartilage, because it contains no perichondrium. The fibrocartilage develops much like other ordinary connective tissue—fibroblasts produce matrix and then differentiate into chondrocytes. Fibrocartilage fills areas between hyaline cartilage and other connective tissues and is found near joints, ligaments, tendons, and in intervertebral discs. Four categories of fibrocartilage have been identified, each with a specific function: intra-articular, connecting, stratiform, and circumferential.

• **Intra-articular fibrocartilage** is found within joints, such as the wrist and knee, as well as in the temporomandibular and sternoclavicular joints. In these joints, where frequent movement and potential impacts occur, the fibrocartilage acts as a cushion. Intra-articular fibrocartilages are flattened plates that are interposed between the joint surfaces and held in position by ligaments and tendons that connect to the edges of the fibrocartilage. The surfaces of these intra-articular fibrocartilages, however, are free of connections and help to prevent friction between the moving joints. Furthermore, intra-articular fibrocartilages act as spacers to fill the gap between joints, improve joint geometry, and protect the surfaces of the underlying articular cartilage. Menisci are a common form of intra-articular fibrocartilage.

• **Connecting fibrocartilage** occurs at limited-motion joints, such as intervertebral discs. These fibrocartilage plates allow the surfaces of the adjacent vertebral bodies to move slightly with respect to each other (read more about intervertebral discs in chapter 8).

• **Stratiform fibrocartilage** forms layers over bone, where tendons may act, and can also be an integral part of the tendon surface. When a muscle contracts and a tendon is forced to slide over a bony surface, friction is minimized by interposing stratiform fibrocartilage between the bone and tendon. Common sites for stratiform fibrocartilage to be found include the lateral malleolus, where the peroneus longus and tibialis posterior tendons traverse, as well as the parapatellar fibrocartilage on the medial patella or within the intertubercular sulcus beneath the biceps brachii tendon (Durham and Dyson 2011).

• **Circumferential fibrocartilage** acts as a spacer in the joints of the hip and shoulder (e.g., glenoid and acetabular labrum). Circumferential fibrocartilage is ring-shaped and thus protects only the edge of the joints and improves the bony fit.

Tendons and Ligaments

Regularly organized fibrous tissues, such as tendons, ligaments, and aponeuroses, are called **dense regular connective tissue**. In each of these, the tissue is primarily composed of collagen fibers running in parallel bundles and extracellular matrix components. Fibroblasts are the principal cells in these tissues. These tissues have great tensile strength but are able to resist stretching (tensile) forces primarily in one direction parallel to the fiber line.

Tendons are white, collagenous, flexible bands that connect muscle to bone. Figure 2.13 shows the generic structure of a tendon. The building blocks of a tendon are the tropocollagen molecules, which generally are aligned in parallel rows to form a microfibril. Subsequently, the microfibrils aggregate into parallel bundles to form subfibrils and then fibrils. Fibrils are gathered into fibers and then fascicles bound together by a loose connective tissue (**endotendineum**), which permits relative motion of the collagen fascicles and supports blood vessels, nerves, and lymphatics (Woo et al. 2000). Tendon fascicles are grouped into the tendon proper. When a tendon is slack (no tensile load), fascicles take on a microscopically crimped or wavy appearance. As a tensile load is applied, the wavy pattern is straightened.

As is evident from the description of the collagen fiber organization in tendon, the major component of tendon is type I collagen, which accounts for about 86% of the dry weight of a tendon (Woo et al. 2000). Elastic fibers are present in small quantities in the matrix of tendons.

The surface of the tendon can be covered with an epitendineum, usually seen as a tendon sheath, to act as a pulley and direct the path around sharp corners, such as in the flexor tendons of the hand. When tendons are not enclosed with the epitendineum

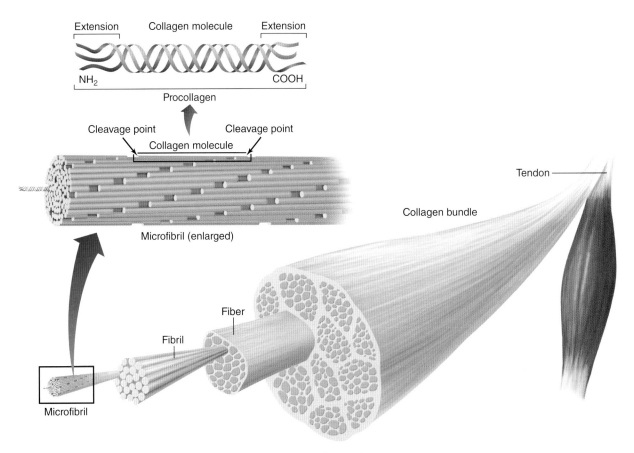

FIGURE 2.13 Schematic representation of the hierarchy of a tendon.

and move in a relatively straight line, a loose areolar connective tissue (**peritenon**) envelops the tendon. The peritenon contains blood vessels and nerves to serve the tendon.

The insertion of tendon into bone (**osteotendinous junction**) is classified as direct or indirect. The direct insertion is characterized by four layers (zones) with a gradual transition from tendon to unmineralized fibrocartilage, to mineralized fibrocartilage, and finally to bone (figure 2.14). Cells within the tendon are tenocytes, whereas those in the fibrocartilage are fibrochondrocytes and those in the mineralized fibrocartilage are osteocytes. The indirect insertion is characterized by an interface made up of three layers: tendon, **Sharpey's fibers,** and bone.

At the opposite end of the tendon, where connective tissue meets muscle tissue, is the **myotendinous junction** (also called **musculotendinous junction**), a specialized region of longitudinal membranous invaginations between the muscle and tendon tissues. Its serrated appearance increases the surface

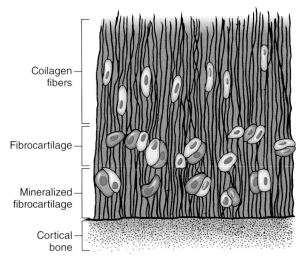

FIGURE 2.14 Osteotendinous junction schematic of transition zones of progressively stiffer tissues (tendon, fibrocartilage, mineralized fibrocartilage, cortical bone).

area and reduces stress on the junction during the contractile force transmission. The strength of the myotendinous junction depends both on the properties of the adjoining structures and on the orientation of forces across the junction. Junctions that are loaded in shear stress, with the force being parallel to the membrane surface, are stronger than junctions with a large tensile component perpendicular to the membrane (Tidball 1991).

Aponeuroses are fibrous, ribbonlike membranes similar in composition to tendons. These structures are sometimes called *flattened tendons*. For example, the palmar aponeurosis encloses the muscles of the palm of the hand. Aponeuroses are whitish in appearance because of the presence of collagen. The fibers of aponeuroses run in a single direction and thus differ from dense irregular fibrous connective tissue (e.g., fascia).

Ligaments are dense regular connective tissue structures that join bone to bone. The primary function of ligaments, like tendons, is to resist tensile forces along the line of the collagen fibers and constrain movement of limbs to maintain joint integrity and geometry. Ligaments are classified and named according to several criteria, including attachment sites (coracoacromial), shape (deltoid), function (capsular), position or orientation (collateral, cruciate), and composition (elastic). Ligaments can also be **intracapsular** (located within the joint capsule), **capsular** (appearing as a thickening of the capsule structure), or **extracapsular** (extrinsic to the capsule).

Joint ligaments have a structure that is similar to tendon, but whereas collagen fibril bundles in tendons are typically aligned parallel to each other (in line with the pull of the muscle), the collagen fibril bundles in ligaments may be oriented in parallel, obliquely, or even in a spiral arrangement. Thus, ligaments are inherently weaker than tendons and do not withstand higher stresses. The geometry of the collagen fibril bundles in ligaments is specific to a ligament's function. Microscopically, the color of collagenous ligaments is a duller white than tendon because of the slightly greater percentage of elastic and reticular fibers found between the collagen fiber bundles. Darker areas indicate less overlap between collagen bundles.

The ligament insertion to bone is either direct or indirect (Lo et al. 2003; Woo et al. 2000). The direct attachment is comparable to the specialized collagen fibers (Sharpey's fibers) that attach tendon to bone. The indirect route is one in which the collagen fibers from the ligament blend with the fibrous periosteum of the bone.

Fibroblasts are the principal cells in ligaments, whereas the main fibrous component of the extracellular matrix is type I collagen (36% of wet weight). Several other types of collagen are also found in ligaments. Proteoglycans are present, although fewer than in articular cartilage. Because almost two-thirds of a ligament is composed of water, the proteoglycans (which are hydrophilic) may play a role in the mechanical behavior of a ligament, helping withstand stress similarly to articular cartilage.

Joint ligaments, such as those in the knee, contain several sensory receptors (i.e., Ruffini corpuscles, Pacinian corpuscles, Golgi tendon organs, and free-nerve endings) that are capable of providing the nervous system with information about proprioception, pressure, and pain. Nevertheless, the exact neurosensory role of ligaments and receptors in joint proprioception is controversial and continues to be studied. After synthesizing anatomical, neurophysiological, and mechanical data, with a particular focus on the sensory receptors of the knee joint ligaments, Kim and colleagues (1995) and Solomonow (2004) concluded that ligaments may provide sensory information about changes in the stiffness of muscles around the knee joint. In this way, ligaments can have an important function in regulating the stability of the knee joint.

Yellow elastic ligaments are less common in the body than collagenous ligaments. Parallel elastic fibers, which predominate in elastic ligaments, are surrounded by loose connective tissue. Elastic ligaments in humans include the vocal cords and the ligamentum flavum of the vertebrae. A classic example of an elastic ligament in animals is the ligamentum nuchae of cattle, which helps the animal hold up its head while grazing.

Fascia is a category of **dense irregular connective tissues** that do not logically fall into the categories of tendon, aponeurosis, or ligament. The principal fibers in fascia are collagenous, although some elastic and reticular elements also exist. Fascia contains loosely and randomly interwoven meshlike fibers and is usually found in layers or sheaths around organs, blood vessels, bones, and cartilage as well as in the dermis of the skin. It provides firm support for muscles. The fibers in fascia traverse in different directions and, in some cases, in different planes (as in the dermis). Because of this organization, fascia withstands stretching in many directions. Examples of fascia include the thoracolumbar fascia on the inferior back deep to the latissimus dorsi muscle and the plantar fascia on the plantar aspect (sole) of the foot.

Case Studies in Ankle and Knee Sprains

Sprains are injuries to ligaments usually caused by sudden overstretching, with varying grades that depend on the degree of stretching or rupture. Sprains can occur in many joints, most commonly the ankle, knee, finger, and wrist. Typically, the symptoms associated with sprains are related to those of inflammation and include pain, swelling, and loss of function.

ANKLE ORTHOTICS AND SPRAINS

The most common form of injury in running and jumping sports is inversion sprain, a stretching or rupture of the weaker tendons on the lateral aspect of the hindfoot. If a person has had a previous ankle sprain, a subsequent sprain is much more likely to happen.

To reduce the number of ankle sprain injuries, some professionals advocate the use of **taping** or semirigid **orthotics**. Taping has advantages and disadvantages—although prophylactic taping can effectively reduce excessive ankle inversion before exercise, in many cases its restraint is lost during an exercise bout. It can also be expensive and requires a skilled individual to apply the tape. Semirigid ankle orthotics have been proposed as a substitute for taping. Few prospective studies, however, have evaluated the effectiveness of ankle orthotics for reducing or preventing ankle sprains.

One such study by Surve et al. (1994) reported results of a comprehensive, prospective study of adult male soccer players over the course of 1 year. Players with a previous history of ankle sprain and those with no previous history of ankle sprain were identified. Each player was then randomly assigned to an orthotic group or a control group (no orthotic or taping). Thus, four groups of players were studied, comprising more than 500 players. Injury was defined as any sprain that occurred during a scheduled match or practice that caused the soccer player to miss the next game or practice. Marked differences occurred among the groups during the 1 year of play. The principal finding was that the application of a semirigid ankle orthotic resulted in a fivefold reduction in the incidence of ankle sprains in players with a previous history of ankle sprains. An ankle orthosis, however, did not significantly alter the incidence of ankle sprains in soccer players who had never sprained their ankles before. Supporting those results, a systematic review by Dizon and Reyes (2010) combined most of the available data and compared the effectiveness of taping and bracing. They found a 67% to 71% reduction in ankle sprains with the use of external orthotic support, with neither taping or bracing being more effective than the other.

Although many people suggest that the positive effects of an external support orthotic are primarily attributable to mechanical support that limits excessive inversion and eversion of the ankle, only the athletes who had previously sprained their ankles received positive benefits from wearing the orthotic. Why this difference? Hertel and Corbett (2019) proposed a new model of chronic ankle instability, which described how tissue injury after an acute ankle sprain may lead to a collection of interrelated pathomechanical, sensory–perceptual, and motor–behavioral impairments that influence a person's clinical outcome. They integrated the findings proposed by Surve and colleagues (1994), which suggested that proprioceptive defects can happen after an ankle sprain because of damage to sensory receptors in the ligaments of the ankle, impairing the ankle's reflex stabilization. The application of an external orthotic may have stimulated mechanoreceptors to improve proprioceptive function of the previously injured ankle, rather than just provide mechanical support.

LOSS OF ACL CAN ALTER NEUROMOTOR CONTROL PATTERNS

After tearing the anterior cruciate ligament (ACL) in the knee joint, 75% of affected individuals alter their patterns of neuromuscular control to accommodate changes in function (Berchuck et al. 1990). In a seminal study, Berchuck and colleagues (1990) found that when an activity such as walking requires the quadriceps to be active while the knee is flexed between 0° and 45°, the contraction of the quadriceps tends to move the proximal end of the tibia anteriorly, thereby straining the anterior cruciate ligament. If a person does not have an anterior cruciate ligament, however, what can he or she do to avoid the forward motion of the tibia on the end of the femur?

In analyzing the gait of patients with ACL-deficient knees, Berchuck and colleagues (1990) reported that patients reduced contraction of their quadriceps during the stance phase of walking, using a so-called

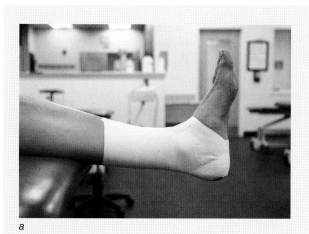
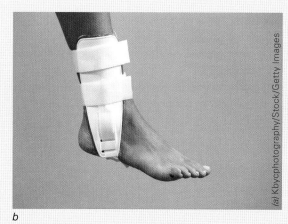

a   b

(a) Closed basket weave taping for the ankle. *(b)* Ankle brace.

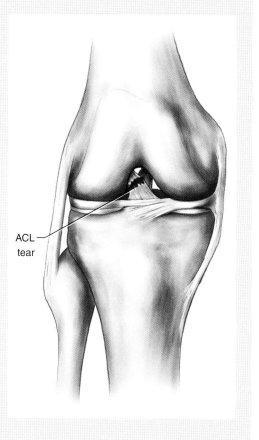

quadriceps-avoidance gait. The patients also may have increased the action of the hamstring muscles to pull back on the tibia during stance, but that was not measured.

But if these patients avoided using the quadriceps to prevent collapse of the knee during midstance, then how did they maintain an extended knee? Why didn't their knees collapse? Apparently the patients learned to increase the amount of hip extensor activity to compensate for the reduction in knee extensor activity. Interestingly, the patients walked with quadriceps-avoidance gait on both their ACL-deficient side and on the other (normal) knee.

The researchers suggested that after ligament injury there is a reprogramming of the locomotor process so that excessive anterior displacement of the tibia is prevented. A systematic review by Slater et al. (2017) showed that these compensatory measures persist following ACL reconstructive surgery. Even if an athlete is granted clearance to return to sports and physical activity following reconstruction, their gait patterns do not appear to normalize over time, suggesting that the current approach to rehabilitation and assessment before return to activity is not adequately identifying individuals with dysfunctional movement patterns. How this abnormal function affects the long-term outcome and the likelihood of posttraumatic osteoarthritis remains unknown.

ACL tear

Muscle Tissue

The final type of tissue, **muscle**, can be divided into three categories: smooth, cardiac, and skeletal. Muscle tissue is derived from mesoderm. All three types of muscle cells perform the specialized tasks of conductivity (excitability through bioelectricity) and **contractility** (ability to shorten and produce force).

Smooth muscle is not striated and is not considered under voluntary control. Rather, contrac-

tion is mediated by paracrine (local) or endocrine (hormonal) signals. It is found in the walls of tubes in the arterial, intestinal, and respiratory systems. Smooth muscle is innervated by both sympathetic and parasympathetic nerves to control constriction and dilation.

Cardiac muscle has structural and functional characteristics of both skeletal and smooth muscle. Cardiac muscle is striated in appearance but is not under voluntary control. Cardiac muscle cells form a functional **syncytium** (multinucleated mass of cytoplasm resulting from a fusion of cells), where muscle cells contract simultaneously, and the tissue acts electrically as though it were a single cell.

Skeletal muscle is also called **striated** muscle, because its fibers exhibit cross striations and appear striped due to its microscopic structure. These cells are multinucleated, facilitating larger amounts of protein synthesis due to the larger size of a muscle cell and fibers (Moffatt and Cohen-Fix 2019). Skeletal muscle is under voluntary control. Because of the contractility of skeletal muscle cells, they are the prime executors of the peripheral nervous system's motor division. Skeletal muscle will be the primary focus in the following sections.

Contractile proteins and a network of connective tissue are the two basic elements of muscles. Fibrous connective tissues within the muscle belly and those that blend with the tendon provide important functional stiffness, which enhances the transmission of force. Significant cellular interactions direct a muscle's physiological response, but muscle adaptation and injury are best described by considering the mechanics of a muscle's functional units.

Microstructure and Function

The structure of skeletal muscle is diagrammatically presented in figure 2.15. The connective tissue surrounding the entire muscle is called the **epimysium**, and the bundles of muscle fibers (fascicles) are surrounded by the **perimysium**. Each individual

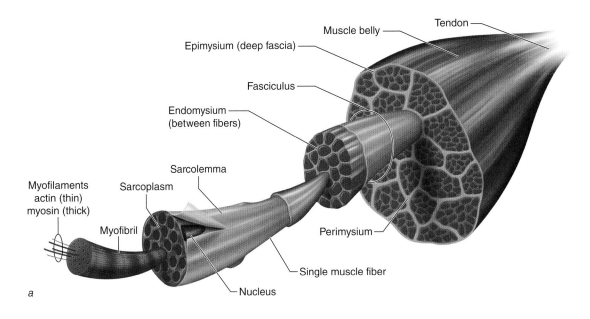

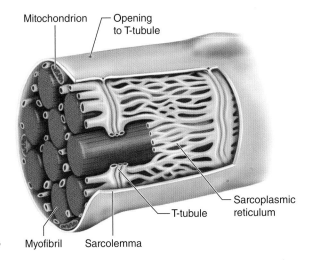

FIGURE 2.15 The structural composition and organization of *(a)* skeletal muscle tissue and *(b)* a muscle fiber.

muscle fiber is surrounded by **endomysium**. A skeletal muscle **fiber** is composed of hundreds of contractile proteins called **myofibrils**. Each myofibril is composed of two contractile **myofilaments**: an alpha-helical thin filament (**actin**), and a dual-chained thick filament (**myosin**). The myofibril has a microscopically striated (striped) appearance with transverse bands of repeated units called **sarcomeres**. The striations are created by the overlapping of myosin and actin filaments.

An array of other proteins (e.g., titin and nebulin) are present within a sarcomere and can contribute to the structure and passive properties of the sarcomere. **Titin** is a large protein that spans from the Z disc to the M band of a sarcomere, anchoring myosin to the Z disc (figure 2.16). It is generally accepted that titin acts as a spring to develop tension as the sarcomere is stretched and may act to center the thick filament within the sarcomere when forces on each side of the sarcomere are unequal. Just as titin is to myosin, **nebulin** anchors actin to the Z discs.

In the **sliding filament theory** of muscle contraction, muscle length shortens with the shortening of individual sarcomeres. The cross-bridge cycle interactions between the actin and myosin filaments allow for an increase in the overlap between the actin and myosin fibers and thus a decrease in overall sarcomere length. Figure 2.16 depicts the sliding filament theory of muscle contraction and shows a schematic of a contracted and extended sarcomere. During muscle contraction, sarcomere length decreases, which results in coiling of the I-band part of titin (Tskhovrebova and Trinick 2010). Simultaneously, interfilament spacings increase, which is likely to reorient or stretch Z- and M-line proteins. During extension, sarcomere length increases and interfilament spacings decrease. That extends titin and releases tension on the Z- and M-line proteins. Overextension of muscle results in the unraveling of titin polypeptide, as well as compression and reorientation of Z- and M-line proteins.

The process of muscular contraction commences with a neural **action potential**. Action potentials travel through the ventral horn of the spinal cord down motor neurons that are connected to muscle fiber membranes (neuromuscular junction or **synapse**). At that synapse, acetylcholine is released from the presynaptic terminal and binds to receptors on the postsynaptic terminal. The binding of acetylcholine to the postsynaptic membrane increases that membrane's permeability to sodium (Na^+). If the depolarization of that membrane attributable to Na^+ exceeds a certain threshold (lower than neuronal threshold potential), the action potential will propagate down the length of the muscle fiber. That action potential is transmitted to the interior of the muscle fiber by specialized cell membrane invaginations called **transverse tubules** (T-tubules). Depolarization leads to a conformational change in a dihydropyridine (DHP) receptor and a ryanodine receptor on the sarcoplasmic reticulum, a calcium-storing organelle within the muscle cell. Calcium is released from the sarcoplasmic reticulum and then binds to specialized sites on a protein called troponin. That triggers a conformational change on a long ropelike protein called tropomyosin, on which troponin is located. Although tropomyosin normally inhibits cross-bridge formation in the relaxed state, calcium-troponin binding removes the inhibition, and the sarcomeres are ready to contract. When a muscle is relaxing, a protein called sarco/endoplasmic reticulum calcium ATPase (SERCA), on the sarcoplasmic reticulum, pumps calcium back into the organelle, dropping intramuscular calcium levels so no binding can occur.

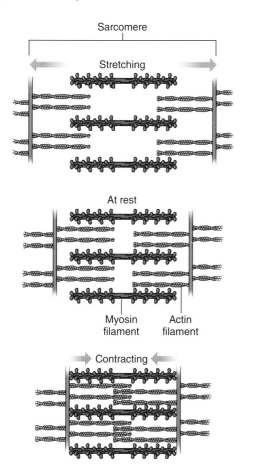

Sarcomere

Stretching

At rest

Myosin filament   Actin filament

Contracting

FIGURE 2.16 Sarcomere structure at various degrees of extension: stretching, at rest, and contracting.

Figure 2.17 illustrates the major states of interactions between myosin and actin during the cross-bridge cycle. The breakdown of bound adenosine triphosphate (ATP) into adenosine diphosphate (ADP) and inorganic phosphate (P_i) with the enzyme adenosine triphosphatase (ATPase) energizes the myosin head. The detachment of ADP from the myosin head provides the energy required to create a configurational change that slides the actin filament past the myosin filament, forming a **cross-bridge**. The myosin portion of the cross-bridge binds to a fresh ATP molecule that facilitates detachment of the cross-bridge and thus prepares the cross-bridge for another cycle.

Muscle fibers vary in length and can shorten to approximately one-half of their resting length. Human skeletal muscle contains three fiber types that have different functional characteristics, arising from the differences between myosin isoforms and speed of ATP hydrolysis, the rate-limiting step in muscle contraction. Garrett and Best (2000) pro-

vided a summary of the three types of muscle fibers and their physiological, metabolic, and structural characteristics (table 2.3). Most muscles in the body are a mixed variety containing a combination of muscle fiber types.

Type I muscle fibers tend to have slower contraction and relaxation times and are very fatigue resistant. Their motor unit size is typically small with a high capillary density. They mostly derive ATP through oxidative phosphorylation. Type II muscle fibers can be subdivided into types IIA and IIB (sometimes called IIX). Type IIA fibers have combined properties of type I and type IIB fibers. They are mostly fast twitch yet have oxidative tendencies, produce higher contraction speeds and force than type I fibers, and are more resistant to fatigue than type IIB fibers. They have a larger motor unit size and relatively high capillary density. Type IIB muscle fibers are fast-twitch fibers and use glycolytic metabolic processes. They are the most fatigable but have the highest contraction speeds and

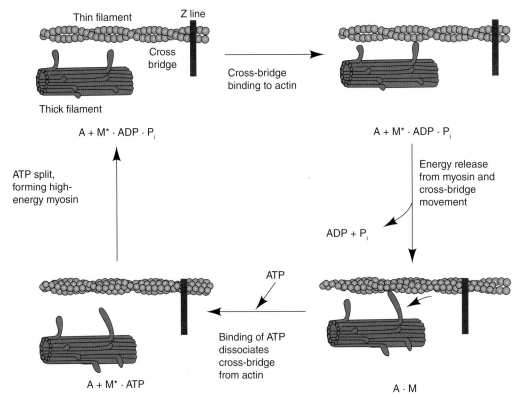

FIGURE 2.17 Schematic illustration of the cross-bridge cycle. When the muscle is at rest, the attachment site on the thin filament is covered by the tropomyosin–troponin complex. Adenosine triphosphate (ATP) is bound to the myosin cross-bridge, leaving the myosin head at rest. When the muscle is activated, calcium concentration increases in the sarcoplasm and calcium (Ca^{2+}) binds to troponin, thereby causing a configurational change that exposes the actin binding site. The cross-bridge attaches to actin and goes through a configurational change. The hydrolysis of ATP into adenosine diphosphate (ADP) and inorganic phosphate (P_i) excites the myosin head, leaving it close in proximity to actin prior to attachment. The detachment of ADP causes the myosin head to slide, resulting in contraction (i.e., movement of the thin past the thick filaments). Subsequently, a new ATP attaches to the cross-bridge and the cross-bridge can detach from the thin filament and is ready for a new interaction with another attachment site on the thin filament.

TABLE 2.3   Characteristics of Human Skeletal Muscle Fiber Types

	Type I	Type IIA	Type IIB
Other names	Red fibers, slow twitch (ST), slow oxidative (SO)	Intermediate (white) fibers, fast twitch (FT), fast oxidative glycolytic (FOG)	White fibers, fast glycolytic (FG)
Speed of contraction	Slow	Intermediate	Fast
Strength of contraction	Low	Intermediate	High
Fatigability	Resistant to fatigue	Moderately fatigable	Rapidly fatigable
Aerobic capacity	High	Intermediate	Low
Anaerobic capacity	Low	Intermediate	High
Motor unit size	Small	Larger	Largest
Capillary density	High	Intermediate	Low

Adapted by permission from W.E. Garrett, Jr. and T.M. Best, "Anatomy, Physiology, and Mechanics of Skeletal Muscle," in *Orthopaedic Basic Science*, edited by S.R. Simon (Park Ridge, IL: American Academy of Orthopaedic Surgeons, 1994), 100.

the greatest contractile strength. Their motor unit size is the largest of the three, but their capillary density is relatively low.

Muscle fibers with the same biochemical profiles tend to have similar force-producing characteristics. A muscle fiber shortening to one-half of its length will have the same force characteristics whether it is long or short, because the sarcomeres are in series. Increasing the number of muscle fibers in parallel, however, increases the absolute force of the muscle.

One important aspect of muscle architecture is the muscle fibers' angle of pennation. Longitudinal or fusiform muscles have muscle fibers lying parallel to the line of pull of the tendon. These fibers pull in a straight line, and the full magnitude of the force is directed along the tendon's line of action. An example of a skeletal fusiform muscle is the biceps brachii. The fibers of pennate muscle (unipennate, bipennate, or multipennate), conversely, arise at an oblique angle to the line of pull (usually considered as a straight line along the tendon). Thus, only a portion of the force generated by the contracting fiber is transmitted along the tendon. Pennation of the fibers allows the number of fibers to increase without significantly increasing the muscle's diameter. Although only one component of the muscle fiber force is used effectively to move the tendon, the advantage of the unipennate muscle system is that an increased number of sarcomeres can work in parallel to increase the effective force of the muscle

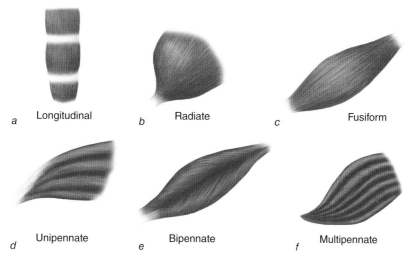

a Longitudinal	*b* Radiate	*c* Fusiform
d Unipennate	*e* Bipennate	*f* Multipennate

FIGURE 2.18   Effect of muscle fiber pennation. In the longitudinal, radiate, and fusiform muscles *(a, b, c)*, all the force generated within the muscle fiber is directed as a resultant force through the long axis of the tendon. The advantage of this arrangement is an increased range of motion (excursion of the tendon end with respect to muscle fiber excursion). By comparison, the unipennate, bipennate, and multipennate muscle fibers are directed at angles off-axis with respect to the tendon *(d, e, f)*. Thus, the force generated within the muscle has a force component that pulls off-axis with respect to the tendon, whereas the force component in parallel with the tendon provides a force component aligned with the intended direction.

through increased cross-sectional area (figure 2.18). Examples of pennate muscles include the extensor digitorum of the hand (unipennate), rectus femoris of the thigh (bipennate), and deltoid of the shoulder (multipennate).

Motor Units

The fundamental neuromuscular unit is the **motor unit** (figure 2.19). Motor units consist of a motoneuron (cell body) located within the spinal cord, its axon, and the muscle fibers that it innervates at the motor end plates. When the neuron depolarizes, all the muscle fibers in the motor unit contract as one (**all-or-none principle**). Muscle tension can be increased by sending action potentials to the muscle more frequently (increasing stimulation rate) and by recruiting additional motor units. Recruiting additional motor units is the more potent mechanism for initial force development; only at higher force levels does increasing the firing frequency assume a prominent role.

In addition to the neural determinants of force, a muscle's force output can be altered by the length

of the muscle when contraction is initiated and by the velocity of contraction. Force, velocity, and length are interrelated variables that affect a muscle's mechanical response. These relations are usually summarized as **force–velocity relation** and **length–tension relation** curves (figure 2.20). Length and velocity are not independent of each other; they are both related to force. The maximal tension can be generated when a muscle is forcibly lengthened while it attempts to shorten (eccentric action), due to the restoring force of titin proteins adding to the concentric force production of sarcomere contraction. Tension declines as an active muscle shortens (concentric action) due to fewer binding sites being available. Maximal strength in rapid eccentric muscle action exceeds the maximum in isometric work, and the strength is even less in concentric muscle action.

Skeletal muscle–tendon units also have inherent passive properties that affect force output. The tension developed in a muscle–tendon unit is transmitted to the skeleton from an integrated blend of muscle cells and fibrous connective tissue, including the sarcoplasm, sarcolemma, and endomysium. The other major load-carrying connective tissues in the

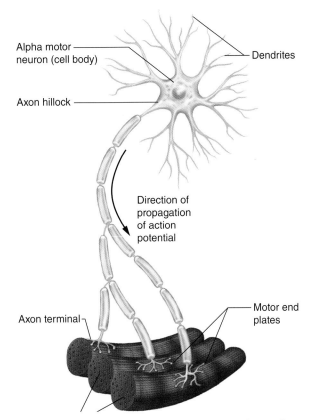

FIGURE 2.19 Single motor unit. A motor unit consists of the motoneuron (cell body) with its accompanying axon and the total number of muscle fibers innervated by that neuron.

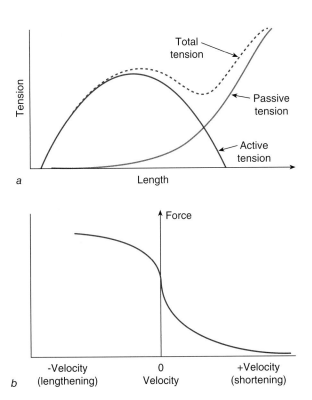

FIGURE 2.20 (a) Skeletal muscle length–tension curve and (b) skeletal muscle force–velocity curve.

muscle–tendon unit include the tendon and the collagen fibers that permeate the muscle belly. Some of these passive structures function in series with the active muscle cells, whereas others function in parallel. The terms **series-elastic component** and **parallel-elastic component** are derived from these functions. Together, the two components account for the passive tension properties of muscle, which can be important in muscle mechanics. As Åstrand and colleagues (2003) noted, a given tension in a muscle–tendon unit can be produced at a lower metabolic energy cost with eccentric than concentric muscle actions because of the mechanical energy that can be stored in the elastic components (titin).

Activated cross-bridges within the myofibrils exhibit a resistance to stretching, thus generating an internal force that is often termed *muscle stiffness*. Measured as change in force per change in length, stiffness is a property of muscle believed to operate over length changes and to have functional significance during locomotion and other movements.

Arthrology

Arthrology, or the classification of joints and joint motion, focuses on the classes, types, and examples of various joints in the human body. The words **articulation** and **joint** are used synonymously to describe the junction of two or more bones at their sites of contact. Some joints allow free movement (e.g., hip and knee joints), whereas others allow little or no movement between the connecting bones (e.g., sutures of the skull). Tables 2.4 through 2.6 organize joints by structure and action.

Joints are divided into those with or without a joint cavity. Synarthrodial (immovable) and amphiarthrodial (slightly movable) joints do not have a cavity. Diarthrodial (movable) joints typically have a joint cavity and are usually analyzed in movement-related injuries. For example, the knee joint is a frequently injured diarthrodial joint. A cross section of a knee joint, illustrating its many complex components, is provided in figure 2.21.

TABLE 2.4 Summary of Joint Structure and Movement of the Head, Neck, and Trunk

Joint	Structural classification	ALL MOVEMENTS BEGIN FROM ANATOMICAL POSITION		
		Movement	Plane	Axiality and planarity
Intercranial	Suture	None		
Temporomandibular	Synovial (condyloid)	Elevation Depression Protraction Retraction	Sagittal Transverse	Biaxial, biplanar
Atlanto-occipital	Synovial (hinge)	Flexion Extension	Sagittal	Uniaxial, uniplanar
Vertebral column: atlantoaxial	Synovial (pivot)	Rotation right Rotation left	Transverse	Uniaxial, uniplanar
C2-L5	Vertebral bodies: Symphysis Articular processes: Synovial (plane)	Flexion Extension Hyperextension Lateral flexion right Lateral flexion left Rotation right Rotation left	Sagittal Frontal Transverse	Triaxial, triplanar
Costovertebral	Synovial (plane)	Gliding		Nonaxial, nonplanar
Sternomanubrial	Symphysis	Sternal angle increase Sternal angle decrease		Nonaxial, nonplanar

Reprinted by permission from W.C. Whiting, *Dynamic Human Anatomy,* 2nd ed. (Champaign, IL: Human Kinetics, 2019).

TABLE 2.5   Summary of Joint Structure and Movement of the Upper Extremity

		ALL MOVEMENTS BEGIN FROM ANATOMICAL POSITION		
Joint	**Structural classification**	**Movement**	**Plane**	**Axial/ Planarity**
Sternoclavicular (shoulder girdle)	Synovial (ball and socket)	Anterior rotation Posterior rotation Upward rotation Downward rotation Abduction Adduction	Sagittal Frontal Transverse	Triaxial, triplanar
Acromioclavicular	Synovial (plane)	Gliding		Nonaxial, nonplanar
Glenohumeral (shoulder)	Synovial (ball and socket) [starting with shoulder flexed 90°]	Flexion Extension Hyperextension Abduction Adduction Internal (medial) rotation External (lateral) rotation Horizontal abduction (horizontal extension) Horizontal adduction (horizontal flexion)	Sagittal Frontal Transverse	Triaxial, triplanar
Elbow	Synovial (hinge)	Flexion Extension	Sagittal	Uniaxial, uniplanar
Radioulnar	Proximal: Synovial (pivot) Middle: Syndesmosis Distal: Synovial (pivot)	Pronation Supination	Transverse	Uniaxial, uniplanar
Radiocarpal (wrist)	Synovial (condyloid)	Flexion Extension Hyperextension Radial deviation (abduction) Ulnar deviation (adduction)	Sagittal Frontal	Biaxial, biplanar
Intercarpal	Synovial (plane)	Gliding		Nonaxial, nonplanar
Carpometacarpal	Synovial (plane)	Gliding		Nonaxial, nonplanar
Metacarpophalangeal	Thumb: Synovial (saddle) 2–5: Synovial (condyloid)	Flexion Extension Hyperextension Abduction Adduction	Frontal (2–5) Sagittal Sagittal (2–5) Frontal	Biaxial and biplanar
Interphalangeal	Synovial (hinge)	Flexion Extension	Sagittal	Uniaxial, uniplanar

Reprinted by permission from W.C. Whiting, *Dynamic Human Anatomy*, 2nd ed. (Champaign, IL: Human Kinetics, 2019).

TABLE 2.6 Summary of Joint Structure and Movement of the Pelvis and Lower Extremity

Joint	Structural classification	Movement	Plane	Axial/Planarity
		ALL MOVEMENTS BEGIN FROM ANATOMICAL POSITION		
Sacroiliac	Synovial (plane)	Gliding		Nonaxial, nonplanar
Pubic symphysis	Symphysis	Distraction; separation during childbirth		
Pelvic girdle (movement of pelvis relative to femur)	Synovial (ball and socket)	Anterior tilt Posterior tilt Lateral tilt right Lateral tilt left Rotation right Rotation left	Sagittal Frontal Transverse	Triaxial, triplanar
Hip (movement of femur relative to pelvis)	Synovial (ball and socket)	Flexion Extension Hyperextension Abduction Adduction Internal (medial) rotation External (lateral) rotation	Sagittal Frontal Transverse	Triaxial, triplanar
	[starting with hip flexed 90°]	Horizontal abduction (horizontal extension) Horizontal adduction (horizontal flexion)	Transverse	
Patellofemoral	Synovial (plane)	Gliding		Nonaxial, nonplanar
Tibiofemoral (knee)	Synovial (bicondyloid)	Flexion Extension Internal (medial) rotation External (lateral) rotation (with knee flexed)	Sagittal Frontal	Biaxial, biplanar
Ankle	Synovial (hinge)	Dorsiflexion Plantarflexion	Sagittal	Uniaxial, uniplanar
Subtalar	Synovial (plane)	Inversion Eversion	Frontal	Uniaxial, uniplanar
Intertarsal	Synovial (plane)	Gliding		Uniaxial, uniplanar
Tarsometatarsal	Synovial (plane)	Gliding		Nonaxial, nonplanar
Metatarsophalangeal	Synovial (condyloid)	Flexion Extension Hyperextension Abduction Adduction	Sagittal Transverse	Biaxial, biplanar
Interphalangeal	Synovial (hinge)	Flexion Extension	Sagittal	Uniaxial, uniplanar

Reprinted by permission from W.C. Whiting, *Dynamic Human Anatomy,* 2nd ed. (Champaign, IL: Human Kinetics, 2019).

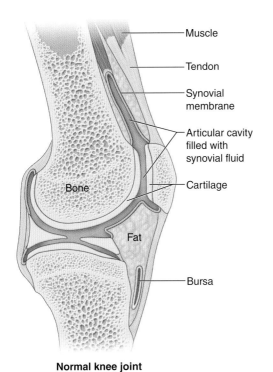

Muscle

Tendon

Synovial membrane

Articular cavity filled with synovial fluid

Cartilage

Bone

Fat

Bursa

Normal knee joint

FIGURE 2.21 A sagittal plane cross section of an adult human knee.

How does such a complex diarthrodial joint develop? To answer this question, we return to the description of the somite-stage embryo provided in the embryology section earlier in this chapter. After the appearance of the limb buds (26- to 28-day embryo), a group of mesenchymal cells coalesces within the developing limb to form a **blastema** (Lo et al. 2003). The blastema is the foundation material that produces the capsule, ligaments, synovial lining, and menisci of the joint. The adjoining bones at this stage are cartilage models that are undergoing endochondral ossification. At the juncture between two of these cartilage–bone models, the interzonal mesenchyme condenses and forms an articular disc (primitive joint plate). The central cavity within the developing joint emerges at about 10 weeks. This cavity ultimately becomes the synovial cavity, which will contain the synovial fluid that assists with joint lubrication.

The development from blastema to definable skeletal elements happens between weeks 4 and 10 in the developing human embryo. Many stimuli can influence the development of joints. Movement appears to be one of the important factors and may result from the extrinsic hydrodynamic forces that act in utero or from the nascent actions of the developing skeletal muscle tissues in the limb.

Chapter Review

Key Points

- Musculoskeletal tissues (i.e., bone, cartilage, tendons, ligaments, skeletal muscle, and joints) allow and can facilitate bodily motion. Motion is created through articulations that can include complex interactions with all musculoskeletal tissues that begin to take form very early during embryological development. All musculoskeletal tissues have structural subcategories.

- Muscle is a force-producing tissue and acts on bones through tendons to control movement. Collagenous bands that tether bones together (ligaments) and fibrocartilaginous discs (menisci) can passively control the relative motion of articulating bones.

- Cartilage covering the bone segments within joints provides suitable surfaces for joint lubrication.

- This chapter emphasized the complexity of these tissues and sets the stage for understanding the potential of these tissues to respond to stimuli, including exercise, training, and injury. This information was presented with broad strokes. There are excellent and extensive sources available to provide the fine details of tissue anatomy and histology, and you are encouraged to explore those details.

Questions to Consider

1. You're giving a lecture to a young audience on the dynamic nature of biological tissues, and someone makes the comment, "I always thought that bone was hard and lifeless." Provide arguments to convince the audience member to the contrary.

2. Consider a musculotendinous unit (e.g., calf muscles and the calcaneal [Achilles] tendon). Describe the embryological processes for each component of the unit (i.e., muscle and tendon).

3. Biological tissues work in concert to complete the many tasks and satisfy the functional needs of the human organism. Each tissue has unique characteristics that distinguish it from other tissues. Describe the unique characteristics of muscle, nervous, epithelial, and connective tissues.

4. Describe the steps involved in bone growth and development, and describe several potential impediments to normal, healthy bone growth.

5. Describe what is meant by the *structure–function relation* of biological tissues. Provide specific examples that illustrate this concept.

6. List and explain the factors that affect the amount of force a muscle can produce.

Suggested Readings

Embryology and Development

Iannotti, J.P., S. Goldstein, J. Kuhn, L. Lipiello, F.S. Kaplan, and D.J. Zaleske. 2000. The formation and growth of skeletal tissues. In *Orthopaedic Basic Science* (2nd ed.), edited by S.R Simon. Park Ridge, IL: American Academy of Orthopaedic Surgeons.

Pettifor, J.M., and H. Juppner. 2003. *Pediatric Bone: Biology and Diseases*. London: Academic Press.

Sadler, T.W. 2004. *Langman's Medical Embryology* (9th ed.). Philadelphia: Lippincott Williams & Wilkins.

Histology

Cormack, D.H. 1987. *Ham's Histology* (9th ed.). Philadelphia: Lippincott.

Fawcett, D.W., and R.P. Jensh. 2002. *Bloom and Fawcett: Concise Histology* (2nd ed.). London: Hoddar Arnold.

Garner, L.P., J.L. Hiatt, J.M. Strum, T.A. Swanson, S.I. Kim, and A.S. Schneider. 2002. *Cell Biology and Histology* (4th ed.). Philadelphia: Lippincott Williams & Wilkins.

Bone

Bostrom, M.P.G., A. Boskey, J.J. Kaufman, and T.A. Einhorn. 2000. Form and function of bone. In *Orthopaedic Basic Science* (2nd ed.), edited by S.R. Simon. Park Ridge, IL: American Academy of Orthopaedic Surgeons.

Hall, B.K. ed. 2005. *Bones and Cartilage: Developmental and Evolutionary Skeletal Biology*. London: Elsevier/Academic Press.

Martin, R.B., D.B. Burr, and N.A. Sharkey. 1998. *Skeletal Tissue Mechanics*. New York: Springer.

Cartilage

Mankin, H.J., V.C. Mow, J.A. Buckwalter, J.P. Iannotti, and A. Ratcliffe. 2000. Articular cartilage structure, composition and function. In *Orthopaedic Basic Science* (2nd ed.), edited by S.R. Simon. Park Ridge, IL: American Academy of Orthopaedic Surgeons.

Mow, V.C., A. Ratcliffe, and A.R. Poole. 1992. Cartilage and diarthrodial joints as paradigms for hierarchical materials and structures. *Biomaterials* 13: 67-97.

Tendon and Ligament

Woo, S.L.-Y., K.-N. An, C.B. Frank, G.A. Livesay, C.B. Ma, J. Zeminski, J.S. Wayne, and B.S. Myers. 2000. Anatomy, biology, and biomechanics of tendon and ligament. In *Orthopaedic Basic Science* (2nd ed.), edited by S.R. Simon. Park Ridge, IL: American Academy of Orthopaedic Surgeons.

Skeletal Muscle

Garrett, W.E., Jr., and T.M. Best. 2000. Anatomy, physiology, and mechanics of skeletal muscle. In *Orthopaedic Basic Science* (2nd ed.), edited by S.R. Simon. Park Ridge, IL: American Academy of Orthopaedic Surgeons.

Jones, D.A., J. Round, and A. de Haan. 2004. *Skeletal Muscle, from Molecules to Movement*. Edinburgh, UK: Churchill Livingstone.

Lieber, R.L. 2002. *Skeletal Muscle Structure, Function & Plasticity* (2nd ed.). Philadelphia: Lippincott Williams & Wilkins.

MacIntosh, B.R., P. Gardiner, and A.J. McComas. 2006. *Skeletal Muscle: Form and Function* (2nd ed.). Champaign, IL: Human Kinetics.

Tskhovrebova, L., and J. Trinick. 2010. Roles of titin in the structure and elasticity of the sarcomere. *Biomedical Research International* 2010:612482. https://doi.org/10.1155/2010/612482

Classic Reference

Simon, S.R., ed. 2000. *Orthopaedic Basic Science* (2nd ed.). Park Ridge, IL: American Academy of Orthopaedic Surgeons.

Thompson, D.W. 1992. *On Growth and Form*, edited by J.T. Bonner (abridged ed.). Cambridge: Cambridge University Press. (Originally published 1917)

Basic Biomechanics

Mechanics is the paradise of the mathematical sciences because by means of it one comes to the fruits of mathematics.

Leonardo da Vinci (1452-1519)

OBJECTIVES

- To identify the major areas of biomechanics relevant to human movement: movement mechanics, fluid mechanics, joint mechanics, and material mechanics
- To explain biomechanics concepts and measures, including linear and angular motion, center of gravity, stability, mobility, and movement equilibrium
- To explain concepts of movement mechanics, including kinematics, kinetics, force, pressure, lever systems, torque (moment of force), Newton's laws of motion, work, power, energy, momentum, and friction
- To explain concepts of fluid mechanics, including fluid flow, fluid resistance, and viscosity
- To explain concepts of joint mechanics, including range of motion, joint stability, joint mobility, lever systems, and joint reaction force
- To explain concepts of material mechanics, including stress, strain, stiffness, bending, torsion, viscoelasticity, and material fatigue and failure
- To describe various model types and model selection criteria
- To describe rheological, finite-element, and complex musculoskeletal models

As noted by comedian Jerry Seinfeld, "To me, if life boils down to one thing, it's movement. To live is to keep moving." And to move is to keep living. Movement *is* essential to life. Life processes such as blood circulation, respiration, and muscle contraction require motion, as do activities such as walking, running, jumping, bending, and grasping. Consider how the human organism seeks, consciously or not, to move. When you sit in a chair, for example, do you remain motionless? Hardly. You cross and uncross your legs, slouch, squirm, and slide to create some degree of movement. Children provide perhaps the best evidence of the inherent nature of humans to move. They never seem to stop moving. Even as we age and slow down, movement remains a quintessential element of our being.

In times past, movement meant survival. Those not able to move—or move rapidly enough—often met with injury or death. Although we no longer have to escape from predators (except on rare occasions), our ability to move can still serve us well in avoiding dangerous situations (e.g., dodging an oncoming vehicle). Therefore, limited movement, whether as a result of disability or a sedentary lifestyle, may directly or indirectly contribute to our susceptibility to injury as well as contribute to deleterious health effects, such as cardiovascular disease, diabetes, and cancer

In mechanical terms there are two basic forms of movement: (1) **linear motion** (also called **translational motion**), in which a body moves along either a straight line (**rectilinear motion**) or a curved line (**curvilinear motion**), and (2) **angular motion** (also called **rotational motion**), in which the body rotates about an **axis of rotation** (figure 3.1). Although there are theoretically an infinite number of axes about which a body can rotate, only a few are of practical interest in discussing movement of human body segments (figure 3.2). As we discuss biomechanics in this chapter, note that we often refer to an object as a **body**. The word *body* in this context is taken to mean any collection of matter. It may refer to the entire human body, a body segment (e.g., thigh or upper arm), or any other collected mass (e.g., a block of wood).

Many of the movements performed by living organisms are a combination of both linear and angular motion. Simultaneous linear and angular motion is termed **general motion**. Consider, for example, the movement of a person's thigh during walking, which combines linear motion in a forward direction with angular motion as it rotates about the hip joint axis in alternating phases of flexion and extension.

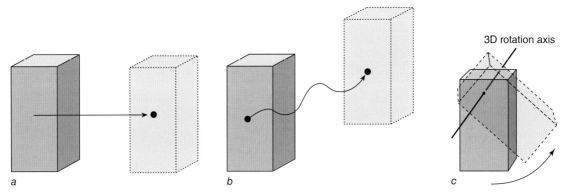

FIGURE 3.1 Linear and angular motion. *(a)* Rectilinear (straight line) motion, *(b)* curvilinear motion, and *(c)* angular (rotational) motion.

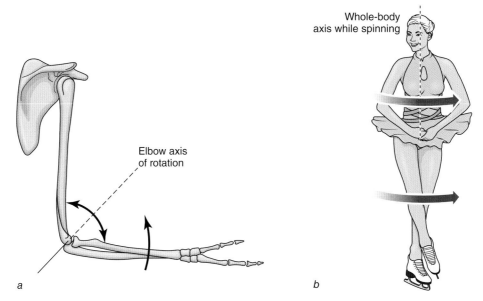

FIGURE 3.2 Examples of anatomical axes of rotation. *(a)* Elbow flexion and extension about the elbow's axis of rotation. *(b)* Ice skater's whole body rotating about a longitudinal (vertical) axis.

The movement of an inanimate object can also exhibit combined motion. The flight of a basketball shot toward the rim demonstrates both linear motion (the curved path, or arc, of the ball) and angular motion (the backspin of the ball). As we explore the mechanical concepts in this chapter, the notions of linear and angular motion recur often. Combinations of these two simple movement forms result in the wide and nearly endless variety of human movement patterns.

Human movement can be viewed from several perspectives. One perspective considers how mechanical factors that produce and control movement work inside the body (**internal mechanics**) and affect the body from without (**external mechanics**). Examples of internal mechanical factors include the forces produced by muscle action and the stability provided by ligaments surrounding joints. External mechanical factors include gravity, friction, and other external forces, such as a foot striking the ground or a falling brick hitting the top of one's head.

Another important perspective on movement involves the difference between describing a movement versus identifying the forces involved in producing or controlling the movement. The description of the temporal (timing) and spatial aspects of movement, without regard to the forces involved, is known as **kinematics**. The assessment of movement with consideration of the forces involved is called **kinetics**.

Kinematics

Kinematics involves five primary variables:

1. Temporal (timing) characteristics of movement
2. Position or location
3. Displacement (describing what movement has occurred)
4. Velocity (a measure of how fast something has moved or is moving)
5. Acceleration (an indicator of how quickly the velocity has changed)

The last four variables (position, displacement, velocity, and acceleration) can be expressed in linear or angular form, giving rise to the general descriptors of linear kinematics and angular kinematics. Keep in mind that displacement, velocity, and acceleration are all **vector** measurements, which have both magnitude and direction.

We can further assess kinematics according to whether the motion is viewed two-dimensionally (*planar kinematics*) or three-dimensionally (*spatial kinematics*). The essential terminology and formulations for planar kinematics are described in the following sections and summarized in figure 3.3.

- *Time.* The first kinematic variable, **time**, provides a measure of the duration of a particular event. Noting that a person's right foot is in contact with the ground for 450 milliseconds (ms or msec) during a single step is a simple example of a temporal kinematic measure. The duration (Δt) of force application associated with acute musculoskeletal injuries is typically quite short and may last only a fraction of a second. This short time interval necessarily results in high loading rates. As we'll see later, loading rate is an important factor in determining a tissue's mechanical response to applied forces.

- *Position.* The position of the body plays a critical role in determining the likelihood of injury. Forces applied to an arm that is hyperextended and externally rotated, for example, will cause a different injury pattern than the same forces applied to an arm that is flexed and internally rotated at the moment of force application. Similarly, a force applied to the top of one's head when the neck is flexed will result in different injuries than if the same force is applied to the head while the neck is hyperextended. The position of a body segment can be described qualitatively (e.g., arm is abducted) or quantitatively (e.g., forearm is positioned with the elbow flexed 45°). The position of a specific point, or landmark, on the body can be specified quantitatively using, for example, either Cartesian (x,y) coordinates or polar (r,θ) coordinates (see figure 3.3).

- *Displacement.* The vector measure of movement from one location to another is called **displacement**. Linear displacement (Δd) is measured as a straight-line vector from the starting position (A) to the ending position (B), regardless of the path taken. The **distance**, a scalar quantity, measures how far the body has moved along any given path in getting from A to B. A body rotating about an axis experiences **angular displacement** ($\Delta\theta$), which is measured by the number of degrees (or radians) of rotation (e.g., the knee flexed through an angular displacement of 35°). A direct relation exists between the linear and angular measures of distance and displacement, as shown in figure 3.4a.

- *Velocity.* **Velocity** is a measure of the time rate of displacement. The average **linear velocity** (v) is given by the quotient of linear displacement (Δd) divided by Δt. **Angular velocity** (ω) is

	Linear		Angular	
	Symbol	Formula or relation	Symbol	Formula or relation
Time	t	$t_2 - t_1 = \Delta t$	t	$t_2 - t_1 = \Delta t$
Position	(x, y)	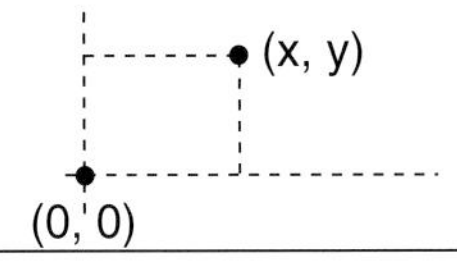 $\bullet\ (x, y)$ $(0, 0)$	(r, θ)	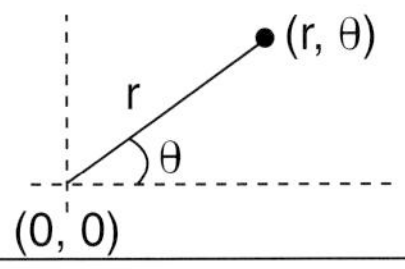 $\bullet\ (r, \theta)$ $(0, 0)$
Displacement (x-direction only)	d	$d = x_2 - x_1$ $x_1 \bullet \xrightarrow{\ d\ } \bullet\ x_2$	θ	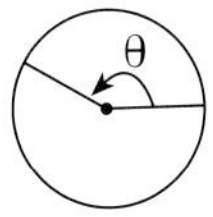
Average velocity	$\bar{v}$	$\bar{v} = \dfrac{d_2 - d_1}{t_2 - t_1} = \dfrac{\Delta d}{\Delta t}$	$\bar{\omega}$	$\bar{\omega} = \dfrac{\theta_2 - \theta_1}{t_2 - t_1} = \dfrac{\Delta\theta}{\Delta t}$
Instantaneous velocity	v	$v = \dfrac{dx}{dt} = \dot{x}$	ω	$\omega = \dfrac{d\theta}{dt} = \dot{\theta}$
Average acceleration	$\bar{a}$	$\bar{a} = \dfrac{v_2 - v_1}{t_2 - t_1} = \dfrac{\Delta v}{\Delta t}$	$\bar{\alpha}$	$\bar{\alpha} = \dfrac{\omega_2 - \omega_1}{t_2 - t_1} = \dfrac{\Delta\omega}{\Delta t}$
Instantaneous acceleration	a	$a = \dfrac{dv}{dt} = \ddot{x}$	α	$\alpha = \dfrac{d\omega}{dt} = \ddot{\theta}$

FIGURE 3.3 Terminology and formulas for planar kinematics.

calculated by dividing the angular displacement ($\Delta\theta$) by the change in time (Δt). A direct relation exists between the linear and angular measures of velocity (figure 3.4*b*). In common usage, the terms *velocity* and *speed* often are used interchangeably. In mechanical terms, however, they have distinct— although related—meanings. Velocity is a vector quantity (magnitude and direction), whereas **speed** is a **scalar** (magnitude only) measure. The speed of a runner might be 5 m/s. To transform the movement

measure to velocity, we must indicate the running direction—for example, 5 m/s due north.

A distinction also needs be drawn between *average* and *instantaneous* values. Average velocity measures the mean value of velocities over a period of time. For example, if a jogger runs at 1.79 m/s for 1 hour, followed by 1 hour running at 2.23 m/s, the jogger's average velocity for the 2-hour period is 2.01 m/s. Instantaneous velocity, in contrast, measures the velocity at a specific instant in time. Using

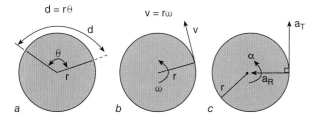

FIGURE 3.4 Relation between linear and angular measures. *(a)* Linear distance (*d*) moved along the circumference of a circle (radius = *r*) equals $r \cdot \theta$. *(b)* Linear velocity (*v*) of a point on the circumference of a circle equals $r \cdot \omega$. *(c)* Linear tangential acceleration (a_T) of a point on the circumference of a circle equals $r \cdot \alpha$. Radial acceleration (a_R) equals v^2/r. (Note: Angular measurements of θ, ω, and α in these equations must be expressed in units of radians (rad), rad/s, and rad/s^2, respectively).

the previous example, after 30 minutes of running, the jogger would have an instantaneous velocity of 1.79 m/s. After 90 minutes, the jogger would have an instantaneous velocity of 2.23 m/s.

• *Acceleration.* **Acceleration** measures the time rate of change in a body's velocity. **Linear acceleration** (*a*) is measured as the change in linear velocity (Δv) divided by the change in time (Δt). Similarly, **angular acceleration** (α) is the change in angular velocity ($\Delta \omega$) divided by change in time (Δt). As was the case with linear and angular velocity, a direct relation exists between the linear and angular measures of acceleration (figure 3.4*c*). Many musculoskeletal injuries are acceleration related. Rapid acceleration or deceleration of the head, for example, can result in concussive injury to the brain. Linear acceleration often is expressed in units of g, where 1 g is the acceleration created by the earth's gravitational pull (-9.81 m/s^2). Thus, a boxer's head hit with a force of 5 g would be accelerated at five times the acceleration caused by gravity.

Kinetics

Description is an important first step in analyzing any movement. Kinematic analyses, however, are limited to describing the spatial geometry and timing of movement without considering the forces involved. Because force is a causal agent in movement, kinetics (the study of forces and their effects) is an area worthy of our consideration. Keep in mind that the following force-related concepts are interrelated, and to consider each of them in isolation limits their applicability and our ability to analyze injury biomechanics.

Linear Kinetics

If the applied forces are large enough to overcome a body's resistance to movement, the body moves linearly. Linear kinetics examines the relation between a body's resistance to a change in its linear state of motion and the effect of applied forces.

Mass, Inertia, and Force

The quantity of matter in a body is its **mass**. Mass is measured in SI units (Système international d'unités); that is, in kilograms (kg). Common sense suggests that the greater an object's mass, the more difficult it is to move. **Inertia** is the resistance to a change in a body's state of linear motion and describes the tendency of a body to remain at rest or in uniform motion in a straight line (i.e., constant velocity) until acted upon by an external force (see Newton's first law of motion later in this chapter). To move an object that is at rest, we must overcome its inertia, or its tendency to remain stationary.

Force is the most fundamental mechanical element involved in injury. **Force** is defined as the mechanical action or effect applied to a body that tends to produce acceleration, or more simply as a "push or pull." The standard SI unit of force is the **newton** (N), defined as the force required to accelerate a 1 kg mass at 1 meter per second in the direction of the force (1 N = 1 kg $\cdot$ m $\cdot$ s^{-2}). In the British Imperial system of measurement, the unit of force is the pound (lb). One pound equals 4.45 N; thus, a person weighing 180 lbs would weigh 801 N.

In preparation for a more general discussion of force, we introduce the concept of an **idealized force vector**. Consider, for example, the forces acting on the head of the femur during the process of standing up: An infinite number of force vectors could be distributed over the articular surface. We can, however, create a single force vector—an *idealized force vector*—that represents the net effect of all the other vectors, essentially idealizing the situation through simplification. In creating a model with a single vector from which calculations and evaluations can be made, we lose information about the actual distribution of the forces across the surface. Nonetheless, this concept of an idealized force vector is useful in many situations, as noted shortly.

Forces inherent to injury analysis are those that act in or upon the human body. Among these are gravity (which accelerates objects downward at ~9.81 m/s^2); friction; the impact of the feet, hands, or body on the ground; the impact of objects col-

The Kilogram: Past, Present, and Future

The standard (SI) unit of mass is the kilogram (also spelled *kilogramme*). The kilogram (kg) has been defined in several ways since its first definition in 1793 as the "mass of 1 litre of water." In 1795, the gram (1/1000 of a kilogram) was defined as the mass of one cubic centimeter of water at the melting point of ice. The Metre Convention, signed in 1875, led to the production of the International Prototype of the Kilogram (IPK) in 1879. For nearly 140 years, the original prototype stood as the standard kilogram.

A new definition of the kilogram was agreed upon by the 26th General Conference on Weights and Measures (CGPM) in November 2018 and implemented on May 20, 2019. The kilogram (kg) is now defined using three fundamental physical constants: (1) Planck's constant h ($6.62607015 \times 10^{-34}$ J·s), (2) c (the speed of light), and (3) Δv_{cs} (a specific atomic transition frequency).

Note: The term *kilogram* also is used in some instances as a unit of force, rather than mass. In these cases, it is designated as *kgf* (in contrast to *kgm* for kilogram mass). When used as a unit of force, 1 kgf = 2.2 pounds.

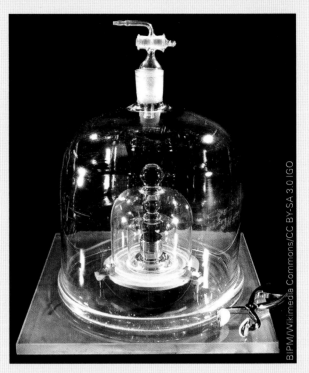

The original prototype kilogram mass, a platinum-iridium cylinder, is stored in a vault at the International Bureau of Weights and Measures (BIPM) in Sèvres, France.

BIPM/Wikimedia Commons/CC BY-SA 3.0 IGO

---

liding with the body (e.g., thrown ball or bullet); musculotendinous forces; ligament forces acting at joints; and compressive forces exerted on long bones of the lower extremities.

In injury-causing situations, seven factors combine, often in complex ways, to determine the nature of the injury, the tissues injured, and the severity of the injury:

1. Magnitude (How much force is applied?)
2. Location (Where on the body or structure is the force applied?)
3. Direction (Where is the force directed?)
4. Duration (Over what time interval is the force applied?)
5. Frequency (How often is the force applied?)
6. Variability (Is the magnitude of the force constant or variable over the application interval?)
7. Rate (How quickly is the force applied?)

In the human body, rarely does a single force act in isolation. Much more common are cases involving multiple forces. To aid in analysis, it is useful to categorize multiple forces as *force systems*. Types of force systems include **linear**, **parallel**, **concurrent**, and **general force systems** (figure 3.5*a*-3.5*d*). A special case of force application is a **force couple**, which is composed of two oppositely directed parallel forces that tend to create rotation about an axis (figure 3.5*e*).

The engineering approach uses a free-body diagram for biomechanical analysis of a force system. A **free-body diagram (FBD)** is simply a graphic representation of all the forces acting in a system. Figure 3.6 depicts a FBD for a simple biomechanical application. Note that the effect of gravity is represented as a single vector, another example of an idealized force vector. In actuality, gravity acts on each small element of body mass.

Center of Mass and Center of Gravity

When an idealized force vector is developed, many vectors are reduced to a single vector. A similar pro-

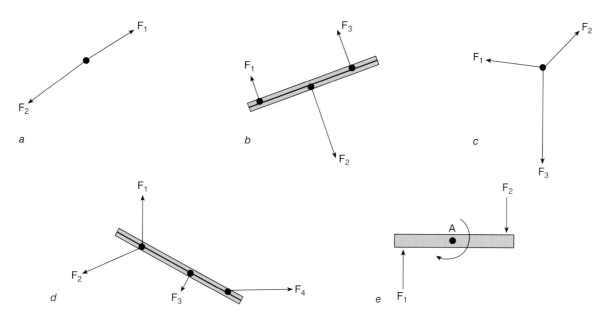

FIGURE 3.5 Force systems. *(a)* Linear force system. *(b)* Parallel force system. *(c)* Concurrent force system. *(d)* General force system, the designation given to a force system that does not fall under one of the classifications *a* through *c*. *(e)* Force couple; parallel and oppositely directed forces F_1 and F_2 cause rotation about axis A.

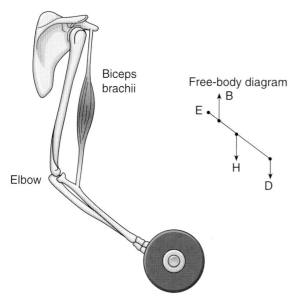

FIGURE 3.6 The free-body diagram (FBD) *(right)* represents the forces acting on the upper extremity while a subject is holding a dumbbell in the hand *(left)*. Gravity creates force (weight) vectors for the dumbbell (*D*) and forearm and hand (*H*). The biceps brachii creates a muscle force represented by the vector (*B*). All force vectors tend to cause rotation about the elbow joint axis (*E*).

cess can be applied to the mass of a body by reducing its distributed mass to a single point (**point mass**) that represents the entire body. Again, this type of simplification will facilitate analysis, but with a loss of information related to the spatial distribution of the mass about the single (point) mass.

For any body, there exists a point at which, if concentrated into a point mass, it would move exactly the same as it would in its distributed state; this known as the **center of mass** (or *centroid*) or **center of gravity**. Even though there is a technical distinction between the center of gravity and the center of mass of a body, in practical terms they are located at the same point, and therefore we use the terms interchangeably.

The center of mass alternatively may be defined as the point about which a body's mass is equally distributed. The center of gravity also acts as a balance point, such as when a food server places their hand at the center of gravity of a tray full of dishes and balances the tray overhead.

The human body's center of mass typically is located within the body's boundaries (figure 3.7*a*), but this may not always be the case (figure 3.7*b*).

Pressure

Because many injuries occur as a result of one object impacting another, it is important to know how the force of impact is distributed across the surface being contacted. A sharp object contacting the skin with 300 N of force will likely have a different effect (e.g., penetration) than a blunt object impacting the skin with a similar force (e.g., contusion). A funda-

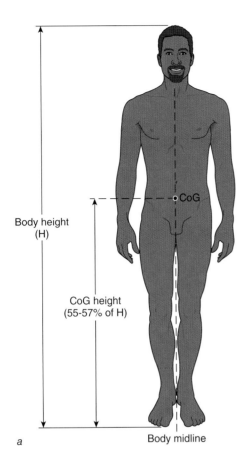

Body height (H)

CoG height (55-57% of H)

CoG

a

Body midline

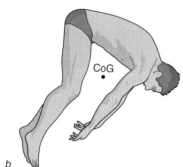

CoG

b

FIGURE 3.7 *(a)* Center of gravity location in the human body in anatomical position. *(b)* Center of gravity located outside the body when the body is in a bent-over, or pike, position, as during a gymnastic maneuver or dive.

Reprinted by permission from W.C. Whiting, *Dynamic Human Anatomy*, 2nd ed. (Champaign, IL: Human Kinetics, 2019).

$$p = F/A \qquad \text{(3.1)}$$

where p = pressure, F = applied force, and A = area of contact. The standard unit of pressure, the **pascal** (**Pa**), is equal to a 1 N force applied to an area 1 meter square ($1 \text{ Pa} = 1 \text{ N/m}^2$). In injury situations, the pressures exerted on body structures can be quite high and are often expressed with a unit of **megapascal** (**MPa**), which is equal to a 1 N force applied to an area 1 millimeter square ($1 \text{ MPa} = 1 \text{ N/mm}^2$).

Angular Kinetics

Angular kinetics examines the relation between a body's resistance to a change in its angular state of motion and the effect of applied torques. Its major concepts include moment of force and moment of inertia.

Moment of Force (Torque)

In the case of linear motion, force is the mechanical agent creating and controlling movement. For angular motion the agent is known as a *moment of force*, **moment** (M), or **torque** (T), and is generally defined as the effect of a force that tends to cause a change in a body's state of angular position or motion (figure 3.8). More specifically, *torque* typically refers to the twisting action (torsion) created by a force, as seen in turning a screwdriver, or torsional loading of the lower leg (tibia) in a skiing fall. *Moment* relates to the rotational (e.g., knee extension) or bending action (e.g., pole vault) of a force. Despite this technical distinction, the two terms are often used interchangeably in biomechanics.

The mathematical definitions of moment and torque are the same. The magnitude of a moment or torque is equal to the applied force times the shortest (perpendicular) distance from the axis of rotation to the line of force action. This perpendicular distance is known as the **moment arm**, **torque arm**, or **lever arm**. The standard unit of moment (torque) measurement comes from the product of the two terms: *force* (N) times *moment arm* (m). The resulting unit is a newton-meter (N·m).

For a force acting at a right angle to the body being rotated, the moment arm is the distance d (figure 3.9*a*), and the magnitude of the moment (M) is given by this equation:

$$M = F \cdot d \qquad \text{(3.2)}$$

If the force F in figure 3.9*a* was 175 N, for example, and was acting at a distance d of 1.2 m from the axis, the moment (torque) created would equal $F \cdot d$, or $M = 175 \text{ N} \cdot 1.2 \text{ m} = 210 \text{ N·m}$.

mental principle of injury mechanics dictates that as the area of force application increases, the likelihood of injury decreases, and vice versa.

The measure of force and its distribution is **pressure**, defined as the total applied force divided by the area over which the force is applied. In equation form,

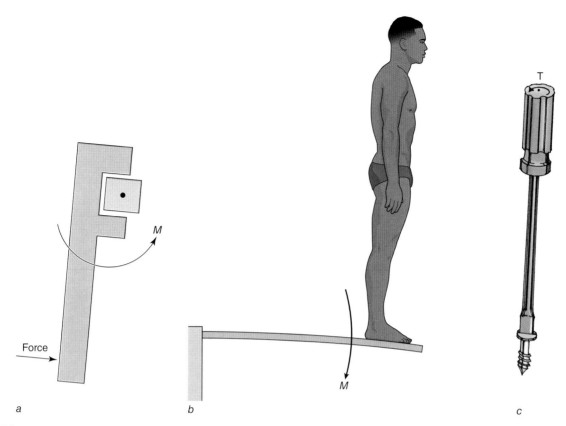

FIGURE 3.8 Applied examples of moment of force (*M*) or torque (*T*). *(a)* Force applied to a wrench creates a moment to turn a nut on a bolt. *(b)* The body weight of a diver creates a moment that bends the diving board. *(c)* Torque shown by the twisting acting of a screwdriver.

Reprinted by permission from W.C. Whiting, *Dynamic Human Anatomy,* 2nd ed. (Champaign, IL: Human Kinetics, 2019).

In cases where the force is not acting perpendicularly to the segment, the moment arm is smaller and is calculated using the appropriate trigonometric function as shown in figure 3.9*b*. The magnitude of the moment (*M*) in this case is

$$M = F \cdot d \cdot \sin(\beta) \text{ or } M = F \cdot d \cdot \cos(\theta) \qquad (3.3)$$

If the same 175 N force as in the preceding example was acting at an angle $\beta = 35°$ (as shown in figure 3.9*b*), the moment arm would be $d' = d \cdot \sin(\beta) = 1.2 \text{ m} \cdot 0.574 = 0.688 \text{ m}$. The moment created now is $M = F \cdot d' = 175 \text{ N} \cdot 0.688 \text{ m} = 120.4 \text{ N·m}$.

Closer examination of equation 3.2 reveals several principles that are important when applying torque concepts to injury biomechanics. First, there is an obvious interaction between the force and the moment arm that directly affects the magnitude of the applied torque. To increase the moment, we have the following options:

- Increasing the force while holding the moment arm constant

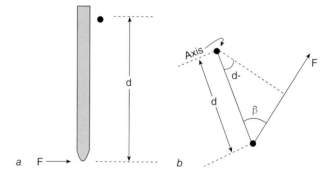

FIGURE 3.9 Moment (torque) arm. *(a)* When the force acts perpendicularly to the segment, the moment arm is the distance *d*. The moment is given by equation 3.2. *(b)* When the force acts at an angle (β) to the segment of length *d*, the moment arm $d' = d \cdot \sin(\beta)$. The moment in this case is given by equation 3.3.

- Increasing the moment arm while holding the force constant
- Increasing both the force and the moment arm

- Decreasing the force while increasing the moment arm more than proportionally so that the net effect is an increase in moment

- Decreasing the moment arm while increasing the force more than proportionally so that the net effect is again an increase in moment

To decrease the moment, we have only to reverse the logic in each of these five cases.

A second moment-related concept, although simple in statement, is powerful in its application. That is, when a force is applied through the axis of rotation, no moment is produced. This concept follows directly from the moment equation $M = F \cdot d$, where d = moment arm. If the force passes through the axis, the moment arm is zero, and hence no moment is produced. This creates the potential for a situation in which body tissues are exposed to extremely high forces but with no moment created. Compressive forces acting through the center of a vertebral body, for example, will cause no vertebral rotation but will increase the likelihood of a compressive fracture.

A third moment concept arises from the fact that in many instances, only a portion of the applied force is involved in producing a moment, as can be seen in the two examples in figure 3.10. In the first situation (figure 3.10*a*), the weight attached to the foot (F_w) can be broken into two force components: F_r, which causes rotation about the knee joint axis and is termed the **rotatory component** of force, and F_d, whose line of action passes through the joint axis and contributes nothing to the moment about the

knee. F_d acts to pull the segment away from the joint axis and is thus referred to as a *distracting, dislocating,* or **destabilizing component** of force. Similarly, in figure 3.10*b*, the biceps force (F_b) has a rotatory component (F_r). In contrast to the previous example, however, the component (F_s) passing through the axis is directed toward the axis and is called a **stabilizing component** of force.

A fourth moment concept arises from many real situations in which more than one moment is applied to the system. The system's response is based on the **net moment** (also called **net torque**) or the result of adding together all the moments acting about the axis. A simple glenohumeral abduction exercise provides an example (figure 3.11). Gravity, acting on the arm and the dumbbell, creates a moment about the glenohumeral axis of rotation that tends to adduct the arm. The magnitude of this moment (M_1) is given by

$$M_1 = W_a \cdot d_a + W_b \cdot d_b \tag{3.4}$$

where W_a = weight of the arm and hand, d_a = moment arm (distance from the glenohumeral axis of rotation to the arm's center of gravity), W_b = weight of the dumbbell, and d_b = moment arm (distance from axis to dumbbell's center of gravity). By convention, moments tending to create clockwise rotation are designated as negative (–) moments. Moments in the counterclockwise direction are positive (+). M_1 is therefore a negative moment.

If M_1 was the only moment acting on the system, the arm would immediately adduct under

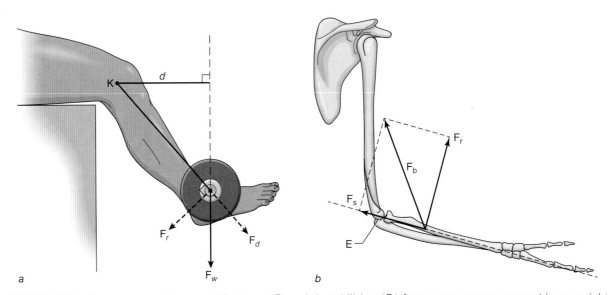

FIGURE 3.10 Components of force. *(a)* Rotatory (F_r) and destabilizing (F_d) force components created by a weight (F_w) secured to the foot of a person performing a leg extension exercise about the knee joint axis (*K*). *(b)* Rotatory (F_r) and stabilizing (F_s) force components created by the biceps brachii (F_b) during elbow flexion about the elbow axis (*E*).

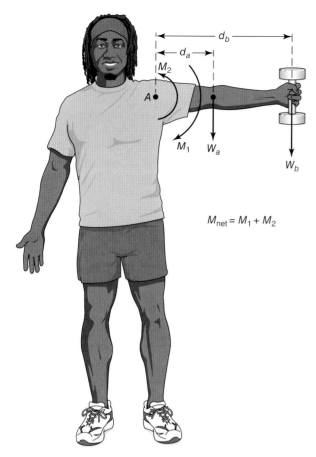

$$M_{net} = M_1 + M_2$$

FIGURE 3.11 Net joint moment. The net moment (M_{net}) of the combined moments created by $M_1 + M_2$. The weight of the arm (W_a) and dumbbell (W_b) combine to create an adductor moment (M_1) acting about the glenohumeral joint axis A. The force of the glenohumeral abductor muscles creates an abductor moment (M_2) to counteract M_1. (M_1 acts in a clockwise direction and thus creates a negative moment. Conversely, M_2 acts counterclockwise and is positive.)

Reprinted by permission from W.C. Whiting, *Dynamic Human Anatomy*, 2nd ed. (Champaign, IL: Human Kinetics, 2019).

the effect of gravity. However, the glenohumeral abductor muscles acting about the glenohumeral joint create a moment (M_2) acting in the opposite direction, which is termed a **countermoment** or **countertorque**. The countermoment in this example is a positive (counterclockwise) moment and will tend to abduct the arm. The movement that results depends on the relative magnitudes of M_1 and M_2. By adding the two moments together, we create a net moment (M_{net}):

$$M_{net} = M_1 + M_2 \tag{3.5}$$

In this example we have three possible scenarios: (1) If M_1 is equal to M_2, then $M_{net} = 0$ and the arm

remains in its horizontal position; (2) if $M_1 > M_2$, then $M_{net} < 0$, and the arm will adduct; (3) if $M_1 < M_2$, then $M_{net} > 0$ and the arm will abduct. The resulting movement thus depends on the net moment acting at the joint about which the movement occurs.

Moment of Inertia

Just as bodies resist change in their state of linear motion (inertia), they also tend to resist changes to angular forms of movement. The term used to describe this resistance to a change in angular state of motion or position is **moment of inertia**. There are three types of moment of inertia corresponding to the three forms or configurations of angular movement: rotation, bending, and torsion.

A body at rest and with a fixed axis (e.g., a pendulum) will resist being moved rotationally, just as a body that is already rotating at a constant angular velocity (ω) will tend to maintain that angular velocity and will resist a change in its velocity. The measure of this resistance to change in a body's state of angular motion (rotation) is termed **mass moment of inertia** (I). Recall that the magnitude of resistance in the case of linear movement was determined by the mass of the object. In the case of angular movement, the magnitude of the resistance is determined by the mass and the mass's distribution with respect to a specified axis of rotation. For a point mass, the mass moment of inertia is defined as

$$I = m \cdot r^2 \tag{3.6}$$

where m = mass of the body and r = distance from the axis of rotation to the point mass (figure 3.12). For a distributed mass, such as a limb segment, the mass moment of inertia is

$$I = \int m_i \cdot r_i^2 \tag{3.7}$$

where m_i = mass of the ith point mass and r_i = distance of the ith point mass from the axis of rotation. As the mass is moved farther from the axis, the resistance, or mass moment of inertia, increases as a function of the square of the distance moved.

The other two types of moment of inertia (area moment of inertia and polar moment of inertia) are explained in later sections.

Kinetic Concepts and Measures

Several kinetic concepts are important in our discussion of injury biomechanics. These include Newton's laws of motion, equilibrium, work and power, energy, momentum, collisions, and friction. These concepts are discussed in the following sections.

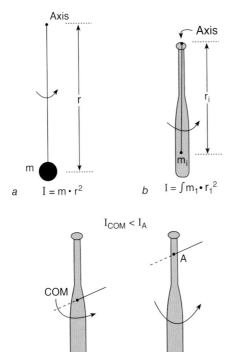

FIGURE 3.12 Moment of inertia. *(a)* Moment of inertia (*I*) for a point mass equals the product of the mass (*m*) and the square of the distance (*r*) from the axis to the mass (equation 3.6). *(b)* A baseball bat illustrates a distributed mass with an axis shown in the handle end of the bat. The moment of inertia for a distributed mass is given by equation 3.7. *(c)* The moment of inertia (I_{com}) of any body (e.g., a baseball bat) about an axis through its center of mass is less than the moment of inertia (I_A) for the same body about an axis at point A because more of the mass is farther away from the axis in the second case.

Newton's Laws of Motion

Among Sir Isaac Newton's (1642-1727) many scientific contributions, perhaps most profound and enduring are his laws of motion, which form the basis for classical (Newtonian) mechanics:

- *Law of inertia.* The **first law of motion** states that a body at rest or in uniform linear motion (moving in a straight line at a constant velocity) will tend to remain at rest or in uniform motion, unless acted upon by an external force. A body at rest or in uniform angular motion (moving about an axis at a constant angular velocity) will tend to remain at rest or in uniform motion, unless acted upon by an external torque.

- *Law of acceleration.* The **second law of motion** states that a force (*F*) acting on a body with mass (*m*) will produce an acceleration (*a*) proportional to the force, or mathematically $F = m \cdot a$. Angularly, a torque (*T*) applied to a body will produce an angular acceleration (α) proportional to the torque, or mathematically $T = I \cdot \alpha$ (where *I* = mass moment of inertia).

- *Law of action and reaction.* The **third law of motion** states that for every action there is an equal and opposite reaction.

Several examples show how these laws play a role in determining the mechanisms of performance and injury (figure 3.13). For example, a cervical whiplash mechanism during frontal impact (figure 3.13*a*) is

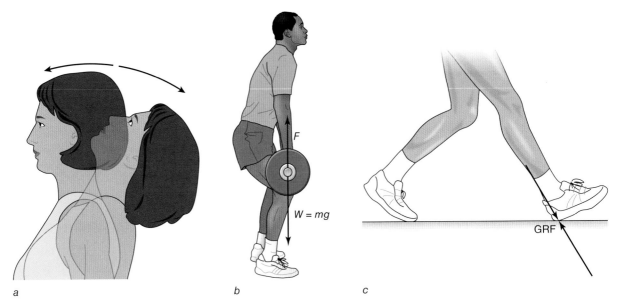

FIGURE 3.13 Newton's laws of motion. *(a)* First law of motion applied to a whiplash mechanism. *(b)* Second law of motion involved during a weightlifting movement. *F* = force applied by the weightlifter; *W* = weight; *m* = mass; *g* = acceleration attributable to gravity. *(c)* Third law of motion exemplified by the ground reaction force created when a runner's foot strikes the ground.

Hip Joint Moments

Hip joint injuries are, unfortunately, quite common, especially in older adults. Structural features of the hip such as the relation of the femoral neck and head to the long axis of the femur can increase the risk of hip fracture. Normally, the angle between the long axis and the neck is about 120°. However, abnormal angles can alter the mechanical loading of the proximal femur. In a condition called **coxa vara**, this angle is smaller than normal; in **coxa valga**, the angle is greater than normal. When the bone is loaded, as during the stance phase of gait, compressive forces act on the femoral head. Because these forces are offset from the long axis of the femoral diaphysis, *cantilever bending* occurs. This produces a moment about an axis (shown as *A* in the figure). In coxa vara, the moment arm (d_r) is longer than in the normal condition (d_n). For a given force (*F*), the coxa vara moment (M_r) is greater than normal (M_n). In contrast, the deviation in coxa valga results in a shorter moment arm ($d_l < d_n$) and, hence, a smaller moment ($M_r > M_n > M_l$). Larger moments create greater stresses in the bony tissue.

   If there is an area of relative weakness in the femur, as in an osteoporotic patient, the likelihood of bone fracture increases. With this potential mechanism of injury, an older woman, for example, on occasion may break her hip and fall, instead of the more common case in which she falls and breaks her hip.

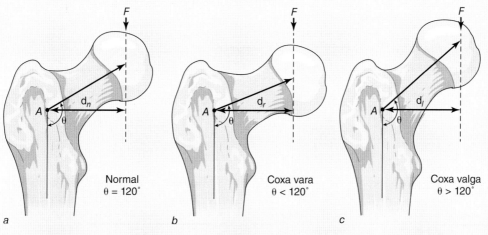

Normal
θ = 120°

Coxa vara
θ < 120°

Coxa valga
θ > 120°

a   *b*   *c*

Structural geometry of the femur: *(a)* normal, *(b)* coxa vara, and *(c)* coxa valga.

simply a consequence of the first law of motion. Just before impact, the automobile and its seat-belted and shoulder-harnessed driver are moving at a constant velocity. At impact, the outside force abruptly decelerates the vehicle and the belted occupant's body. However, for a brief interval the head obeys the first law of motion and continues in its uniform motion (straight ahead). Resistance forces provided by neck structures rapidly decelerate the head, causing violent flexion of the cervical spine. The head then rebounds into hyperextension. This flexion–extension pattern is typical of many whiplash-related injuries and is explained by Newton's first law.

   In the second example (figure 3.13*b*), the weightlifter must exert considerable force to accelerate the bar upward. Newton's second law of motion determines the magnitude of the acceleration in response to the applied force, $F = m \cdot a$. More detailed application of the laws of motion allows us to estimate the forces acting at various joints throughout the body. If these forces exceed the ability of the body's structures to tolerate load, injury occurs.

   In the third example (figure 3.13*c*), the marathon runner's feet contact the ground many thousands of times. At each contact, Newton's third law comes into play. The force that the foot exerts on the ground is equally and oppositely resisted by the ground; this is called **ground reaction force** (GRF). Increasing the magnitude and frequency of the GRF increases the chances of injury.

Equilibrium

The word *equilibrium* implies a balanced condition. From a mechanical standpoint, **equilibrium** exists when forces and moments are each balanced. Equilibrium exists for a body at rest or for one moving with constant linear and angular velocities; the net force (ΣF, where the Greek letter sigma means "sum of") and net moment (ΣM) acting on the body are both equal to zero. A body at rest is in a state called **static equilibrium**. In spatial terms (three-dimensional space), for a body in static equilibrium the following equations must be satisfied in two dimensions (planar):

$$\sum F_x = 0 \quad \sum F_y = 0 \quad \sum M = 0 \tag{3.8}$$

and in three dimensions (spatial):

$$\sum F_x = 0 \quad \sum F_y = 0 \quad \sum F_z = 0 \tag{3.9}$$

$$\sum M_x = 0 \quad \sum M_y = 0 \quad \sum M_z = 0$$

where F_x, F_y, and F_z are the forces in the x, y, and z directions, respectively, and M_x, M_y, and M_z are the moments about the x, y, and z axes, respectively.

Bodies in motion and experiencing external forces and moments are in **dynamic equilibrium** and must adhere to the following equations. In two dimensions (planar):

$$\sum F_x = m \cdot a_x \quad \sum F_y = m \cdot a_y \quad \sum M = I \cdot \alpha \tag{3.10}$$

In three dimensions (spatial):

$$\sum F_x = m \cdot a_x \quad \sum F_y = m \cdot a_y \quad \sum F_z = m \cdot a_z \tag{3.11}$$

$$\sum M_x = I_x \cdot \alpha_x \quad \sum M_y = I_y \cdot \alpha_y \quad \sum M_z = I_z \cdot \alpha_z$$

where a_x, a_y, and a_z are the linear accelerations of the center of mass in the x, y, and z directions, respectively; α_x, α_y, and α_z are the angular accelerations about the x, y, and z axes, respectively; and I_x, I_y, and I_z are the mass moments of inertia about the x, y, and z axes, respectively.

Work and Power

The term **work** is used in many ways, including reference to physical labor ("I'm working hard"), physiological energy expenditure ("I worked off 100 calories"), or an occupation ("I went to work"). In mechanical terms, work has a specific meaning. **Mechanical work** is performed by a force acting through a distance in the direction of the force. By definition, **linear work** (W) is a scalar measure equal to the product of force (F) and the distance (d) through which the body is moved (figure 3.14a):

$$W = F \cdot d \tag{3.12}$$

The standard (SI) unit of work is the joule (1 J = 1 N·m). If the entire force is not acting in the direction of motion (figure 3.14b), then only the component of force in that direction is used to calculate the work done. Figure 3.14b shows a force (F) at an angle (β) above the horizontal. In this case, the work performed is

$$W = F \cdot d \cdot \cos(\beta) \tag{3.13}$$

where F = applied force, d = distance, and β = angle of force above the horizontal.

In the example depicted in figure 3.14c, the work performed in lifting the barbell from point A to point B is equal to the product of the barbell's weight (W_b) and the distance from A to B (d_{AB}). If, for example, the barbell weighed 800 N and was lifted 0.5 m, the work done would be 400 J.

In the previous examples, the force was assumed constant. In real-world situations, however, that often is not the case. Determination of work done by a varying force is more involved, because it must be calculated at successive intervals and requires the use of calculus. The equation becomes

$$W = \int F_x \cdot dx \tag{3.14}$$

In similar fashion, **angular work** ($W_\angle$) is defined as the product of torque (T) times the angle (θ) through which a body rotates. In equation form,

$$W_\angle = T \cdot \theta \tag{3.15}$$

The calculation of work alone often is insufficient to completely describe the mechanics of a body's movement. In many cases, the *rate* of work also is important. The rate of work is termed **power**. **Linear power** (P) is defined as the rate at which linear work is done:

$$P = W / \Delta t \tag{3.16}$$

where W = work performed and Δt = change in time, or the time interval over which the work was done.

Angular power ($P_\angle$) is defined as the rate at which angular work is done:

$$P_\angle = W_\angle / \Delta t \tag{3.17}$$

where $W_\angle$ = angular work performed and Δt = change in time.

Power is expressed in units of **watts** (1 W = 1 J/s). A given amount of work performed in a shorter time will have greater power. Therefore, in the previous barbell example, a person lifting the 800 N barbell 0.5 m in 2 s would perform 400 J of work with a power of 200 W, whereas a lift done in 0.5 s would have the same work (400 J) but a power of 800 W.

Alternatively, linear power may be expressed as the product of force (F) and linear velocity (v):

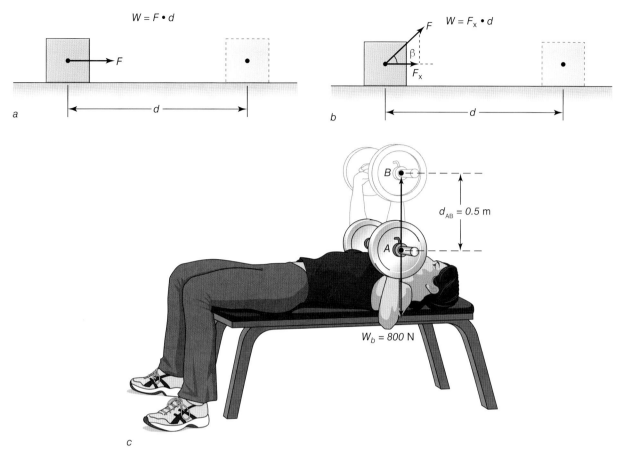

FIGURE 3.14 Mechanical work. *(a)* Linear work (*W*) as the product of force (*F*) and distance (*d*) in the case where the entire force acts in the direction of movement (equation 3.12). *(b)* Linear work performed when only part of the force acts in the direction of movement (equation 3.13). In the case shown, the force (*F*) is directed at an angle β above the horizontal. *(c)* A weightlifter who bench-presses 800 N through a distance of 0.5 m performs 400 J of work.

Reprinted by permission from W.C. Whiting, *Dynamic Human Anatomy*, 2nd ed. (Champaign, IL: Human Kinetics, 2019).

$$P = F \cdot v \tag{3.18}$$

and angular power as the product of torque (*T*) and angular velocity (ω):

$$P_{\angle} = T \cdot \omega \tag{3.19}$$

Equations 3.18 and 3.19 highlight the fact that, to be powerful from a mechanical perspective, one has to be able to generate large forces at high velocities. In other words, a powerful athlete must be both strong and fast. Strength (force) alone is not sufficient; to be powerful, one must be able to generate force and do so quickly.

Energy

In discussing the epidemiology of injury, Robertson (2018) concluded, "The leading source of injury by far is mechanical energy, the characteristics of which have been known since Sir Isaac Newton's

work on the laws of motion in the 17th century. Although Newton's laws of motion do not apply near the speed of light, they are applicable to moving motor vehicles and bullets, or to falling human beings" (p. 18).

As the primary agent of injury, energy is critical to an understanding of injury biomechanics. **Energy**, defined as the capacity or ability to perform work, can assume many forms, including thermal, chemical, nuclear, electromagnetic, and mechanical. Although each form of energy has the potential to cause injury, **mechanical energy** is the one most frequently involved. Mechanical energy is measured in joules (J), the same unit as for mechanical work.

The mechanical energy of a body can be classified according to its **kinetic energy** (energy of motion) or its **potential energy** (energy of position or deformation). Kinetic energy can be either linear (E_k) or angular ($E_{\angle k}$). These two types of kinetic energy are defined, respectively, as

$$E_k = \frac{1}{2} \cdot m \cdot v^2 \qquad (3.20)$$

$$E_{\angle k} = \frac{1}{2} \cdot I \cdot \omega^2 \qquad (3.21)$$

where m = mass, v = linear velocity of the center of mass, I = mass moment of inertia, and ω = angular velocity.

Potential energy can take two forms. **Gravitational (positional) potential energy**, measures the potential to perform work as a function of the height a body is elevated above some reference level, most typically the ground. The equation describing gravitational potential energy is

$$E_p = m \cdot g \cdot h \qquad (3.22)$$

where m = mass, g = gravitational acceleration –9.81 m/s^2), and h = height in meters above a reference level.

The second form of potential energy is **deformational energy**, or **strain energy**, which is energy stored in a body by virtue of its deformation. Common examples of strain energy include a stretched rubber band, a pole vaulter's bent pole, and a drawn bow prior to arrow release. The equation describing the amount of stored energy depends on the **material properties** of the deformable body. In physics, with respect to a linear (Hookean) spring, the stored strain energy equals $(kx^2)/2$, where k is the spring constant and x is the amount of deformation. Tissues and structures in the human body, however, are not entirely linear in their response to loading, and thus no single equation describes the strain energy for these tissues and structures.

Biomechanists studying whole-body or limb segment movement dynamics often assume that each body segment is a rigid (nondeformable) body. When this assumption is made, there is no strain energy component in the system. In these cases, the **total mechanical energy (TME)** = linear kinetic energy + angular kinetic energy + positional potential energy + heat. In biomechanical situations, the heat term is negligible and so is sometimes (as here) omitted from the TME equation. If we use equations 3.20 to 3.22, this TME equation for a body segment (e.g., thigh or forearm) becomes

$$TME = E_k + E_{\angle k} + E_p = \left(\frac{1}{2} \cdot m \cdot v^2\right) + \left(\frac{1}{2} \cdot I \cdot \omega^2\right) + \left(m \cdot g \cdot h\right)$$

$$(3.23)$$

where m = mass of the body segment, v = linear velocity of the body segment's center of mass (COM), I = mass moment of inertia, ω = angular velocity, g = –9.81 m/s^2, and h = height of the relevant body segment's COM.

Consider, for example, a soccer player swinging their leg to kick the ball. Each of the lower-limb segments (thigh, lower leg, and foot) possesses a continuously changing total mechanical energy. Let's focus on the shank (lower leg) to illustrate how to calculate the total mechanical energy of a segment at a given instant. Assume that the shank, with a mass of 2.6 kg and a mass moment of inertia (I) of 0.04 kg · m^2, is rotating with an instantaneous angular velocity of 7.0 rad/s, has an instantaneous linear velocity of 3.5 m/s, and is positioned at a height of 0.38 m above the ground.

By substituting the values given into equation 3.23, we can calculate that the TME for the shank at this instant is 26.6 J. Similar calculations done at successive points in time create an energy profile for the shank as a function of time and show how the energy increases and decreases (i.e., flows) throughout the kick. The same analysis can be done for the thigh and foot to create a complete mechanical energy profile of the lower extremity during a kick, or any other activity.

Two principles governing energy and its effects are important in assessing the effects of energy on injury; each of these principles applies to both linear and angular energy. The first, **conservation of energy**, indicates how much of a system's energy is conserved and how much is gained or lost during a given time period. The more energy conserved, the greater the potential for injury. True conservation results in no net gain or loss in system energy.

The companion principle, **transfer of energy**, is the mechanism by which energy is transferred from one body to another. This can take many forms in the course of human movement. Transfer during a throwing motion can happen as energy moves from a proximal segment (e.g., upper arm) to a more distal segment (e.g., forearm, hand) as the throw progresses. Transfer of energy can also happen between different bodies (e.g., impact), as in the case of an American football player blocking or tackling an opponent or cars colliding in an automobile crash. Transfer of energy in these cases often results in injury when the energy transferred exceeds the tolerance of tissues in any of the bodies.

Momentum

Momentum measures quantity of motion. An old adage suggests that the bigger they are, the harder they fall. With respect to injury, this maxim can be accurately modified to state that the bigger and faster they are, the harder they hit. This revised maxim embodies the concept of momentum. In mechanical terms, **linear momentum** (*p*) is defined as

$$p = m \cdot v \tag{3.24}$$

where *m* = mass and *v* = velocity of the body's center of mass. Increasing either a body's size (mass) or speed (velocity) will increase its linear momentum.

Similarly, **angular momentum** (*L*), or the quantity of angular motion, is defined as

$$L = I \cdot \omega \tag{3.25}$$

where *I* = mass moment of inertia about the center of mass and ω = angular velocity.

The principles of conservation and transfer apply to momentum the same way they do for energy. **Conservation of momentum** measures how much of a system's momentum, or quantity of motion, is conserved and how much is gained or lost during a given time period. True conservation would imply no net gain or loss in system momentum. **Transfer of momentum** is the mechanism by which momentum is transferred from one body to another, either from one body segment to another (e.g., momentum transfer from the upper arm to the forearm during a throw) or between different bodies (e.g., from the foot to the ball in a soccer kick).

There is a direct relation between an applied force and the change in momentum it creates. Consider a force applied to a particular body over a very short time interval, as is often the case in force-related injuries. Such a force is referred to as an **impulsive force**.

This impulsive force (*F*) relates to momentum in what is termed the **impulse–momentum principle**, which states that the **impulse** equals the change in momentum. In the linear case, the **linear impulse** ($F \cdot \Delta t$) equals the change in linear momentum ($\Delta m \cdot v$).

$$F \cdot \Delta t = \Delta m \cdot v \tag{3.26}$$

where *F* is the impulsive force, Δt is the time period of force application, *m* = mass, and *v* = linear velocity.

In the angular form, **angular impulse** ($T \cdot \Delta t$) equals the change in angular momentum ($\Delta I \cdot \omega$).

$$T \cdot \Delta t = \Delta I \cdot \omega \tag{3.27}$$

where *T* is the impulsive torque (moment), Δt is the time period of torque application, *I* = mass moment of inertia, and ω = angular velocity.

The importance of impulsive force in our exploration of injury can be seen in the following example. Consider a person landing on the ground after jumping from an elevated surface. Would the person rather land on a concrete surface or a padded one? At the instant before ground contact, the person will have a certain momentum (*p*), calculated as the product of the falling velocity (*v*) times the person's body mass (*m*). At the end of the landing, the person's body comes to a stop and, hence, has no momentum. The impulse ($F \cdot \Delta t$) created between the ground and the jumper caused the momentum to change from *p* to zero. If the jumper landed on a concrete surface, the impulse time (Δt) would be very short and the impulsive force (*F*) would be high. In contrast, if the jumper landed on a padded surface, the impulse time would be longer and as a consequence the impulsive force would be lower— certainly the preferred landing surface. Falling from an extreme height (which creates considerable momentum) onto an unyielding surface (which causes high impulsive forces) is a recipe for injury.

Collisions

In many cases, musculoskeletal injuries occur as a result of one object impacting another. In athletic contests, body–body and body–ground impacts are common. In automobile crashes, multiple impacts occur between the various parts of both vehicles and occupants. In slips and falls, an impact occurs between the person and the ground. Because of their impact characteristics, all of these situations have injury potential. Injury happens when the forces applied during an impact exceed the body tissues' ability to withstand the force.

A forceful impact between two or more bodies is known as a **collision**. Collisions have relatively large impact forces acting over a relatively short time interval. In every collision the contacting bodies undergo deformation; that is, their shape (configuration) changes. In some instances, the deformation is negligible (e.g., a collision between two billiard balls), whereas in others the deformation can be considerable (e.g., a forceful blow to a person's abdomen). The deformed body may experience a plastic deformation, an elastic deformation, or a combination of both. In a **plastic deformation**, the body's change in physical configuration is permanent. In an **elastic deformation**, the body recovers from the deformation and returns to its original configuration when the force is removed. The ability of a material to return to its original shape is termed **elasticity** and is an essential characteristic of body tissues.

The nature of the collision between two bodies depends on their relative masses and velocities (both magnitude and direction) and on the material properties of the respective bodies. In theory, collisions occur along a continuum ranging from **perfectly plastic (inelastic) collisions** at one extreme to **perfectly elastic collisions** at the other. In a perfectly plastic collision, the bodies stick together and move with a common velocity after impact with no loss of energy or momentum. In contrast, a perfectly elastic collision involves bodies that rebound away from each other following the collision with no energy or momentum loss.

In real terms, most collisions involving the human musculoskeletal system are **elastoplastic** in nature. The bodies deform, sometimes permanently, and energy is transferred and lost in the collision. The greater the energy involved, the more likely injury will occur and the more severe it will be. In elastoplastic collisions energy is lost, and the relative post-collision velocity between the two bodies decreases. To measure this loss of separation velocity, we introduce the concept of **coefficient of restitution** (*e*), defined as the ratio between the relative post-collision velocity (RV_{post}) of two bodies and their relative pre-collision velocity (RV_{pre}):

$$e = -RV_{post}/RV_{pre} \tag{3.28}$$

The coefficient of restitution can range between 0 and 1. A hard rubber ball dropped onto a hard surface would have an *e* value near 1, indicating little energy loss. A partially deflated basketball, in contrast, would bounce very little and would have an *e* value close to 0. The material properties of the colliding bodies determine where on the collision continuum each impact falls.

Friction

Newton's first law of motion tells us that bodies in motion tend to remain in motion unless acted upon by an outside force. The force may be an abrupt one, such as a collision, or may be a force of lower magnitude and greater duration, such as the force of friction. **Friction** is defined as the resistance created at the interface between two bodies. Frictional resistance results from microscopic irregularities, known as *asperities*, on the opposing surfaces. Asperities tend to adhere to each other, and efforts to move the bodies result in very small resistive (shear) forces that oppose the motion.

In the simple case of a body at rest on a surface, **static friction** resists movement until a force sufficient to overcome the frictional resistance is applied. The magnitude of this static friction (f_s) is given by

$$f_s \leq \mu_s \cdot N \tag{3.29}$$

where μ_s = the coefficient of static friction and N = the component of the contact force that is normal, or perpendicular, to the surface. This **normal force** is also referred to as the **reaction force** (*R*). In the case of a horizontal surface, N equals the weight of the body. For bodies on an inclined surface, N changes as a function of the angle of inclination, becoming lower as the incline becomes steeper.

As the force applied to a body at rest increases, a level is reached at which the static resistance is overcome, and the body begins to slide along the surface. Once the body begins moving, the friction decreases slightly and then is known as **kinetic friction** or **dynamic friction** (f_k) with a dynamic coefficient of friction (μ_k):

$$f_k = \mu_k \cdot N \tag{3.30}$$

The relation between static and dynamic friction is depicted in figure 3.15. Coefficients of sliding friction generally are between 0 and 1, where $\mu = 0$ indicates a frictionless surface.

When an automobile or bicycle is moving, the wheels are free to rotate, and the tires roll along in contact with the road surface. If the tires are prevented from rotating (e.g., when one applies the brakes), the vehicle slides along the road, resisted by sliding friction. Even when rolling, however, friction is present. This rolling resistance is not as obvious as sliding resistance, because rolling resistance is much lower, often by a factor of 100 to 1,000. The actual value of resistance depends on the material properties of the body and surface and on the normal force acting between them.

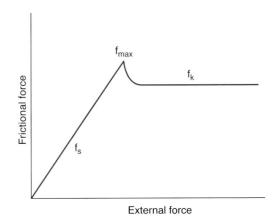

FIGURE 3.15 Relation between static friction and kinetic friction. For an object at rest, static friction (f_s) increases linearly to oppose the externally applied force. When maximum static friction (f_{max}) is reached, the object breaks loose and begins sliding. While sliding, kinetic friction (f_k) resists the movement.

Artificial Turf: Friend or Foe?

Surface friction, especially on playing fields, is a primary variable in injury risk. Higher friction on artificial turf (AT), as compared to natural turf (NT) fields, may improve performance because it allows for greater traction; however, more rapid deceleration may also increase the risk of injury. The research on this topic is mixed, at best. Dragoo et al. (2013) concluded that, between 2004 and 2009, NCAA football players "experienced a greater number of ACL injuries . . . when playing artificial surfaces." (p. 191). However, Steffen et al. (2007) concluded that the "overall risk of acute injuries was similar between artificial turf and natural grass" (p. i33) in young female soccer players. A meta-analysis by Williams and colleagues (2013) concluded that "it appears that the risk of sustaining an injury on AT under some conditions might be lowered compared to NG" (p. 1). In summary, the issue remains equivocal.

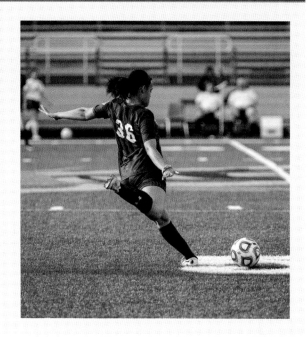

Sliding friction plays a critical role in many injuries. A person walking on a wet, slippery surface, for example, is more likely to slip, fall, and become injured because the wet surface has a lower coefficient of friction than a dry one. Similarly, an individual navigating an icy stretch of sidewalk needs to be careful because of the very low frictional coefficient that ice provides.

In many cases, however, friction works to our advantage. In fact, we would be unable to walk or run without friction acting between our shoes and the ground. Too much friction, however, may contribute to injury. High levels of friction lead to abrupt deceleration, which causes high forces and extreme loading of body tissues. The typically higher friction on artificial surfaces, for example, is assumed to cause more injuries, particularly to the knee and ankle. Caution is warranted in making broad generalizations, however, because the frictional characteristics in a given situation are determined by the interactive effect of many factors such as shoe type, surface wear, type of sport, weather conditions, and the athlete's individual anthropometrics (e.g., height and weight), experience, and skill level.

Our examples so far have focused on friction acting upon a body. Friction also plays an important role within the human body. During normal limb movements, for instance, the friction in joints is extremely low, allowing for freedom of movement

with minimal resistance; details of this low joint friction are presented later in the section on joint mechanics. However, internal friction can also lead to injury, as in the case of a tendon sliding along its tendon sheath. Excessive friction between the tendon and sheath can hasten an inflammatory response and conditions such as tendinitis (see chapter 5).

Fluid Mechanics

A fluid is defined as a substance that has no fixed shape and yields readily to external forces. **Fluid mechanics**, the branch of mechanics dealing with the properties and behavior of fluids (i.e., gases and liquids), assumes an important role in our framework for studying human biomechanics. Areas as diverse as **performance biomechanics** (study of human mechanical function), **biotribology** (study of the friction, lubrication, and wear of diarthrodial joints), **tissue biomechanics** (study of mechanical response of tissues), and **hemodynamics** (study of blood circulation) all rely on the principles of fluid mechanics.

We live and operate in various fluid environments, with air as the principal gas and water as the predominant liquid. The temperature, density, and composition of each fluid contribute to its mechanical properties. We consider these mechanical properties in three broad categories: **fluid flow, fluid resis-**

tance, and viscosity. Flow, resistance, and viscosity are all essential to our understanding of body function and tissue response, and are intrinsically related to the biomechanics of injury:

- *Fluid flow.* This term refers to the characteristics of a fluid, whether liquid or gas, that allow it to change its shape and move, and that govern the nature of this movement. Blood circulating through a coronary artery is a biomechanical example of fluid flow. Fluid flow can exhibit many movement patterns. **Laminar flow** is characterized by a smooth, essentially parallel pattern of movement. **Turbulent flow** exhibits a more chaotic pattern, characterized by areas of turbulence (eddies) and multidirectional movement. Arterial blood flow

provides us with a good example of these differences. The blood flowing in the middle of a large arterial cavity (lumen) would be mostly laminar. Blood flowing along the arterial walls, especially if the wall is atherosclerotic, would experience more turbulent flow. Factors contributing to turbulent flow include the roughness (degree of irregularity) of the surface over which the fluid flows, the diameter of the vessel through which the fluid flows, obstructions, and the speed of flow.

- *Fluid resistance.* Fluids also provide resistance, such as the resistance we might experience while running into a headwind or swimming in a pool. Fluid resistance takes many forms, some of which are advantageous and some of which are detrimental.

Fluid Mechanics of Atherosclerosis

Normal physiological function depends on efficient transport provided by the cardiovascular system. Compromise of this system's efficiency can have harmful, even fatal, consequences. Normal, healthy vessels allow for smooth, unobstructed blood flow with minimal resistance. Fatty (plaque) buildup on vessel walls signals the onset of **atherosclerosis**. As the amount of atherosclerotic plaque increases, the vessel wall becomes rougher and more irregular, and the vessel cavity (lumen) is occluded and, therefore, narrows.

These mechanical changes that accompany plaque accumulation can have serious physiological consequences. Roughened arterial walls increase the turbulence of the blood flow and increase resistance. Narrowing of the arterial lumen also increases resistance to flow. The increase in resistance can be dramatic for even small degrees of narrowing. Mathematically, the resistance (R) is inversely proportional to the fourth power of the lumen's radius (r), or $R = 1/r^4$. Thus, reduction in radius to one-half normal size, for example, produces a 16-fold increase in resistance. The heart, which must pump much harder to force blood through the narrowed lumen, is at risk for serious and deleterious long-term effects.

The injury that atherosclerosis inflicts on vessel walls can have catastrophic consequences if left untreated. For example, when a piece of plaque becomes dislodged from an arterial wall and blocks blood flow, the situation can become life-threatening. Such a blockage in a coronary artery is termed a myocardial infarction, or heart attack.

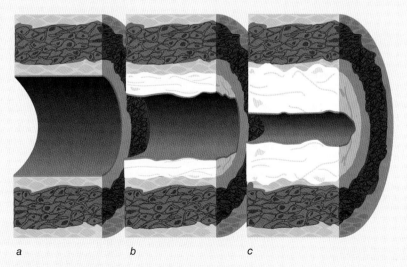

Stages of atherosclerosis: *(a)* normal artery, *(b)* partially blocked artery, and *(c)* significantly blocked artery.

Examples of the positive effects of fluid resistance include **buoyant force**, which allows a person or object to float in water (according to **Archimedes' principle**, which states that the magnitude of the buoyant force equals the weight of the displaced liquid); **lift** and **drag forces**, which assist in keeping an object in flight (aerodynamics) or allow a person to swim (hydrodynamics); and **magnus forces**, which affect the trajectories of objects spinning through the air. Negative effects of fluid resistance are evident in the extra physiological work expenditure required of a cyclist riding into the wind or by the severe and unpredictable forces acting on an airplane during a storm.

• *Viscosity.* Viscosity, which may be considered "fluid friction," is the property of a fluid that enables it to develop and maintain a resistance to flow dependent on the flow's velocity (rate of flow). This viscous effect and its dependence on velocity can be seen in a familiar example. When you move your hand slowly through water, the resistance is minimal. Increasing the speed of movement markedly increases the resistance. Because all biological tissues have a fluid component (usually water), logic dictates that a tissue's response to mechanical loading will include a viscous component. For example, the response of tendon and ligament to stretch will vary depending on the rate of stretch created by the applied load and its temperature. Details of this rate-dependent response will be considered later.

Joint Mechanics

Many of the estimated 360 articulations (joints) in the human body allow us to move. Because many injuries involve joint structures, a study of their mechanical characteristics is essential to our discussion of injury biomechanics. No two joints are structurally the same; each has its own distinct combination of tissues, tissue configuration, and movement potential. This variety of joint structure and function results in many complex injuries, which we explore in subsequent chapters.

The body's major articulations (e.g., hip, knee, and elbow) are diarthrodial (synovial) joints containing synovial fluid that serves lubricative, shock absorptive, and nutritive functions. In its lubricative role, synovial fluid reduces friction in the joint to extremely low levels. In fact, studies have estimated the static frictional coefficient (μ_s) in synovial joints at about 0.01, and kinetic frictional coefficient (μ_k) as low as 0.003. By comparison, ice sliding across ice has

a μ_k of between 0.02 and 0.09. This minimal friction plays an important part in the durability (i.e., lack of wear) of normal articular cartilage. The lubrication mechanisms acting in synovial joints are complex and not completely understood. These mechanisms are detailed in chapter 4.

Movement analysis depends on proper description of the joint motions that constitute each movement pattern. Joint motions are defined with respect to **anatomical position**. In this position, the body is referenced according to three mutually perpendicular planes: sagittal, frontal, and transverse (figure 3.16). Primary joint motion typically occurs in one of these movement planes. For example, knee flexion from anatomical position occurs in the sagittal plane, glenohumeral abduction happens in the frontal plane, and hip internal (medial) rotation occurs in the transverse plane (table 3.1). Movements confined to a single plane often appear restricted and robotic. Full expression of the wide variety of human movement depends on our ability to move unconstrained in three dimensions.

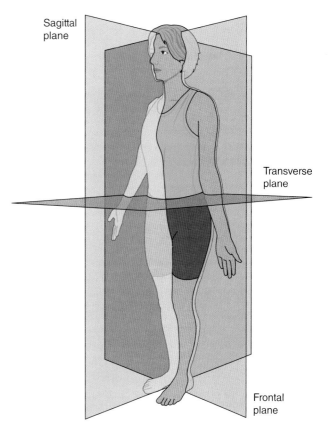

FIGURE 3.16 Three primary movement planes shown for a person standing in anatomical position. These planes are the transverse (horizontal), frontal (coronal), and sagittal (midsagittal or median) planes. These names are given to any plane parallel to the ones shown.

TABLE 3.1   Summary of Primary Joint Motions and Planes of Action

Joint	Joint motion	Plane of action*
Hip	Flexion–extension Abduction–adduction Internal–external rotation	Sagittal Frontal Transverse
Knee	Flexion–extension	Sagittal
Ankle	Plantarflexion–dorsiflexion	Sagittal
Shoulder	Flexion–extension Abduction–adduction Internal–external rotation Horizontal flexion–extension	Sagittal Frontal Transverse Transverse
Elbow	Flexion–extension	Sagittal
Radioulnar	Forearm pronation–supination	Transverse
Wrist	Flexion–extension Ulnar–radial deviation	Sagittal Frontal
Intervertebral (spine)	Flexion–extension Lateral flexion Rotation	Sagittal Frontal Transverse

*Planes of action for movements begun from anatomical position.

Mobility and Stability

Each joint in the body has a **range of motion (ROM)** throughout which the joint normally operates. This ROM determines a joint's mobility. The magnitude of allowable ROM is specific to both the joint and the person. Joints with an ability to move in more than one plane have ROMs specific to each particular plane of movement. ROMs vary considerably from one person to another, and thus individual measurement is the surest method of determining accurate joint ROM (table 3.2). Intrinsically related to ROM is the notion of **joint stability**, defined as "the ability of a joint to maintain an appropriate functional position throughout its range of motion" (Burstein and Wright 1994, p. 63). Maintenance of joint stability depends on cooperative action of the nervous, muscular, and skeletal systems as well as supporting structures (e.g., joint capsule, ligaments).

Injuries often occur when a joint exceeds its normal ROM (e.g., when an elbow hyperextends), which raises the question of what determines normal ROM. Joint ROM is determined by the combined effects of

- the shape of the articular surfaces and their geometric interaction (degree of bony fit);
- the restraint provided by ligaments, joint capsule, and other periarticular structures; and
- the action of muscles around the joint.

When the limits imposed by these stabilizing factors are exceeded, normal ROM is violated, and the tissues may experience injury-producing forces.

One way of viewing joint stability is the joint's ability to resist dislocation. Stable joints have a high resistance to dislocation. Unstable joints tend to dislocate more easily. Joints can be classified along a mobility–stability continuum, which specifies that joints that have a tight bony fit or numerous ligamentous and other supporting structures or that are surrounded by large muscle groups will be very stable and relatively immobile. Joints with a loose bony fit, limited extrinsic support, or minimal surrounding musculature tend to be very mobile and unstable. One exception to this categorization is the hip joint, which is both very mobile—with large ROM potential across all three primary planes—and very stable, as seen by the rarity of its dislocation.

Lever Systems

Most motion at the major joints results from the body's structures acting as a system of levers. A **lever** is a rigid structure, fixed at a single point, to which two forces are applied at two points. One of the forces is commonly referred to as the **resistance force**; the other is termed the **applied force** or **effort force**. The fixed point, known as the **axis**, **pivot**, or **fulcrum**, is the point about which the lever rotates.

TABLE 3.2   Average Ranges of Motion (ROM) of Joints

Joint	Joint motion	ROM[a]
Hip	Flexion	90°-125°
	Extension	10°-30°
	Abduction	40°-45°
	Adduction	10°-30°
	Internal (medial) rotation	35°-45°
	External (lateral) rotation	45°-50°
Knee	Flexion	120°-150°
Ankle	Plantarflexion	20°-45°
	Dorsiflexion	15°-30°
Shoulder	Flexion	130°-180°
	Extension	30°-80°
	Abduction	170°-180°
	Adduction	50°
	Internal (medial) rotation[b]	60°-90°
	External (lateral) rotation[b]	70°-90°
	Horizontal flexion (adduction)[b]	135°
	Horizontal extension (abduction)[b]	45°
Elbow	Flexion	140°-160°
Radioulnar	Forearm pronation (from midposition)	80°-90°
	Forearm supination (from midposition)	80°-90°
Cervical spine	Flexion	40°-60°
	Hyperextension	40°-75°
	Lateral flexion	40°-45°
	Rotation	50°-80°
Thoracolumbar spine	Flexion	45°-75°
	Hyperextension	20°-35°
	Lateral flexion	25°-35°
	Rotation	30°-45°

[a]ROM for movements made from anatomical position (unless otherwise noted). Averages reported in the literature vary, sometimes considerably, depending on method of measurement and population measured. [b]Movement from 90° abducted position.

In the human body, these three components are typically an external force, a muscle force, and a joint axis of rotation, such as when one is performing an elbow curl exercise to lift a dumbbell (Resistance) using the biceps brachii (Force) about the elbow joint axis (figure 3.17c).

These lever system components may be spatially related to one another in three configurations, giving rise to three classes of levers. Distinctions among the classes are determined by the location of each component relative to the other two (figure 3.17). In a **first-class lever**, the pivot-point axis is located between the resistance and the effort force. A **second-class lever** has the resistance located between the effort force and the axis, whereas a **third-class lever** has the effort force between the resistance and axis. Joints in the human body are predominantly third-class levers, with some first-class levers and few second-class lever systems.

Lever systems in the human body perform two important functions. First, they increase the effect of an applied force, because the applied force and the resisting force have different moment arms. In a first-class lever, for example, increasing the moment arm on the side of the applied force increases the effective force seen on the other side of the pivot point, in the same way that a leverage advantage is gained by using a bar to pry a large rock loose from the ground.

The second function of levers is to increase the effective speed (or velocity) of movement. During

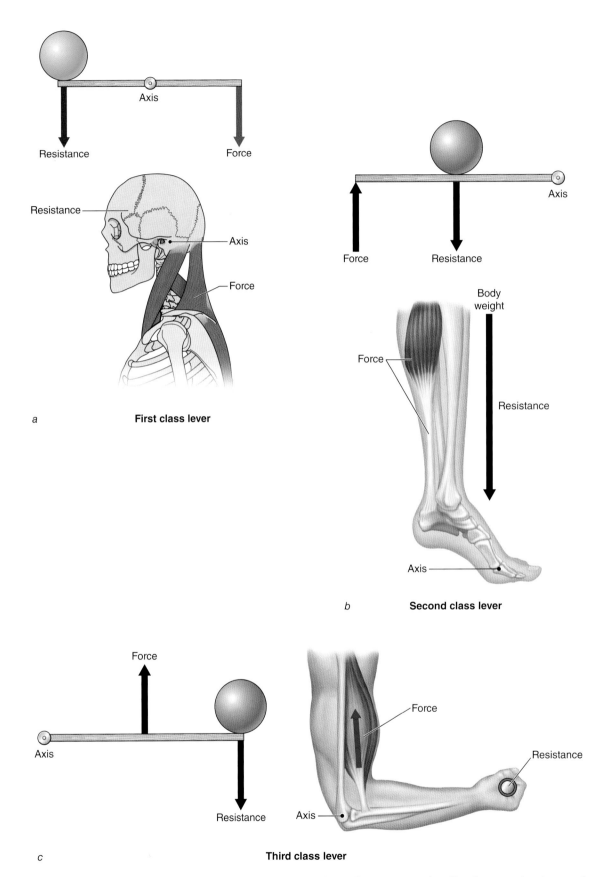

FIGURE 3.17 Lever systems. Simple lever systems comprise three elements: an axis, effort force, and resistance force.

Reprinted by permission from W.C. Whiting, *Dynamic Human Anatomy,* 2nd ed. (Champaign, IL: Human Kinetics, 2019).

knee extension (figure 3.18), a given angular displacement ($\Delta\theta$) produces different linear displacements of points x and x' on the lower leg. Similarly, if the knee is extended at a constant angular velocity (ω), the linear velocity of point x' will be greater than that of x. Thus, by increasing the lever arm distance from x to x', we have increased the linear velocity of movement. The human body effectively uses both the force and speed advantages provided by lever systems in accomplishing the many tasks it performs daily. As expected, these force and speed enhancements can play a role in injury occurrence and prevention as well.

Moment of Force (Torque) and Joint Motion

We defined *moment of force*, or *torque*, as the effect of a force tending to cause rotation about an axis. With respect to joint function, moments created by the action of skeletal muscles are the essential element in controlling joint motion. In figure 3.19a, the muscle force F acts at a perpendicular distance (moment arm = d) from the elbow joint axis E, producing a moment $M = F \cdot d$. In static situations such as this, calculation of the moment is straightforward.

In real-life cases involving joint motion, however, the calculation is much more complex. Consider each component of the moment calculation: The magnitude

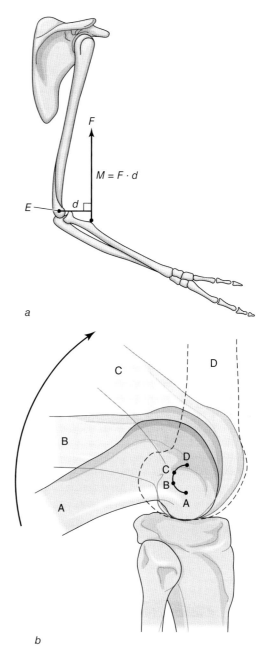

a

b

FIGURE 3.19 Moment production at a joint and instantaneous joint center of rotation. *(a)* Biceps brachii muscle force (F) with a moment arm (d) producing a moment of force (M) about the elbow joint axis (E). *(b)* Structural asymmetries result in movement of the instantaneous joint center with respect to the bones constituting the joint. Movement of the instantaneous joint center is shown for the knee as the joint extends from a flexed position (A) to full extension (D).

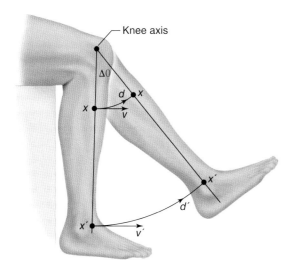

FIGURE 3.18 Knee extensor mechanism acting as a lever system. For a given angular displacement ($\Delta\theta$), the curvilinear displacement (d') for point x' will be greater than the displacement (d) for point x. Similarly, for a given angular velocity (ω), the linear velocity (v') for point x' exceeds the velocity (v) of point x.

Reprinted by permission from W.C. Whiting, *Dynamic Human Anatomy*, 2nd ed. (Champaign, IL: Human Kinetics, 2019).

of muscle force F typically varies and is determined by a combination of factors, including the muscle's length, velocity, level of neural activation, and fatigue, along with the external resistance that the system is experiencing. Changes in any or all of these factors directly influence the amount of muscle force produced.

As the joint moves through its ROM, the musculotendinous line of action (i.e., direction of pull) changes continuously, thus affecting the moment arm distance. Because joints in the human body are not perfect hinge joints, the location of the axis of rotation relative to the bony structures at any instant in time (**instantaneous joint center**) changes as well (figure 3.19b). These changes in muscle force, line of action, and moment arm result in a continuously varying moment of force.

The asymmetry of joint motion that accounts for movement of the instantaneous joint center motion is caused by a combination of three movements: rotation, sliding, and rolling. In rotation, the motion is purely angular, with rotation about a fixed axis (figure 3.20a). Sliding joint motion occurs when one articulating surface moves linearly relative to the other (figure 3.20b). Rolling results in angular joint movement combined with linear displacement of the axis of rotation (figure 3.20c).

Joint Reaction Force Versus Bone-on-Bone Forces

Repeated high-force loading of articular surfaces—such as those occurring at the knee during running or jumping—may lead to joint injuries (e.g., meniscal tears, articular cartilage degeneration). Actual measurement of these forces can be a complex undertaking, and thus mathematical models (discussed later in this chapter) are often used to estimate these joint loads. The net effect of muscle and other forces acting across a joint is called the **joint reaction force** (**JRF**); examples are depicted in figure 3.21a. The

JRF is not the same as the actual bone-on-bone force (figure 3.21b). Although measurement of actual bone-on-bone force is complex and beyond the scope of this text (see, e.g., Bergmann et al. 2018; D'Lima et al. 2013; Kirking et al. 2006; Rudert et al. 2014; Stansfield et al. 2003; Westerhoff et al. 2009; Winter 2009), valuable information can be gained from in vivo force-sensing transducers implanted in human joints.

Material Mechanics

Our discussion so far has focused on external mechanics, or the effect of external forces on the movement of bodies. In this section we shift our attention to the internal mechanics of structures, focusing on the internal response of materials to externally applied loads.

In previous sections we considered bodies as if they were rigid structures whose size and shape do not change when loads are applied. This approach, known as **rigid-body mechanics**, is useful when we examine movement characteristics. Rigid-body formulations make certain assumptions about the body, including nondeformability, fixed center of mass, and homogeneity of the composite material. Although biological tissues are deformable, viewing body segments as rigid bodies is a reasonable approximation in fields of inquiry such as movement mechanics. In examining the biomechanics of injury, however, we also need to explore the mechanics of deformable solids, because injury mechanisms often result in considerable tissue deformation.

Biological materials such as tissues exhibit many properties that influence each material's response

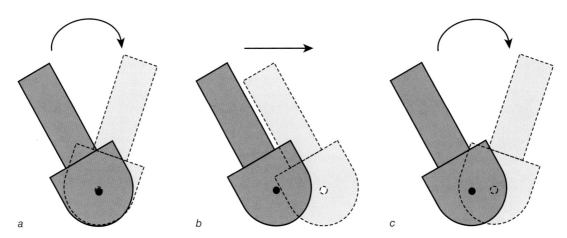

FIGURE 3.20 Components of joint motion: *(a)* rotation, *(b)* sliding, and *(c)* rolling.

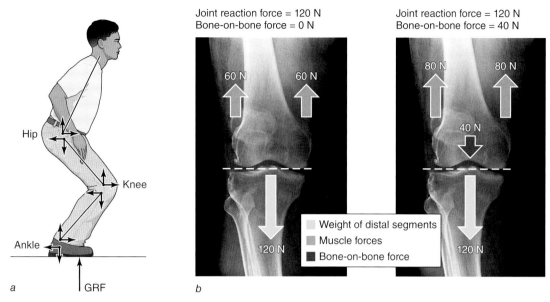

Joint reaction force = 120 N
Bone-on-bone force = 0 N

Joint reaction force = 120 N
Bone-on-bone force = 40 N

FIGURE 3.21   *(a)* Joint reaction forces. Equal and opposite joint reaction forces (in accordance with Newton's third law) act at the ankle, knee, and hip joints in a squatting position with each joint in a flexed position. These joint reaction forces develop in response to the ground reaction force (GRF). *(b)* Joint reaction force vs. bone-on-bone force.

to loading and, hence, the likelihood and severity of injury. Among these material properties are size, shape, area, volume, and mass. Additional properties derived from these fundamental ones include **density** (ratio of mass to volume) and center of mass. The tissue's **structural properties**, discussed in the previous chapter, are also important factors in describing tissue mechanical response.

Tissue Response to Loading

In an earlier section we described internal and external mechanics. Consistent with that distinction, we can describe forces as being either internal forces (i.e., forces acting within the body) or external forces (i.e., forces acting on the body from without). An externally applied force is called a mechanical **load**. There are three principal load types: **compression** (compressive load), **tension** (tensile load), and **shear** (shear load) Compressive loads tend to push the ends of a body together, tensile loads tend to pull the ends apart, and shear loads tend to produce horizontal, or parallel, sliding of one layer over another.

Load Deformation and Stiffness

When a load is applied to a deformable body, the body changes shape or configuration, although sometimes imperceptibly (e.g., bone). This absolute change in shape or dimension is termed **deformation**. Tensile loads create elongation in the material;

compressive loads shorten (or compress) the material; and shear loads cause a sliding or angulation in the material (figure 3.22). Deformation typically is measured in absolute units (e.g., a tendon was stretched, or elongated, by 5 mm). Note that *absolute measure* refers to measurement of things in known amounts with standard units (e.g., weight = 82 kg; distance = 3 m). *Relative measure*, in contrast, refers to measurement of something compared to another thing, or estimating things proportionally to one another (e.g., percent, times body weight).

Each material or tissue has a characteristic relation between load and deformation that is graphically depicted by a **load–deformation (L–d) curve** (figure 3.23). The slope of the linear portion of the L–d curve measures the tissue's **stiffness** (often represented by *k*). Curves with a steeper slope represent stiffer materials. The opposite, or inverse, of stiffness is known as **compliance** (1/*k*). The terms *stiffness* and *compliance* are used as relative terms, meaning that a material is not absolutely stiff or compliant; rather one material is stiffer, or more compliant, than another.

Stress and Strain

Any body, when loaded, develops an internal resistance to the external load. In the case of a small rubber band, this resistance is minimal. In contrast, a steel bar provides considerable resistance. This

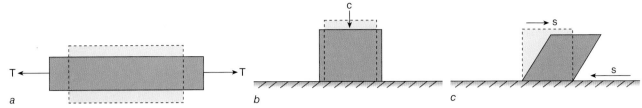

a   *b*   *c*

FIGURE 3.22 Mechanical loading. External loads change the shape of a material. This deformation can manifest as *(a)* elongation, or tensile deformation; *(b)* compression, or compressive deformation; or *(c)* angulation, or shear deformation. Dashed lines indicate unloaded condition. Solid lines indicate loaded condition.

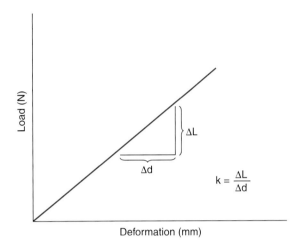

FIGURE 3.23 Relation between the load and deformation when a force is applied to a tissue or structure. Stiffness (*k*) is measured by the slope (ΔL/Δd) of the linear portion of the load–deformation curve.

internal resistance to an axial load is common to all materials and in mechanics is called **stress** (σ). Axial, or normal, stresses are categorized as either **compressive stress** (i.e., resistance to being pushed together) or **tensile stress** (i.e., resistance to being pulled apart). The magnitude of the normal stress is

$$\sigma = F/A \qquad (3.31)$$

where *F* = magnitude of the axial load and *A* = internal cross-sectional area over which the load is distributed. Because stress is calculated as the ratio of force to area, it is classified as a relative measure.

Those forces acting parallel, or tangential, to the applied load create **shear stress** (τ):

$$\tau = F/A \qquad (3.32)$$

The standard (SI) unit of stress is the *pascal* (Pa), defined as 1 N distributed over 1 m² (1 Pa = 1 N/m²). To avoid possible confusion, note that although both pressure (*p* = *F/A*) and stress (σ = *F/A*) are defined as force divided by area, the area (*A*) is different

between the two. Pressure is an *external* measure of the force divided by the surface area over which the force is distributed (see equation 3.1). Stress is an *internal* measure of the force divided by the cross-sectional area of the tissue. As with pressure, the megapascal (1 MPa = 1 N/mm²) is a commonly used unit for stress when applied to tissue mechanics.

Earlier, we defined *deformation* as the change in shape or configuration of a body. **Mechanical strain** (ε) provides another measure of shape change, but in contrast to deformation, which is measured in absolute units (e.g., mm), strain is measured in relative terms. Strain is measured as the change in dimension divided by the unloaded dimension and, therefore, is technically dimensionless. Strain is typically reported as mm/mm (or inch/inch) or as a percent (%) strain:

strain (%) = (dimension change)/
(unloaded dimension) × 100   **(3.33)**

For example, an unloaded tissue of length 50 mm that is elongated by 3 mm has a deformation of 3 mm and a percent strain of (3 mm)/(50 mm) × (100) = 6%. Compare that with an unloaded tissue of length 100 mm that is elongated by 6 mm. This tissue has a deformation of 6 mm, twice that of the first example, but has an identical 6% strain. Strain measures allow for comparison of tissues with unequal dimensions.

Deformations in biological tissues such as bone are so small that their strain is measured in units of microstrain (με), which is (10⁻⁶). A measured strain of 0.001 (0.1%) would be equal to 1000 με.

As with load and deformation, a direct relation exists between stress and strain, and the consequences of this relation in a tissue determine its susceptibility to injury. Compressively loaded bone, for example, develops high resistance while deforming very little. Skin, in contrast, deforms considerably more at substantially lower forces. The strain responses of tendon, ligament, and cartilage fall somewhere between these two. Plotting stress as a function of strain (figure 3.24*a*) allows us to visualize the σ–ε relation. The figure shows linear σ–ε curves for two materials labeled A and B. A closer look at the curves reveals several important relations. For a given stress (σ_o), material B exhibits more strain than material A, which is evident as $\varepsilon_B > \varepsilon_A$. Conversely, for a given strain (ε_o), material A develops a greater stress than material B, as demonstrated by $\sigma_A > \sigma_B$ (figure 3.24*b*).

The stress–strain (σ–ε) relation can be summarized in a single measure as the ratio of the two values. This ratio is termed the **modulus of elasticity**, or **elastic modulus** (*E*), also known as **Young's modulus**. Stiff materials such as bone have a steeply sloped σ–ε curve and a high *E* value. More compliant materials such as skin have flatter σ–ε slopes and lower *E* values.

Thus far we have considered only the linear σ–ε relation. Linear materials are said to operate according to Hooke's law, which posits that stress and strain are linearly related; that is, the resulting strain is directly proportional to the developed stress. Mathematically, Hooke's law is expressed by

$$\sigma = E \cdot \varepsilon \tag{3.34}$$

The mechanical response of biological tissues typically is not linear throughout its physiological range, attributable largely to nonlinear characteristics created by the tissue's fluid component.

Loading Types

Recall from earlier discussion the seven factors involved in force application: magnitude, location, direction, duration, frequency, variability, and rate. These factors are fundamental determinants of loading response. The type of loading also plays a primary role in the response of biological tissues. We focus now on various types of loading.

Uniaxial Loading

The simplest form of force application, **uniaxial loading**, refers to forces applied along a single line, typically along a primary axis of the structure. For any uniaxially loaded material, the location and direction of the force will determine how each of the three loading types (tension, compression, and shear) presents.

As the magnitude of applied load increases, the tissue eventually is unable to withstand the loading and fails (i.e., tears apart or ruptures). The level of force at which **failure** occurs (**ultimate load**) defines the tissue's **structural strength**. The concept of structural strength has obvious implications as we examine failure characteristics of tissue in injury situations.

A homogeneous material will respond the same irrespective of the direction of loading. Biological tissues, however, are generally not homogeneous (i.e., their structure varies throughout the tissue), and as a result the direction of force application is an essential factor in the loading response. A material exhibiting a direction-dependent response is termed **anisotropic**. As an example, consider a long bone undergoing uniaxial compression. The structural strength for a compressive load along the longitudinal axis is much greater than the structural strength for a force directed perpendicular to the long axis. That anisotropic effect largely results from the bone's structure, wherein the osteons in the cortical bone of the diaphysis are aligned with

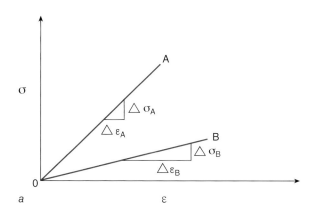

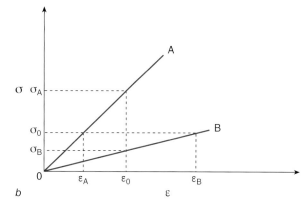

FIGURE 3.24 Relation between mechanical stress (σ) and strain (ε). *(a)* Linear stress–strain (σ–ε) curves for two materials. The slope (Δσ–Δε) of each line measures each material's modulus of elasticity (*E*). *(b)* The relative *E* of the materials determines their response to loading. For a given stress level (σ_o), material B shows more strain than material A.

the long axis of the bone and are designed to accept compressive loads.

Biological tissues can exhibit linear behavior through certain loading ranges but typically are nonlinear through other parts of their normal, or physiological range. Such nonlinearities result in a generalized σ–ε curve (figure 3.25).

Consider a tissue experiencing a gradually increasing tensile load. At low loads, with commensurate low stress levels, the σ–ε response is linear (Hookean). The proportional response continues until point B in figure 3.25. At stresses greater than σ_B, the response becomes nonlinear. Point B, therefore, is known as the **proportional limit** (or **linear limit**). As the stress continues to increase, we reach point C, known as the **elastic limit**. At stresses less than σ_C, the material is elastic (i.e., returns to its original shape when the load is removed). At stresses greater than σ_C, the material is no longer elastic and experiences permanent plastic deformation (or plastic strain), shown in figure 3.26. When the load is removed, stress decreases, and the material shortens. Because the tissue has exceeded its elastic limit, the tissue is no longer able to return to its original shape (point A). Instead, it deforms to an unloaded length at point P. The difference between points A and P is the amount of plastic deformation, or **permanent set**.

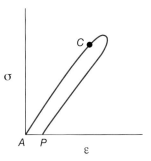

FIGURE 3.26 Permanent set (AP) created by stress exceeding the elastic limit at point C.

Point D in figure 3.25 is approached as stress continues to increase in response to increasing external loads. Point D is known as the **yield point**, at and above which there begins a brief region of relatively large strain for little increase in stress (i.e., increased compliance). This yielding phenomenon is characteristic of many biological tissues. Further increase in stress eventually brings the material to its ultimate stress (σ_E), or **material strength**, at which complete failure begins to occur. Some amount of fiber failure can occur prior to reaching σ_E. Upon reaching σ_E, complete failure is imminent. Because the failure of most tissues is not instantaneous, the actual completion of failure may occur at a stress level below σ_E, at what is termed the **rupture point** (**F**), at a stress level of σ_F. The actual σ–ε curves for specific tissues vary in their response characteristics and may not exactly mirror the curve presented in figure 3.25. Chapter 4 presents detailed discussion of the differences for bone, cartilage, tendon, and ligament.

Two other important mechanical parameters shown in figure 3.27 are measures of energy stored by the tissue and the tissue's dimensional change. On the L–d curve, the area under the curve represents the **energy to failure** (an absolute value measured in joules). The dimensional change is termed the **deformation to failure** (measured in absolute units, such as millimeters). Comparable measures are found on the σ–ε curve in figure 3.25. The area under the curve is the **strain energy density**, a measure of the relative strain energy stored by the tissue prior to failure, and the dimensional change is termed **strain to failure** (ε_F), a relative measure of how much the tissue has deformed to the point of failure.

When a compressive load is applied to an object (e.g., a ball), the resulting deformation compresses

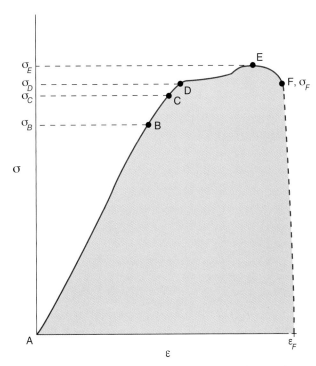

FIGURE 3.25 Generalized stress–strain (σ–ε) curve for biological tissues.

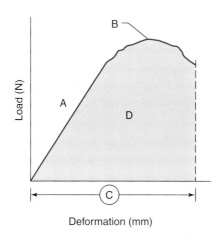
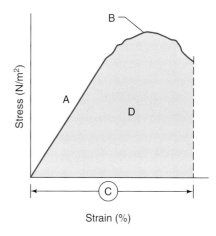

Units	Load-deformation	Stress-strain
	Absolute	Relative
A-Slope of linear portion of curve	Stiffness	Elastic modulus (E) or Young's modulus (Y)
B-Highest point on curve	Ultimate (maximum) load or structural strength	Ultimate (maximum) stress or material strength
C-Change in dimension	Deformation at failure	Strain at failure
D-Area under curve	Energy at failure	Strain energy density

FIGURE 3.27 Comparison of a load–deformation curve versus a stress–strain curve and related measures.

the object in the direction of the load (figure 3.28*a*). At the same time, an accompanying deformation happens perpendicular to the axial load. This distortion is a tensile deformation, and the ball in this example gets wider. This simple case is an example of **Poisson's effect**, which says that when a body is subjected to a uniaxial load and its dimension decreases in the axial direction, its perpendicular (or transverse) dimension increases. Poisson's effect applies in the opposite sense as well. A body experiencing a tensile load shows an increase in its axial dimension and a decrease in its transverse dimension (figure 3.28*b*). The quantitative measure of this effect is given by **Poisson's ratio** (v):

$$v = -\left(\frac{\varepsilon_t}{\varepsilon_a}\right) \qquad (3.35)$$

where ε_t = transverse strain and ε_a = axial strain.

Similar to the two-dimensional case just presented, Poisson's effect also occurs in three-dimensional space, with transverse strains occurring in two dimensions in response to a uniaxial load in the third dimension (figure 3.28*c*).

Multiaxial Loading

We have so far considered only the simple case of uniaxial loading. In most real-life situations, however, the forces applied to a body are multidimensional, and hence an understanding of **multiaxial loading** and its effects is essential. An analysis of multiaxial loading uses the same stress and strain concepts just discussed and extends them into two- and three-dimensional space. Although the biaxial and triaxial responses are illustrated for tensile loading only, the concepts are equally applicable to compressive loading and to force vectors with reversed orientation. The following formulations are for linearly elastic materials.

Biaxial (Two-Dimensional) Loading Responses

Consider a three-dimensional body (figure 3.29) with sides of length X', Y', and Z' that is subjected

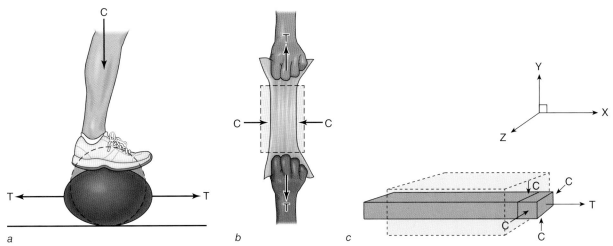

FIGURE 3.28 Poisson's effect. *(a)* An applied compressive load causes tensile stress and strain perpendicular to the applied load. *(b)* An applied tensile load results in compressive stress and strain perpendicular to the applied load. *(c)* Poisson's effect shown for a three-dimensional case in which tension T applied in direction X causes contraction C in directions Y and Z. Dashed lines indicate conformation prior to loading. Solid lines indicate conformation while loaded.

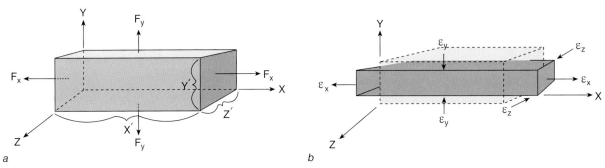

FIGURE 3.29 Biaxial loading. *(a)* Applied forces in the *X* and *Y* direction (*F$_x$* and *F$_y$*, respectively) load the material biaxially. *(b)* Elongation caused by *F$_x$* and the resulting perpendicular contraction in the *Y* and *Z* directions. Dashed lines indicate conformation prior to loading. Solid lines indicate conformation while loaded.

to axial forces F_x and F_y. The stresses produced in the *X* and *Y* directions are as follows:

$$\sigma_x = \frac{F_x}{A_x} = \frac{F_x}{(x' \cdot z')} \tag{3.36}$$

$$\sigma_y = \frac{F_y}{A_y} = \frac{F_y}{(x' \cdot z')} \tag{3.37}$$

The *X*-direction stress (σ_x) will, according to Poisson's effect, cause deformation in all three directions. Elongation in the *X* direction and contraction in the *Y* and *Z* directions are shown in figure 3.29*b*. By applying equations 3.34 and 3.35, we obtain *X*- and *Y*-direction strains attributable to σ_x:

x direction: $\varepsilon_{x\sigma x} = \dfrac{\sigma_x}{E}$ $\tag{3.38}$

y direction: $\varepsilon_{y\sigma x} = -v \cdot \varepsilon_{x\sigma y} = -v \cdot \dfrac{\sigma_x}{E}$ $\tag{3.39}$

We similarly obtain *Y*- and *X*-direction strains attributable to σ_y:

y direction: $\varepsilon_{y\sigma y} = \dfrac{\sigma_y}{E}$ $\tag{3.40}$

x direction: $\varepsilon_{x\sigma y} = -v \cdot \varepsilon_{y\sigma y} = -v \cdot \dfrac{\sigma_y}{E}$ $\tag{3.41}$

To obtain the combined effect of σ_x and σ_y, we add the strain effects just calculated. The net strains in the *X* and *Y* directions are then

$$\varepsilon_x = \varepsilon_{x\sigma x} + \varepsilon_{x\sigma y} = \left(\frac{\sigma_x}{E}\right) - v \cdot \frac{\sigma_y}{E} \tag{3.42}$$

$$\varepsilon_y = \varepsilon_{y\sigma y} + \varepsilon_{y\sigma x} = \left(\frac{\sigma_y}{E}\right) - v \cdot \frac{\sigma_x}{E} \tag{3.43}$$

We have presented two normal stresses, σ_x and σ_y. As previously described, a tangential, or shear, stress (τ) is also created. In the case of biaxial loading, shear stress (τ_{xy}) is created as shown in figure 3.30*a*.

Triaxial (Three-Dimensional) Loading Responses The addition of a third axial force in the

Z direction complicates the conceptual model only slightly, whereas the mathematical aspects of the model become quite involved. Focusing on the conceptual application (figure 3.31), we now have

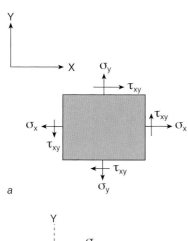

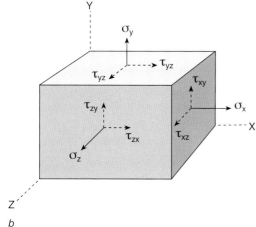

b

FIGURE 3.30 Shear stresses in response to biaxial and triaxial loading. *(a)* Shear stress (τ_{xy}) created by biaxial loading. Because of equilibrium conditions, $\tau_{xy} = \tau_{yx}$. *(b)* Triaxial tensile stresses (σ_x, σ_y, σ_z), shown as solid vectors, result in shear stresses (τ_{xy}, τ_{yz}, τ_{zx}), depicted as broken-line vectors. Equilibrium constraints dictate that $\tau_{xy} = \tau_{yx}$, $\tau_{yz} = \tau_{zy}$, and $\tau_{zx} = \tau_{xz}$.

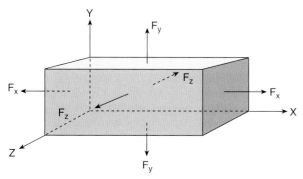

FIGURE 3.31 Triaxial loading. Applied forces in the *X*, *Y*, and *Z* directions (F_x, F_y, and F_z, respectively) load the material triaxially.

- *Fx*, which creates $\sigma x = Fx/(y' \cdot z')$ and produces elongation in the *X* direction and contraction in the *Y* and *Z* directions
- *Fy*, which creates $\sigma y = Fy/(x' \cdot z')$ and produces elongation in the *Y* direction and contraction in the *X* and *Z* directions
- *Fz*, which creates $\sigma z = Fz/(x' \cdot y')$ and produces elongation in the *Z* direction and contraction in the *X* and *Y* directions

The equations for resultant strains seen in triaxial loading are

$$\varepsilon_x = \frac{1}{E} \cdot [\Sigma_x - v \cdot (\Sigma_y + \Sigma_z)] \tag{3.44}$$

$$\varepsilon_y = \frac{1}{E} \cdot [\Sigma_y - v \cdot (\Sigma_x + \Sigma_z)] \tag{3.45}$$

$$\varepsilon_z = \frac{1}{E} \cdot [\Sigma_z - v \cdot (\Sigma_x + \Sigma_y)] \tag{3.46}$$

The shear stresses (τ_{xy}, τ_{yz}, τ_{zx}) produced in triaxial loading are shown in figure 3.30*b*.

Bending

So far we have discussed axial loading. Two other types of loading happen frequently in the human body: bending and torsion.

Any structure that is relatively long and slender (e.g., long bone) may be considered a **beam** in mechanical terms. Any force, force component, or moment acting perpendicular to the longitudinal axis of such a beam will tend to deflect, or bend, the beam.

In **bending**, the material on the **concave** (inner) surface of the structure experiences compressive stress, whereas that on the **convex** (outer) surface is subject to tensile stress (figure 3.32*a*). These tensile and compressive stresses are maximal at the outer surfaces of the beam, with the material closer to the middle experiencing less stress than at the surfaces. The line along which neither compressive nor tensile stress exists is known as the **neutral axis**.

Each force acting on the beam may create a moment in the beam. The sum of these moments is referred to as the **bending moment** (M_b), which creates different stress levels in the beam that vary with the distance from the neutral axis. At a distance *y* from the neutral axis (figure 3.32*b*), a normal stress (σ_x) is created with a value given by

$$\sigma_x = (M_b \cdot y)/I \tag{3.47}$$

where M_b = bending moment, *y* = distance from neutral axis, and *I* = area moment of inertia of the cross-sectional area about the neutral axis. The **area** moment of inertia (I) measures the resistance to bending, and its value depends on the cross-sectional shape of the structure. The area moment of inertia for common shapes is depicted in figure 3.33.

The area moment of inertia (I) for a solid cylinder is measured by

$$I = (\pi \cdot r^4)/4 \tag{3.48}$$

where r = the radius of the cylinder.

The area moment of inertia (I) for a hollow cylinder is measured by:

$$I = [\pi\,(r_o^4 - r_i^4)]/4 \tag{3.49}$$

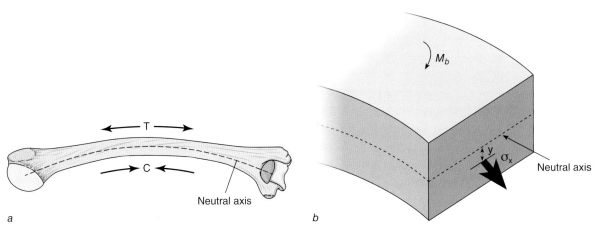

FIGURE 3.32 *(a)* Material stresses in response to bending. Bending creates compressive stress (C) on the concave (inner) surface and tensile stress (T) on the convex (outer) surface. Maximal stress happens at the surfaces, with lower stress levels toward the center of the bent object. A neutral axis exists along which there are no tensile or compressive stresses present. *(b)* Bending moment. A beam subjected to a bending moment (M_b) develops a normal stress (σ_x) as given by equation 3.47.

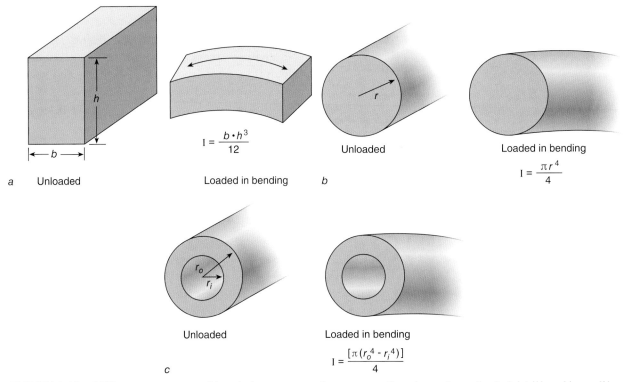

FIGURE 3.33 *(a)* The area moment of inertia for a rectangular cross section depends on the height (h) and base (b) dimensions of the cross section. *(b)* The area moment of inertia for a solid cylinder (equation 3.48) depends on the radius (r). *(c)* For a hollow cylinder (tube), the area moment of inertia (equation 3.49) depends on the outer radius (r_o) and the inner radius (r_i).

where r_o = outer radius and r_i = inner radius of the cylinder.

In instances when shear forces are acting on a beam, shear stresses are created that are maximal at the neutral axis and zero at the surfaces (figure 3.34). The magnitude of this shear stress (τ) is given by

$$\tau = (Q \cdot V)/(I \cdot b) \tag{3.50}$$

where Q = the first moment of the area about the neutral axis, V = shear force, I = area moment of inertia, and b = width of the cross section.

Two common bending modes seen in biomechanical cases are **three-point bending** and **four-point bending** (figure 3.35a and b). A boot-top skiing injury mechanism illustrates three-point bending (figure 3.35c), whereas the forces acting on a barbell produce four-point bending (figure 3.35d).

The failure differences between these two modes are important when considering injury mechanisms. In three-point bending, failure occurs at the middle point of force application (figure 3.36a). In contrast, failure in four-point bending occurs at the weakest point between the two inner forces, not necessarily at the midpoint (figure 3.36b).

An important combined loading mode is **cantilever bending**, in which a force offset from the longitudinal axis creates both compression and bending. Cantilever bending (figure 3.37) occurs in a loaded femur when compressive forces are applied

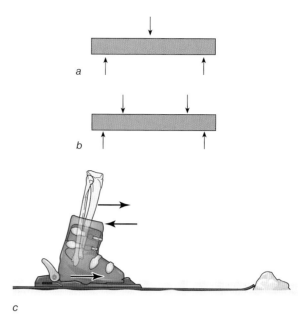

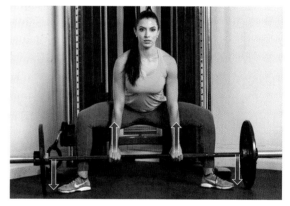

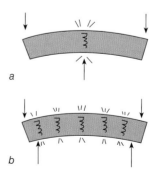

FIGURE 3.35 Three- and four-point bending. *(a)* Three-point bending caused by the action of three parallel forces. The middle force is in the direction opposite to the outer two forces. *(b)* Four-point bending caused by two pairs of parallel forces. The inner pair is in the direction opposite the outer pair. *(c)* Skiing boot-top fracture exemplifies three-point bending. *(d)* An athlete lifting a barbell creates a four-point bending system.

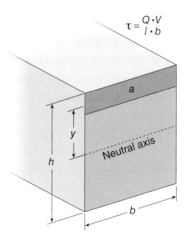

FIGURE 3.34 Shear stress in response to bending. The magnitude of the shear stress (τ) is given by equation 3.50. V = vertical shear force (obtained from a shear force diagram or from static analysis), Q = area moment (calculated as the product of the shaded area a and the distance y from the neutral axis to the centroid of area a), I = moment of inertia of the total cross section (see figure 3.33a), b = width of cross section.

FIGURE 3.36 Failure attributable to bending. *(a)* Failure (fracture) caused by three-point bending happens at the middle point of force application. *(b)* In four-point bending, failure (fracture) happens at the weakest point between the two inner forces, not necessarily at the midpoint.

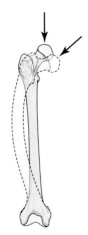

FIGURE 3.37 Compressive loading offset from the longitudinal axis creates a combined loading situation (compression and bending) known as cantilever bending. Solid lines indicate conformation prior to loading. Dashed lines indicate conformation while loaded.

to the femoral head, creating a bending moment in the diaphyseal bone shaft combined with axial compressive effect (e.g., Poisson's effect).

Torsion

Any twisting action applied to a structure results in **torsion**, as seen in the simple example of unscrewing a lid from its jar. Although torsional concepts are applicable to both cylindrical and noncylindrical structures, we limit our mathematical formulations to solid, circular shafts because of the complex mathematics necessary to explain torsional loading of noncylindrical structures. The following torsion formulations are based on assumptions of tissue isotropy, linear elasticity, and structural homogeneity.

Earlier we presented two types of moment of inertia: *mass moment of inertia* (resistance to rotation about a fixed axis) and *area moment of inertia* (resistance to bending of a beam about its neutral axis). A third form of angular resistance is involved when torsional loads are applied to a body. The internal stresses developed in response to the torsional loading produce resistance to the applied torque. This resistance to torsional loading about the longitudinal axis is termed **polar moment of inertia** (J), and its magnitude for a solid cylindrical shaft (figure 3.38a) is

$$J = (\pi \cdot r^4)/2 \tag{3.51}$$

where r = radius of the shaft. For a hollow cylindrical shaft (figure 3.38b), such as a long bone, the polar moment of inertia (J) is

$$J = [\pi \cdot (r_o^4 - r_i^4)]/2 \tag{3.52}$$

where r_o = outer radius of the shaft and r_i = inner radius.

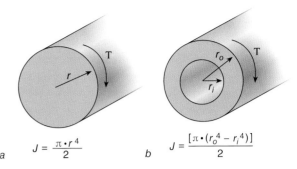

$$a \quad J = \frac{\pi \cdot r^4}{2} \qquad b \quad J = \frac{[\pi \cdot (r_o^4 - r_i^4)]}{2}$$

FIGURE 3.38 Polar moment of inertia. Resistance to an applied torque, measured by the polar moment of inertia, for *(a)* a solid shaft and *(b)* a hollow cylindrical shaft.

Torsion creates stresses throughout the shaft with the magnitude of shear stress (τ) being a function of shaft radius (r), applied torque (T), and polar moment of inertia (J) (figure 3.39a), expressed as

$$\tau = (T \cdot r)/J \tag{3.53}$$

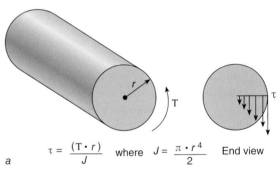

$$a \quad \tau = \frac{(T \cdot r)}{J} \quad \text{where} \quad J = \frac{\pi \cdot r^4}{2} \quad \text{End view}$$

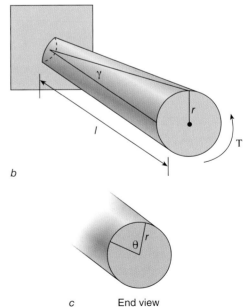

FIGURE 3.39 Torsional loading. *(a)* Shear stress (τ) developed in response to torsional loading (T) (equation 3.53), where r is the radius of the cylinder and J is the polar moment of inertia. *(b)* Shear strain (γ) created by torsional loading (T). *(c)* Angle of twist (θ).

The resulting shear strain (γ) is shown in figure 3.39*b*. The ratio of shear stress (τ) to shear strain (γ) is called the **shear modulus of elasticity** (*G*):

$$G = \tau/\gamma \qquad (3.54)$$

The angle of twist (θ) shown in figure 3.39*c* is given by

$$\theta = (T \cdot l)/(G \cdot J) \qquad (3.55)$$

where *T* = applied torque, *l* = shaft length, *G* = shear modulus of elasticity, and *J* = polar moment of inertia.

Several important generalizations emerge from an examination of torsional loading:

- The larger the radius of the shaft, the more resistance it creates and the more difficult it is to deform.

- The stiffer the material or structure being loaded, the harder it is to deform in torsion.

- In addition to shear stress, torsion produces normal stresses (tensile and compressive) in the form of helical stress trajectories (figure 3.40*a*). These stresses are maximal at the outer surfaces and may result in spiral failure lines (figure 3.40*b*), as seen in a spiral fracture of a tibia loaded in torsion.

Viscoelasticity

As noted in the discussion of fluid mechanics, the mechanical response of a material depends on its constituent matter, which in the case of biological tissues usually has a fluid component. This viscous element provides resistance to flow and affects the stress–strain (σ–ε) relation. The stress response is a function of both the strain and the strain rate ($\dot{\varepsilon}$). Such tissues are said to be **strain-rate dependent**. Tissues with conjoint properties of viscosity (i.e., strain–rate dependency) and elasticity (i.e., ability to return to original shape when load is removed) are termed **viscoelastic**. In viscoelastic tissues, an increasing strain rate steepens the slope of the σ–ε curve and increases the tissue's stiffness.

Purely elastic (i.e., nonviscous) materials subjected to load will deform according to their particular L–d or stress–strain (σ–ε) relation and store energy in the process. When the load is removed, the stored strain energy is returned, and the tissue returns to its original shape with no energy loss by retracing the L–d path traversed during loading (figure 3.41*a*). No biological tissue, however, is purely elastic.

Viscoelastic tissues, in contrast, lose energy to heat during deformation, and the return following unloading is retarded, or delayed, resulting in a return path different from the initial path during loading (figure 3.41*b*). This delayed return is termed

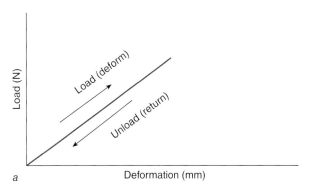

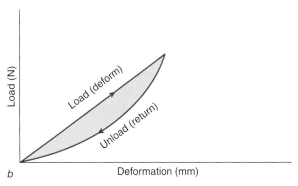

FIGURE 3.41 *(a)* Perfectly elastic materials return along the same load–deformation path and therefore lose no energy. *(b)* Viscoelastic materials exhibit a delayed return response (hysteresis) and lose energy (heat) during the deformation–return cycle. The shaded area within the hysteresis loop measures the energy loss.

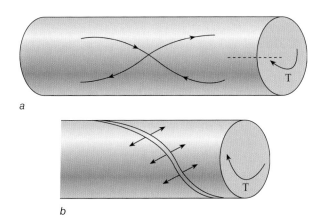

FIGURE 3.40 Helical stress trajectories. *(a)* Applied torque (*T*) creates helical (spiral) stress lines. *(b)* When the stresses exceed the material's threshold, tensile failure happens along the helical stress trajectories. This fracture pattern is seen in spiral fractures of long bones.

hysteresis. The **rate of elastic return** is determined by the material properties, in particular the amount of viscous resistance. Materials that quickly return to their original shape are termed **resilient**; those that return more slowly exhibit a **dampened response**, or **damping**. The path of a loading–unloading cycle graphed on a L–d curve creates a characteristic pattern known as a **hysteresis loop**. The area within the hysteresis loop (shaded area in figure 3.41b) represents the energy lost during the loading–unloading cycle.

Viscous effects also are responsible for a characteristic **biphasic response** in biological tissues. When loaded, viscoelastic tissues exhibit an immediate mechanical response (first phase), followed by a delayed second phase. We explore two common biphasic, time-dependent phenomena associated with biological tissues. The first of these, **creep response**, is seen when a tissue is subjected to a *constant load*. At initial loading, the tissue deforms rapidly (first phase) until the specified constant force level is reached. Instead of maintaining this deformation under the constant load, the tissue continues to deform (second phase), or creep, as it approaches an asymptotic deformation plateau (figure 3.42).

The second phenomenon, seen in viscoelastic tissues subjected to constant deformation, is the **stress-relaxation response** (also called **force-relaxation response**). A tissue stretched (or compressed) to a given length (first phase) and then held at that length develops an initial resistance, or stress. While being maintained at the constant deformation (second phase), the stress decreases, or relaxes, as shown in figure 3.43a.

The creep and stress-relaxation responses are *strain-rate dependent* (i.e., the mechanical response

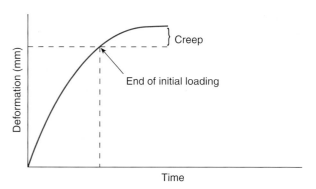

FIGURE 3.42 Mechanical creep in response to constant load. After an initial deformation while the load is initially applied, the material further deforms (creeps) to an asymptotic value while maintained at a constant load.

depends on the rate of deformation). This is shown for the stress-relaxation curve in figure 3.43b. With increased strain rate ($\dot{\varepsilon}_2$), the tissue is stiffer (i.e., steeper σ–ε slope), and the peak stress (σ_{max}) is higher and occurs sooner than with the slower strain rate ($\dot{\varepsilon}_1$).

Material Fatigue and Failure

Materials, including biological tissues, that are subjected to repeated loads above a certain threshold experience material **fatigue** and exhibit a decreased ability to withstand applied forces. Continued loading of a fatiguing material leads to eventual material failure. The number of loading cycles that may occur before failure may range from a few, as in the case of repeatedly bending a paper clip, to many millions.

An important fatigue-related concept, known as the **initial-cycles** or **first-cycle effect**, implies that the mechanical response seen in initial loading cycles may differ from the response seen during later loading cycles. This effect is shown in the σ–ε relations

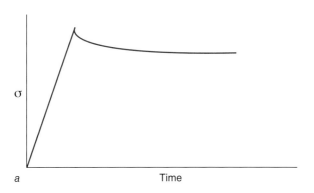

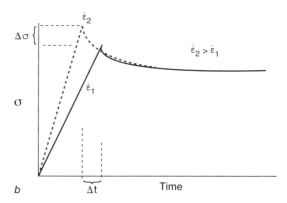

FIGURE 3.43 (a) Stress-relaxation response to constant deformation. The initial deformation elicits a stress (σ) response. Once the material reaches and maintains its constant deformation, the stress decreases (relaxes) to a constant level. (b) The effect of strain rate on the stress-relaxation response. At the higher strain rate ($\dot{\varepsilon}_2$), the maximum stress is greater (by Δσ) and reaches this peak stress earlier (by Δt).

depicted in figure 3.44. We see a gradual shift in tissue behavior from the initial cycles to later ones. Reasons for this shift include temperature fluctuation, fluid shift, and viscous response characteristics.

The susceptibility to tissue failure is determined in large part by how the stresses generated in response to loads are distributed throughout the material. If the stress is equally distributed, as in a smooth, homogenous solid, there is less chance of failure. If the stress is concentrated at a specific location, the likelihood of failure at that point increases. Stress concentration tends to occur at locations of **material discontinuity** within the tissue. These discontinuities create **stress risers** (also called *stress concentrations* or *stress raisers*), or points of focused stress. Examples of stress risers include tissue interfaces (e.g., osteotendinous and myotendinous junctions) and interruptions to tissue continuity (e.g., fracture sites, bone screw insertion points).

The material response prior to failure can vary considerably. Some materials (e.g., glass or bone) deform very little before failure and are described as **brittle**. Other materials (e.g., putty or elastic ligament) undergo considerable deformation before failing and are called **ductile**. Caution must be taken not to confuse the strength of a material with its brittleness or ductility. Brittle materials, for example, may possess high strength (e.g., steel) or may fail quite easily (e.g., chalk).

Various theories have been advanced to explain material failure, but the critical point is that biological tissue failure is inextricably linked to severe injury. Greater insight into a tissue's mechanical behavior may lead to more specific strategies to control or reduce injury.

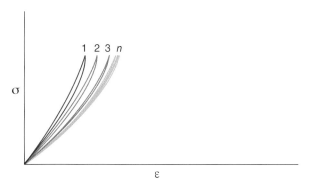

FIGURE 3.44 First-cycle or initial-cycles effect. Schematic representation of the different σ–ε responses seen in early loading cycles compared with later cycles when the response settles into a steady-state pattern.

Biomechanical Modeling and Simulation

A **model** is defined as a representation of one or more of an object's or system's characteristics. One of the primary goals of *modeling* is to improve, often through idealization and simplification, our understanding of the system or phenomenon being studied. Virtually every field of endeavor uses models in some way. Engineers and architects construct miniature versions of machines and buildings before constructing the real structure; economists create elaborate models to represent how the financial markets behave; psychologists construct models of human behavior. Simulations are intrinsically related to models, so much so that the two terms are often—erroneously—used interchangeably. The distinction is that a model uses equations to describe a system, whereas a **simulation** uses a validated model to perform experiments to address questions related to a system and its operation.

Biomechanical models typically exist in one of two forms: a physical model or a mathematical (or computer) model. Many of these models have the potential to provide valuable insights into the mechanisms of injury. Physical models in biomechanics are perhaps best exemplified by crash-test dummies, which have generated valuable data to improve vehicle occupant safety.

The biomechanics literature is replete with examples of computer models. These models use mathematical equations as the language of expression to characterize aspects of the system being modeled. In biomechanics, mathematical models have addressed movements such as walking, running, jumping, and throwing, along with more sport-specific movement patterns in swimming, diving, track-and-field events, gymnastics, ice skating, golf, and other sports. Recent biomechanical models have probed areas as diverse as muscle force production, meniscal dysfunction, arterial hemodynamics, prosthetic design, and foot placement during gait.

Why use modeling over other means of investigation, such as direct experimentation? First, mathematical models prove useful in situations that are not easily duplicated in real life. For obvious reasons, studies involving high-speed collisions or musculoskeletal injuries are not tenable using human subjects. Computer models provide a means of manipulating potential injury conditions without risk. Second, models allow investigators to

Crash-Test Dummies Are No Dummies

Anthropometric models, commonly known as crash-test dummies, are much more than friendly reminders for us to buckle our seat belts. The data they provide about the body's response to collision have proved invaluable in making automobiles safer. Countless lives have been saved through innovations these dummies have pioneered. State-of-the-art versions are much more than lifeless masses; current models use sophisticated instrumentation that allows measurement of body velocities, accelerations, impact forces, and much more. The effective designs of current passive restraint systems, airbags, crumple zones, side-impact reinforcements, collapsing steering columns, and safety windshields are in large part products of information generated from crash-test dummies.

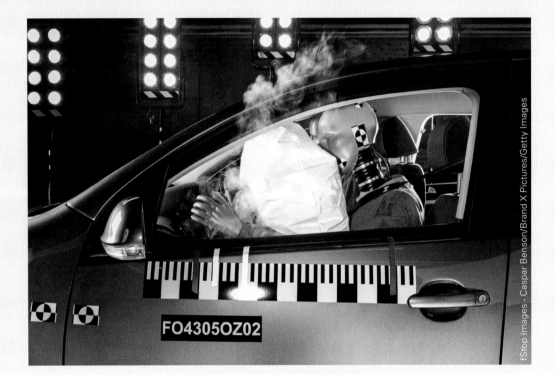

fStop Images - Caspar Benson/Brand X Pictures/Getty Images

FO4305OZ02

make changes in a system that could not be accomplished readily by an organism operating in a real environment. A human running, for example, would be unable to modulate his or her performance to produce specific changes in ground reaction forces at each step. A model of the runner, however, could easily produce these forces through appropriate inputs and can be used to predict the response of the system across a range of values.

The third reason for using models is time. Time-consuming direct experimental paradigms can be simulated in a fraction of the time required for direct experimentation. The continuing development of sophisticated mathematical models in recent decades parallels advances in computing power, allowing the implementation of complex models that would have been computationally intractable in the past.

Model Selection Criteria

Once the decision is made to create a model of a device, object, or system, the next step is to select the most appropriate type or class of model. Proper selection of model type depends largely on the questions being posed. An important caveat is that model complexity is directly related to the difficulty of model formulation and interpretation.

Biomechanical model selection relies on many considerations. These criteria are not mutually exclusive but rather are complementary. The human body can be studied at many levels, ranging from molecular to whole body. The questions being addressed by the model dictate whether the model is a molecular, cellular, tissue, organ, segmental, or whole-body formulation.

Because body tissues subjected to external loads will deform to varying extents, different structural types can be modeled. Tissues experiencing measurable deformation are best modeled using a **deformable-body model**. Tissues exhibiting negligible deformation or bodies assumed to be nondeformable (e.g., limb segments) can be represented by a **rigid-body model**. Structures considered without regard to their molecular characteristics are best examined using a **continuum mechanical model**. A contrasting view of a structure according to its component parts is best considered with a **discrete-element** or **finite-element model**.

The level of system motion determines whether the appropriate model is a **static model** (e.g., assessing the loads on the low back while in a bent-over position), a **quasi-static model** (e.g., patellofemoral joint loads during a slow squat), or a **dynamic model** (e.g., ankle joint moments during a vertical jump).

Most human body functions are inherently nonlinear across their physiological ranges. Thus, even though linear models are easier to formulate and manipulate, more complex nonlinear models often are the models of choice. The complexity of the process being modeled dictates the level of mathematical sophistication required for its formulation. Some simple systems may only require algebraic calculations for their solution, but complex systems may be assessable only through advanced mathematics. Another aspect affecting model selection is whether the system is fully determined (i.e., **deterministic model**) or comprises functions based on certain probabilistic behaviors (i.e., **stochastic model**).

Activities involving movement in a single plane, or primarily in a single plane (e.g., walking), can be represented by a two-dimensional **planar model**. Most human movements, however, occur in multiple planes and require a more complex three-dimensional **spatial model**.

If actual forces and moments (i.e., kinetics) are measured and used in a model to predict the details of movement (kinematics), this is termed a **forward solution** or **direct solution** approach. In contrast, using measured kinematics (velocities and accelerations) to predict the kinetics (forces and moments) is referred to as an **inverse solution** approach. This second approach, sometimes called **inverse dynamics**, is useful when the movement characteristics are measurable but measuring the actual forces or moments (torques) is either very difficult or impossible. Inverse dynamics models are commonly used in biomechanics to estimate internal forces and moments at joints. Direct measurements of muscle forces and joint torques are difficult at best, and inverse dynamics techniques provide a noninvasive means of estimating these values.

All models are simplifications of the actual situation being modeled. Simplification, however, does not necessarily imply simplicity. Even with simplification, models can be quite complex, and with available computer processing power increasing exponentially, there is a temptation to create extremely complex models. How complex a model is needed? Hubbard (1993) provides sage advice: "Always begin with the simplest possible model, which captures the essence of the task being studied" (p. 55).

Elements of a model often are idealized representations of real-life variables, in much the same way an idealized force vector (discussed earlier in this chapter) is representative of many force vectors. When a system component is idealized, however, information about its actual functional properties is lost. The ability of a model or simulation to achieve its purpose is only as good as the data that it receives as input.

A stable model can maintain its validity over an appropriate range of values and conditions. The predictive ability and, therefore, the usefulness of any model are related to the accuracy with which variables can be specified over a range of values. The critical issue becomes how well the model predicts values between known data points (**interpolation**) and beyond the ranges of known values (**extrapolation**).

Biomechanical modeling is a useful tool for exploring many areas of human function, particularly in describing and evaluating human movement. Modeling has yet to reach its full potential in assessing the biomechanics of injury and holds much promise. As technological capabilities increase, we must maintain our focus on the mechanical and physiological processes of interest and not become distracted by mathematical sophistication.

Tissue Models

Our discussions of material mechanics and tissue structure (chapter 2) have highlighted the viscoelastic nature of tissues such as bone, tendon, ligament, and cartilage. The details of these tissues' mechanical characteristics are presented in chapter 4, but it is instructive at this point to examine the viscoelastic properties of tissue in some modeling applications.

Rheological Models

Rheology is the study of the deformation and flow of matter. Given that all body tissues have a fluid component and therefore have viscous (flow-related) characteristics, we introduce the concept of a **rheological model**, which has been used extensively to examine the mechanical behavior of human tissues.

Rheological models of tissue interrelate stress (σ), strain (ε), and strain rate ($\dot{\varepsilon}$) of biological tissues. They use three model components that, although having no direct association with actual tissue structural elements, allow us to examine tissue response to loading. These three model components are the linear spring, the dashpot, and the frictional element (figure 3.45). In normal situations, internal friction is negligible compared with other forces and so is often omitted from rheological models of biological tissues.

The **linear spring** represents the elastic properties of the tissue, assuming that the material deforms and returns to its original shape linearly with respect to the applied force and the deformation. The relation between the spring's stress (σ) and strain (ε) is given by equation 3.34, where E is the modulus of elasticity, or Young's modulus.

The fluid component of biological tissues dictates a loading response that is strain-rate dependent. The **dashpot** models this viscous contribution to the overall response. If the fluid's stress–strain rate response is linear, the fluid is termed a **Newtonian fluid**. The following equation indicates the dashpot's linear relation:

$$\sigma = \eta \cdot \dot{\varepsilon} \tag{3.56}$$

where η = the proportionality coefficient relating stress and strain rate.

Researchers can use linear springs (or nonlinear springs) and dashpots as building blocks in constructing composite models with the goal of accurately predicting the response of real tissues. Two standard combinations of linear spring and dashpot are the **Kelvin–Voight model** (spring and dashpot in parallel) and the **Maxwell model** (spring and dashpot in series). These models and their loading responses are shown in figure 3.46. Neither of these models is directly applicable for modeling tissue behavior, but combining them with other components produces models with good predictive abilities. A simple, standard solid model and a classic complex model (Viidik 1968) are depicted in figure 3.47. If we vary the coefficients E_i and η, the models can be fine-tuned to provide an accurate representation of a tissue's response to loading.

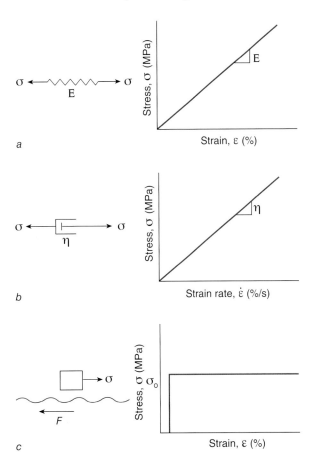

FIGURE 3.45 Rheological model components: *(a)* linear spring, *(b)* dashpot, and *(c)* frictional element.

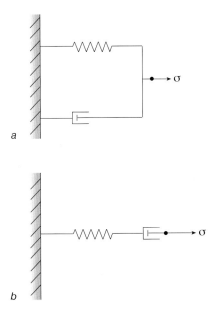

FIGURE 3.46 Rheological models. *(a)* Kelvin–Voight model, with spring and dashpot in parallel. *(b)* Maxwell model, with spring and dashpot in series.

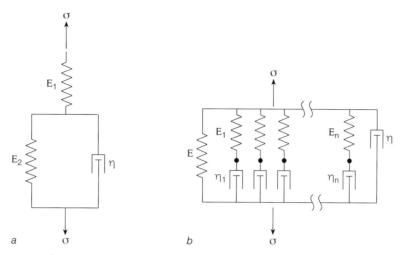

FIGURE 3.47 Examples of rheological models. *(a)* Standard solid model. *(b)* Complex model.

Finite-Element Models

The finite-element (FE) method originated in the mid-1950s as a tool to assist engineers in the design of structures. The FE approach often requires lengthy and complex calculations and, therefore, became tractable only with advances in computer technology. Originally, its use was restricted to experts specializing in FE methods who used large, mainframe computers to solve problems. As computer size decreased and speed increased, FE methods became more accessible to nonspecialists via commercially available FE program packages. Originally used in aerospace engineering (primarily by NASA), FE methods gradually found their way into other areas of structural analysis in mechanical and civil engineering. Biomechanists have found finite-element modeling to be a valuable tool for investigating a wide range of biological problems, such as designing artificial hip joints.

Finite-element modeling uses simple shapes, known as *elements* (building blocks), which are assembled to form complex geometrical structures (meshes). The elements are connected at points known as *nodes*. In a model, a finite number of elements (or shapes) are connected at nodes to form a mathematical representation of a structure such as bone (figure 3.48). As forces are applied to the model or as the model is deformed, elaborate equations predict the structure's stress and strain responses to loading. The complexity of a finite-element model is determined by the imagination of its creator, the level of mathematical sophistication, and the available computing power.

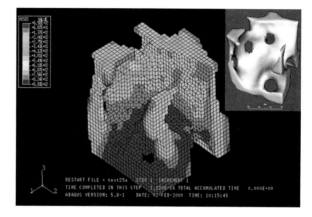

FIGURE 3.48 Finite element model of trabecular bone.
Image by Ronald Zernicke and Steven Boyd.

Recent and ongoing research combines finite-element modeling with other technologies (e.g., imaging techniques) to create sophisticated models to characterize complex musculoskeletal systems. For example, Blemker and Delp (2005) developed a three-dimensional finite-element model using magnetic resonance images to describe moment arms of fibers within specific muscles (psoas, iliacus, gluteus maximus, and gluteus medius). Such efforts improve the accuracy of musculoskeletal computer models and allow researchers to answer emerging questions about how the human body functions.

A number of open-source programs, such Open-Sim (Seth et al. 2018) and FEBio, are available for researchers to use finite-element modeling techniques to investigate topics across the spectrum of biomechanical problems.

Chapter Review

Key Points

- Four major areas of biomechanics form the foundation for an understanding of musculoskeletal injury: movement mechanics, fluid mechanics, joint mechanics, and material mechanics.

- From a mechanical perspective, human movement depends on effective integration of linear and angular motion, center of gravity positioning and control, stability, mobility, and equilibrium.

- The primary mechanical agents involved in injury are force and energy. These two mechanical variables and related measures (e.g., work, power, and torque) explain the mechanics of injury.

- Human movement and susceptibility to musculoskeletal injury are governed by Newton's three laws of motion.

- The fluid component in musculoskeletal tissues governs tissue responses to loading (e.g., viscoelasticity and biphasic response) and, hence, plays an important role in the mechanics of injury.

- Biological tissue responses can be described using engineering variables such as load—deformation, stress—strain, and related measures.

- Mechanical models are used to represent the human body at all levels (i.e., from molecular to whole body) and are useful in explaining tissue response to loading and mechanisms of injury.

Questions to Consider

1. Many engineering texts present linear mechanics and angular mechanics in separate chapters. From a biomechanical perspective, why is it important to consider linear and angular mechanics simultaneously?

2. Explain the relation between muscle force (chapter 2) and muscle torque (chapter 3).

3. Describe the importance of Sir Isaac Newton's contributions to our understanding of mechanics, and specifically of the biomechanics of musculoskeletal injury.

4. Explain how the principles of fluid mechanics apply to cardiovascular disease.

5. Consider a person jumping down and landing from a platform 1 m above the ground. What movement strategies might the jumper employ to reduce injury risk at landing? What mechanical principles are being applied in devising an effective landing strategy?

6. Describe three detailed examples that illustrate the role of friction in the biomechanics of injury.

7. Describe the utility of using both absolute and relative measures to explain tissue response to loading and injury potential.

8. List and briefly describe what factors should be considered in selecting the type of model to be used for assessing a biomechanical problem.

9. When a long bone is bent until it fractures, what factors will determine the bone's resistance to bending and the location of eventual fracture?

Suggested Readings

Aaron, R., ed. 2021. *Orthopaedic Basic Science* (5th ed.) Park Ridge, IL: American Academy of Orthopaedic Surgeons.

Bartlett, R. 2014. *Introduction to Sports Biomechanics: Analyzing Human Movement Patterns* (3rd ed.). Abingdon-on-Thames, England: Routledge.

De, S., W. Hwang, and E. Kuhl, eds. 2015. *Multiscale Modeling in Biomechanics and Mechanobiology*. New York: Springer.

Enoka, R.M. 2015. *Neuromechanics of Human Movement* (5th ed.). Champaign, IL: Human Kinetics.

Flanagan, S.P. 2018. *Biomechanics: A Case-Based Approach* (2nd ed.). Burlington, MA: Jones & Bartlett Learning.

Hall, S.J. 2019. *Basic Biomechanics* (8th ed.). New York: McGraw-Hill.

Hamill, J., K.M. Knutzen, and T.R. Derrick. 2021. *Biomechanical Basis of Human Movement* (5th ed.). Baltimore: Lippincott, Williams & Wilkins.

Hamilton, N., W. Weimar, and K. Luttgens. 2007. *Kinesiology: Scientific Basis of Human Motion* (11th ed.). New York: McGraw-Hill.

Kaufman, K. 2021. Biomechanics of the skeletal system. In *Orthopaedic Basic Science*, edited by R. Aaron. Park Ridge, IL: American Academy of Orthopaedic Surgeons.

Levangie, P.K., C.C. Norkin, and M.D. Lewek. 2019. *Joint Structure and Function: A Comprehensive Analysis* (6th ed.). Philadelphia: F.A. Davis.

Limbrunner, G., C. D'Allaird, and L. Spiegel, eds. 2015. *Applied Statics and Strength of Materials* (6th ed.). London: Pearson.

Martin, R.B., D.B. Burr, N.A. Sharkey, and D.P. Fyhrie. 2015. *Skeletal Tissue Mechanics* (2nd ed.). New York: Springer.

McGinnis, P.M. 2021. *Biomechanics of Sport and Exercise* (4th ed.). Champaign, IL: Human Kinetics.

Mow, V.C., and R. Huiskes, eds. 2005. *Basic Orthopaedic Biomechanics and Mechano-Biology* (3rd ed.). New York: Lippincott, Williams & Wilkins.

Nigg, B.M., and W. Herzog, eds. 2007. *Biomechanics of the Musculo-skeletal System* (3rd ed.). New York: Wiley.

Nordin, M., and V.H. Frankel. 2012. *Basic Biomechanics of the Musculoskeletal System* (4th ed.). New York: Lippincott, Williams & Wilkins.

Whiting, W.C. 2019. *Dynamic Human Anatomy* (2nd ed.). Champaign, IL: Human Kinetics.

book

Tissue Mechanics
and Injury

Tissue Biomechanics and Adaptation

The form . . . of matter . . . and the changes of form which are apparent in . . . its growth . . . are due to the action of force(s).

D'Arcy Thompson (1860-1948)

OBJECTIVES

- To explain the biomechanical behaviors of the human musculoskeletal system
- To highlight form and function of load-bearing tissues such as bone, tendon, ligament, cartilage, and muscle
- To link comprehensive knowledge of tissue adaptation to its environment with tissue biomechanical function and injury

Building on the tissue anatomy already presented in chapter 2 and the biomechanical principles detailed in chapter 3, here we review viscoelastic properties and adaptive responses of the multiple tissue types within the human musculoskeletal system (e.g., bone, articular cartilage, tendon, ligament, and skeletal muscle). These tissues exhibit complex mechanical behaviors, such as a stress-relaxation response to constant strain, creep at constant stress, hysteresis under cyclic loading, strain-rate dependency, and cyclic stress fatigue. Skeletal muscle, in addition to these passive phenomena, also has active force, length, and velocity properties that are unique and synergistic. Information about the mechanical properties and behaviors of musculoskeletal tissues has been gathered using in vitro, in situ, and in vivo methods.

Knowledge of the adaptive capabilities of musculoskeletal tissues is as important to understanding injury as knowledge of their biomechanical function. Although **homeostasis** is a tenet of physiology, when we examine that tenet more closely we see that the more typical status of these tissues is a continually changing mosaic—tissues in the body are constantly adapting in response to internal and external stimuli to maintain equilibrium. **Adaptation** is a natural, form-function interaction and can be defined as the "modification of an organism or its parts that makes it more fit for existence under the conditions of its environment" (Merriam-Webster 2003).

Throughout a person's life span, dramatic physiological changes and adaptations occur in bone, cartilage, tendon, ligament, and muscle. Factors such as physical activity, immobilization (e.g., with a cast or brace), or diet can profoundly affect the quality and quantity of load-bearing connective tissues. For each musculoskeletal tissue, we first review the biomechanical properties and then summarize each tissue's adaptive capabilities.

Biomechanics of Bone

Bone's role is to support the body, protect internal organs, provide levers for movement, and store minerals. There are two major types of bone—cortical (compact) bone and trabecular (spongy or cancellous) bone. Eighty percent of the weight of the human skeleton comes from cortical bone, which is dense and forms the outer covering of bones. Cortical bone is composed of the typical osteon structure described in chapter 2. Trabecular bone is spongy, giving rise to its moniker, and makes up the interior of most bones. This bone is more porous and is composed of beams and struts (**trabeculae**) that are aligned in the directions of stress to best resist tissue damage. Trabecular bone has lower calcium content and density than cortical bone. In turn, trabecular bone has greater water content and is a

In Vitro, in Situ, or in Vivo?

Accurate testing and measurement of mechanical properties are essential to understand tissue function and responses, but the act of measuring, in itself, can change a tissue's behavior. The challenge facing scientists who study the properties of biological tissues is highlighted by a statement by C.J.H. Nicolle: "Error is all around us and creeps in at the least opportunity. Every method is imperfect" (in Beveridge 1957, p. 115).

The methodological approaches for studying the full range of joints, tissues, or tissue constituents fall broadly into three categories: in vitro, in situ, and in vivo. Each successive category gets closer to measuring tissue behaviors as they exist in the body—although each has its own respective merits and disadvantages.

In vitro literally means "within a glass," but in the generic sense, in vitro refers to testing done in an artificial environment. The specimen—from whole bones to cells—is usually immersed in a physiological buffer solution maintained at body temperature, but the environment is artificial. In vitro fertilization is a common example of a procedure accomplished outside the body's organs.

One advantage of in vitro tests is that direct measurements can be taken. One disadvantage, however, is that the in vitro method is invasive—a tissue is removed from the body and its normal environment. The cells no longer have their native chemical and physical connections to the surrounding tissues and fluids, and therefore respond differently in a petri dish (Nickien et al. 2018).

In situ means "in its normal place," or confined to the site of origin. One advantage of in situ preparations is that some elements of the natural environment are preserved in the testing. Notably, much of the information available on skeletal muscle properties has been gathered through in situ techniques. During in situ experiments to record skeletal muscle contractions, a muscle's natural neurovascular supply can remain intact, the orientation of the muscle with respect to its bony attachments can be maintained, and the muscle temperature can be kept within the physiological range. Although this method is closer to natural, certain components of the test environment are still artificial. The properties are determined under constrained conditions and not in the freely moving organism. Examples of in situ testing may involve dissected or plastinated models, in which the targeted structure is still located in its naturally occurring state while the testing occurs in laboratory conditions.

In vivo indicates that the testing is done within the living body, and this approach might appear to be the best. However, obtaining accurate in vivo data is technically challenging. Even if the data are recorded successfully, the implanted transducers can affect the measurements being taken, or a person's movements may be altered because of the Hawthorne effect (i.e., modification of behavior by persons being studied due to their awareness of being observed or recorded). Furthermore, ethical concerns must be addressed, especially when trying to manipulate and measure responses of musculoskeletal tissues in humans. A few investigators have recorded in vivo muscle–tendon forces (Gregor et al. 1991) or bone strains (Burr et al. 1996) in humans, but the great majority of in vivo experiments involving musculoskeletal tissues have been conducted with animal models.

better subject for bone remodeling, at a rate of 26% turnover per year compared to 3% for cortical bone (Oftadeh et al. 2015).

Cortical (Compact) Bone

The mechanical behavior of cortical (compact) bone can be assessed in a variety of ways. The method of testing should be selected to best approximate the way the bone is loaded during a given activity. Because bone is usually loaded from multiple directions (multiaxially) and responds differently based on the direction (anisotropy), it is difficult to uniquely test each condition in which bone is loaded. As a way to simplify the testing scenario, cortical bone can either be treated as an elastic beam of uniform dimension and tested in three- or four-point bending, or a bone sample of known dimensions can be tested in uniaxial compression or tension.

In a typical bone bending test (figure 4.1), as a tissue (bone) is initially loaded, the load–deformation curve is concave toward the load axis and resembles an exponential function. This **toe region** (i.e., initial curvilinear portion at the start of the loading) is

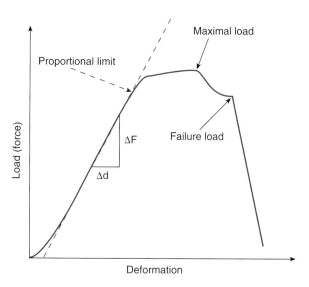

FIGURE 4.1 Example of a load–deformation curve from a sample of cortical bone that is being tested in three-point bending. In three-point bending, the flexural rigidity of the bone is calculated as $(L^3/48) \cdot (\Delta F/\Delta d)$, where L is equal to the distance between the two supporting points on which the bone rests and $(\Delta F/\Delta d)$ is the slope of the force–deformation curve in the linear region. Flexural rigidity is the product of the elastic modulus (E) and the cross-sectional area moment of inertia (I) of a tissue (e.g., bone). When the value of flexural rigidity increases, the bending strength of the bone to resist bending also increases.

characterized by the tissue, initially slack, becoming taut. As the load increases, deformation increases in a relatively linear fashion, resembling Hooke's law (see chapter 3). Consistent with Hooke's law, all deformation in this **elastic region** can be reversed with internal restoring forces, and the tissue will not be damaged. The slope of this **linear region** is related to the bone's **flexural rigidity** or elastic modulus, a measure of tissue (e.g., bending) stiffness. The yield point, or proportional limit (see figure 4.1), marks the end of the elastic region and the transition into the **plastic region**. As the response of bone moves into the region of *plastic deformation,* smaller and smaller increases in load will produce greater and greater increases in deformation and structural damage to the tissue. If the applied load is removed just after the transition to plastic deformation (but before maximal and failure loads are reached), the tissue does not return to its original (preloaded) configuration. Instead, the tissue takes on a permanent set—it remains bent or deformed. A typical bone loading test (figure 4.1) reveals a unique point known as the **maximal load**, where additional stress can be placed upon the bone past the proportional limit in the plastic region. After this point, excess loading causes hairline fractures and loss of structural integrity, leading to loss of load resistance. At the end of the plastic region—denoting the end of the load–deformation curve—is the point of ultimate failure. At that point, the tissue has been deformed to maximal capacity and further loading will permanently disrupt the tissue (e.g., bone fracture). These load–deformation tests can be used to determine the material properties of soft tissues as well, prompting similar curves with different elastic moduli and ultimate failure points; these will be explored in a later section.

Flexural rigidity, load behaviors, and stored energy (area under a load–deformation curve) are *structural properties* of the bone. If the geometry (shape) of the bone sample is known, then the *material properties* of the bone can be calculated. **Material properties** refer to the mechanical quality of the bone. The elastic modulus and stresses (force per unit area) at the proportional limit and at the maximal and failure points are examples of the bone's material properties.

The distinction between structural and material properties can be easily recognized by considering the diaphyses of a femur and a phalanx. The obviously larger femoral diaphysis is able to carry substantially greater loads than the smaller phalanx, and thus the structural properties (e.g., maximal load and bending stiffness) of the femur will be much greater than those of the phalanx. The cortical bone within the femur and phalanx, however, could have very similar composition, and thus, if their differences in size were removed (normalized), the material properties of the two bones may be very similar (e.g., maximal stress, calculated as force per unit area).

Understanding the importance of bone shape and geometry leads us to consider how the area moment of inertia (I) influences the structural properties of bone during bending. Take a moment to consider the following: Imagine an oak plank that is 2 m long, 5 cm thick, and 30 cm wide, supported only at either end. If you stand on the plank at midlength, the board is being loaded in three-point bending. When you stand on the flat side of the board, you will easily bend the board as it sags under your weight. If, however, you rotate the board 90° so you balance on the 5 cm edge, the board will be much stiffer, and it will sag much less.

This potent effect of bone cross-sectional geometry can be seen in the three scenarios illustrated in figure 4.2. Assume that you are testing tubular long bones of three different cross-sectional shapes in three-point bending. The examples in figure 4.2a and b have the same periosteal diameter, but the example in figure 4.2a has a medullary cavity (hollow core), whereas the example in figure 4.2b has no medullary cavity (solid bone). Figure 4.2c shows a slightly larger periosteal diameter of 2.5 centimeters and a relatively large medullary cavity (a thin-walled, tubular bone). The three-point bending load is applied identically across scenarios (figure 4.2d). As seen in table 4.1, these shape differences generate pronounced differences in area moment of inertia and bending behaviors. The bone cross-sectional areas in figure 4.2a (2.95 cm^2) and figure 4.2b (3.14 cm^2) are more than 66% greater than the cross-sectional area of the large tubular bone shown in figure 4.2c (1.77 cm^2). At the same time, because the area moment of inertia (see figure 3.33) is related to the amount of bone and the distribution of the bone about the bending axis, the thin-walled, tubular bone (figure 4.2c) has an area moment of inertia that is substantially greater (>40%) than either example a or b. In figure 4.2a and c, area $= \pi \cdot (r_o^2 - r_i^2)$, and area moment of inertia $(I) = [\pi \cdot (r_o^4 - r_i^4)]/4$ (see equation 3.49). In figure 4.2b, which has no medullary (marrow) cavity, area $= \pi \cdot r_o^2$ and area moment of inertia $(I) = \pi \cdot r^4/4$ (see equation 3.48). Thus, if the same bending load is applied to each of the bones, approximately 13% more stress would be developed within both the smaller tubular bone (figure 4.2a) and the solid bone (figure 4.2b) than in the large tubular bone (figure 4.2c).

For examples a through c, during three-point bending (d), the stress (σ) developed in the bone is $\sigma = MC/I$, where M = moment, C = distance from center of cross section to periosteal surface (outer radius), and I = area moment of inertia of the cross section. $M = (F/2) \cdot L$, where F = 20N, and L = 20 cm.

Changing the ratio of the periosteal-to-endosteal diameters alters the bending stiffness of a long bone without adding large amounts of bone mass. The theoretical implications and potential optimization of the structural features of the wall thickness of tubular bones were explored in a classic paper by Currey and Alexander (1985).

Extensive data on the material properties of cortical bones of many species (including human) have been reported by Croker, Reed, and Donlon (2016). In addition to a wide assortment of human

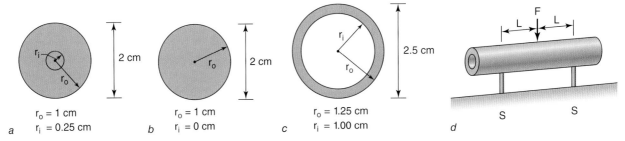

FIGURE 4.2 Cross-sectional geometry affects bending behavior of tubular (*a* and *c*) and solid (*b*) bone of different dimensions, where r_o = outer (periosteal) radius and r_i = the inner (endosteal) radius of long bone. (*d*) Three-point bending loads being applied to the bone samples. F = applied force; S = positions of supports under bone sample; L = distance between applied force F and each support S.

TABLE 4.1   Cross-Sectional Geometry and Bone Bending Behavior

	Example *a*	Example *b*	Example *c*
Outer (periosteal) radius (r_o)	1.00	1.00	1.25
Inner (endosteal) radius (r_i)	0.25	0.00	1.00
Bone area (*A*), cm²	2.95	3.14	1.77
Area moment of inertia (*I*), cm⁴	0.78	0.79	1.13
Force (*F*), N	20.0	20.0	20.0
Stress ($\sigma = MC/I$), N/cm²	256	253	221

cortical bones (e.g., humerus, radius, femur, and tibia), bone samples from a range of animals have also been reported (e.g., kangaroos, sheep, juvenile pigs, greyhound dogs, and cattle). The data from Croker and colleagues (2016) expanded the pioneering studies by Yamada (1973), who reported that the average ultimate tensile stress for the long bones of limbs from humans 20 to 39 years of age ranged between 120 and 150 MPa. Later studies (Martin et al. 2015) of the ultimate tensile stress in cortical bone reported nearly the same range (e.g., 108-130 MPa). In terms of ultimate compressive stress, the human femur had the greatest value (up to 166 MPa in persons 20-39 years of age), followed by the tibia and then the humerus. The lowest ultimate compressive stress values were found in the fibula, ulna, and radius—although even those three bones had an average ultimate compressive stress greater than 115 MPa. Compared with human cortical bone, the mechanical properties of cortical bone from a host of species have been studied extensively (Currey 1988, 2002, 2003a, 2003b, 2005).

Currey's comparative osteological results reveal that a bone's calcium content and porosity can explain about 80% of the variation seen in a bone's elastic modulus (stiffness). Sampling 28 bones from 17 species of mammals, birds, and reptiles, Currey (1988) reported that bone's maximal strain and the mechanical work under the stress–strain curve are sharply decreased with excessive mineralization.

Cortical bone is an anisotropic material, and thus bone's elastic modulus and strength depend on the orientation of the collagen–mineral matrix. Bone has a grain associated with its structure, similar to wood. The bone or piece of wood has a much greater elastic modulus and strength when a compressive load is applied along the long axis (in line with its grain) than when applied at right angles to the

long axis (shear force perpendicular to the grain). In contrast, if you apply loads from any direction to an **isotropic** metal (e.g., stainless steel), the elastic modulus and strength are the same in all directions.

Poisson's ratio (v) is the other parameter used to quantify a bone's elastic behavior. This effect was previously illustrated in figure 3.28 and mathematically defined in equation 3.35. The ratio v is previously illustrated in figure 3.28 and mathematically defined as

$$v = -\left(\frac{\varepsilon_t}{\varepsilon_a}\right)$$

Bone has a relatively high Poisson's ratio (v ≤ 0.6), much higher than found in metals.

Toughness is a measure of a tissue's ability to absorb mechanical energy. Cortical bone is considered to be tough because it is able to absorb a great deal of mechanical energy before it fractures. Bone is also a relatively ductile (malleable) material. If a metal is ductile, it can be hammered into thin sheets without breaking. A gold nugget, for example, can be flattened into a wafer-thin foil. Bone, of course, is not as ductile as gold, but it can be deformed to some extent without fracture. As discussed in chapter 3, the opposite of ductile is *brittle*. With increasing age, bones have a tendency to become less ductile, more brittle, and more fragile.

Finally, cortical bone is viscoelastic—that is, it exhibits strain-rate sensitivity, creep behavior, hysteresis, and fatigue. Some mechanical properties of cortical bone are very sensitive to differing strain rates. As a bone is loaded more and more rapidly, its ultimate strength increases at a faster rate than does its elastic modulus, it can store more potential energy, and it is stiffer. *Fatigue* is the loss of strength and stiffness that occurs in materials subjected to repeated cyclic loads. Although bone can withstand substantial stresses when loaded only once, as the

What if Bones Were Solid Beams Rather Than Thin-Walled Tubes?

Two renowned biologists, Currey and Alexander (1985), hypothesized that the mechanical design of tubular long bones suggests that there may be an optimal ratio of diameter to cortical thickness for thin-walled bones. It is generally accepted that the tubular structure of most limb bones ensures that they will be lighter without sacrificing strength or stiffness. But does that notion hold across a wide range of species?

In assessing the concept of an optimal ratio, Currey and Alexander considered the counterbalancing of relative bone mass against structural properties, such as yield (or fatigue) strength, ultimate (or impact) strength, and stiffness. By measuring the limb bones of 56 species of mammals, birds, and reptiles (including some extinct), the researchers generated results showing why tubular, marrow-filled (long) bones appear to be an effective design for bones that undergo substantial bending loads—such as the bones of limbs.

Currey and Alexander calculated the ratio of cross-sectional radius (C) to the thickness of the bone cortical shell (t). They predicted that if marrow-filled bones were basically tubular structures of minimal mass and optimal strength, then the C/t ratio would be 2.3. By comparison, if stiffness were the criterion for bone design, then C/t would be 3.9.

To better understand the mechanical effects of the different-sized tubular bones, compare the three long bones for which we contrasted cross-sectional geometry and stresses in three-point bending (figure 4.2a-c). In the following table, we provide values for their cross-sectional radius (C), cortical thickness (t), and the ratio C/t. The larger diameter and thinner walled bone (Figure 4.2c) has the much larger C/t ratio.

Interestingly, chickens trained by running on a treadmill also demonstrated a shift toward Currey and Alexander's predicted strength-optimal C/t ratio for a weight-bearing limb bone (Loitz and Zernicke 1992; Matsuda et al. 1986). Adult roosters were exercised on a treadmill for 1 hour per day, 5 days per week for 9 weeks, at 70% and 75% predicted maximal aerobic capacity (Loitz and Zernicke 1992) and had an average C/t of 2.3 in their tarsometatarsal bones—precisely the values predicted by Currey and Alexander (1985).

Why is that important? Consider the following. Currey calculated that when a horse gallops at 54 km/h, about 50% of its power is used to accelerate and decelerate the bones of its limbs, and a 10% decrease in limb bone mass would generate a 5% power savings. That savings could be significant in the context of natural selection (escape from a predator) or even in a thoroughbred horse race.

	Example *a*	Example *b*	Example *c*
Radius (*C*), cm	1.00	1.00	1.25
Cortical thickness (*t*), cm	0.75	1.00	0.25
Radius/thickness (*C/t*)	1.33	1.00	5.00

Note: See figure 4.2 for sketches and dimensions of these examples.

number of cyclic loads increases, the ultimate tensile stress of the bone decreases and further loading cycles of higher magnitude can lead to stress responses. In bone, fatigue has been attributed to microscopic cracks (microcracks) that develop within and between the osteons (Martin et al. 2015). In healthy bone, if damage is not excessive, remodeling resorbs the material around microcracks, and new bone is deposited. However, if the damage is excessive and the normal remodeling process cannot keep up with the repair, macroscopic failure (fractures) can happen. For example, among distance runners, stress fractures are commonly associated with fatigue due to repetitive impact stresses about the long axis of the bone (Crowell and Davis 2011).

Trabecular (Cancellous) Bone

The latticework organization of trabecular bone is diverse, and the apparent density and architecture of trabecular bone have potent effects on their elastic modulus and strength. The elastic modulus of trabecular bone can vary from 10 to 2,000 MPa, in contrast to cortical bone, which has an elastic modulus around 13 to 17 GPa.

Comparative Properties of Bone

From the perspective as a biologist, Currey viewed the structure–function relation of bones as it relates to natural selection. For example, in 1979 Currey assessed the mechanical properties of three types of bones from three different specimens—a deer's (Cervus elaphus) antler, a cow's (Bos taurus) femur, and a fin whale's (Balaenoptera physalus) tympanic bulla. The bones served very different functions, and consequently demonstrated very different mechanical properties.

Because the principal functions of the red deer's antlers are for display and dueling, **impact strength** is an important property for winning the fight. Currey found a high impact resistance in the antlers but a simultaneously low elastic modulus (perhaps to account for shock absorption) and relatively low bending strength.

The fin whale's tympanic bulla, in contrast, had the highest mineral content and highest elastic modulus of the three bones. Currey described the bulla as "quite rocklike to handle" and about the size of a fist. Like the auditory ossicles in the human ear, the tympanic bulla of the fin whale is securely protected in the skull from the outside world. Stiffness (high modulus) would be a very important property to ensure that sound waves are transmitted with fidelity for accurate hearing. The fracture strength of the fin whale's bulla therefore is less important, and there is a natural blend of form and function in this bone. The cow's femur, on the other hand, has an elastic modulus, impact strength, and bending strength that are all rather high but not extreme.

Significant Implications of Bone Microcracks

When mechanical properties of a material such as bone are compromised, it can be said that the material is damaged. Because microcracks usually develop within the interior of cortical bone, they are hard to see in situ. Using microscopy, Zioupos and Currey (1994) visualized the three-dimensional distributions of microcracks in cortical bone and found that the cracks were associated with regions of high stress. The microstructure (grain) of the bone affected the magnitude and direction of propagation of microcracks within the bone, and microcracks were most likely to occur in the most highly mineralized parts of the bone (perhaps due to a greater brittleness associated with mineralization). Why are these microcracks significant? As we know, bone has both elastic and plastic responses. In the plastic region, even with decreasing load levels during continuous and cyclic loading, there is an increasing amount of deformation—the bone becomes damaged and increasingly compliant. Dispersed microcracks may weaken bone and decrease its structural stiffness.

The porous spaces between trabeculae (beams) are typically filled with red marrow, which can play an important part in the load-bearing capabilities of trabecular bone. Impact-speed tests have shown that the strength and elastic modulus are dramatically greater in specimens of trabecular bone with bone marrow present than those with the marrow removed before the test. This "stiffening" effect of the marrow is minimal, however, at physiological rates of loading. Nevertheless, with or without the marrow, trabecular bone exhibits the previously mentioned viscoelastic effects because its fundamental building block is viscoelastic lamellar bone (as exists in cortical bone).

Adaptation of Bone

Bone is a dynamic tissue that is exquisitely adapted to multiple internal factors (e.g., systemic calcium or hormone levels) and external factors (e.g., mechanical loads) that can affect its structure, composition, and quantity. The capacity of bone to adapt its structure to imposed loads has become known as **Wolff's Law**, after the 19th-century surgeon who stated that "Every change in the form and function of . . . bone[s] or of their function alone is followed by certain definite changes in their internal architecture, and equally definite secondary alterations in their external conformation, in accordance with mathematical laws" (Martin et al. 2015).

Among the concepts that arose in the 19th century and that are now incorporated into Wolff's law are the optimization of bone strength with respect to bone weight, trabecular alignment with the lines of principal stress, and the self-regulation of bone structure by cells responding to mechanical stimuli (Martin et al. 2015; Weinkamer et al. 2019).

Events that signal changes in bone are classified as either modeling or remodeling. **Modeling** is the addition (formation) of new bone, whereas **remodeling** involves resorption and formation or reformation of existing bone. Differences between modeling and remodeling of bone are summarized in table 4.2.

Modeling can happen at various rates and is a continuous process that can occur on any bony surface to produce a net gain in bone. During modeling, osteoclasts and osteoblasts are not active along the same surface; resorption can occur along one cortex while deposition occurs along another. The specific stimulus that initiates modeling remains unclear. Modeling happens mainly during the growing years (e.g., endochondral ossification). The ability of bone to adapt to mechanical loading is greater during growth than after maturity, but limited modeling can still happen after skeletal maturation (Suva et al. 2005).

Skeletal remodeling, the resorption and replacement of existing bone, triggers a mobilization of minerals stored in the bone and consequent shuttling into the blood (resorption). Hydroxyapatite can be mobilized in response to a low serum calcium level and circulating hormone levels, inclusive to parathyroid hormone (PTH), calcitriol (vitamin D_3), calcitonin, sex hormones, thyroid hormone (T_3 and T_4), growth hormone, and glucocorticoids. Resorbed minerals, such as calcium and phosphate, can be used to repair skeletal microdamage or to balance mechanical and mass needs of the skeleton (Sid-

diqui and Partridge 2016). The sequence of remodeling events can be remembered as **activation–resorption–formation**. The first step in remodeling is activation of osteoclasts to resorb existing bone. New bone is deposited by osteoblasts that follow the resorptive front of osteoclasts. Deposition of new bone takes three times longer than resorption, which translates into a 1-week time lapse between resorption and formation (Martin et al. 2015).

Lanyon (1987) described functional remodeling as an "interpretation and purposeful reaction" to a bone's strain state, allowing for adaptation to both increased and decreased strains. "Functional strains are both the objective and the stimulus for the process of adaptive modeling and remodeling" (Lanyon 1987, pp. 1084-1085). Rubin and Lanyon (1985) proposed that if functional strains are too high, the incidence of damage and probability of failure increase. If strains are too low, the metabolic cost of maintaining the unnecessary bone mass is high, and bone is resorbed (e.g., a proposed mechanism for the loss of bone mineral density following prolonged space flight). Thus, functional strain appears to be a relevant parameter to control. A question remains, however: To which attribute or combination of attributes of strain (magnitude, rate of application, frequency, distribution, or gradient) does bone have the greatest sensitivity?

Development and Maturation

Much of the accumulated information about the relation between bone growth and bone mineral acquisition is summarized in figure 4.3. From birth to early adolescence, although a wealth of bone modeling and growth happens in both the axial and appendicular (limb) skeleton, the differences between sexes in **bone mineral content (BMC)** are negligible. At about 13 years of age, the bone min-

TABLE 4.2 Bone Modeling and Remodeling

	Modeling	Remodeling
Timing	Continual changes and adaptation during growth and throughout the life span	Episodic renewal, involving processes of activation–resorption–formation
Osteoclasts and osteoblasts	Located on different surfaces	Located on the same surfaces
Changes to bone shape and size	Yes	Variable
Surfaces affected	All surfaces	20% of surfaces
Sequence and activation	Systemic	Localized activation–resorption–formation

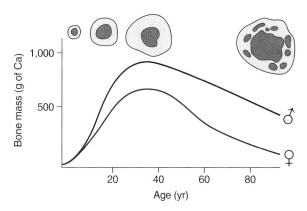

FIGURE 4.3 Relations among bone mass, age, and sex. The ordinate (bone mass) is represented by the total grams of calcium (Ca) in the skeleton.

Adapted by permission from F.S. Kaplan et al., "Form and Function of Bone," in *Orthopaedic Basic Science,* edited by S.R. Simon (Park Ridge, IL: American Academy of Orthopaedic Surgeons, 1994), 167.

eral content for boys and girls diverges, with boys having a greater rate of gain than girls following the pubertal growth period (figure 4.3).

Usually about 1 year after the peak rate of longitudinal growth, or **peak height velocity (PHV)**, the peak rate of gain in BMC occurs. The associations between linear growth and bone accrual during human development (i.e., PHV and BMC) were revealed in the longitudinal data collected from 5 clinical centers over a period of 7 years, as reported by McCormack and colleagues (2017). Their results included over 2,000 healthy children, adolescents, and young adults, comprising males and females in both African American and non-African American populations, with the participants ranging from 5 to 19 years at the start of the data collection. The PHV of boys occurred between 13.0 and 13.4 years of age, versus 11.0 and 11.6 years of age for girls. In comparison, the age of peak acquisition of whole body BMC was 14.0 years for boys and 12.1 to 12.4 years for girls. Thus, in the interval between the time of PHV and the rapid gain in BMC, there is a period of relative bone weakness with a greater chance of fracture. A bone's resistance to fracture is typically a reflection of lean body mass, because the skeleton must support the weight of the tissues laying atop it. Underweight children typically have lower BMC than their peers, increasing fracture risk due to inability to withstand high external forces. Additionally, obese children have a greater fracture incidence, due to an increased proportion of weight not attributed to lean body mass and greater internal

forces acting upon the bones that are unaccounted for (Vaitkeviciute et al. 2014). Growth and sex hormones are mainly responsible for the rapid increases in BMC (Suva et al. 2005).

As longitudinal growth begins to slow during late adolescence, about 90% of adult BMC has already been deposited. Maximal BMC is attained between 20 and 30 years of age. Furthermore, generally neither bone mineral content nor **bone mineral density (BMD)** increases after the age of 30 for men or women. At skeletal maturity, men have greater BMC than women, and most of that difference is because of men's thicker cortical bone.

By the fifth decade, bone mass begins to decline. Both men and women lose cortical bone at about the same rate, but women lose trabecular bone much more rapidly than men—especially following menopause. Between the ages of 40 and 50, men will lose up to 0.75% of total bone mass yearly, whereas women can lose bone at more than twice that rate. In the few years immediately following menopause, the annual rate of bone loss in some women can be as much as 3% (Bostrom et al. 2022).

Reaching maximal bone mass in adolescence and early adulthood, therefore, is crucial for reducing the effects of bone loss and reducing fracture risk later in life. Suggestions for optimizing bone mineral acquisition during the growing years include making a lifelong commitment to weight-bearing physical activity at an early age, engaging in a variety of vigorous daily activities of short duration as opposed to prolonged repetitive activity, doing activities that increase muscle strength and work all large muscle groups, and avoiding immobility (Suva et al. 2005).

Nutrition

Nutrition has potent effects on bone growth and remodeling, and therefore on bone quality and mechanical properties. We will now discuss a few of the nutritional factors that can influence bone quality and quantity: calcium, vitamin D, protein, fats, and sugar.

Normally, the body's bone–mineral balance is regulated by the synergistic actions of vitamin D metabolites, parathyroid hormone, and calcitonin—substances that influence the dietary absorption of calcium, bone mineral resorption and deposition, and the renal secretion and resorption of calcium and phosphorus. Of the total-body calcium, about 99% is found in the skeleton, with the remaining 1% circulating in the extracellular fluid (Bostrom et al. 2022; Ross et al. 2011). Calcium compounds (e.g., hydroxyapatite) constitute more than half of the mass of bone. Because calcium is excreted throughout the day, adequate calcium intake is vital for bone health. Bones with diminished bone mineral content may be more prone to fractures.

Vitamin D, dietary protein, phosphorus, fiber, and fats all can affect calcium absorption. Vitamin D is a fat-soluble molecule that can be stored in body fat. Synthesis of vitamin D involves a chemical reaction involving the integumentary system, cholesterol, and solar ultraviolet B light rays. Thus, stores of vitamin D primarily depend on the amount of time the skin is exposed to the sun and on the size of the exposed area. For this reason, there is higher incidence of population-wide vitamin D deficiency among those living further from the equator (Kopiczko 2014). A relatively small fraction of the body's vitamin D stores also comes from the diet. Vitamin D_3 (calcitriol) helps to increase calcium absorption from the intestinal tract; thus, a person deficient in vitamin D poorly absorbs dietary calcium and increases the risk of fracture in osteoporosis and can lead to osteomalacia (Kopiczko 2014; Staud 2005).

Dietary protein has a significant effect on urinary calcium handling (Ashizawa et al. 1997; Darling et al. 2009). Protein deficiency can lead to decreased levels of calcium in the urine (hypocalciuria) and reduced calcium absorption in the intestine (Hengsberger et al. 2005; Ross et al. 2011). Conversely, excessive dietary protein can result in greater renal calcium loss and the development of negative calcium balance (Giannini et al. 2005). Protein deficiency has been implicated in the genesis of osteopenia (reduced bone mass) in malnourished humans (Darling et al. 2009; Deprez and Fardellone 2003) and animals (Bourrin et al. 2000).

For optimal bone health, excessive ingestion of saturated fats and refined sugar must be avoided, because both can have negative effects on the body's ability to absorb calcium. High levels of dietary fatty acids reduce the amount of dietary calcium absorbed in the intestine and thereby lead to lower calcium levels in bones (Liu et al. 2004). High levels of sugar cause excess acidity, which causes calcium resorption as a protective mechanism to balance the highly regulated pH level of the blood, because calcium derivatives can be reduced as a base.

Female Athlete Triad

Whether dealing with the rapid bone growth during puberty or loss of bone during menopause, sex hormones have a potent effect on bone health. For females, estrogen is important in building and maintaining the skeleton, and it is apparent that highly intensive training by young female athletes can lead to deleterious effects on the skeleton and reproductive system as a result of disturbances in normal menstrual cycles.

In sports such as gymnastics, ballet, running, and figure skating, there are numerous examples of young female athletes who experience no menstruation (**amenorrhea**) or only intermittent and irregular menstruation (**oligomenorrhea**) as a consequence of altered hormone and low body fat levels. With the lower estrogen levels that accompany amenorrhea and oligomenorrhea, these young athletes may not achieve as great of a peak bone mass as they would have experienced with normal levels of estrogen. If this is coupled with calorie-restricted diets to reduce body weight, there is a further danger of slipping into what is termed the **female athlete triad**, a mesh of interrelated symptoms that includes disordered eating, disrupted hormone levels (and accompanying menstrual dysfunction), and increased risk of poor bone quantity and quality. A comparison of the vertebral mineral mass of amenorrheic elite athletes and cohorts with normal menstrual function found that the amenorrheic athletes had up to 25% less mineral mass than the women with normal menstrual function, suggesting that estrogen deprivation has a powerful effect on trabecular mineral mass (Marcus et al. 1985).

Not only are these young female athletes at potentially greater risk of osteoporosis in later years, but they also have a likelihood of developing stress fractures in their late teenage years and early 20s (Zernicke et al. 1994). Among the multiple factors that could contribute to lower-extremity stress fractures in elite intercollegiate runners, one of the most significant predictors of stress fracture was how much time elapsed between beginning serious, high-intensity training and the runner's first menses. Those runners who had been regularly training longer before their first menses (and whose first menses may also have been delayed by heavy training) had a significantly greater chance of suffering a stress fracture while they were running at the intercollegiate level.

Interestingly, high-intensity and high-impact loading activities (even though they may disrupt normal hormonal balance in young females) may partially counterbalance the full effects of the menstrual disturbances (Bailey et al. 1996). For example, Robinson and colleagues (1995) reported that although 47% of the young female gymnasts they studied were either oligomenorrheic or amenorrheic, these gymnasts had greater bone mineral density than either a cohort of runners or control females with normal menses. According to Bailey and colleagues (1996, p. 256), the data suggested that high-impact loading activities in female athletes with disrupted menstrual function can have a "sparing effect [on bone mineral density] at weight-bearing sites but not to the same extent at non-weight-bearing sites."

Use Versus Disuse

Exercise and physical activity can stimulate bone remodeling, but how exercise affects the skeleton is profoundly complex. Exercise intensity, skeletal maturity, type of bone (trabecular or cortical), and anatomical location (axial or extremity bones) can all influence the response of specific bones to exercise (Lieberman et al. 2003).

Use

The following five points summarize current knowledge of the relations between physical activity and bone mass (Lorentzon et al. 2005):

1. Growing bone responds to low or moderate exercise through significant addition of new cortical and trabecular bone, with periosteal expansion and endocortical contraction.

2. Moderate to intense physical training can generate modest increases (1%-3%) in BMC in men and premenopausal women. In young adults, very strenuous training can increase BMC of the tibia by up to 11% and its bone density by 7%. Some evidence shows that exercise can also add bone mass to the postmenopausal skeleton, although the amounts are modest and site specific. After 1 to 2 years of intensive exercise, increases as high as 5% to 8% can be found, but are usually less than 2%.

3. There exists a threshold of activity above which some bones respond negatively by suppressing normal growth and modeling activity.

4. The long-term benefits of exercise are retained only by continuing to exercise.

5. The amount of bone mass that can be achieved appears to depend primarily on the initial bone mass, suggesting that individuals with extremely low initial bone mass may have more to gain from exercise than those with moderately reduced bone mass.

In the adult skeleton, regular prolonged exercise can increase the skeletal mass of involved limbs (Bass et al. 2005; Lee 2019; Lorentzon et al. 2005; Suva et al. 2005), cortical thickness (Hiney et al. 2004; Howe et al. 2011; Specker et al. 2004) and bone mineral content (Engelke et al. 2006; Iwamoto et al. 2004; Korpelainen et al. 2006; Senderovich and Kosmopoulos 2018). If, for example, a person participated in a sport such as tennis for many years, greater bone density would be expected in the radius and the ulna of the dominant arm.

Disuse

Disuse-related changes in bone are commonly associated with bed rest, immobilization, or space flight. Without normal loading, resorption substantially increases and deposition of bone decreases because of the high metabolic cost of maintaining bone structure accompanied by little to no functional strains. In some cases, bone resorption can increase dramatically in a very short period of time (Loitz-Ramage and Zernicke 1996).

In humans, the adverse effects of reduced loading on bone have been highlighted by the substantial skeletal degeneration and calcium loss that can occur in space flight (Iwamoto et al. 2005). The loss of bone density may not be as dramatic in the non-weight-bearing bones (e.g., radius and ulna), but weight-bearing trabecular bones (e.g., calcaneus, tibia, and femur) are highly sensitive to the lack of normal loads experienced during microgravity (Doty 2004; Oganov 2004).

Because disuse changes are dramatic and immobilization may be necessary in some instances, it is important to understand to what extent these changes can be reversed by remobilization. To examine this issue, a study (Tuukkanen et al. 1991) reported the effects of 1 or 3 weeks of immobilization followed by 3 weeks of remobilization in rats. The researchers examined the tibia and the femur; after 3 weeks of immobilization, the bone ash weights decreased as much as 12% compared with nonimmobilized controls. After a period of remobilization, the tibia recovered 62% of its mineral mass, whereas the femur regained only 38% of the lost mineral mass. Their research showed that mineral loss caused by immobilization can be reversed to

The Question of Diminishing Returns

Are there thresholds above which there is a diminishing return in adding new bone in response to greater and greater exercise? One facet of that question was examined by MacDougall and colleagues (1992) at McMaster University.

These researchers investigated the relation between the amount of running and bone mineral mass in adult male runners. Using dual-photon absorptiometry, they examined the bone density of the trunk, spine, pelvis, thighs, and lower legs of 22 sedentary controls and 53 runners who were grouped by their weekly mileage as follows: 5 to 10, 15 to 20, 25 to 30, 40 to 55, and 60 to 75 miles per week. The ages (20–45 years) and dietary habits of the runners were similar. In this cross-sectional study, the researchers found no significant differences in bone density measurements, except in the lower legs. The bone mineral density of the lower legs of runners in the 15- to 20-miles-per-week group was significantly greater than that of the control or 5- to 10- miles-per-week groups. Interestingly, the researchers found no further increase in bone mineral density in the lower legs of runners who covered more than 20 miles per week. Indeed, there was a tendency for decreased bone mineral density for runners who covered 60 to 75 miles per week, perhaps due to maladaptations from fatigue. These high-mileage runners had bone mineral density that was no different from that of the sedentary controls.

Their data suggested that the amount of running may influence bone mineral density and bone thickness in weight-bearing bones, but that there also may be a threshold effect for those adaptations—both at the high and low ends of the loading spectrum. Other investigators have found similar lower bone mineral densities in the vertebrae (Bilanin et al. 1989) and the legs (Ormerod et al. 1988) of very high-mileage male runners compared with normal subjects and weightlifters. In the aggregate, these studies suggest that there is an upper limit for exercise beyond which bone mechanical integrity may stop increasing and actually decrease. In fact, excessive exercise has been known to cause osteoporosis when high trauma rates exceed the rate of remodeling (Hetland et al. 1993; O'Brien 2001).

Is Exercise Enough?

More than three decades ago, Snow-Harter and Marcus (1991) posited that the efficacy of exercise in preventing and treating osteoporosis was unclear, summarizing what was known at that time by answering the following questions (p. 381):

- Can exercise maximize peak bone mass?
- Can exercise forestall or reduce age-related bone losses?
- Does exercise enhance bone mineral density in people with existing osteoporosis?
- Can exercise supersede estrogen replacement therapy during the postmenopausal years?

With some qualifications, we now know the answer is "yes" to the first three questions, but the answer to the fourth question still remains unclear today. Estrogen replacement (i.e., hormone therapy, or HT), which is known to inhibit osteoclast activity, has been approved by the U.S. Food and Drug Administration for prevention of bone loss and osteoporosis in postmenopausal women (NHTPSAP, 2017), and no incontrovertible evidence exists that exercise alone is as effective as HT alone, or as HT plus exercise for maintaining bone mass and reducing the fracture risk for postmenopausal women (Maddalozzo et al. 2007; Mehta et al. 2021). Aggregate data (Mehta et al. 2021) show a significant risk reduction of all fractures in postmenopausal women undergoing combined HT. Thus, the recommendation is to use an individualized approach of combined HT and exercise when treating symptomatic menopausal women, with periodic reevaluation that includes a precision medicine approach to determine the best type, dose, formulation, and route of administration to meet treatment goals (Mehta et al. 2021).

some extent, but that the recovery does not occur as rapidly as the loss of bone. Furthermore, the degree of recovery is related to the length of immobilization (Loitz-Ramage and Zernicke 1996). For these reasons, early remobilization is recommended in the management of orthopedic injuries.

Biomechanics and Adaptation of Other Connective Tissues

Whereas articular cartilage functions primarily under compressive loads, ligaments and tendons function primarily under tensile loads. The extracellular matrix composition of ligaments and tendons is specially formulated for those specific tasks. However, there are special cases where specialized structures must function under both compressive and tensile loads. A classic example of this is the Achilles tendon, which connects the calf muscles to the heel and has both a region capable of bearing tension and another that is subjected to compressive forces.

Articular Cartilage Biomechanics

Understanding the synergy among collagen fibers, proteoglycans, and synovial fluid is essential for understanding the mechanical behavior of articular cartilage. Mow and colleagues (1992, p. 67) conducted pioneering studies of articular cartilage function and mechanics, stating that normally these components "perform their functions so well that we are often not even aware of their existence nor the functions they provide until injury strikes or arthritis develops."

Load Response

Type II collagen is the principal fibrous protein in hyaline cartilage. Figure 4.4 shows how collagen fibers are recruited as a tensile load is applied—whether in articular cartilage, ligament, or tendon. Similar to a bone's response to mechanical loading (figure 4.1), initially (toe region) the fibers are partially relaxed and wavy in appearance. As the tensile load continues to increase (linear region), the fibers straighten and become taut. If the load is increased even further, individual fibers begin to tear, and finally large groups of fibers fail in tension (failure).

We usually think of a tensile load applied to tissue as the tendency to pull the tissue apart. With a straight tendon, a simple tensile load is easy to envision. With articular cartilage, however, recall

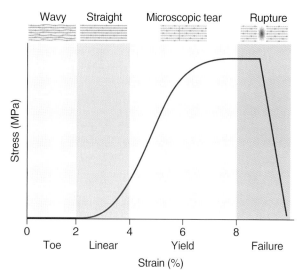

FIGURE 4.4 Recruitment of collagen fibers (in articular cartilage, ligament, or tendon) as a tensile load is applied to the tissue fibers.

that collagen changes its orientation throughout the depth of the cartilage to resist loads from multiple directions. The fibers of the superficial tangential zone are oriented parallel to the surface of the joint, whereas in the middle region the fibers are more randomly arranged. In the deepest layer, the radially directed fibers penetrate into the underlying bone.

Tension is applied to the collagen fibers in the cartilage matrix in many ways. Shear forces can be generated along the surface of the articular cartilage as the two bone ends move past each other. The surface collagen fibers can be deformed in this way (superficial tangential zone). Also, recall that the negatively charged and hydrophilic proteoglycan aggregates (aggrecan) repel each other and draw water into the extracellular matrix. Thus, the cartilage has a natural tendency to swell, and this tendency is resisted by the matrix collagen. A homeostatic equilibrium, therefore, develops because of cartilage's swelling pressure and the tensile restraint of the collagen fibers.

The creep response, or gradual lengthening of a tissue as a constant load is applied, causes extracellular fluid to release from the matrix. After time, the cartilage reaches a stable compression deformation, or equilibrium strain. If the compressive load is released, the lost fluid is drawn into the matrix by the hydrophilic proteoglycans (Mow et al. 1992). Cartilage filled with water is easier to compress, and cartilage densely packed with charged glycosaminoglycan is more resistant to compression.

The cyclic loading and unloading of cartilage allow for a dynamic flow of fluid (with accompanying nutrients and waste products) into and out of the tissue. Thus, cyclic loading of cartilage can be beneficial for normal matrix and cell health. Excessive loading, however, can be destructive to the matrix.

Lubrication Mechanisms

Diarthrodial joint surfaces have remarkably low coefficients of friction attributable in part to the synovial fluid found in the cavities of synovial joints. Synovial fluid lubricates and cushions the tissues of the joint during movement. Articular cartilage also contributes significantly to joint lubrication by means of cartilage's intrinsic properties and fluid flow. The coefficient of friction for articular cartilage in human diarthrodial joints ranges from 0.01 to 0.04. By comparison, the coefficient of friction for ice sliding on ice at 0 °C ranges between 0.02 and 0.09, and the coefficient of friction for glass sliding on glass is 0.90.

How is this elegant system of lubrication achieved? Several hypotheses have been proposed, but the definitive answer is unknown. Two principal types of lubrication mechanisms have been proposed: boundary and fluid film. **Boundary lubrication** happens when a layer of molecules adheres to each of the two surfaces that glide past each other. **Fluid-film lubrication** exists when two nonparallel surfaces move past each other on a thin layer of fluid. The fluid wedge is trapped between the two moving surfaces and maintains a distance between the two surfaces. If the two moving surfaces are nondeformable, this produces a subtype of fluid-film lubrication called **hydrodynamic lubrication**. If one or both of the surfaces are deformable (e.g., isotropic and linear elastic), this second subtype is called **elastohydrodynamic lubrication**. That latter type of lubrication commonly is used to model the lubrication in diarthrodial joints, because articular cartilage is a deformable substance (Lo et al. 2012; Mow et al. 1992).

Additional theories of cartilage fluid-film lubrication have been proposed (Lo et al. 2012). One mechanism has been called **squeeze-film lubrication**. In this model, the two surfaces move at right angles to each other, as might happen in the knee joint at the instant of heel strike in walking. The weight of the body tends to bring the distal femur and proximal tibia closer together as the knee joint compresses, and synovial fluid is forced laterally out of the cartilage to produce a fluid interface between the two surfaces. This type of lubrication would be effective only for a short duration and would be more apparent with heavier loads.

Additionally, **boosted lubrication** is a potential mechanism that blends elastohydrodynamic and squeeze-film types of lubrication. Boosted lubrication may occur, for example, in the knee joint during the stance phase of walking or running. As the femoral and tibial articular surfaces assume load and slide past each other, the articular cartilage of both surfaces is deformed, forcing matrix fluid into the space between the surfaces. This dynamic fluid flow increases the fluid's viscosity, which in turn boosts the effectiveness of the lubricating fluid film.

Articular Cartilage Adaptation

Articular cartilage is highly adapted for its purpose in synovial joints. As with many load-bearing connective tissues, articular cartilage requires a certain amount of use to provide optimal function. If the cartilage is used too little (e.g., immobilization) or too much (e.g., excessive loading), the quality of cartilage breaks down. The active loading and unloading of articular cartilage may facilitate the diffusion of nutrients through the cartilage matrix, which is avascular (e.g., nonhealing) in the adult. As described later, cartilage does adapt, but in many cases the adaptation is degenerative, leading to osteoarthritic changes to the joint.

Development and Maturation

Immature articular cartilage looks quite different from adult cartilaginous tissue; it is blue-white in color and is comparatively thicker. The thickness appears to be a function of the substantially greater number of chondrocytes in young cartilage, which are found on the articular surfaces and in the epiphyseal plates of bones.

Besides the morphological differences in young versus older articular cartilage, a substantial difference is found in the biochemistry of articular cartilage as a function of age. The relative water content in immature articular cartilage is substantially greater than in the adult. Proteoglycan content in articular cartilage is highest at birth and diminishes slowly throughout growth, and collagen concentration therefore increases with maturity. The protein core and the glycosaminoglycan chains are longer in immature articular cartilage, and with advancing age, synthesis of proteoglycan decreases. The average length of the proteoglycan protein cores within articular cartilage and fibrocartilage (e.g., intervertebral disks) decreases with age (Mankin et al. 2022; Singh et al. 2009). With the shorter protein cores and diminished number of glycosaminoglycan chains, as a person ages, the resilience and mechanical properties of articular cartilage can be significantly reduced.

Use Versus Disuse

In both animals and humans, exercise causes articular cartilage to swell (Walker 1996). Prolonged exercise in animals may produce chondrocyte **hypertrophy**, an increase in the pericellular matrix surrounding the chondrocyte as well as in the number of cells per unit of cartilage (Englemark 1961). These effects are already evident after brief bursts of exercise, but long-term exercise produces a lasting change in the cartilage. In some studies, mechanically loaded chondrocytes responded positively by displaying increased proteoglycan and protein biosynthesis in cartilage explants (Jin et al. 2001; Musumeci 2016). However, other studies have shown that increased loading causes wear and tear on articular cartilage (Chen et al. 2003; Musumeci 2016), displaying decreased synthesis and increased degradation, particularly with excessive loading. These changes may lead to osteoarthritis, the most common joint disease in humans and the leading cause of chronic disability in older adults. Osteoarthritis is discussed in further detail in chapter 5.

At the other end of the spectrum, if the loading of articular cartilage is substantially reduced, the cartilage can also significantly atrophy, or degenerate. When cartilage is left unloaded for substantial lengths of time, there can be a reduction in the synthesis and amount of proteoglycans within the cartilage, an increased fibrillation of the surface of the cartilage, and a decrease in the size and amount of the aggregated proteoglycans. Similarly, the mechanical properties of articular cartilage are degraded with prolonged immobilization. Cartilage that has been immobilized deforms much more rapidly when compressed, as fluid rapidly exudes from the matrix. All of the biochemical and biomechanical changes that occur in articular cartilage as a consequence of immobilization are partially, if not completely, reversible after remobilization of the joint (Mankin et al. 1994; Musumeci 2016).

Thus, articular cartilage can be compromised by too little or too much loading. A lack of stress or excessive stress can negatively affect articular cartilage, but the normal physiological zone of cyclic loading can optimize cartilage health.

Tendon and Ligament Biomechanics

The average ultimate tensile stress of tendons and ligaments ranges between 50 and 100 MPa. The *ultimate load* (i.e., maximal tension prior to failure) is related to the cross-sectional area of the tendon or ligament. Ultimate loads in tendons, for example, can be extremely high, particularly in tendons such as the Achilles or patellar tendon. As discussed in chapter 6, the patellar tendon of a competitive weightlifter was able to withstand an estimated 14.5 kN (more than 17.5 times the body weight of that Olympic weightlifter) before rupturing (Zernicke et al. 1977).

Like bone and articular cartilage, both tendon and ligament exhibit viscoelastic behaviors such as cyclic and static force stress-relaxation (figure 3.43), hysteresis (figure 3.41*b*), and creep (figure 3.42). By comparison, bone is more sensitive to changes in strain rate; nonetheless, the mechanical responses of both tendons and ligaments exhibit moderate strain-rate sensitivity. For example, if a tendon is stretched at a high strain rate, its stiffness will be greater than if it is stretched at a lower strain rate. This differential effect of strain rate on bone and ligament can influence which structure is injured based on the rate of load application. If the tensile load is applied very quickly, it is more likely that the ligament will fail, whereas if the load is applied slowly, it is more likely that a piece of bone at the ligament attachment site will fail (avulsion fracture).

A classical stress–strain curve for ligament collagen fibers loaded in tension was shown in figure 4.4. At low stresses (toe region), the crimp (waviness) of the collagen fibers begins to disappear as slack diminishes. As the collagen fibers straighten, linearity develops, and the material's elastic (Young's) modulus E can be measured. As noted earlier, the elastic modulus (E) is the slope of the linear region of the stress–strain curve (σ–ε). Note that the strains in the toe and linear regions are relatively small (0%-4% strain).

Near the end of the linear loading (elastic) region, some of the collagen fibers may exceed their load-bearing capacity and rupture. If the load (stress) was removed at that point, there would be a partial failure of the tendon or ligament, but the remaining intact fibers of the structure might still be able to carry out the load-transmission function. The partial tear may induce an inflammatory response, and subsequent healing eventually will form scar tissue (chapter 5). If the tensile stress is increased even further, however, the remaining fibers of the tendon or ligament will fail.

Like bone, a ligament or tendon has a specific geometry that affects its structural mechanical behavior. Figure 4.5a and b depicts two situations that highlight how ligament (or tendon) size could affect its mechanical function in the body. In figure 4.5a, we show two ligaments of equal fiber length but different cross-sectional areas. As a tensile load is applied to each of the ligaments, ligament 2A—with twice the cross-sectional area—will have double the tensile strength and stiffness of ligament A; however, the elongation at failure (rupture) will be the same in both ligaments.

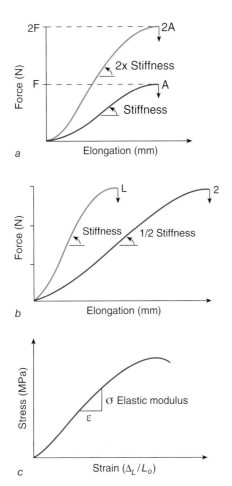

FIGURE 4.5 Effects of a ligament's (a) cross-sectional area (A = original area; 2A = double original area) and (b) original length on its structural properties (L = original length; 2L = double original length). (c) The normalizing effect of stress and strain calculations to estimate the material properties of ligaments of various sizes; Young's modulus (E) is calculated as stress divided by strain (E = σ/ε).

Adapted from Butler et al. (1978).

Figure 4.5b shows two ligaments with same cross-sectional area (same number of collagen fibers in parallel); however, ligament 2L is twice the original (resting) length of ligament L. If a similar load is applied to each ligament, ligament 2L will have one-half the stiffness and twice the elongation at failure as ligament L, but because they have the same cross-sectional area, the structural strength is the same for both ligaments.

Figure 4.5c shows that all four of these ligaments—even with different geometries—can have the same material properties, such as elastic modulus (E). That is because the material properties of stress, strain, and elastic modulus are determined from values that are characteristic to the molecular composition of ligamentous tissue.

Tendon and Ligament Adaptation

Several decades ago, tendons and ligaments were considered to be passive and inert cords for transmitting loads. Since then, research has revealed the marked adaptive abilities of these fibrous connective tissues.

Development and Maturation

The mechanical properties and composition of tendons are greatly influenced by age. Prior to skeletal maturity, tendons and ligaments are slightly more viscous (resistant to structural changes) and are relatively more compliant (moveable with muscle contraction; Frank 1996). With increasing age, the stiffness and elastic modulus increase within the linear range up until the point of skeletal maturity, and then these properties remain relatively constant (Woo et al. 2022). In middle age, the insertional attachments of ligaments or tendons into bone begin to weaken, viscosity begins to decline, and the collagen becomes more highly cross-linked and less compliant (Couppé et al. 2009; Frank 1996; Woo et al. 2022). With age, bones also become more fragile, and the insertion between a ligament or tendon and the bone becomes a much weaker link. As a result, avulsion fractures—in which a piece of bone pulls away from its attachment site—become more common as aging progresses.

Use Versus Disuse

Dense, fibrous connective tissues, such as ligaments and tendon, are sensitive to both training and disuse (Galloway et al. 2013; Taylor et al. 2004; Woo et al. 2004). With exercise, normal tendons and ligaments adapt to the greater loads by becoming larger or by changing their material properties to become stronger per unit area (Galloway et al. 2013; Kasashima et al. 2002; Kjaer 2004).

Normal, everyday activity (without training) is apparently sufficient to maintain about 80% to 90% of ligament's mechanical potential (Frank 1996; Galloway et al. 2013). The primary effects of exercise on ligaments are increased structural strength and stiffness, with the potential to increase both by up to 20% (figure 4.6). In comparison to the baseline control, exercise can moderately enhance the structural and mechanical properties of ligaments over time (up to 40%), whereas immobilization has a dramatic negative effect within 8 to 12 weeks (e.g., see the red curve illustrating the rapid loss of ligament mechanical properties with immobilization in figure 4.6). After stopping immobilization (red curve) and initiating remobilization and rehabilitation (blue curve), there can be a rapid recovery of the ligament properties. The recovery of a formerly immobilized ligament's insertion site to bone, however, has a relatively slower recovery rate.

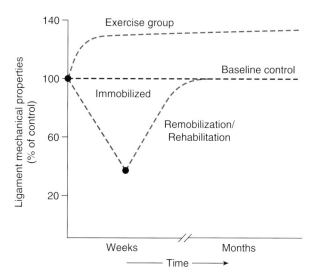

FIGURE 4.6 Ligament responses to exercise, immobilization, and remobilization in comparison to normal (control) ligaments. This figure incorporates experimental data from Woo and colleagues (1987) with theoretical and computationally derived data reported by Wren and colleagues (2000) to illustrate how the mechanical properties (e.g., maximal tensile strength) of a normal (control) ligament are affected by an exercise program compared to a sequence of immobilization and remobilization/rehabilitation interventions. Three experimental data sets are presented: (1) baseline normal control (black), (2) exercise intervention (blue), and (3) immobilization intervention (red) followed by rehabilitation/remobilization (blue).

Adapted from Woo (1987) and Wren (2000).

Exercise generally increases the strength of the bone–ligament junction (Doschak and Zernicke 2005). Tipton and colleagues (1975) concluded that endurance training is the most effective form of exercise to increase the strength of the bone–ligament junction.

Fewer quantitative data are available about the exercise-related adaptations of tendon than are available for ligaments. Data suggest that exercise can increase the number and size of collagen fibrils and increase the cross-sectional area of tendons compared with the tendons of sedentary controls (Galloway et al. 2013; Kasashima et al. 2002). Exercise can also lead to increased collagen synthesis (Galloway et al. 2013; Kjaer 2004) and an increased number of fibroblasts in growing tendons (Benjamin and Hillen 2003; Galloway et al. 2013).

Load deprivation or joint immobilization produces a rapid deterioration in ligament biochemical and mechanical properties, partly due to atrophy, which causes a net loss in ligament strength and stiffness (Frank 1996; Galloway et al. 2013; Mullner et al. 2000). Immobilization or disuse decreases the glycoprotein and water content of ligaments, increases the nonuniform orientation of the collagen fibrils, and increases reducible collagen cross-links (Akeson et al. 1987; Galloway et al. 2013). Collagen turnover rates increase with immobilization, so the ratio of new collagen to old increases in immobilized ligaments (Galloway et al. 2013; Harwood and Amiel 1992). Furthermore, decreases occur in the total collagen mass (Harwood and Amiel 1992) and stiffness (Kjaer 2004; Palmes et al. 2002) of ligaments. The effect of immobilization or disuse is dramatic and rapid. With immobilization, major deterioration happens within a few weeks as ligament cells produce an insufficient quantity of ligamentous material, which in turn contributes to the structural weakening of the ligament complex (Frank 1996). At the same time, there is an osteoclast response at the bone–ligament junction that decreases the strength of the insertional bone.

Similarly, Achilles tendon rupture without repair leads to calf muscle atrophy. These findings suggest that Achilles tendon ruptures should be surgically repaired soon after injury and early mobilization implemented to reduce range of motion loss, increase blood supply, and reduce the degree of muscle atrophy, especially in athletes (Galloway et al. 2013; Sorrenti 2006).

Overuse tendon injuries account for nearly 7% of musculoskeletal disorders within the United States.

These include tendinopathies of the Achilles (calcaneal), extensor carpi radialis brevis, and patellar tendons. Accompanying these tendinopathies are changes in tenocyte and collagen fibril morphology, inflammation, apoptosis (cell death), and neurovascular changes associated with microtearing and inflammatory responses within the tendon in question (Galloway et al. 2013).

Biomechanics of Skeletal Muscle

The fundamental properties of muscle are linked to force, length, and velocity. In chapter 2 we reviewed muscle contractile dynamics (figures 2.15 and 2.16) and length–tension and force–velocity relations (figure 2.20).

The fundamental mechanical events of a muscle contraction relate to twitch properties, unfused tetanic contraction, and tetanus. A single twitch develops in a muscle when the muscle is stimulated once. If another stimulus arrives to depolarize the muscle before it completely relaxes, the stimuli have an additive effect, and the force produced in the muscle is greater than with a single twitch. That is referred to as temporal summation. As the volleys of stimuli (impulses) arrive faster and faster, the tension developed in the muscle will continue to increase until—at maximal stimulation—the muscle is in **tetany** (or **tetanus**) and a steady maximal tension is achieved. If the stimulation rate is slightly less than maximum, then fluctuations in the tension are seen; this is called **unfused tetanic contraction**. When generating excessive loads, these motor units are typically recruited asynchronously, so as to not spur a tetanic contraction each time the muscle is recruited (Dean et al. 2014).

The total force developed in a skeletal muscle is proportional to the number of active cross-bridges in parallel, whereas the rate at which force can be developed in a muscle is proportional to the number of sarcomeres in series. As such, increasing muscle cross-sectional area through resistance training augments the recruitment of contractile proteins, such as actin and myosin, into each individual muscle cell, resulting in proportionally more cross-bridge connections, increasing force production.

To induce muscle cell hypertrophy, a threshold stimulus must be reached to induce adaptation in expression of contractile proteins, which will lead to subsequent muscle enlargement. This phenomenon is based on the training principle of **progressive overload**, which states that muscles worked close to their force-generating capacity will increase in strength (Lorenz et al. 2010; McArdle et al. 2001). Resistance training programs are thus developed on the basis of exercise volume (a product of sets, repetitions, and loads associated with the specific exercise), frequency (number of exercise bouts per week), and intensity (usually measured as a percentage of a one repetition maximum) (Lorenz et al. 2010; Macaluso and De Vito 2004; Wackerhage et al. 2019). The key is that the loads progressively increase to provide an adequate stimulus throughout the entire training regime. A learning effect, which involves improvements in motor skill coordination and level of motivation, causes rapid improvement in performance during weeks 1 and 2. During weeks 3 and 4, muscle strength increases without a corresponding increase in muscle size (Macaluso and De Vito 2004; Schoenfeld et al. 2019). These improvements are mainly attributable to neural adaptations, such as intermuscular coordination (efficient communication and coordination between agonist and antagonist muscle groups), intramuscular coordination (number of motor units recruited and the synchronization of motor units), and an increased neural drive from the central nervous system. Beyond 6 weeks, muscle hypertrophy occurs both within the whole muscle (5%-8% increase in size) and within the muscle fibers themselves (25%-35% increase) (MacDougall 2003; Schoenfeld et al. 2019). For skeletal muscle, this phenomenon occurs without **hyperplasia** (cell division) (McCall et al. 1999).

Upon microtearing of skeletal muscle caused by **resistance training**, a local inflammatory response leads to the activation and fusion of local support cells, called *satellite cells*, which are mitotically quiescent myoblasts located between sarcolemma (or the muscle fiber and its extracellular matrix). On physical stimulation, insulin-like growth factor-1 (IGF-1) found circulating in the extracellular matrix is able to react with satellite cells, causing them to divide. The resulting daughter cells then fuse with the underlying muscle fiber, adding nuclei, cytoplasm, and proteins to the existing fiber. Because the number of nuclei within the muscle fiber increases, contractile protein synthesis can be up-regulated, and hypertrophy of the muscle cell results (Chakravarthy et al. 2000; Ehrhardt and Morgan 2005; Kadi et al. 2005; Yin et al. 2013). As a result of hypertrophy, muscle cross-sectional area increases, and capillary and mitochondrial density decreases as a result of a dilution effect (Baldwin and Haddad 2002; Parry et al. 2020).

Adaptation of Skeletal Muscle

Skeletal muscle is capable of enormous adaptation, as can be readily appreciated by contrasting the muscular development of an Olympic gymnast or weightlifter with the wasted muscles of an individual who has been bedridden for years. The type of training influences the type of muscle adaptation due to local adaptations specific to the muscle fibers being used. Endurance training enhances a muscle's oxidative potential, whereas resistance training increases a muscle's myofibrillar diameter and contractile power. For example, type I and type IIA muscle fiber (with oxidative capabilities) adaptations may include increased myoglobin and mitochondrial enzyme biosynthesis, whereas type IIB muscle fibers (with glycolytic capabilities) may show increased glycolytic enzyme biosynthesis and lactate buffering capability (Parry et al. 2020; Platt 2005).

Development and Maturation

As explained in chapter 2, skeletal muscle cells are derived from the mesoderm (Brand-Saberi 2005; Tajbakhsh 2003; Yin et al. 2013). The typical muscle fiber type in the early fetus is a primitive fast-twitch fiber (Bandy and Dunleavy 1996). As the neurological and muscular systems mature, histochemically and metabolically distinct fiber types begin to emerge (Buckingham et al. 2003). Williams and Goldspink (1981) indicated that, although their development is incomplete, the gross number of muscle fibers in the body is probably set at birth. Thus, continued muscle growth is the result of the increase in fiber size (in both width and length) and maturation. After the first year of life, a genetic, individual-specific distribution of fast-twitch and slow-twitch fibers begins to emerge in the musculoskeletal system, the ratio of which predisposes the individual for better performance toward certain types of physical activity. The developmental addition of sarcomeres and hypertrophy of muscle fibers continue until growth ceases and adult fiber size is reached at approximately 15 years of age.

Although a bone has growth plates that allow it to extend in a longitudinal direction, the length associated with skeletal muscle growth is usually derived from the addition of sarcomeres in series to the muscle fibers, primarily in the region of the myotendinous junction. If a muscle–tendon unit is stretched, additional sarcomeres are typically added at the region of the myotendinous junction (Garrett and Best 2022). In terms of functional adaptation, the myotendinous junction is an active and very dynamic—and injury-prone—region. Surprisingly, little is known about how the myotendinous junction adapts to training. With overload training, there is no change in the relative junctional angle between the myofibril and the collagen at the myotendinous junction, which may mean that its strength capacity is near optimal (Tidball 1983). Thus, adaptation at the myotendinous junction may be related to changes in the quality of the collagen and sarcolemmal membrane rather than to changes in the morphology of the junction. Research also suggests that resistance training also may cause greater invagination and evagination of the sarcoplasm to increase muscle–tendon contact to facilitate a more efficient force transfer (Pimentel Neto et al. 2020).

Compared with the amount of information on muscle adaptation in adults, the data related to muscle adaptation in children are sparse. Bandy and Dunleavy (1996) reported that in prepubescent boys who underwent a program of progressive resistance training, muscle strength increased without any appreciable change in cross-sectional area. The researchers suggested that the increased strength was a result of improved coordination and neural control of muscle groups responsible for the movements as opposed to changes in fiber size. Over a person's life span, maximal strength in men and women is reached between the ages of 20 and 30 years, about the same time that the cross-sectional area of muscle and bone mineral content is greatest. Strength level tends to plateau through the age of 50, followed by a decline in strength that accelerates by 65 years of age and beyond.

The loss of strength accompanying aging may be related to the loss of muscle mass associated with the atrophy and reduction in number of muscle fibers. Typically, the fast-twitch muscle fibers degenerate at a faster rate than slow-twitch muscle fibers as aging progresses. Nevertheless, skeletal muscles of older adults (≥60 years) still respond to progressive resistance training with increases not only in performance and strength, but also in muscle mass and muscle fiber size, particularly in fast-twitch fibers. This increase or maintenance of strength may have significant consequences for maintaining neuromotor coordination and for reducing falls and injury from 13% to 40% (Bandy and Dunleavy 1996; Li et al. 2016).

Sex-Related Effects

Before the onset of puberty, sex differences in athletic performance are not obvious; the muscular strength of girls and boys is essentially equal. However, girls do not experience a significant change in muscle mass during puberty. Flanagan and colleagues (2015) reported changes in strength characteristics between pubescent boys and girls from fourth to fifth grade (i.e., ages 9.6-10.6). They found that, although boys were stronger than the girls in fourth grade, the girls improved more during the course of the study and had similar strength values to boys in fifth grade. Others have reported further strength differences during growth and development, with girls being approximately 90% as strong as boys from 11 to 12 years of age, and decreasing to 85% at ages 13 to 14 (Komi 2003). By the ages of 15 to 16, girls are typically 75% as strong as boys. Note that these data following the pubertal years currently focus on biological sex differences.

These diverging strength values are consistent with the differences in body composition that exist between men and women in the adult range. For example, the average percentage muscle mass (per total body mass) for a conditioned female athlete is about 23%, whereas in the conditioned male athlete it is 40%. The average percentage fat (per total body mass) for conditioned women is in the range of 10% to 15%, whereas in conditioned men it is less than 7%. For the unconditioned woman, the average percentage body fat is 25%, whereas for the unconditioned man it is closer to 15%. Similarly, there are differences in average heart size; in adult women the heart is 10.7 cm in diameter, whereas in adult men it is 12.1 cm in diameter. Average total lung capacity for adult women is 4,200 ml versus 6,000 ml for men; the average vital lung capacity for women is 3,200 ml, whereas in men the value is closer to 4,800 ml (Åstrand et al. 2003).

The relative proportions of muscle fiber types are similar in men and women, but the total cross-sectional area of women's muscles is only about 75% that of men, which accounts for the differences in overall strength (Cureton et al. 1990; Haizlip et al. 2015). Strength differences between men and women are greater in the upper extremities than in the lower extremities (Chen et al. 2012; Hakkinen 2002); women, however, are able to gain relative strength similarly to men (Cureton et al. 1990; Gentil et al. 2016).

Wilmore (1979) indicated that although men have greater upper-body muscle strength, elite female athletes are nearly equivalent to their male counterparts in strength per unit size and muscle fiber type. Ikai and Fukunaga (1968), who examined the strength of muscle elbow flexors in men and women in comparison to muscle size, found that there is little or no difference in the relative strength of men and women. The force-producing capability of a muscle fiber is independent of sex (Bandy and Dunleavy 1996). There is some indication that men and women can increase strength to a similar degree following resistance training, but muscle hypertrophy seems to be less pronounced in women. One of the factors that may contribute to the greater hypertrophy in men is their testosterone level, which has a potent anabolic function in building muscle tissue. Although individual differences in testosterone production exist, serum testosterone levels in men are 20 to 30 times higher than that of women, partly due to testosterone being the primary sex hormone driving male development (Haizlip et al. 2015; Linnamo et al. 2005).

Use Versus Disuse

The specificity principle of exercise training states that skeletal muscle adaptation is specific to the imposed demands of the exercise. Two common training modes are *resistance training* (or *strength training*) and *endurance training* (Garrett and Best 2022). Because resistance training was discussed in the section on skeletal muscle biomechanics, this section focuses on endurance training.

Training to increase muscle endurance involves a different challenge to the muscle than does strength training, and different adaptations will occur. **Endurance training** enhances the muscle's capability to utilize energy rather than its size. An important element is the increase in oxidative metabolism associated with the mitochondria, which increase in size, number, and density in endurance-trained skeletal muscles. With endurance training, the metabolic pathways adapt to a more effective use of fatty acids for fuel instead of glycogen—for example, through greater biosynthesis of enzymes involved in fatty acid cleavage (esterases), citric acid cycle, oxidative phosphorylation, and membrane transport (carnitine shuttle). Different muscle fiber types respond differently to endurance training, although the oxidative capacity of all three fiber types can increase with endurance training.

Dietary intake can also affect the endurance capacity of muscle. Glycogen, which is a polymer of glucose stored in muscle fibers and the liver, is used extensively in exercises of moderate to high intensity. Intense exercise requires anaerobic glycolytic metabolism for rapid energy availability to fuel muscle contraction, whereas prolonged exercise requires greater oxidative metabolism of carbohydrates for sustenance. If high quantities of carbohydrates are eaten prior to competition, muscle and liver glycogen stores can provide maximal energy availability for both intense and prolonged contractions.

The opposite of hypertrophy is atrophy. This decrease in the size of muscle tissue can result from several causes, such as immobilization, bed rest, aging, or a sedentary lifestyle after a period of high-intensity training. The clinical signs of atrophy include decreases in muscle circumference and cross-sectional area, strength, and endurance. The decreases in strength and endurance become the principal concerns during rehabilitation after injury or when resuming training. The changes in fiber size that occur with atrophy are most likely related to a decreased rate of structural and functional protein synthesis and an increased rate of protein degradation (catabolism). With immobilization and disuse, the atrophy that occurs in skeletal muscle is more likely to affect the more tonically recruited slow-twitch (type I) fibers than the fast-twitch (type II) fibers.

Chapter Review

Key Points

- For load-bearing connective tissues such as bone, cartilage, tendon, ligament, and muscle, form and function are inextricably linked.

- All of these tissues are able to adapt to their environment to a greater or lesser extent.

- The integrated mechanical, biochemical, hormonal, and molecular abilities of these tissues to adapt favorably to environmental influences are the primary attribute of healthy tissues.

- The inability of these tissues to adapt to excesses (either high or low) is a leading factor associated with degradation and injury.

Questions to Consider

1. The chapter begins with a quote by D'Arcy Thompson (1860-1948) stating that "the form . . . of matter . . . and the changes of form which are apparent in . . . its growth . . . are due to the action of force(s)." Based on your understanding of the chapter, assess the correctness of Thompson's statement.

2. Compare and contrast the conventional concept of homeostasis (physiological steady state) with what the text alternatively describes as "continually changing equilibrium."

3. Describe the difference between *structural properties* and *material properties* and the functional consequences of that difference.

4. Explain the advantages and disadvantages of a long bone's hollow structure.

5. Compare and contrast the *modeling* and *remodeling* of bone.

6. An inverted-U model often applies to concepts in human performance (e.g., in physiology, biomechanics, or psychology). Such a model predicts that the optimal effect is achieved by some moderate level of stimulus, and that lower or higher stimulus levels result in diminished effects. Select a biological tissue and explain how an inverted-U model helps describe its response to loading.

7. Explain why a multidisciplinary approach is warranted in treating an athlete diagnosed with the female athlete triad.

8. What training recommendations would you give to someone who wants to maintain healthy musculoskeletal tissues?

Suggested Readings

Bone

Bostrom, M.P.G., A. Boskey, J.J. Kaufman, and T.A. Einhorn. 2022. Form and function of bone. In *Orthopaedic Basic Science* (5th ed.), edited by R. Aaron. Park Ridge, IL: American Academy of Orthopaedic Surgeons.

Dull, P. 2006. Hormone replacement therapy. *Primary Care* 33: 953-963.

Howe, T.E., B. Shea, L.J. Dawson, F. Downey, A. Murray, C. Ross, R.T. Harbour, L.M. Caldwell, and G. Creed. 2011. Exercise for preventing and treating osteoporosis in postmenopausal women. *Cochrane Database of Systematic Reviews* 2011(7): 1-167.

Iwamoto, J., T. Takeda, and Y. Sato. 2005. Intervention to prevent bone loss in astronauts during space flight. *The Keio Journal of Medicine* 54(2): 55-59. doi:10.2302/kjm.54.55

Oftadeh, R., M. Perez-Viloria, J.C. Villa-Camacho, A. Vaziri, and A. Nazarian. 2015. Biomechanics and mechanobiology of trabecular bone: A review. *Journal of Biomechanical Engineering* 137(1): 0108021-01080215. doi:10.1115/1.4029176

Articular Cartilage

Mankin, H.J., V.C. Mow, J.A. Buckwalter, J.P. Iannotti, and A. Ratcliffe. 2022. Articular cartilage structure, composition and function. In *Orthopaedic Basic Science* (5th ed.), edited by R. Aaron. Park Ridge, IL: American Academy of Orthopaedic Surgeons.

Tendon and Ligament

Curwin, S.L. 1996. Tendon injuries: Patho-physiology and treatment. In *Athletic Injuries and Rehabilitation*, edited by J.E. Zachazewski, D.J. Magee, and W.S. Quillen. Philadelphia: Saunders.

Maffuli, N., P. Renström, and W.B. Leadbetter. 2005. *Tendon Injuries: Basic Science and Clinical Medicine.* London: Springer.

Woo, S.L.-Y., K.-N. An, C.B. Frank, G.A. Livesay, C.B. Ma, J. Zeminski, J.S. Wayne, and B.S. Myers. 2022. Anatomy, biology, and biomechanics of tendon and ligament. In *Orthopaedic Basic Science* (5th ed.), edited by R. Aaron. Park Ridge, IL: American Academy of Orthopaedic Surgeons.

Skeletal Muscle

Alexander, R.M. 2003. *Principles of Animal Locomotion.* Princeton, NJ: Princeton University Press.

Biewener, A.A. 2003. *Animal Locomotion.* Oxford, UK: Oxford University Press.

Flanagan, S., C. Dunn-Lewis, D. Hatfield, L. Distefanso, M. Fragala, M. Shoap, M. Gotwald, J. Trail, A. Gomez, J. Voler, C. Cortis, B. Comstock, D. Hooper, T. Szivak, D. Looney, W. DuPont, D. McDermott, M. Gaudiose, and W. Kraemer. 2015. Developmental differences between boys and girls result in sex-specific physical fitness changes from fourth to fifth grade. *Journal of Strength and Conditioning Research* 29: 175-180.

Garrett, W.E., Jr., and T.M. Best. 2022. Anatomy, physiology, and mechanics of skeletal muscle. In *Orthopaedic Basic Science* (5th ed.), edited by R. Aaron. Park Ridge, IL: American Academy of Orthopaedic Surgeons.

Herzog, W. 2000. *Skeletal Muscle Mechanics: From Mechanisms to Function.* Toronto: Wiley.

Lieber, R.L. 2002. *Skeletal Muscle Structure, Function, & Plasticity* (2nd ed.). Philadelphia: Lippincott Williams & Wilkins.

Concepts of Injury and Healing

Kindnesses are easily forgotten; but injuries!—what worthy (person) does not keep those in mind?

William Makepeace Thackeray (1811-1863)

OBJECTIVES

- To establish an overview of injury mechanisms, principles of injury, and contributing factors to injury occurrence
- To examine the pathological and healing pathways involved in injury to tissues of the musculoskeletal and nervous systems

When assessing injury, most people first ask, "How did it happen?" Accurately answering this query involves establishing a cause-and-effect relation between the events surrounding the injury and the injury itself. In biomechanical terms, this is the *mechanism of injury*. Mechanism, in this context, is defined as the fundamental physical process responsible for a given action, reaction, or result. Retrospective and accurate identification of injury mechanisms is essential for diagnosis, effective treatment, and prevention of future injuries.

Most people have experience in identifying injury mechanisms. Consider, for example, a basketball player who, in descending from a jump shot, lands on an opponent's foot and crumples to the floor in pain. Her coach rushes over and asks, "What happened?" The player grimaces and responds, "I twisted my ankle." In simple terms, the player specified the mechanism of her injury. Knowledge of the

mechanism provides the coach, athletic trainer, and physician with insights that can help determine the proper course of action.

Now imagine an elderly man found lying on a sidewalk one January night. Responding paramedics, after checking vital functions, determine that the man is in no immediate danger, although he is in considerable pain. The man indicates that he slipped on an icy patch of sidewalk and landed on his tailbone and hands. Again, by describing the mechanism of the fall, the man gives paramedics valuable information to help them determine how to proceed. With further questioning, more details of the fall will emerge.

Trained professionals can translate the simple description of an injury, as illustrated in the preceding examples, into more discipline-specific terms. A physician, for instance, may explain a twisted ankle as rapid loading of the lateral aspect of the ankle and foot, with possible injury to the anterior talofibular and calcaneofibular ligaments. A biomechanist might approach a slip and fall from a mechanistic perspective, focusing on the coefficient of friction at the foot–ground interface and the velocity of the body at the instant of ground contact. In both cases, the practitioner uses knowledge of the mechanism of injury to establish a cause-and-effect relation.

The description of an injury mechanism depends in part on the perspective of the person involved. Physicians, athletic trainers, coaches, supervisors, physical therapists, and the injured party undoubtedly will describe the mechanism of an injury differently, each being correct from their perspective.

Overview of Injury Mechanisms

Although sometimes a single mechanism is responsible for an injury, mechanisms often act in combination. Accurate identification of the mechanisms of injury is important for appropriate diagnosis, treatment, and rehabilitation. Many of these mechanisms have been alluded to in our earlier discussions and are explored in the next section and in subsequent chapters.

Mechanisms should not be confused with the related but different concept of *predisposing* or *contributory factors*. Mechanisms establish a cause-and-effect relation. Contributory factors increase or decrease the likelihood of occurrence and the level of the effect; these factors are discussed in detail later in this chapter.

The mechanisms responsible for injury are many and varied, and there is no single system for categorizing them. Categorization of injury mechanisms is based on mechanical concepts, tissue responses, or a combination of the two. From a sports medicine perspective, for example, one classification system identifies seven mechanisms of injury: contact, dynamic overload, overuse, structural vulnerability, inflexibility, impact, and rapid growth (Leadbetter 2001). Another source lists crushing deformation, impulsive impact, skeletal acceleration, energy absorption, and the extent and rate of tissue deformation as causal mechanisms (Committee on Trauma Research 1985).

From another perspective, one could view every injury mechanism as a variation of overload. In chapter 3, we defined *load* as the application of an external force to a body and identified seven factors that characterize forces, and hence loads: magnitude, location, direction, duration, frequency,

variability, and rate. Body tissues continuously experience loads during normal activity with no obvious injury. Typical and noninjurious loads are said to be within a **physiological range**. The probability of injury increases when loads exceed the physiological range. If the tissue being loaded is already damaged by previous injury or disease, its physiological range will be reduced.

Use refers to normal functional loading, whereas repeated overload is *overuse*. Many injuries (e.g., tendinitis, carpal tunnel syndrome) are called **overuse injuries** because they result from repeated overloads with insufficient time for recovery. Specific examples of overuse injuries are described in chapters 6 through 8.

Overuse injuries exemplify a broad class of conditions that are caused by repeated application of force. Such injuries are **chronic injuries** (also known as **cumulative trauma disorders** or **repetitive stress syndromes**). Injury also can result when a single overload exceeds a tissue's maximal tolerance; these are called **acute injuries**. Chronic and acute injuries are usually distinguishable, but may also be related. For example, chronic loading (overuse) may weaken a tissue, lower its maximal strength, and increase the likelihood of an acute injury. Thus, for example, a person with chronic inflammation of the calcaneal (Achilles) tendon has an increased risk of acute tendon rupture.

Principles of Injury

The mechanical *how* and *why* of injury are the keystones of our approach; therefore this section presents principles of injury important to later discussions of specific injury mechanisms.

Injury Terminology

In the context of musculoskeletal biomechanics, we defined *injury* as damage to body tissues caused by physical trauma. Injury biomechanics has its own vocabulary that draws heavily from medicine and mechanics. Although agreement exists on most definitions, some exceptions may lead to confusion and lack of clarity (e.g., see discussion of valgus and varus in chapter 6).

Confusion also arises when nonspecific, catch-all terms—what O'Donoghue (1984) called "wastebasket" terms (p. 591)—are used to describe an injury or group of injury conditions. For example, *tennis elbow, shin splints, jumper's knee, Little League elbow,* and *whiplash injuries* are nebulous terms that have minimal clinical or biomechanical utility. Although some use these common but vague descriptors, we discourage their use and encourage more specific and appropriate terminology.

Injury Severity

Every injury is unique; although injuries may be similar to one another, they are never exactly the same. This presents challenges in assessing injuries and classifying their severity. Although all categorization systems create discrete groupings and assign similar characteristics to all injuries in that group, injuries actually occur on a continuum (figure 5.1). Thus, although two different head injuries categorized as mild concussions may share similar characteristics, they are not identical injuries. Diagnosis and treatment must remain specific to each injury based on its own characteristics.

Nonetheless, clinical classification schemes are useful in assigning general or common characteristics to similar injuries. Many such schemes exist, based on the tissues (e.g., bone vs. ligament) and body regions (e.g., head vs. leg) involved. A typical three-level classification system for ligament injury, for example, specifies the structural involvement, physical signs, and level of dysfunction (mild, moderate, and severe) (Leadbetter 1994).

Classification of Ligament Injury Severity

- *Grade 1.* Mild, with minimal microscopic fiber tears. At evaluation no visible injury, local tenderness, and the joint remains stable. Functional loss is minimal and lasting a few days.
- *Grade 2.* Moderate, with partial tissue damage (e.g., fiber tears). At evaluation visible swelling, marked tenderness, and potential instability are present. Functional loss is up to 6 weeks (may require protective bracing).

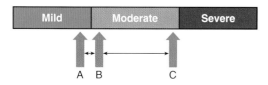

FIGURE 5.1 Severity of injury continuum. Injuries A and B are close to each other on the continuum of injury, but are classified differently (i.e., A is considered *mild*, B is considered *moderate*). In contrast, injuries B and C are far apart on the injury continuum, but both are classified as *moderate* based on discrete classification.

- *Grade 3.* Severe, with complete tear or rupture. At evaluation significant swelling, marked tenderness, and joint instability are present. Functional loss is indefinite, with a minimum of 6-8 weeks.

Injury severity is linked to the amount of damage experienced by the tissue. In mild and moderate injuries, the tissue structure typically is minimally or partially disrupted. The damaged tissue is still able to accept loads, although of smaller magnitudes than before the injury. In cases of complete failure, the tissue's continuity is totally disrupted, and load transmission is not possible. In some cases appearances can be deceptive; a tissue may appear to be intact and capable of load acceptance, but in reality the fibers are disrupted and possess little or no ability to transmit loads.

In addition to general severity classifications, systems have been proposed for specific structures, such as the anterior talofibular ligament (Cai et al. 2017), medial collateral ligament (Makhmalbaf and Shahpari 2018), and acromioclavicular joint separations (Gorbaty et al. 2017).

Related to understanding of classification systems are two concepts, *level of dysfunction* and *progression of injury*:

- *Level of dysfunction.* Some injuries are simply annoying and relatively trivial. These injuries do not limit function appreciably, and they heal quickly. Increasing injury severity, however, produces greater dysfunction. At the extreme are catastrophic injuries that result in permanent disability or death.

- *Progression of injury.* Relatively minor injuries that are ignored may, with repeated loading or insult, progress to more severe injuries. Delayed, improper, or inadequate treatment also may contribute to progression to a more serious injury. Athletes or workers may try to do too much too soon after injury. A minor injury, given inadequate time to heal, may progress to a more debilitating level.

Injury Type

Several important distinctions help define injury type:

- *Primary versus secondary injury.* **Primary injury** refers to an injury that is a direct, immediate consequence of trauma. A skull fracture from blunt trauma and a torn medial collateral knee ligament from a violent lateral impact are examples of primary injuries. A **secondary injury** can surface some time after the initial trauma (i.e., temporally delayed). In cases of traumatic head impact, for example, primary brain injury can occur as a direct and immediate result of the impact, whereas delayed (or secondary) brain injuries, such as diffuse axonal injury and local or regional ischemia (localized decrease in blood flow to a tissue), may not appear until hours or days after the initial trauma.

Alternatively, a secondary injury can develop as an accommodation to, or as compensation for, a primary injury. When an injured person alters their movement patterns in response to the pain or dysfunction of a primary injury, the altered movements redistribute loads through other joints in the body. These changes in loading can generate injury remote from the primary injury in what is termed a compensatory injury. An individual with a twisted ankle, for example, may alter their gait and place unaccustomed loads on both ipsilateral and contralateral joints and tissues. These sites, not accustomed to these redistributed forces, may develop secondary injuries while compensating for the original injury.

- *Chronic versus acute injury.* Injuries can result from a single insult (acute injury) or from long-term, repeated loading (chronic injury). Continuing chronic insults to tissues may lead progressively to degenerative conditions that set the stage for an acute injury.

- *Microtrauma versus macrotrauma.* Chronic injury can begin as microscopic damage to a tissue's structure. For example, the damage could be microscopic tendon fiber tears or bone microcracks (microtrauma). Repeated loading can exacerbate the injury, and eventually the injury becomes macroscopic. If left untreated, tendon microtears presage eventual tendon rupture (macrotrauma). Similarly, X-ray findings of a patient complaining of a dull ache in the foot may be negative because of the microscopic nature of the bone cracks, but

continued loading may eventually progress into a stress fracture.

Tissue Structure

The mechanical response of biological tissue depends largely on the tissue's noncellular structural makeup, including its constituent material, orientation, density, and connecting substances. Bone, for example, with its mineral latticework and collagen fibers, is designed to transmit compressive, shearing, and tensile loads of high magnitude. Any change in the relation between structure and load, as might occur in an osteoporotic bone or in a bone experiencing abnormal and unaccustomed loading, increases the likelihood of bone injury.

Similarly, the collagen fibers of tendon and ligament afford them exceptional load-bearing capacity parallel to the fiber orientation. Because of the anisotropic nature of these tissues, off-angle forces may expose them to a greater risk of injury. The complex, synergistic relationship between tissue structure and loading behavior has important consequences for proper function and potential injury.

When different tissues form a functional unit, the weakest-link phenomenon typically occurs during an injury. This means that when a structure is mechanically loaded, initial failure will happen at the weakest link in the structural chain. In the human body, the factors that contribute to determining the weakest link are many, interrelated, and often not easily identified or well understood.

Contributory Factors

Simply stated, injury happens when an imposed load exceeds the tolerance (i.e., load-carrying ability) of a tissue or structure. However, establishing the determinants of injury are anything but simple. Among the determinants are myriad contributory factors that increase or decrease injury risk and severity. The following are examples of contributory factors.

Compensatory Injury

One notable example of indirect secondary injury happened to Dizzy Dean, a Hall of Fame baseball pitcher. In the 1937 All-Star Game, the right-handed Dean's left big toe was broken after being struck by a line-drive hit. Rather than wait until the toe healed completely, Dean returned to action too soon, altering his pitching mechanics to accommodate the pain caused by the toe injury. In doing so, Dean suffered a career-ending injury to his pitching shoulder. Dean was the unfortunate victim of a secondary compensatory injury, now sometimes called Dizzy Dean Syndrome.

• *Age*. During our formative years, our tissues are growing and developing. Later, tissues may begin to degenerate and lose strength, compliance, density, and energy-carrying capacity. Acute injuries are more common in younger people, but as we age, chronic injuries happen more often, as do unintentional injuries (e.g., from slips and falls). When discussing age as a contributory factor, it is important to distinguish between **chronological age** and **physiological age**. The former is based on calendar years, whereas the latter is based on the physiological quality of the tissues. A 60-year-old person, for example, may have tissues with better physiological and mechanical properties than those of a 45-year-old. Although generalities are routinely used to describe aging responses, each person's response is unique and may be quite different from another person's response.

• *Sex*. Sex-specific differences in structure, hormones, sociology, activity patterns, and many other measures dictate that one sex may be at greater or lesser risk of injury than the other in certain circumstances. The number of fatalities from unintentional injury is higher for men in all categories except for strangulation, ignited clothing, falls from the same level, and certain types of poisoning. The male-to-female fatality ratio for injuries from machinery is 20:1, motorcycling 10:1, firearms 7:1, and suffocation 2:1 (Anderson et al. 2004). Similar ratios exist for nonfatal injuries as well. Women, however, are not at less risk in all areas. For example, as discussed in a later section, women are more likely than men to suffer the consequences of osteoporosis. Osteoporotic bone has decreased density and diminished strength and is more susceptible to fracture.

• *Genetics*. Genetic factors influence tissue matrix composition and are implicated in the predisposition toward certain injuries, including intervertebral disc and rotator cuff degeneration, carpal tunnel syndrome, and tendon ruptures.

• *Physiological status and physical condition*. A person's physical condition is a primary factor in their chances of sustaining an injury. The fitter the person is, the less likely they are to be injured. If injury does occur, a better-conditioned person likely will have a less severe injury and will recover more quickly.

• *Nutrition*. Diet provides the raw materials to build, sustain, and repair the body's tissues and therefore plays an indirect yet essential role in injury biomechanics. Tissue homeostasis depends on remediating nutritional deficiencies, excesses, or imbalances.

• *Psychological status*. Psychological parameters can influence the incidence of injury. These factors include stress levels, inattention, distraction, fatigue, depression, excitation, human error, risk evaluation, personality factors, and coping resources.

• *Fatigue*. Physical and mental fatigue increases the likelihood of injury because it compromises muscle strength, coordination, mental attentiveness, and concentration. Fatigue-related injuries tend to happen later in an activity period; for example, truck drivers were found to have three times the risk of crash involvement after 6 hours of driving compared with the first 2 hours and to be asleep at the wheel or inattentive in 45% of commercial vehicle crashes (Bunn et al. 2005). Athletes also tend to show greater risk of injury during the latter stages of a practice session or game. For example, skiing-related injuries are more likely to happen later in the day after multiple runs down the mountain.

• *Environment*. Numerous environmental factors contribute to injury, including location (indoors vs. outdoors, urban vs. rural), weather conditions (temperature, humidity, visibility), time of day or night, terrain (flat vs. inclined, smooth vs. rough, slippery vs. sticky), altitude, and activity (work vs. recreation).

• *Equipment*. Equipment often plays a central role in injury, either in prevention, causation, or both. Equipment can include clothing, pads or protective devices, and implements such as tools, machinery, or computers. Apparel can be protective, especially in environments likely to produce injury. Implements such as bulletproof vests, helmets, and shields aid in injury prevention as well. Equipment also can be associated with acute injuries (e.g., finger severed in machinery) or chronic injuries (e.g., carpal tunnel syndrome caused by long-term, repetitive typing).

The same piece of equipment can both protect a person from and contribute to injury. A hockey player's helmet and pads, for example, protect the head and body from direct impact. However, the helmet and pads may also contribute to heat stress (by decreasing thermoregulatory capacity and increasing heat production and retention) and to cervical injury if the helmet fits improperly; helmets also can inflict injury on another player if that player is hit with the top of the helmet.

- *Human interaction.* Interactions among people can be social, occupational, or competitive, as seen in sports. Whenever people interact, the potential for injury exists. The possibility of injury may be remote at a dinner party, for example, but becomes a prime factor in a rugby match.

- *Previous injury.* Following any serious injury, elements of the injury can persist, whether physically or psychologically. Repaired tissues are often not equal to their preinjury condition and for many reasons may be more susceptible to a subsequent injury. A person's psychological status following injury may be affected as well, as shown by a reluctance to perform certain movements even when an injury is fully healed.

- *Disease.* Many diseases increase the risk of injury. For example, an **osteosarcoma** (malignant bone tumor) weakens bone, atherosclerosis damages arterial walls, and diabetes predisposes one to peripheral neuropathies and skin ulcers, particularly on the plantar surface of the foot.

- *Drugs.* Whether used for recreational or medical purposes or as ergogenic aids, drugs can affect the body's tissues and alter performance so that risk of injury is changed. In addition, these chemical agents may also indirectly contribute to an injury because of their systemic effects.

  - Recreational drugs, either legal (e.g., alcohol) or illegal (e.g., cocaine), may increase the risk of musculoskeletal injury (Chikritzhs and Livingston 2021; Miller et al. 2001; Taylor et al. 2010). Use of drugs (e.g., heroin, morphine, barbiturates, or alcohol) is associated with all types of violence and accidents as diverse as automobile collisions, gunshot wounds, and shaken baby syndrome.

  - Medical drugs can be obtained over-the-counter or by prescription and include everything from **nonsteroidal anti-inflammatory drugs (NSAIDs)**—for example, aspirin and ibuprofen—to prescription painkillers (opioids), asthma medications, and many others. The use of medications may increase injury risk, such as when drugs increase reaction times, impair vision, or alter a driver's judgment.

  - The use of drugs as performance-enhancing (ergogenic) aids has become more insidious and widespread, most noticeably in competitive sports. **Ergogenic** refers to the work-generating or power-generating potential of these aids, which can include a host of substances or treatments that purportedly improve a person's physiological performance or remove the psychological barriers associated with more intense activity (Ellender and Linder 2005). Many pharmacological aids have been banned by official sports federations because of the unfair advantage they give athletes during training and competition and because of the negative side effects that can occur, including a greater risk of injury. For example, anabolic steroids (e.g., oral or injectable forms of synthetic testosterone that facilitate increased body size and muscular strength) have permeated many sports at every level, from high school to the Olympic and professional levels. Besides risking overuse or acute muscle–tendon injuries associated with the heightened training that may accompany anabolic steroid use, individuals who take anabolic steroids may experience other side effects, including acne vulgaris, increased sex drive and aggression, mood disturbances, cardiomyopathy, atrial fibrillation, and hepatic dysfunction (Hartgens and Kuipers 2004). Anabolic steroid use has also been associated with increased risk of tendon ruptures, based largely on animal studies. Evidence in humans is mostly anecdotal and equivocal (Jones et al. 2018).

- *Inadequate rehabilitation.* After sustaining an injury, delaying even limited activity for too long or returning to extremely high levels of activity too soon can result in further damage. Although inflammation—a primary response to joint and tissue injury—is a necessary step in the healing process (as described more fully later in this chapter), it can lead to joint pain, which carries the potential for tissue atrophy as a consequence of inactivity and lack of motion. On the other hand, if an inflamed tissue continues to be overused, there is a risk of developing a more serious injury.

Once inflammation is controlled, the body must rebuild tissue that has been disrupted. The optimum rate at which activity is resumed can be gauged by paying attention to signs of regression or robustness. If tasks that were once challenging become significantly easier, it is time to challenge the tissue more; if symptoms of pain or weakness increase, it may be time to consider scaling back temporarily. Without such management, the tissue can be reinjured—and sometimes the secondary damage is even more serious than the original problem.

• *Anthropometric variability.* People come in many shapes and sizes, and these differences in body dimensions often play a critical role in injury. Anthropometry is the study of comparative measurements of the human body. Anthropometric measures such as height, weight, body composition, muscle mass, and shape (**somatotype**) can play a central role in assessing injury. Obese individuals, for example, are more likely to have knee problems, and this risk increases with age. Anthropometric measures also influence body posture and flexibility (joint range of motion), both of which—either alone or in concert—can affect the risk of injury.

• *Skill level.* The adeptness with which a person performs a task influences the risk of injury. Especially in high-risk activities (e.g., auto racing), the skill level of the performer may be the most important determinant of injury risk. Novice or less skilled performers are more likely to be injured. The opposite may prove true, however, when particularly skilled individuals believe that they are competent to attempt tasks with an unacceptably high risk of injury.

• *Experience.* Closely related to skill level is experience. Although related, skill and experience are not synonymous. An individual may be experienced, having performed a task many times, but remain relatively unskilled. Another person may be naturally gifted with a skill but have little experience at the task. Usually, however, the two factors are closely linked. Experienced performers typically exhibit efficiency of movement, along with sound judgment and decision-making abilities. These all combine to lower injury risk.

• *Pain.* The sensation of pain is fundamental to any discussion of injury. Pain, the body's signal of distress, accompanies most consequential injuries and often is the limiting factor in continued participation in an activity. Pain derives from various biomechanical and inflammatory sources. Pain is one factor used in determining an injury's severity and in prescribing and monitoring the rehabilitation during postinjury therapy. Pain also influences movement patterns (sometimes in serious ways, such as in Dizzy Dean Syndrome). Pain may hinder further activity or preclude participation altogether.

Rehabilitation

Successfully returning an individual to preinjury status depends on the nature of the injury, the person's motivation, the expertise of the rehabilitation therapist, and the sophistication of the available rehabilitation methods.

One of the first priorities in treating musculoskeletal injuries is controlling excessive inflammation. Many effective modalities are used to counteract the inflammatory process, including cryotherapy (e.g., ice, cold compresses, and cooling sprays) and thermotherapy (e.g., moist hot packs, whirlpool baths, heating pads, and ultrasound). An injury may require other types of treatment such as reconstructive surgery or physical therapy.

Sometimes even the best rehabilitation methods are unable to return a person to their preinjury capacity. Severe injury may be permanently disabling or career threatening. On the other hand, rehabilitation has the potential to return a person not only to preinjury condition, but potentially to an even higher level of function.

Inflammation and Entrapment Conditions

Although the physical damage resulting from each injury is unique, the human body has a generalized response to injury that occurs in all cases, regardless of the specific body region or tissues affected. This immediate reaction to injury is termed the *inflammatory response.* Although the inflammatory response is essential to the healing process, it can lead to damage if uncontrolled. Because the inflammatory response often is a contributor to compartment or entrapment syndromes, these pathological conditions are discussed in this section.

Inflammatory Response

The inflammatory response, or **inflammation**, is a generalized process affecting blood vessels and adjacent tissue. Inflammation happens in response to a variety of stimuli, especially injury. The cardinal signs of inflammation were identified long ago by Aulus Cornelius Celsus (30 BC to AD 38). Celsus described the inflammatory response as having *rubor et tumor cum calore et dolore,* or redness and swelling with heat and pain. A fifth sign, *functio laesa,* or functional loss, was added by Galen (AD 129-199) and is often, but not always, present with inflammation as well.

Inflammation can develop in response to an acute injury or may develop from chronic irritation (indicated by the suffix *-itis*), as seen in arthritis, bursitis, or tendinitis. The redness and heat of inflammation are caused by blood vessel dilation and increased flow. Increases in intracapillary hydrostatic pressure and enhanced capillary permeability cause inflammatory swelling. Pain develops from the

Ergonomics and Injury

The economic and personal costs of work-related injuries are staggering. For example, the United States saw a total of 4.64 million work-related injuries requiring medical attention in 2019, resulting in 70,000,000 lost work days and a monetary cost of $171 billion (National Safety Council 2019).

Efforts to reduce these costs fall under the province of **ergonomics** (also called *human factors* or *human engineering*), which

> is the scientific discipline that seeks to understand and improve human interactions with products, equipment, environments and systems. Drawing upon human biology, psychology, engineering and design, Ergonomics aims to develop and apply knowledge and techniques to optimise system performance, whilst protecting the health, safety and well-being of individuals involved. The attention of ergonomics extends across work, leisure and other aspects of our daily lives. (Chartered Institute for Ergonomics and Human Factors, 2022)

Ergonomics seeks to improve the things that people use and the environments in which they work and live. In many ways the problems associated with workplace injuries are more complex than the problems associated with sports-related injuries, and despite the considerable progress that has been made in many areas of injury prevention, challenges remain for the professionals responsible for promoting society's health and well-being.

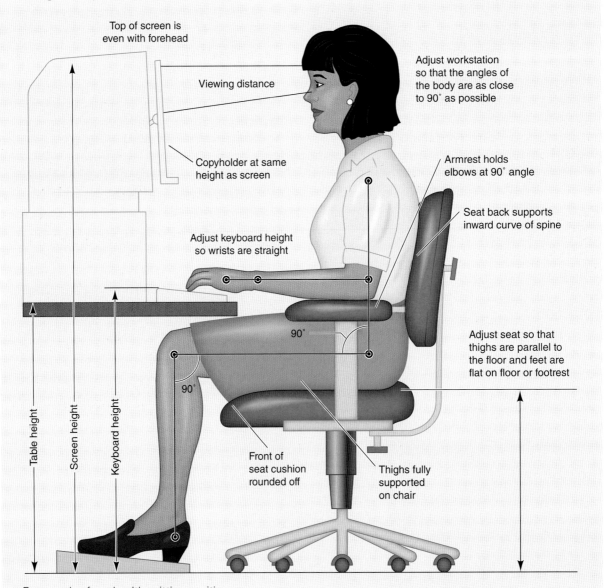

Ergonomics for a healthy sitting position.

swelling-related increase in pressure on nerve endings and is most pronounced when a confined space (e.g., synovial joint) is inflamed. Swelling can limit function and may persist as the damaged tissues heal (e.g., torn ligament or fractured bone). The series of events involved in inflammation is referred to as the *inflammatory cascade* (figure 5.2).

An injury produces a vasoconstrictive response known as the *coagulation phase*. This is followed within minutes by an increase in vascular permeability, which permits the flow of materials from the vessels into the surrounding tissues; this is the *vasodilatory phase*. These moving substances are termed **exudate** and consist of fluid and plasma proteins. Although the edema (swelling) caused by the exudate may contribute to pain, the exudate

has a number of positive functions: It dilutes and inactivates toxins; provides nutrients for inflammatory cells; and contains antibodies, complement proteins, and fibrinogen (a precursor to fibrin, a protein instrumental in the coagulation process).

The inflammatory process is controlled by substances known as *chemical mediators*. This includes the immediately available histamine, as well as other mediators—such as serotonin, bradykinin, prostaglandins, leukotrienes, and plasmin—produced at the site of inflammation or by leukocytes (white blood cells) drawn to the injury site through **chemotaxis** (cellular attraction caused by chemical action).

The chemical mediators of the inflammatory response are joined by cells that perform specific functions. Among these are a class of cells known

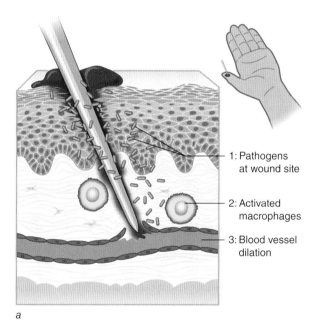

1: Pathogens at wound site

2: Activated macrophages

3: Blood vessel dilation

a

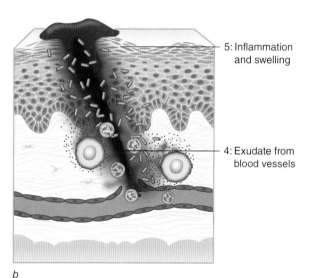

5: Inflammation and swelling

4: Exudate from blood vessels

b

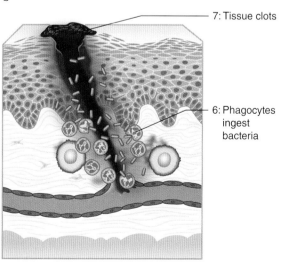

7: Tissue clots

6: Phagocytes ingest bacteria

c

FIGURE 5.2   Inflammatory cascade.

as **phagocytes** (which degrade bacteria and necrotic tissue), the most predominant of which are polymorphonuclear neutrophils, responsible for **phagocytosis** (the engulfing and destruction of particulate matter by phagocytes) and defense against fungal and bacterial infections. Several immune system cells—for example, accessory cells and lymphocytes (B cells, T cells, and NK cells)—also assist in defending against foreign substances (collectively known as *antigens*).

Inflammation is the body's first line of defense against insults such as those imposed by injury. The details of the process are complex and in some cases unknown. A detailed discussion of inflammation is beyond the scope of this text. A comprehensive presentation of inflammation is presented in a four-volume set by Cavaillon and Singer (2018).

But for all the complexity of the inflammatory process, "it seems . . . that the more we learn about inflammation, the simpler its message becomes: Our cells and humors defend the self against invisible armies of the other. We call our losses 'infection' and our victories 'immunity'" (Weissmann 1992, p. 5).

Entrapment Conditions

The fundamental mechanical relation between mass and volume plays a central role in various entrapment conditions, also called *compartment* or *impingement syndromes*. The common element of all such conditions is the ratio of mass and volume, or density, and its mechanical consequences on biological tissues. Increasing the density of material within a confined space—either by increasing the mass or decreasing the volume (or both)—increases the pressure exerted on the boundaries of the space and on the material within the space. This increase in pressure is transmitted to all structures within the enclosed space.

The pressure–density relation and its physiological effects can be seen in many instances of musculoskeletal injury, some of which are detailed in the following chapters. Included in the wide array of these conditions are carpal tunnel syndrome, glenohumeral impingement syndrome, skeletal muscle compartment syndromes, synovial joint swelling, and cerebral edema. All are either caused or aggravated by the mechanical relations among mass, volume, and pressure.

The affected spaces may be compartments of the body completely enclosed in inextensible fascia, joint capsules, or narrow apertures defined by bony tunnels through which vascular and neural tissues pass, such as the carpal tunnel or the thoracic outlet. The causes of entrapment conditions include fractures, casts, prolonged limb compression, car-crash related injuries, burns, hemorrhage, and intravenous drug use.

In biological systems, the structures affected typically are muscles, nerves, and circulatory vessels. Pressure on nerves is felt as tingling, numbness, or pain. Pressure on circulatory vessels results in decreased arterial or capillary perfusion or restricted venous return. In the case of compartment syndrome, because the fascia that encloses the compartment does not stretch, even a small amount of bleeding inside the compartment can increase the pressure dramatically. Tissues that rely on proper neural and circulatory supply will be deleteriously affected if the syndrome is not treated promptly—even to the extent of nerve damage and muscle death. As noted previously, such situations are often either caused or worsened by inflammation—in particular, the swelling that accompanies the inflammatory response. In many cases, the affected system becomes involved in a positive feedback loop, with increases in pressure causing restricted outflow, which in turn further increases pressure.

Our comments on injury thus far have applied generally to most biological tissues and structures. In addition, each tissue possesses unique characteristics determined by its own structure and function. The following sections examine some of the characteristics of the major tissues involved in musculoskeletal and neural injury.

Bone Injuries

The essential role of bone in providing structural support and protection, facilitating movement, and serving as a site for hematopoiesis (blood cell production) and mineral storage cannot be understated. Injury to bone can compromise any of these functions and interfere with daily routines.

Pathology

The viability of bone as a tissue depends on the proper function of the bone's cellular component and the ability of these cells to produce extracellular matrix and perform other important physiological processes. Any disease or injury that compromises osteocyte performance jeopardizes the structural integrity of both the affected bone specifically and the skeletal system in general. Three conditions that affect bone tissue are described briefly in the following sections. Specific injuries involving these conditions are examined in detail in later chapters.

Osteonecrosis

Osteonecrosis refers to the death of bone cells resulting from cessation of blood flow necessary for normal cellular function. This term is preferred to the commonly used terms **avascular necrosis** (i.e., cell death caused by an absent or deficient blood supply) and **aseptic necrosis** (i.e., cell death in the absence of infection), because it best describes the histopathological processes involved and does not implicate any specific cause (Day et al. 1994).

The mechanisms of compromised circulation that may lead to osteonecrosis are mechanical disruption of vessels, occlusion of the arterial vessels, injury to or pressure on arterial walls, and occlusion of venous outflow. These conditions may result from bone fracture, joint dislocation, infection, arterial thrombosis, or a number of conditions that affect circulatory integrity. Although the bone's noncellular structures (e.g., organic and inorganic matrix) may not be immediately affected, over time they may suffer deleterious effects from the absence of cellular production. A decrease in extracellular matrix production, for example, may result in decreased bone strength and increased likelihood of fracture.

Osteopenia and Osteoporosis

Osteopenia (a loss of bone tissue) is a bone condition classified by having a bone mineral density (BMD) rating that is 1.0 to 2.5 standard deviations below the mean recorded for young, healthy adults. As such, osteopenia is not an injury in itself. However, if left untreated it can lead to the development of osteoporosis and subsequently predispose an individual to fracture (figure 5.3).

Osteoporosis is a Latin-derived term that literally means "bone that is porous." The World Health Organization (WHO, 2006) has defined osteoporosis as a "progressive systemic skeletal disease characterized by low bone mass and micro-architectural deterioration of bone tissue, with a consequent increase in bone fragility and susceptibility to fracture." Clinically, osteoporosis is operationally defined by a BMD rating more than 2.5 standard deviations below normative bone density values (figure 5.3). Osteoporosis was identified as a prominent public health issue more than 70 years ago and has been the subject of extensive research and scientific debate ever since. Histological, radiological, and clinical evidence has clearly demonstrated that progressive

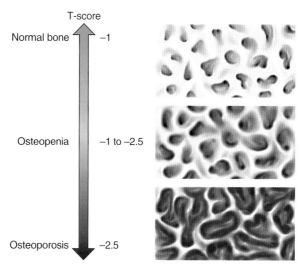

FIGURE 5.3 Normal, osteopenic, and osteoporotic bone.(With respect to bone density, standard deviation [SD] often is referred to as a T-score.)

bone loss begins in the fourth decade of life, and the rate of loss increases with advancing age (figure 5.4).

Osteoporosis predominantly affects trabecular bone and the endosteal surface of cortical bone and is marked by reduced bone mineral mass and changes in bone geometry, leading to an increased probability of fractures, primarily of the hip, spine, and wrist. Progressive loss of bone mass can be a function of the normal aging process or can be caused by other disease processes. Furthermore, the amount of bone mass at one site in the body is not necessarily correlated with bone mass at other sites.

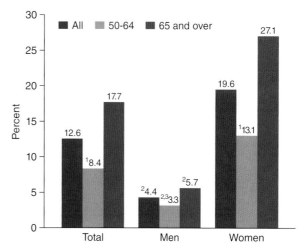

FIGURE 5.4 Osteoporosis prevalence as a function of age and sex.

Reprinted from N. Sarafrazi, E.A. Wambogo, and J.A. Shepherd, "Osteoporosis or Low Bone Mass in Older Adults: United States, 2017–2018," *NCHS Data Brief*, no. 405 (2021).

Both men and women experience some loss of bone mass as part of normal aging, but osteoporosis progresses much more rapidly in postmenopausal women. After the age of 30, men typically lose bone mass at approximately the same rate for the remainder of their lives. In women, however, the loss of bone increases significantly for about 5 years after menopause and then slows to a more gradual loss. Just after menopause, the rate of bone mass loss in women is up to 10 times faster than in men of the same age (Reginster et al. 2006).

Identifying the precise causes and pathogenic mechanisms involved in both the onset and the progression of osteoporosis is a multifactorial problem that continues to challenge researchers. Postmenopausal estrogen deficiency is but one of the factors involved in osteoporosis risk, making this condition a useful example of the complexity of analyzing injury-contributing factors. Other major contributory factors include inadequate nutritional absorption (e.g., low vitamin D and calcium levels), lack of physical activity, weight loss, cigarette smoking, excessive alcohol consumption, air pollution, stress, history of falls, older age, sex, white ethnic background, family history (genetics), chronic use of certain medications, and comorbidity of certain conditions (Pouresmaeili et al. 2018). The conditions associated with osteoporosis include the following:

- Alcoholism
- Cancer
- Celiac disease
- Corticosteroid treatment
- Diabetes
- Disordered eating
- Immobilization
- Gastric reflux
- Kidney or liver disease
- Lupus
- Malabsorption syndromes
- Menstrual dysfunction
- Multiple myeloma
- Osteogenesis imperfecta
- Rheumatoid arthritis
- Smoking

The World Health Organization has stated that the number of hip fractures primarily associated with osteoporosis will increase by more than 300%

in the next 30 to 40 years. In China, estimated osteoporosis-related fractures will double by 2035 (Si et al. 2015). With the average age of the population increasing, osteoporosis will undoubtedly continue to be a major public health concern and will provide fertile ground for research in the coming decades, especially in the areas of stem cell therapy, gut microbiome dynamics, and other interventions to slow the progression or reverse the course of osteoporosis.

Clinically, fracture risk most frequently is assessed using FRAX®, a model developed at the University of Sheffield, UK (Kanis et al. 2008). The model uses algorithms based on clinical risk factors and femoral neck bone mineral density (BMD) to calculate the 10-year probability of fracture (https://www.sheffield.ac.uk/FRAX/).

Fracture

The injury most commonly associated with bone is **fracture**, derived from the Latin *fractura*, meaning "to break." Although the term *fracture* is also used to describe disruption to cartilage and the epiphyseal plate, it is most closely associated with breaks in the structural continuity of bony tissue. In a simple sense, fracture occurs when an applied load exceeds the bone's ability to withstand the force. The many factors involved in specifying the loading conditions and the response characteristics of the loaded bone, however, make the study of fracture mechanics anything but simple.

The fracture resistance of bone is determined by both the material properties of bone as a tissue and the structural properties of bone as an organ. Fracture resistance is influenced by the complex interaction of viscoelastic characteristics (e.g., strain rate), bone geometry (e.g., cross-sectional dimensions), anisotropic effects (e.g., microstructural orientation with respect to the loading direction), and bone porosity (Hipp and Hayes 2003).

The nature of bone loading determines in large part the potential for injury and the type of fracture produced. An acute traumatic fracture may occur in response to a single, large-magnitude loading, as occurs in a violent collision. Alternatively, fractures may result from repeated application of lower-magnitude forces (chronic loading), as is characteristic of a metatarsal stress fracture resulting from excessive running or jumping.

A fracture at the specific site of force application is termed a **direct injury**. When the fracture is remote from the location of force application, it is an **indirect injury.** Indirect injuries result from force transmission through other tissues. An example of indirect injury is when a force applied to a tendon or ligament is transferred to its bony attachment site and causes an **avulsion fracture** at that location, meaning that a piece of bone is pulled away from its insertion site.

Fracture risk also depends on the type of bone being loaded. Cortical (compact) bone, because of its relatively low porosity (i.e., high density), is more fracture resistant than less dense trabecular (cancellous) bone. Factors that increase bone density also increase bone strength and thus decrease fracture risk. Conversely, factors that contribute to decreased bone density increase the risk of bone injury. Various fracture types are shown in figure 5.5.

Fractures often are classified according to their mechanism of injury. However, they can be classified or described in various other ways, including those presented by Salter (1999):

• *Injury site.* Fractures may be classified according to their location, such as diaphyseal, epiphyseal, or metaphyseal fractures.

• *Extent of injury.* Fractures may be either **complete** or **incomplete**, depending on whether the damage completely or only partially traverses the bone structure, respectively.

• *Configuration.* When there is only a single fracture line, the shape of the line may be either transverse, oblique, or spiral. When there is more than one fracture line, the fracture may be classified as a **comminuted** (shattered bone from high-energy impact) or **butterfly fracture.**

• *Fragment relations.* Fractures may be either **undisplaced** or **displaced.** In the latter case, the displacement of bone fragments may occur in many ways, including angulation, rotation, distraction, overriding, impaction, or sideways shifting.

• *Environmental relations.* Fractures that remain within the body's internal environment, even if displaced, are termed **closed fractures.** Those penetrating the skin and resulting in exposure of bone to the external environment are **open fractures.** For obvious reasons, open fractures pose a much greater risk of infection than do closed fractures. Closed and open fractures historically have been called *simple* and *compound fractures*, respectively. However, this terminology misrepresents the nature of the fractures and can be misleading. Many clinicians and other professionals, therefore, discourage the use of *simple* and *compound* as fracture descriptors, preferring *closed* and *open*.

• *Complications.* Some fractures are accompanied by few, if any, complications. Many, however,

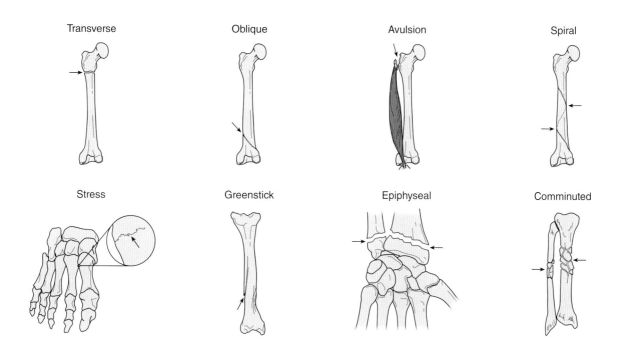

FIGURE 5.5 Fracture types.

have complications that may be immediate (e.g., skin, vascular, neurological, muscular, or visceral injury), early (e.g., tissue necrosis, infection, tetanus, pneumonia), or late (e.g., osteoarthritis, growth disturbances, posttraumatic osteoporosis, or refracture).

• *Etiological factors.* In some cases, fracture is preceded by conditions that predispose a bone to injury. Examples of predisposing etiological factors are repetitive-use microfractures that precede stress fractures and inflammatory disorders, bone disease, congenital abnormalities, and **neoplasms**.

• *Combination injuries.* Bone fracture may be associated with or caused by other injuries, such as multiple fractures and fracture–dislocation injuries. Another combination condition results from the "connectedness" of tissues. Forces applied to an osteotendinous junction, for example, can produce a tendon injury, bone fracture, or both. The weakest-link phenomenon predicts that if the bone is stronger, the tendon will be strained. Conversely, if the tendon is relatively stronger, the bone will experience an avulsion fracture. Here, the viscoelastic properties of bone and tendon come into play. If the injury load is applied slowly, the bone is more likely to experience an avulsion fracture, whereas the tendon is more likely to tear if the load is applied rapidly.

Healing

Fracture healing can be divided into three phases: inflammation, reparative (initial union of the bony ends), and remodeling of the callus. Immediately following injury, a **hematoma** (pool of blood) develops around the fracture site (figure 5.6). Within 3 days, mesenchymal cells arrive in the area and produce a fibrous tissue that envelops the fractured bone ends and begins to form the new periosteum. Until this point, stable fractures (which tend not to displace) and unstable fractures (which tend to slip out of place after reduction and immobilization) react similarly, but between 3 and 5 days after the fracture the degree of stability influences subsequent healing steps. Microscopic examination of the fibrous tissue reveals that the tissue is well vascularized in a stable fracture, but poorly vascularized in an unstable fracture.

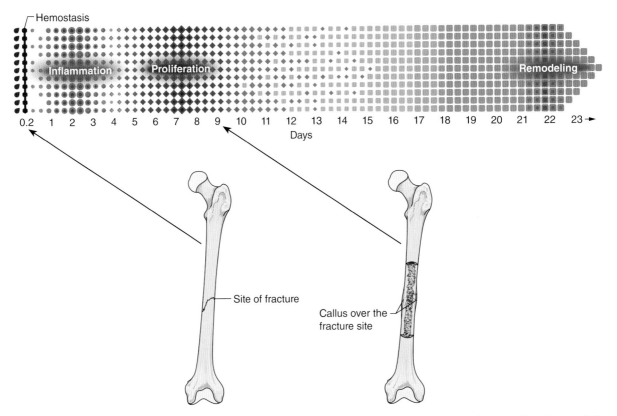

FIGURE 5.6 Bone fracture healing. Inflammatory phase (~days 0-4), reparative phase (~days 5-11), and remodeling phase (~day 12 and beyond).

Where the fibrous tissue meets the original bony cortex—in both stable and unstable fractures—new trabeculae are formed by osteoblasts lying on the old bone surface. In a stable fracture, new bone forms along the periosteal surface of the fibrous layer and spans the fracture site. In an unstable fracture, new bone also forms along the periosteal surface of the fibrous material but does not span the fracture line. In humans, minimal periosteal bone formation occurs at this point in healing, and periosteal union is further delayed. As bony trabeculae continue to form, the bony collar becomes more compact, and the periosteum thickens.

In the gap between the bony ends (rather than along the periosteal surface), the first cells to invade after injury (approximately day 9) are macrophages, followed by fibroblasts and capillaries. Macrophages remove cell and matrix debris, whereas the fibroblasts generate the structural matrix for cells and vessels. Osteoblasts begin bone deposition by 2 weeks post fracture, and bony union across the fractured ends is established (optimally) by 3 weeks. If the bone adjacent to the fracture site dies secondary to disruption of its blood supply at the time of fracture, osteoclasts may be present to resorb the dead tissue. Otherwise, osteoclasts are not routinely present in all fractures.

In small gaps (<0.01 mm) or where fracture ends contact and strain is below 2%, primary bone healing is via direct Haversian remodeling: Osteoclasts resorb a cone of bone, osteoblasts deposit new Haversian bone, and osteocytes maintain the new bone after mineralization. In 0.01 to 0.03 mm gaps (too large for Haversian remodeling but too small for cells to move), osteoclasts may resorb the bone to increase the gap width. Osteoblasts later arrive to lay down disorganized lamellae across the gap. The disorganized bone is then remodeled.

When strain is between 2% and 10%, as in an unstable fracture, periosteal bone formation continues from the old bone ends toward the fracture line, but across the fracture line (where the fibrous material is avascular) chondrocytes proliferate and lay down a cartilage matrix. In a sequence identical to that which happens during endochondral ossification of long bones, the cartilage bridging the fracture ends is gradually replaced by bone. In humans, good stability is achieved by 6 weeks. With the improved stability, blood vessels and fibroblasts proliferate in the fracture gap.

Remodeling of the fracture callus begins as soon as the fracture site gains stability. The dynamics of this remodeling are similar to those of Haversian remodeling: Old bone is resorbed by osteoclasts, and new bone is deposited by osteoblasts. The process is vigorous in the area where the periosteal callus meets the surface of the old bone. Prior to remodeling, this line is clearly visible, but after remodeling, the junction is indistinguishable between the old bone and the callus.

Injuries to Other Connective Tissues

Articular cartilage, fibrocartilage, tendon, and ligament are specialized connective tissues that support and protect the body. They are characterized by a dense collagenous matrix and specialized cells, although each has a unique composition and function. For example, articular cartilage is composed principally of type II collagen and chondrocytes and is avascular. It functions principally by being compressed. Tendons and ligaments are primarily composed of fibroblasts surrounded by type I collagen, and although they are hypovascular, they have a significant neurovascular component. These two tissues are designed to bear tensile loads. Just as their compositions and functions vary, so too does their response to injury and healing.

Articular Cartilage

The articular surfaces of bones in synovial joints are, with few exceptions, covered with a thin (1-5 mm) layer of hyaline articular cartilage. This layer serves several important functions, including load distribution, joint surface protection, and minimization of friction and wear.

Injury

Injury to articular cartilage can severely compromise normal joint function and, in advanced cases, may necessitate joint replacement. Experimental data suggest that excessive joint loading leads to three types of articular damage:

1. Loss of cartilage matrix macromolecules, alteration of the macromolecular matrix, or chondrocyte injury (any or all of these can occur with no detectable disruption of the tissue)

2. Isolated damage to the articular cartilage itself in the form of **chondral fracture** or **flap tears**

3. Injury to the cartilage and its underlying bone, a condition known as an **osteochondral fracture**

Osteoarthritis

Osteoarthritis (OA)—sometimes referred to as degenerative joint disease (DJD)—is a disorder of synovial joints, particularly those with load-bearing involvement, and is characterized by deterioration of the hyaline articular cartilage and bone formation on joint surfaces and at the joint margins (figure 5.7).

OA is a progressive condition, initially characterized by softening of articular cartilage attributable to a decrease in matrix proteoglycan content. The degenerative process is characterized by cartilage fibrillation, cell loss, **chondromalacia** (cartilage softening), loss of elastic support, and disruption of the collagen framework (Fulkerson et al. 1987; Horton et al. 2005). These structural alterations increase the susceptibility of the articular cartilage to shearing loads and thereby predispose it to injury. Subsequently, the cartilage thins and its surface becomes rougher with characteristic pitting, fissuring, and ulceration. The cartilage damage results in enzyme release that causes further breakdown. Advanced cartilage degeneration is accompanied by subchondral bone necrosis and bony outgrowths of ossified cartilage (osteophytes) formed at the joint margin. The severity of OA is typically graded according to the degree of joint space narrowing, osteophyte formation, sclerosis, and joint deformity.

In describing the pathogenesis of osteoarthritis, Brandt (1992) stated,

[Osteoarthritis] develops in either of two settings: (1) the biomaterial properties of the articular bone and cartilage are normal, but excessive loads applied to the joint cause the tissues to fail, or (2) the applied load is physiologically reasonable, but the biomaterial properties of the cartilage or bone are inferior. In general, the earliest progressive degenerative changes in [osteoarthritis] happen at those sites within the joint that are subject to the greatest compressive loads. (pp. 75-76)

The exact cause of osteoarthritis is unknown. It is likely that there is no single cause or common final pathway, but rather a variety of factors that contribute to the end stage of osteoarthritis. It may be initiated by mechanical trauma and attendant chemical process alterations, especially excessive joint laxity attributable to previous ligament injury (Mankin et al. 1994). For example, rupture of the anterior cruciate ligament frequently leads to the development of knee osteoarthritis (Friel and Chu 2013). Among other factors that may contribute are heredity; alterations in chondrocyte activity; and changes in humeral-, synovial-, and cartilage-derived chemical mediators (e.g., interleukin-1).

In addition, tissues within the musculoskeletal system are highly interrelated, and common inflammatory pathways have been implicated in the pathogenesis of a variety of conditions (e.g., OA, osteoporosis, and tendinopathy) (Collins et al. 2018; Hoy et al. 2014; Smith et al. 2014). Functionally, impaired muscle integrity, persistent atrophy, and lipid accumulation in muscle are risk factors for OA (Lee et al. 2012). Indeed, metabolic syndrome (a cluster of conditions that includes obesity, hypertension, and elevated blood glucose and lipids) has been associated with OA tissue damage (Farnaghi et al. 2017).

OA has been etiologically described as being either (1) primary, or **idiopathic** (of unknown origin); or (2) secondary, resulting from identifiable conditions such as trauma, metabolic disorders (e.g., calcium pyrophosphate dihydrate deposition

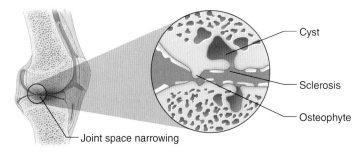

FIGURE 5.7 Osteoarthritis in the knee showing joint space narrowing (inset), sclerosis of the bony end plates, cysts, and osteophytes at the joint margins.

disease or diffuse idiopathic skeletal hyperostosis), existing inflammatory conditions, or crystalline diseases. Among the factors implicated in the pathogenesis of osteoarthritis are obesity, genetics, endocrine and metabolic disorders, joint trauma, and activity patterns determined by a person's occupation or choice of recreation. Epidemiological evidence suggests that up to 90% of the population show some degree of osteoarthritic involvement by the age of 40, although in many cases with no clinical symptoms.

Although the causes of primary OA remain elusive, classifying OA as idiopathic may be a misnomer. In summarizing the evidence from a number of studies, Harris (1986) concluded that in the large majority of cases reported as primary OA of the hip, mild and unrecognized developmental abnormalities (e.g., acetabular dysplasia and pistol-grip deformity) were the likely causal factors. Subsequently, Tanzer and Noiseux (2004) reconfirmed that repetitive anterior femoroacetabular impingement often gives rise to anterior groin pain, labral tears, and chondral damage, which usually ends with the development of arthritis. Thus, a large proportion of OA is misclassified as primary OA.

In cases of OA with known cause, mechanical overuse plays a prominent role. This overuse can be acute (e.g., traumatic injury) or chronic (e.g., repeated heavy lifting). The mechanism of injury in chronic conditions is often related to occupation. For example, the incidence of OA among farmers has been linked to heavy lifting, walking on rough ground, and prolonged tractor driving. As expected, occupation-related OA has also been reported in the knees and spines of coal miners and the hands of cotton mill workers.

Somewhat surprisingly, obesity is not strongly associated with the onset of OA at the hip but rather may be more involved in the progression of already established OA (Croft et al. 1992). That contrasts with the knee joint, where obesity, along with repeated use and previous injury, is a strong risk factor for the occurrence of OA (Collins et al. 2018; Felson et al. 1988).

OA is also strongly associated with advancing age. Radiological evidence of OA is rare in individuals younger than 25, but by age 75 almost all persons exhibit some evidence of OA in their hands and about half show some degree of OA in their feet (Lawrence et al. 1989). The onset of OA at specific joints varies, occurring earliest at the metatarsophalangeal joints, next at the wrist and spine, the interphalangeals and first carpometacarpal, the tibiofemoral, and lastly in the hip. The reasons for this sequential appearance are unclear, but anatomical ultrastructural, biophysical, and biomechanical changes are likely involved. The development of OA is determined by a person's genetic predisposition to OA, abnormalities in the joint, and patterns of mechanical loading and use. The precise relation among these biological and mechanical factors largely remains a mystery, and identification of the specific mechanisms is a challenge.

Healing

When significant damage occurs to articular cartilage, repair with new hyaline cartilage rarely takes place. The inability of articular cartilage to repair defects of any significant size is attributed to its lack of blood vessels and relative lack of cells. This inability of articular cartilage to effect substantial self-repair contributes to osteoarthritis.

Fibrocartilage

Fibrocartilage, composed of dense bundles of collagen fibers, serves as a transitional tissue at osteotendinous and osteoligamentous junctions, facilitating the distribution of forces at attachment sites and lowering the risk of injury. Fibrocartilage is also found in certain joints as a **meniscus**, an interposed fibrocartilage pad that acts as a shock absorber and a wedge at the joint periphery, thus improving the structural fit of the joint. Menisci are found in the joints of the tibiofemoral (knee), acromioclavicular, sternoclavicular, and temporomandibular joints. Meniscal injuries at several of these joints are discussed in later chapters. The fibrocartilaginous labrum in the glenohumeral joint serves similar functions as the meniscus.

Fibrocartilage also is found in the outer layers (annulus fibrosus) of the intervertebral discs. Injury to the fibrocartilage of the annulus fibrosus plays a central role in the mechanisms of low back pain caused by herniated intervertebral discs (see chapter 8). Healing of injured fibrocartilage is limited by the tissue's hypovascularity.

Tendon

As the structure responsible for force transfer from skeletal muscle to bone, tendon is a critical link in the musculoskeletal system. Injury to tendinous structures can restrict or even prevent normal movement and function. The connective structure of tendon creates three structural zones: (1) the

Advances in Joint Replacement

The debilitating pain of advanced osteoarthritis of the hip and knee can severely limit mobility. Joint replacement surgery (**arthroplasty**), in which the damaged structures are replaced by artificial materials, provides remarkable pain relief and restores function in most cases (Merola and Affatato 2019). Because of the load-bearing responsibilities of the lower extremities, it is not surprising that the hip and knee are the leading arthroplastic sites. In light of continued advances in biomaterials and surgical techniques, the advent of computer-assisted designs, and an aging population, the number of arthroplasties will continue to increase dramatically. For example, the American Academy of Orthopaedic Surgeons (AAOS) estimates that by 2030, total knee replacements in the United States will increase by more than 180% (1.28 million), and total hip replacements will increase by more than 170% (635,000) (AAOS 2018).

Total hip replacement (THR) involves excision of the femoral head and part of the neck and enlargement of the acetabulum. A metallic femoral prosthesis is then inserted into the medullary canal of the femur and may be cemented into the canal using methyl methacrylate. An alternative, cementless technique uses a prosthesis with porous structure that encourages bony ingrowth, although the success of cementless prostheses remains a subject of debate. In resurfacing, a more rarely used technique, the neck and head of the femur are not removed. The prosthesis is designed so that it fits like a cap on the head of the femur and a matching cup fits precisely into the groove of the acetabulum.

Although traditional THR is reasonably successful among older and relatively inactive individuals, it may offer less optimal long-term outcomes among active younger patients. Revision surgery may be necessary to repair damage from a previous surgery, and is most commonly caused by infection and less often by fracture and instability.

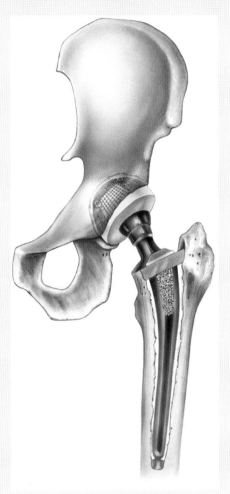

MedicalArtInc/iStock/Getty Images

Over the last two decades, improvements in technology, robotic design, and surgical technique have contributed to better outcomes in joint replacement surgery. Moving forward, a "new generation of robotic systems is being introduced into the arthroplasty arena, and early results with unicompartmental knee arthroplasty and total hip arthroplasty have demonstrated improved accuracy of placement, improved satisfaction, and reduced complications" (Jacofsky and Allen 2016, p. 2353).

body of the tendon itself (tendon substance), (2) the connection of tendon with bone (osteotendinous junction), and (3) the connections with its accompanying muscle (myotendinous junction, shown in figure 5.8).

Pathology

Tendon injury may result from a direct insult, such as when tendons of the hand or fingers are lacerated by knives, saws, or other sharp implements.

Tendinous injury also may be indirect, resulting from excessive tensile loads applied to the tendon structure. Attempted transmission of loads exceeding the ultimate strength of fibers (or the whole tendon) leads to tendon injury.

Injuries to musculotendinous units are termed **strains** (not to be confused with *mechanical strain*, discussed in chapters 3 and 4). Like many tissue injuries, tendon injuries are categorized according to their severity. Mild strain is characterized by

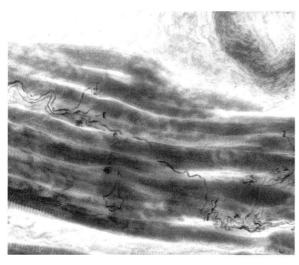

FIGURE 5.8 Transmission electron micrograph of the myotendinous junction.

Jlcalvo/Dreamstime.com

negligible structural disruption, local tenderness, and minimal functional deficit. Moderate strain exhibits partial structural defect, visible swelling, marked tenderness, and some loss of stability. Severe strains have complete structural disruption, marked tenderness, and functional deficits that typically necessitate corrective surgical intervention.

Severe tendon strain (complete rupture of the tendon's structure) is often preceded by undetected tissue damage that existed before the specific incident of rupture. Such cases have been termed *spontaneous tendon ruptures* and are typically seen in middle-aged people engaged in strenuous activities. The injured often have no history of injury or any prior recognized distress. These spontaneous tendon ruptures occur unexpectedly and are accompanied by a popping sensation. Postinjury examination during surgery often identifies preexisting pathology, suggesting that previously undetected tendon degeneration and other pathologies may facilitate spontaneous failure (Kannus and Józsa 1991; Longo et al. 2007; Woo et al. 1994). Examples of spontaneous ruptures in the calcaneal (Achilles) and patellar tendons are described in chapter 6.

Repetitive overloading of a tendon may lead to an inflammatory response, or **tendinitis**. The reaction may be acute (in response to a limited session or event) or chronic (a result of repeated overuse). In addition to the tendon itself, related structures that facilitate tendon sliding (e.g., peritenon, tendon sheath, and accompanying bursa) may also become inflamed and subsequently injured.

The terms used to describe tendon and tendon-related conditions vary. The terms *tendinitis* (also spelled *tendonitis*), *tenosynovitis*, *tendinosis*, and others are used by clinicians and researchers in various contexts to describe a variety of conditions; thus, caution is warranted in interchanging these terms. Specific structures under examination must be clearly identified to avoid confusion.

In addition to the tendon substance, the myotendinous junction can also be injured. The structure of the myotendinous junction shows an interdigitation of skeletal muscle fibers with tendinous collagen fibers in a characteristic membrane-folding pattern. This folding pattern reduces stress at the myotendinous junction during muscular contraction, lessening the likelihood of injury.

Injury also occurs at the osteotendinous junction, where the tendon attaches to the cortical bone surface. This attachment frequently features four layers (zones) of increasing mechanical stiffness: tendon, unmineralized fibrocartilage, mineralized fibrocartilage, and bone. These transition zones distribute the tensile forces and reduce the chance of injury.

Healing

A great deal is known about the healing of severed tendons that have been surgically repaired. After an initial inflammatory phase, synthesis of glycosaminoglycans (GAGs) and collagen is triggered in what is termed the *proliferative phase*. These substances are used in restoring the matrix integrity of the tendon. Rest, ice, and immobilization are recommended to avoid additional tissue damage for the first week after a tendon is acutely injured. In the second and third weeks, low cyclic loads applied to the healing tendons may help align the new fibers and strengthen the repairing tendon; this is called the *regenerative* (or *remodeling*) *phase*. In addition, stretching and activation of the muscle–tendon unit may prevent excessive muscle atrophy and joint stiffness. After the third week, progressively increasing the stress on the tendon optimizes the tissue's healing.

Much less is known about the processes and healing responses associated with chronic tendinitis. According to Andarawis-Puri et al. (2015), "Tendinopathies leading to tendon rupture most commonly result from sub-rupture damage accumulation. The underlying mechanisms associate with pathogenesis of tendinopathies are largely unknown" (p. 783).

Ligament

A ligament is a collagenous connective tissue that joins one bone to another. Ligaments protect the integrity of bone-to-bone connections by resisting excessive movements or dislocation of the bones. In that role, ligaments are characterized as passive joint stabilizers.

Pathology

Injury to a ligament, termed a ligamentous sprain, may compromise a ligament's stabilizing ability and impair its ability to restrict joint movements. The severity of the sprain is clinically specified with a three-level scheme, as shown in the *Injury Terminology* section earlier in the chapter. Mild and moderate sprains are most common. Complete ligament tearing (severe sprain) happens in a minority of cases.

Recall that ligaments can be intracapsular, capsular, or extracapsular. The location and attachments of these ligament types help determine their function, their response to mechanical loading, and their susceptibility to injury. Examples in chapters 6 and 7 illustrate these ligament-specific responses in lower- and upper-extremity joints.

The attachment of ligament to bone follows a structure similar to that at the osteotendinous junction. The osteoligamentous junction exhibits transitional zones of fibrocartilage and mineralized fibrocartilage intervening between the ligament and the cortical bone to which it attaches. This zonal structure facilitates load distribution at the ligament attachment sites. Additionally, fibers of the ligament travel relatively parallel to the surface of the bone and gradually blend with the periosteum.

Healing

More than 25 years ago, Frank (1996) outlined the three phases of ligament healing: bleeding and inflammation, proliferation of bridging material, and matrix remodeling. These phases are explained in detail by Leong et al. (2020). In brief, the first phase, an inflammatory response, parallels the description in the preceding section on inflammation. Platelets from the blood promote clotting, a fibrin clot is deposited, growth factors are released to promote the inflammatory cascade, local vessels dilate, acute inflammatory cells infiltrate, and the fibroblastic scar cells arrive on the scene.

The second phase of ligament healing is the generation of a scar matrix. The scar that is produced in phase 2 and eventually remodeled in phase 3, however, is not normal ligament. The collagen fibers in the scar are typically smaller in diameter than in normal ligament, cross-linked, aligned in a more haphazard manner than in normal ligament, and consist of more type III collagen (Woo et al. 2006).

Matrix remodeling constitutes the third phase of ligament healing. In this phase, the scar matrix diminishes in size and becomes less viscous and more dense and organized. The scar, with time, may start to look and function more like an uninjured ligament, but it never becomes the same as a normal, uninjured ligament, in either structure or strength.

Skeletal Muscle

Skeletal muscles are the engines that provide the human body with the power needed to move. They have a unique ability among all the body's tissues to generate force and contract. Their specialized cells allow muscle to produce force (sometimes referred to as *tension*, or tensile load) and to change their shape by shortening, or contracting.

Injury to skeletal muscle is common and can take several forms and involve various mechanisms. As seen in many occupations, sports, and physical activities, skeletal muscles have the capacity to generate high forces (and power) without sustaining injury. But if too much force is transmitted through a muscle–tendon unit, injury is likely to result. Which regions of the muscle–tendon unit are the most likely to be damaged?

Stimulated Versus Passive Muscle

Research has shown that when muscle–tendon–bone units are pulled to failure, tears can happen at bone–tendon junctions, within the muscle belly, or at the myotendinous junctions (McMaster 1933). Later experimental studies confirmed tears in muscle–tendon units at the myotendinous junction (Garrett et al. 1988) or at sites within the muscle cell approximately 0.5 mm from the myotendinous junction (Tidball and Chan 1989).

Much of this work probed the failure characteristics of passive (unstimulated) muscle–tendon units, but two studies (Garrett et al. 1987; Tidball et al. 1993) investigated muscle–tendon failure in stimulated versus quiescent muscle. Garrett and colleagues (1987) compared the biomechanical properties of passive versus stimulated muscle (rabbit extensor digitorum longus) that was rapidly lengthened to failure, finding no significant difference in the amount of lengthening at which the failure happened, regardless of activation state. But when muscles were stimulated, they achieved 14% to 16% greater peak forces at failure than if the muscle was passive. Also, substantially more energy was absorbed to the point of failure in the stimulated than in the unstimulated muscle–tendon units. Garrett and colleagues reported that the site of failure was typically at the myotendinous junction.

Tidball and colleagues (1993) used electron microscopy to locate the specific sites of the muscle–tendon interface that failed in tetanically stimulated versus unstimulated bone–tendon–muscle–tendon–bone units, using a frog semitendinous muscle. The specimens were strained at physiological strain rates to failure, and all failures happened at or near the proximal (tendon of origin) myotendinous junction in both stimulated and unstimulated muscle. Like Garrett and colleagues (1987), Tidball and colleagues (1993) found that the stimulated muscle–tendon units required about 30% more force and about 110% more energy to reach failure. Interestingly, the electron-microscopic analysis revealed systematic differences in the sites of failure, which varied with

the state of activation of the muscle cells at the time of injury. Also, the breaking strength of the Z disc in stimulated muscle differed from unstimulated muscle—suggesting that two load-bearing systems may be in parallel within the Z discs.

Figures 5.9, 5.10, and 5.11, taken from Tidball and colleagues (1993), show clearly the variation in failure site with activation state of the muscle. A transmission electron micrograph (figure 5.9a) illustrates a longitudinal section from an unstimulated muscle, and figure 5.9b illustrates a similar section from a stimulated muscle. In the unstimulated muscle, the site of failure was within the muscle, near the myotendinous junction. Failure happened in a single transverse plane of each cell within Z discs, and other Z discs in the area remained stretched—with residual strains of several hundred percent (figure 5.9a). In contrast, figure 5.9b was taken from

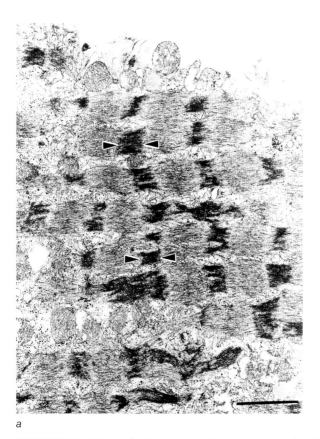
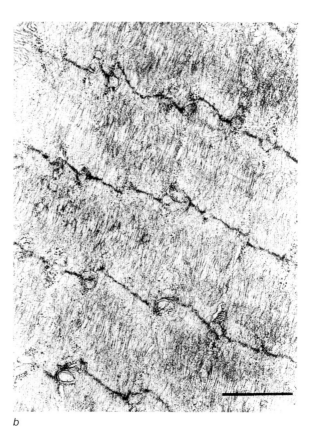

a　　　　　　　　　　　　　　　　　　b

FIGURE 5.9 *(a)* Longitudinal section from an unstimulated muscle loaded to failure. This transmission electron micrograph shows an incomplete tear through a muscle fiber about 80 μm from the site of the complete tear. The Z discs (between the arrowheads) show extensive residual strain. *(b)* Longitudinal section taken through a stimulated muscle that was strained to failure. The site in the photograph is about 100 μm from the failure site. The Z discs are distinct and show no signs of persisting strain. The insert bar (1.5 μm) is the same in both photographs.

(a) Reprinted by permission from J.G. Tidball, G. Salem and R.F. Zernicke, "Site and Mechanical Conditions for Failure of Skeletal Muscle in Experimental Strain Injuries," *Journal of Applied Physiology,* 74 (1993): 1283. *(b)* Reprinted by permission from J.G. Tidball, G. Salem and R.F. Zernicke, "Site and Mechanical Conditions for Failure of Skeletal Muscle in Experimental Strain Injuries," *Journal of Applied Physiology,* 74 (1993): 1285.

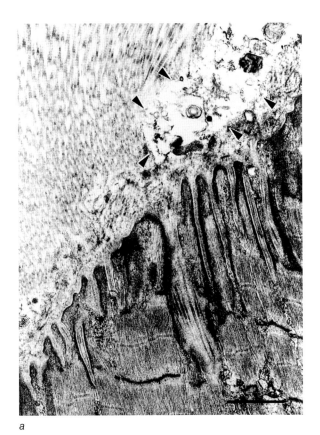

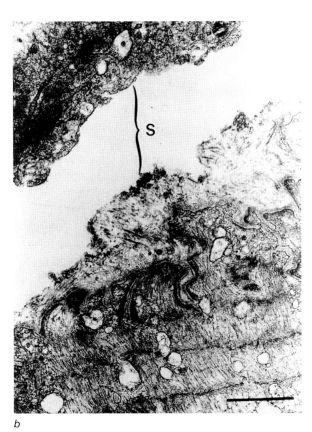

a

b

FIGURE 5.10 Longitudinal section through the myotendinous junction of origin of an unstimulated muscle that was strained to failure. *(a)* Tears existed in the tendon, near the myotendinous junctions (outlined by the arrowheads). Identical-looking tears were found at the myotendinous junctions of both unstimulated and stimulated fibers. The inset bar is 2.0 μm. *(b)* Large separations (S) within the tendon near the myotendinous junctions were observed in some preparations, although complete tears were located in the fibers for these preparations. The insert bar is 2.5 μm.

Reprinted by permission from J.G. Tidball, G. Salem and R.F. Zernicke, "Site and Mechanical Conditions for Failure of Skeletal Muscle in Experimental Strain Injuries," *Journal of Applied Physiology,* 74 (1993): 1285.

a stimulated muscle at a site about 100 μm from the failure site. Here you can see the relatively normal-looking Z discs; they show no residual strains.

When the sites of failure were examined more closely in the unstimulated muscle, tears were found in the tendon near the myotendinous junction (outlined by the arrowheads in figure 5.10*a*). Identical-appearing tears were seen at the myotendinous junctions of both unstimulated and stimulated specimens. Large separations (denoted by S in figure 5.10*b*) were seen within the tendon near the myotendinous junction of an unstimulated muscle. In figure 5.11 (an electron micrograph taken through the myotendinous junction for a stimulated muscle), site of failure (complete separation) is immediately external to the membrane of the myotendinous junction, and no connective tissue appears connected to the junction membrane (see arrowheads).

Types of Injury

A *strain* injury happens when damage is inflicted on a musculotendinous unit. Use of the term *strain* to describe musculotendinous injury is common, but not universally accepted. For example, Mueller-Wohlfahrt et al. (2013) proposed alternative terminology and classification of muscle injuries, concluding that "*Functional muscle disorders* are differentiated from *structural* injuries. The use of the term *strain*—if used undifferentiated—is no longer recommended, since it is a biomechanical term, not well defined and used indiscriminately for anatomically and functionally different muscle injuries. Instead of this, we propose to use the term *tear* for *structural injuries*" (p. 348). Given its broad and continued use, however, we will use the term *strain* in our discussion of musculotendinous injuries.

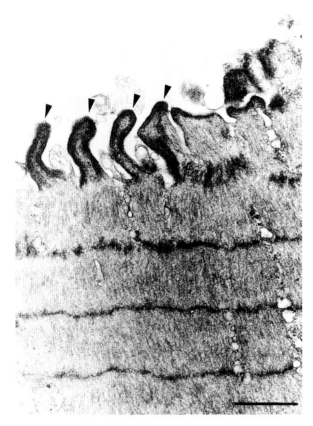

FIGURE 5.11 Longitudinal section through the myotendinous junction of origin of a stimulated muscle that was loaded to failure. The site of complete separation is immediately external to the junctional membrane so that no connective tissue is found associated with the junctional processes (see arrowheads). Inset bar is 2.0 μm.

Reprinted by permission from J.G. Tidball, G. Salem and R.F. Zernicke, "Site and Mechanical Conditions for Failure of Skeletal Muscle in Experimental Strain Injuries," *Journal of Applied Physiology*, 74 (1993): 1284.

The specifics of tendon injury were discussed previously; here we concentrate on three forms of skeletal muscle injury: acute muscular strain, impact injury, and exercise-induced muscle injury.

• **Acute muscular strain** typically results from overstretching a passive muscle or dynamically overloading an active muscle, either in concentric or eccentric action. The severity of tissue damage depends on the magnitude of the force, the rate of force application, and the strength of the musculotendinous structures. Mild strains are characterized by minimal structural disruption and rapid return to normal function. Moderate strains are accompanied by a partial tear in the muscle tissue (often at or near the myotendinous junction), pain, and some loss of function. Severe muscle strains are defined by complete or near-complete tissue disruption and functional loss, as well as marked **hemorrhage** and swelling.

• **Impact injuries** result from a direct compressive impact. Such contact may cause a muscle bruise (contusion), which is distinguished by intramuscular hemorrhage. Muscular contusion commonly occurs in contact sports (e.g., basketball, football, soccer), as when an athlete's thigh has a violent impact with another participant's knee. Repeated mechanical insult to a damaged muscle prior to healing may worsen the injury and lead to serious secondary conditions, such as myositis ossificans (development of an ossified mass within the muscle).

• **Exercise-induced muscle injury** results from connective and contractile tissue disruption following exercise, and is characterized by local tenderness, stiffness, and restricted range of motion. This type of injury, also referred to as **delayed-onset muscle soreness (DOMS)**, typically happens 24 to 72 hours after participation in vigorous exercise, especially following eccentric muscle action in contractile tissue unaccustomed to the activity's demands. Historically, DOMS was thought to be caused by lactic acid accumulation in the muscle, although that theory has been debunked. DOMS is now thought to be primarily a result of microdamage to the muscle tissue (Hotfiel et al. 2018). The symptoms and metabolic events (e.g., pain, swelling, presence of cellular infiltrates, increased lysosomal activity, and increased levels of some circulating acute-phase proteins) attendant to DOMS are similar to those of acute inflammation and suggest a relation between the two (Close et al. 2005).

Although not particularly injurious itself, the common muscle cramp may indicate conditions predisposing to injury. Excessive demands placed on a muscle in such a sustained and often painful spasm may result in muscle strain. The mechanisms of muscle cramps, despite the frequency of their occurrence, are not fully understood. Most cramps occur in a shortened muscle and are characterized by abnormal electrical activity. Many factors have been proposed to cause muscle cramps, including dehydration, electrolyte imbalances, direct impact, fatigue, and lowered levels of serum calcium and magnesium. Cramps happen in many muscles, especially the gastrocnemius, semimembranosus, semitendinosus, biceps femoris, and abdominals, and can be relieved by antagonistic muscle activity or manual stretching of the afflicted muscle. Stretching warrants care because excessive force applied to a muscle in spasm may result in muscle strain.

Joint Injuries

Skeletal articulations (joints), by virtue of their often intricate structure and the complex mechanical loading of multiple tissues involved, are susceptible to injury. Although not well understood in many cases, the dynamics of joint mechanical loading determine the actual injuries that occur. Because numerous joint injuries are examined in detail in subsequent chapters, we limit our discussion here to basic concepts and terminology of joint injury.

When sufficient force is applied to a joint, the articulating bones may become displaced. This results in a complete dislocation (**luxation**) or a partial dislocation (**subluxation**) (figure 5.12). Note that the term *subluxation* can be defined in various ways. For example, the biomechanical definition (used here) refers to a partial, rather than a complete, dislocation. In contrast, clinicians typically apply the term *subluxation* to cases in which a dislocation (either partial or complete) is followed immediately by spontaneous joint **reduction** (i.e., realignment or replacement of the dislocated bone into normal position).

Complete dislocations in particular often are accompanied by additional injuries, including ligamentous sprain and tears of the fibrous joint capsule, along with potential vascular and neural damage.

The inner surface of the joint capsule is lined by the **synovial membrane**, a thin layer of tissue that has negligible biomechanical function but plays an important role in the physiology of both normal and injured joints. Irritation or trauma to the synovium may lead to **synovitis**, a condition with inflammatory symptoms that can in turn limit joint function.

Arthritis refers to inflammation of a joint or a state characterized by joint inflammation. It includes many conditions that have either primary or secondary inflammatory involvement; more than 100 types of arthritis have been identified. Among the major types are those resulting from chronic and excessive mechanical loading (e.g., *osteoarthritis*, described earlier), systemic disease (e.g., **rheumatoid arthritis**), or biochemical imbalances (e.g., **gouty arthritis**). Arthritis may be a primary condition or may develop in response to a noninflammatory insult, as is the case in osteoarthritis. In any case, arthritis and its **sequelae** (aftereffects)

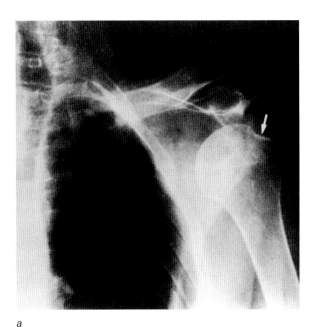

a

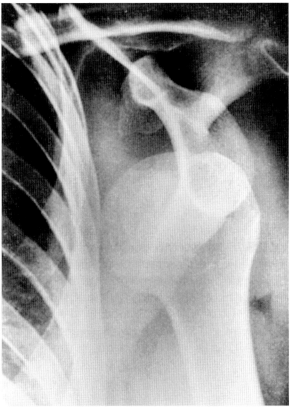

b

FIGURE 5.12   X-ray of *(a)* partial dislocation (subluxation) and *(b)* complete dislocation (luxation).

(a) Reprinted by permission from M.J. Julian and M. Mathews, "Shoulder Injuries," in *The Team Physicians Handbook,* edited by M.B. Mellion (Philadelphia: Hanley & Belfus, Inc., 1990), 320. *(b)* Reprinted by permission from P.G. Gusmer and H.G. Potter, "Imaging of Shoulder Instability," *Clinics in Sports Medicine* 14, no 4: 780.

have the potential to inflict debilitating pain and loss of joint function.

Nonmusculoskeletal Injuries

A wide range of nonmusculoskeletal injuries involve the skin and nervous tissue, which often are affected secondary to musculoskeletal injury.

Skin

Skin forms the outer protective covering for most of the body's surface. As the body's outermost defense, skin is susceptible to a wide variety of injuries.

Pathology

Injury to the skin can take various forms and involve many causal mechanisms, some of which are mechanical in nature. Sufficient friction between the skin and an opposing surface may result in superficial injury such as an **abrasion** (scraping away of the superficial skin layer, usually by mechanical action) or deeper injury such as a **blister** (a fluid-filled structure under or within the epidermis caused by heat, chemical, or mechanical means).

Nonpenetrating skin injury is termed a **contusion**, or bruise, which usually results from a direct, violent impact. Internal hemorrhage can accompany contusion and, in severe cases, be quite debilitating.

Sharp implements that penetrate the skin create **puncture** wounds, which not only damage the dermal and epidermal layers but may, with sufficient penetration depth, injure intervening internal structures as well. The mechanics of puncture injury often result in a wound that appears on the skin surface to be much less severe than it actually is, because the skin often closes on implement removal to obscure deeper damage. The wound often appears to be clean, leaving little visible external evidence of the damage created internally. Jagged tearing of the skin (**laceration**) is characteristic of cut wounds by a knife or other sharp implement, because the mechanism of injury is tearing rather than puncture. The external appearance of a laceration, compared with that of a puncture wound, is usually more indicative of the extent of injury.

Skin exposed to heat, chemical or electrical contact, radiation, or sun overexposure can sustain burn injuries. Minor, first-degree burns are characterized by redness and pain, with damage limited to skin's outer layer (epidermis). Second-degree burns damage the epidermis and underlying second layer (dermis) and exhibit swelling, redness, blisters, and considerable pain. The most severe (third-degree) burns penetrate beneath the skin, with burned areas showing black, white, or brown coloring, potential numbness, nerve damage, and extreme pain.

Healing

Any injury that penetrates the skin, to any depth, carries the risk of infection. Caution is warranted in treating any penetrating injury, however slight, because the damaging effects of infection resulting from an improperly treated injury may far exceed the deleterious effects of the original injury itself.

Given the proximity of venous vasculature to the dermis, skin injuries are often characterized by considerable bleeding (hemorrhage). Facial lacerations, for example, commonly produce effusive bleeding, especially in the areas immediately above (supraorbital) and below (infraorbital) the eye and on the chin.

Skin wounds heal through four overlapping phases: (1) hemostasis, (2) inflammation, (3) proliferation, and (4) maturation (figure 5.13). In the hemostasis phase, the body seeks to stop bleeding through clotting, in which platelets combine with collagen to block blood flow. Thrombin then works to form a fibrin mesh, which stabilizes the clot.

During the inflammation phase, coagulation works to destroy bacteria (through action of neutrophils) and remove debris (through macrophage action) from the injured area. The healing process then progresses to the proliferative phase, during which the wound is filled with granulated connective tissue and new blood vessels. The final phase, maturation, is characterized by reorganization of collagen fibers, along with increased flexibility and strength. The maturation phase can last from a few weeks to two years, depending on the severity of the wound.

Nervous Tissue

Nervous tissue is not classified as a musculoskeletal tissue, but because injury to nervous tissue can directly or indirectly affect the function of musculoskeletal tissues, we present a brief outline of nervous tissue injury.

Injury to nervous tissue has the potential to produce the most debilitating types of dysfunction. Damage to the brain and other supraspinal structures, spinal cord, spinal nerves, or peripheral nerves can affect the most essential of the body's communication systems, impairing or even eliminating sensory and motor processes. Injuries

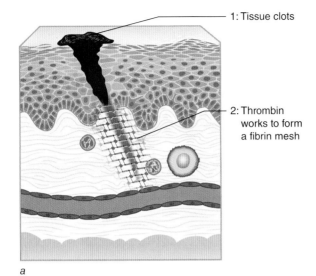

1: Tissue clots

2: Thrombin works to form a fibrin mesh

a

3: Wound is filled with granulated connective tissue and new blood vessels

b

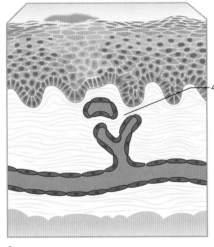

4: Reorganization of collagen fibers

c

FIGURE 5.13 Stages of wound healing: Inflammation, proliferation, and maturation.

to structures of the peripheral nervous system are considered in chapters 6 and 7; examples of injuries to the central nervous system (e.g., cerebral concussion) are presented in chapter 8. As a prelude, a brief review of nervous tissue injury is presented here.

Nerves are cordlike organs that serve as the communication conduits sending information between the periphery and the central nervous system (figure 5.14). Each nerve consists of multiple individual fibers (axons) arranged in parallel bundles. These bundles are enclosed by layers of connective tissue. Each axon is covered by a delicate endoneurial sheath, or **endoneurium**. Axons are grouped into nerve bundles (fascicles) that are surrounded by **perineurium**. Finally, the fascicles collectively form the whole nerve (nerve trunk), which is surrounded by a tough covering of epineurial tissue (**epineurium**).

Nervous tissue can be injured through chemical, thermal, ischemic, or mechanical means; here we focus on only the mechanical means. Mechanical influences on nervous structures can take one of two forms—namely, entrapment or trauma. In the former, nervous tissue becomes compressed within a confined anatomical space or between other anatomical structures. The resulting forces impinge on the nervous tissue and can produce damage and compromise function.

The second form of nerve injury, trauma, results from a direct mechanical insult to the tissue or from forces indirectly applied to the nervous tissue via surrounding structures. Each of the three principal loading types may be present, either alone or in combination. Compressive loading results in pressure, tensile loading creates tissue elongation (which may result in stretch injury), and shear loading may lead to friction-related injury. In entrapment and trauma, the nature of any resulting dysfunction depends on the characteristics (e.g., magnitude and duration) of the mechanical environment at the time of injury.

The severity of injury, based on nerve histopathology, is commonly assessed with a qualitative five-level classification system (Sunderland 1990). The basic elements of these levels are presented here and in figure 5.15:

• The least severe level, first-degree injury, is characterized by the presence of a conduction block. This interruption of nerve signal transmission may be brief, mild, or severe. First-degree nerve injuries do not involve any denervation effects and result in full recovery, although this recovery may take several months. First-degree injury can happen after a pro-

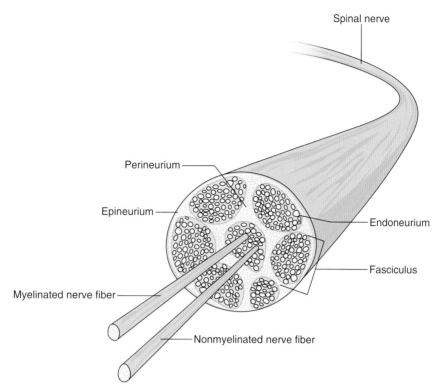

FIGURE 5.14 Structure of a nerve.

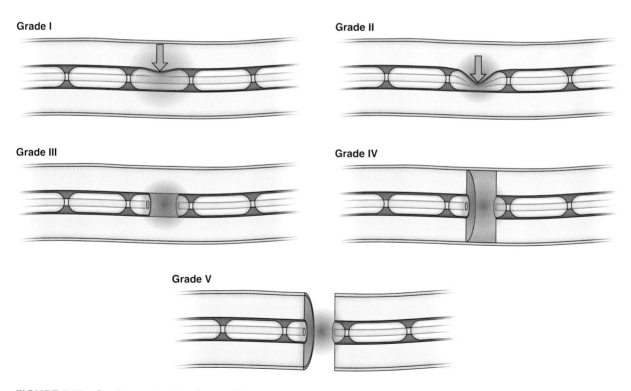

FIGURE 5.15 Grades, or levels, of nerve injury.

longed, low-pressure compression or an acute, high-compression event that results in a conduction block without axonal discontinuity, or **neurapraxia**. Carpal tunnel syndrome is an example of nerve entrapment resulting in a first-degree injury. In this instance, overuse and inappropriate position of the hand and finger flexors result in swelling of the tendons as they pass through the carpal tunnel. In turn, the swelling places pressure on the median nerve, resulting first in tingling or burning in the digits, and then progressing to functional impairment if not treated.

• Second-degree injury involves **axonotmesis**, an interruption of axonal structure, and later Wallerian degeneration (discussed later), but without severance of the nerve's supporting structure. These lesions may result from pinching or crushing mechanisms or from prolonged pressure. During recovery from second-degree nerve injury, nerve regeneration normally occurs. In some cases, injury to the brachial plexus resulting from an excessive stretching of the upper trunk, commonly called a "stinger" or "burner," can result in impaired sensation and motor function of the affected arm.

• Third-, fourth-, and fifth-degree injuries all represent varying degrees of fiber continuity loss (**neurotmesis**) with damage to both the axon and the endoneurial sheath, typically resulting from direct trauma to the tissue such as a knife cut or secondary to a joint dislocation. Third-degree injuries involve damage to the endoneurium, although the epineurium and perineurium remain undamaged. A third-degree injury results in complete loss of sensory and motor function and recovery is possible, although surgery may be required. Fourth-degree nerve injury involves disruption of the endoneurium and perineurium, with only the epineurial tissue remaining to provide structural continuity. Successful recovery seldom occurs spontaneously, and surgical repair is indicated in most cases. Fifth-degree injury, the most severe nerve injury, results in complete severance of the nerve. Regeneration, if it occurs at all, usually is incomplete and disrupted and usually requires surgical repair.

In trauma cases where there is damage to the nerve fiber, the portion of the nerve distal to the injury site may degrade in a process known as **Wallerian degeneration**. These cases involve degeneration of the axon and its myelin sheath, resulting in separation (denervation) between the axon's neuron (nerve cell) and its target organ. The cell's response depends on the location and severity of injury and may either enable a regenerative response or result in cell death.

Any level of compromised sensory or motor function can hasten or exacerbate musculoskeletal injury because impaired afferent (inward) information precludes the central nervous system from generating an appropriate efferent (outward) response. Impaired sensory function, for example, may alter pain sensation, thus retarding the body's warning system and permitting a more severe injury than might occur with normal sensation. This can be seen in the **peripheral neuropathies** commonly found in the feet of persons with diabetes. These neuropathies can lead to foot ulcerations and eventual amputation. Similarly, axonal damage that results in motor impairment can alter muscle recruitment patterns and produce uncoordinated and potentially dangerous movements. For example, a runner with impaired motor control attributable to nervous tissue injury may experience selective muscle weakness that results in altered gait mechanics and consequent musculoskeletal injury.

Chapter Review

Key Points

- This chapter presents key concepts of injury mechanics, terminology, and mechanisms of injury, including mechanical load and overload, use and overuse, and level of dysfunction and progression of injury.

- Injuries are graded based on the degree to which tissues are damaged. Injury severity dictates the level of impairment and the scope of repair and rehabilitation.

- The likelihood and severity of injury depend on myriad contributory factors that interact in complex ways. Each tissue in the body (e.g., bone, cartilage, tendon, ligament, muscle, and nerve) has its own morphological, physiological, and biomechanical characteristics. These inherent differences, combined with the type of injury mechanisms, cause tissue-specific injury patterns and repair processes.

Questions to Consider

1. Select a specific injury that you or someone you know has experienced. Describe the injury, its mechanism(s), and any contributory factors that may apply to the injury you've described.

2. Explain the weakest-link phenomenon as it applies to musculoskeletal injury and what factors may be involved in determining the weakest link for a particular anatomical structure or system.

3. Describe an injury situation in which two or more contributory factors (from those listed in the text or additional ones you identify) interact to further increase or decrease the chance of injury.

4. Describe an example of how a single contributory factor might both increase *and* decrease injury risk.

5. Explain how inflammation provides a "first line of defense" against insult following an injury.

6. Osteoporosis and related conditions (e.g., fall-related fractures) are a growing public health concern. Describe the multifactorial nature of osteoporosis as a public health issue.

7. Select a tissue (e.g., bone, articular cartilage, tendon, ligament) and explain its pathology and healing.

Suggested Readings

Aaron, R. 2021. *Orthopaedic Basic Science: Foundations of Clinical Practice* (5th ed.). Rosemont, IL: American Academy of Orthopaedic Surgeons.

Browner, B.D., J. Jupiter, C. Krettek, and P.A. Anderson. 2019. *Skeletal Trauma: Basic Science, Management, and Reconstruction* (6th ed.). Philadelphia, PA: Elsevier.

Fu, F.H., and D.A. Stone. 2001. *Sports Injuries: Mechanisms, Prevention, Treatment.* Baltimore: Williams & Wilkins.

Hamblen, D.L. 2020. *Adam's Outline of Fractures* (14th ed.). Edinburgh, UK: Churchill Livingstone.

Tornetta, P., III, W. Ricci, C.M. Court-Brown, M.M. McQueen, and M. McKee. 2019. *Rockwood and Green's Fractures in Adults* (9th ed.). Philadelphia: Wolters Kluwer.

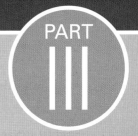

Regional Injuries

Lower-Extremity Injuries

Pain is just something I live with and that is pretty odd for my age, right? . . . There's been a calf I have partially torn two or three times, I broke a rib in 2016, and oh yeah, it turned out my toe was shattered in five pieces after the last Olympics without me knowing. . . . I guess that is it. If you are jumping up in the air all the time, sometimes gravity says no.

Simone Biles (Olympic gymnast)

OBJECTIVES

- To describe the relevant lower-extremity anatomy involved in musculoskeletal injury
- To identify and explain the mechanisms involved in musculoskeletal injuries to the major joints (hip, knee, ankle) and segments (thigh, lower leg, foot) of the lower extremity

Injuries to lower-extremity joints, in particular the knee and ankle, are among the most common of all musculoskeletal disorders. Given the importance of the lower extremities in everyday activities such as walking, running, and maintaining posture, injury to these joints has a significant effect on daily living. The circumstances of lower-extremity injury can vary, ranging from the acute, high-energy trauma of a twisted ankle to the more gradual onset of a metatarsal stress fracture.

The lower-extremity injuries presented in this chapter were selected based on their prevalence and their value in illustrating specific injury mechanisms. Representative injuries are presented for the major lower-extremity joints (hip, knee, and ankle) and the regions spanning those joints (thigh, lower leg, and foot). In addition, we explore anterior cruciate ligament (ACL) injuries in depth, expanding our discussion beyond the mechanisms of injury to describe the ACL's structure and tissue mechanics and explain clinical evaluation, treatment, and rehabilitation. Although space restrictions preclude this level of detail for all injuries, we believe this section to be an instructive tool to show how any injury can be presented in a broader context and in greater detail.

Hip Injuries

The hip joint is formed by articulation of the femur with the pelvic girdle (coxal bone), specifically by the articulating surfaces of the femoral head and the acetabulum (figure 6.1). The bony fit is improved by the acetabular labrum, a fibrocartilage pad

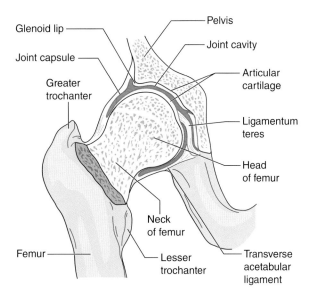

FIGURE 6.1 Structures of the hip joint.

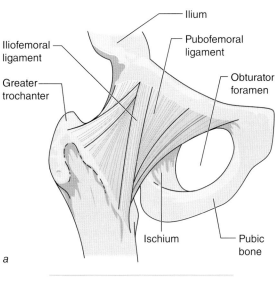

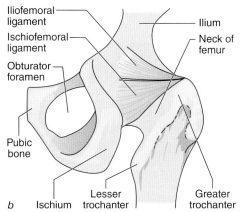

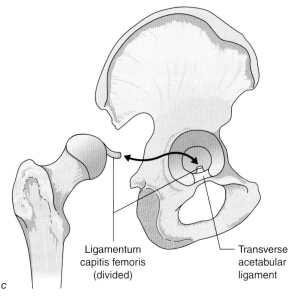

FIGURE 6.2 Ligaments of the hip joint: *(a)* the ilio-femoral and pubofemoral ligaments, anterior view; *(b)* the ischiofemoral ligament, posterior view; and *(c)* the transverse acetabular ligament and ligamentum capitis femoris, anterior view.

attached to the bony rim of the acetabulum. The hip joint is reinforced anteriorly by the iliofemoral ligament, posteriorly by the ischiofemoral ligament, and anteroinferiorly by the pubofemoral ligament (figure 6.2). The ligament of the head of the femur provides limited structural support, serving primarily to contain the vasculature supplying the femoral head. Additional support is provided by the articular joint capsule, whose fibers form a fibrous collar around the femoral neck and help secure the femoral head in the acetabulum.

The hip joint's ball-and-socket configuration permits movements in the three primary planes, referred to as flexion–extension (sagittal plane), abduction–adduction (frontal plane), and internal–external rotation (transverse plane). The muscles responsible for controlling movements about the hip joint are shown in figure 6.3; their actions are summarized in table 6.1. This considerable musculature further stabilizes the hip joint.

In the next two sections, we discuss hip fracture and dislocation. Although these injuries are presented in separate sections, conjoint fracture–dislocation injuries are not uncommon given that most severe hip injuries involve high-energy trauma.

Hip and Pelvic Fractures

Bone fractures in the hip typically result from high-energy trauma such as that associated with falls from heights and automobile crashes. Fracture risk is elevated in persons with fragile bones (e.g., osteoporosis). The incidence of hip fracture is about three times greater among women than men and increases

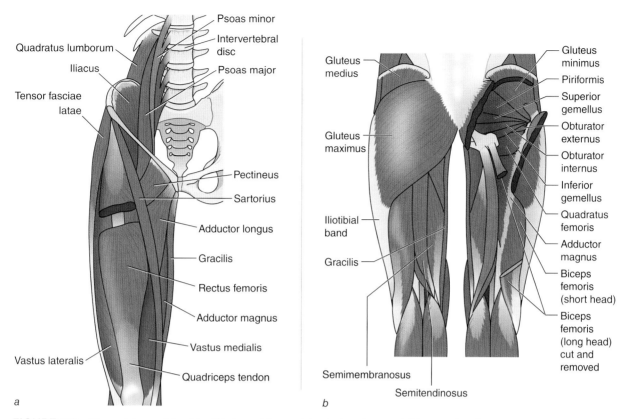

FIGURE 6.3 Musculature of the hip, thigh, and knee: *(a)* anterior view and *(b)* posterior view.

TABLE 6.1 Muscles of the Hip

Muscle	Action
Adductor group Adductor brevis Adductor longus Adductor magnus	Adducts and laterally rotates the thigh
Biceps femoris (long head)	Extends the thigh
Gluteus maximus	Extends and laterally rotates the thigh
Gluteus medius	Abducts and medially rotates the thigh
Gluteus minimus	Abducts and medially rotates the thigh
Gracilis	Adducts the thigh
Iliopsoas (psoas major and iliacus)	Flexes the thigh; flexes the trunk when femur is fixed
Pectineus	Adducts, flexes, and laterally rotates the thigh
Piriformis	Laterally rotates the thigh; assists in extending and abducting the thigh
Rectus femoris	Flexes the thigh
Sartorius	Extends the thigh
Semimembranosus	Extends the thigh
Semitendinosus	Extends the thigh
Tensor fasciae latae	Assists in flexion, abduction, and medial rotation of the thigh

significantly with advancing age (Cummings and Melton 2002; Kanis et al. 2012; Papadimitropoulos et al. 1997). Pelvic fractures, although not nearly as prevalent as femoral fractures, nonetheless present a significant danger (Breuil et al. 2016). Although accounting for only 3% of skeletal injuries, pelvic trauma victims have a high mortality rate, making pelvic trauma "one of the most complex management (issues) in trauma care" (Coccolini et al. 2017, pp. 1).

In motor vehicle crashes, the direction of force largely determines the pattern of injury. Pelvic fractures resulting from severe motor vehicle crashes are significantly more frequent in side-impact collisions, occur at much lower speeds in side impacts than in frontal collisions, and incur high mortality rates from associated injuries (Gokcen et al. 1994). Fracture-related mortality and morbidity are especially problematic for women. Trochanteric soft tissue thickness and total hip bone mineral density are significant determinants of fracture outcome in women with pelvic fractures resulting from side-impact collisions (Etheridge et al. 2005).

Proximal femoral (hip) fractures are a major health concern, with more than 350,000 fractures occurring annually in the United States. Globally, hip fracture affects millions and is a significant cause of morbidity and mortality worldwide (Johnell and Kanis 2004). The statistics are all the more sobering when we consider that an estimated 10% to 30% of hip fracture victims die within a year of injury—not necessarily as a direct result of the fracture, but rather because of chronic conditions (e.g., pneumonia, dementia) that worsen after the injury. Davidson and colleagues (2001), for example, reported a 12-month mortality rate of 26%.

Although there are encouraging projections of a leveling or even decrease in hip fractures among certain populations (Lewiecki et al. 2018; Lofman et al. 2002) and the promise of effective pharmacological therapies (Curtis et al. 2017), worldwide trends point to an increasing number of hip fractures in the foreseeable future, with an estimated overall increase in hip fracture incidence of 1% to 3% per year in most areas of the world for both women and men (Cummings and Melton 2002). Globally, hip fractures are projected to be as high as 4.5 million by 2050 (Veronese and Maggi 2018).

Although hip fractures are relatively rare in young individuals, the likelihood of hip fracture increases markedly with advancing age. Hip fractures are common in older populations. In China, for example, the overall prevalence of hip fracture in

middle-aged and older Chinese adults was reported at 2.36%. Within that population, the prevalence was 1.62% for persons younger than age 50, and 5.42% for those age 70 and up (Ren et al. 2019).

Interestingly, the country-specific risk of hip fracture varies considerably. In a comparison among 63 countries, Kanis et al. (2012) reported a more-than-tenfold variation in hip fracture risk among countries. The lowest risk countries, measured by fractures per 100,000 women per year, included Nigeria (2), South Africa (20), Tunisia (58), and Ecuador (73). The highest fracture rates were found in Denmark (574), Norway (563), Sweden (539), and Austria (501). Among the many risk factors for hip fracture are falls, decreased bone mineral density and bone mass, small body size, decreased muscular strength, physical inactivity, environmental circumstances, drug use, chronic illnesses, and impairment of cognition, vision, and perception (Marks et al. 2003).

Classification and Causes

Proximal femoral (hip) fractures are classified according to their location (figure 6.4). Fractures to the femoral neck are considered intracapsular because that region is proximal to the distal

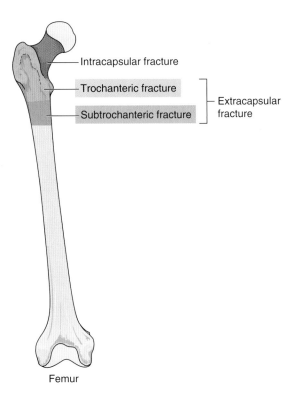

FIGURE 6.4 Classification of hip fractures based on location.

joint capsule boundary. The extracapsular region is subdivided into trochanteric (also known as intertrochanteric) and subtrochanteric areas. Fracture incidence depends on region, with one study reporting 49% of hip fractures occurring in the intertrochanteric region, 37% in the femoral neck (intracapsular), and 14% in the subtrochanteric region (Michelson et al. 1995). Other more recent studies suggest similar incidence rates between the femoral neck and intertrochanteric region (Diaz and Navas 2018; Fox et al. 2000).

Because the area contains large amounts of cancellous bone and good blood supply, extracapsular fractures (both intertrochanteric and subtrochanteric) typically heal well overall, with more complications occurring in the subtrochanteric region. In comparison, the femoral neck and femoral head contain less cancellous bone and relatively poor blood supply, thus intracapsular hip fractures exhibit a higher incidence of avascular necrosis, nonunion, malunion, and degenerative changes (LeBlanc et al. 2014).

Hip fractures in the young usually result from high-energy impacts, most commonly occurring in motor vehicle crashes. These injuries often are associated with hip luxation. The most common mechanism for femoral neck fracture is direct trauma to the hip, as seen in a fall (Lauritzen 1997). A less common mechanism involves a lateral rotation of the leg while the body falls backward. In this case, the femoral neck fractures when the person falls backward with the foot planted on the ground; the iliofemoral ligament secures the femoral neck while the stiffened iliopsoas tendon provides a solid base against which the femoral neck fractures. On rare occasions, young people experience a stress fracture of the proximal femur as a result of repeated loading during strenuous activity.

Hip fractures in older people are associated with falls (discussed in the next section), often caused by tripping or unsteady gait. This association raises an intriguing question: Does hip fracture cause the fall, or does the impact of landing from a fall cause the bone to break? In most cases, the force of impact precipitates the fracture, with only rare instances of a spontaneous fracture causing a fall. Hayes and colleagues (1993) showed that impact on the hip or side of the leg was the strongest determinant of fracture risk in older nursing home residents.

The energy created by a fall is much greater than that necessary to fracture a bone. Because hip fractures occur in fewer than 5% of falls, other tissues obviously absorb considerable energy. This observation is substantiated by the fact that risk of hip fracture is lower in people with a higher **body mass index** (weight/height^2). Robinovitch and colleagues (1995) concluded that although the thicker trochanteric soft tissues in obese people do cushion the fall, this force attenuation is insufficient by itself to prevent hip fracture. Additional absorptive mechanisms (e.g., breaking the fall with outstretched arm or eccentric action of the quadriceps during descent) are likely involved in preventing fracture.

Research suggests that even though osteoporotic bone exhibits diminished strength and increases the likelihood of fracture, the dynamics of the fall may be the dominant component in the incidence of fracture. Dynamic models of sideways falls predict peak trochanteric impact forces ranging from 2.90 to 9.99 kN, which are more than sufficient to cause fracture (van den Kroonenberg et al. 1995). The effects of osteoporosis must therefore be considered in conjunction with bone quality, muscular strength, soft tissue characteristics, and neuromuscular coordination. (Osteoporosis is usually associated more with bone *quantity*, whereas bone *quality* refers to the structural integrity of a given volume of bone.)

Risks and Prevention in Older Persons

Impact force from falling is the predominant mechanism of hip fracture in older persons. Fall risk is a multifactorial problem. Among the many risk factors identified by the CDC (2021) are the following:

Intrinsic Factors
- Advanced age
- Previous falls
- Muscle weakness
- Gait and balance problems
- Poor vision
- Postural hypotension
- Chronic conditions including arthritis, stroke, incontinence, diabetes, Parkinson's, or dementia
- Fear of falling

Extrinsic Factors
- Lack of stair handrails
- Poor stair design
- Lack of bathroom grab bars
- Dim lighting or glare

- Obstacles and tripping hazards
- Slippery or uneven surfaces
- Psychoactive medications
- Improper use of assistive devices

Reducing or eliminating the risk factors associated with falling is the best way to address the continuing health crisis of hip fracture in older people. Numerous strategies can be used, including the following:

- Improving lower-extremity muscle strength
- Improving balance
- Training in safe falling techniques
- Limiting alcohol use
- Using assistive devices
- Using vision and auditory aids
- Using hip pads and energy-absorbing floors
- Using nonskid footwear

More than 50% of falls are caused by tripping (Pavol et al. 1999). Among the factors contributing to falls, especially in older persons, are quick walking pace, forward-leaning posture, and weak back and knee extensor muscles (Pavol et al. 2001). Prevention strategies include improving response time, practicing recovery responses, improving muscular strength, and walking more slowly (Grabiner et al. 2002; Owings et al. 2001; Pavol et al. 1999; Pavol et al. 2001; van den Bogert et al. 2002).

In 1985, Baker wrote that there was no major health problem with more potential for improvement than hip fracture. She hoped that "our generation and those that follow will not be subject to the same likelihood of morbidity, disability, and tragic changes in lifestyle that today characterize falls in the elderly that lead to hip fracture" (Baker 1985, p. 507). Although progress has been made in the decades since Baker's hopeful statement, much remains to be done to further reduce falls and consequent hip fractures.

Hip Dislocation

Hip dislocation (luxation) happens rarely, attributable in large part to the joint's strong ligamentous support and substantial surrounding musculature. In most cases, hip luxation requires tremendous forces, so it should come as no surprise that motor vehicle crashes, falls from heights, and skiing accidents are among the most common causes. Although isolated luxations have been documented, the large forces involved often produce accompanying fracture of the acetabulum, proximal femur, or both.

Force application causing hip dislocation can arise in several ways. Force may be applied to the greater trochanter, flexed knee, foot with ipsilateral knee extended, and, rarely, posterior pelvis (Levin and Browner 1991). Depending on their location and direction, the applied forces tend to translate and rotate the femur. In most cases these forces cause posterior dislocation of the femur relative to the acetabulum.

Automobile crashes have long been the leading cause of hip dislocation, typically with concomitant injuries, most commonly acetabular fracture (Cooper et al. 2018). More than eight decades ago, Funsten and colleagues (1938) coined the term "dashboard dislocation" to describe 20 cases of traumatic dislocation. The mechanism of injury is a violent collision of the occupant's knee against the dashboard (figure 6.5), resulting in posterior hip dislocation and often accompanied by acetabular or, less commonly, femoral fracture. Not surprisingly, the victims of vehicle-related hip luxation invariably are not wearing seat belts.

Although the dashboard impact mechanism has been accepted for decades, however, Monma and Sugita (2001) more recently suggested that the mechanism of traumatic posterior dislocation of the hip (TPDH) involves the brake pedal rather than the dashboard. They hypothesized that in an impending head-on collision, the driver vigorously pushes on the brake pedal with the right hip slightly flexed, adducted, and internally rotated and that force is transmitted from the pedal through the lower extremity to the hip. In support of their hypothesis, the researchers presented evidence of 48 drivers involved in head-on collisions and noted that the right hip was involved in 45 of the cases; 31 cases did not involve knee injuries. Monma and Sugita posited that if the injury mechanism involved the dashboard, more left hip involvement would be found. Their data support a reasonable alternative explanation for TPDH in head-on collisions. Monma and Sugita (2001) suggested that the true mechanism was impossible to discern in actual accidents and may remain elusive, because in an experimental design, crash test dummies cannot actively push the brake pedal. Now more than twenty years later, advances in robotics may make it feasible to answer the question in the not-too-distant future.

In response to Monma and Sugita's hypothesis, Kumar and Parkinson (2002) posed some ques-

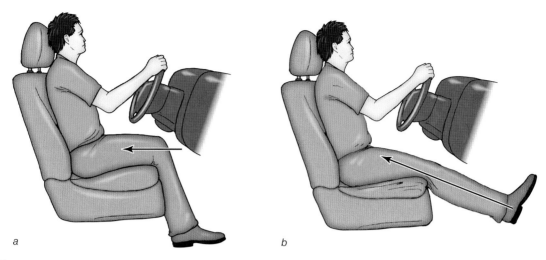

FIGURE 6.5 Mechanisms of hip luxation in a motor vehicle collision. *(a)* Hip and knee joints at 90° of flexion at impact with dashboard. *(b)* Knee fully extended to brace for axially directed impact force that drives femoral head out of the acetabulum posteriorly.

tions for consideration, including the possibility that some drivers may have used their left foot for braking, the potential influence of alcohol or drug use (which might render the driver unable to use the brake pedal), and the nonspecificity of knee injuries in 35% of the patients that may have provided clues as to the mechanisms of injury.

Although automobile collision is the predominant cause of posterior hip dislocation, these injuries have been reported in sporting contexts as well (Chudik et al. 2002). Moorman and colleagues (2003), for example, reported eight subluxations (i.e., partial dislocations) in American football players and identified the most common mechanism as a fall on a flexed, adducted hip. More recently, Bakalakos et al. (2019) described a posterior hip dislocation in a nonprofessional football (soccer) player with accompanying posterior wall fracture of the acetabulum. The mechanism was described "falling on his knee with his hip flexed." Matsumoto and colleagues (2003) also found that, although snowboarders were five times more likely to suffer hip dislocation than skiers, there was a significantly higher incidence of anterior dislocation in skiers and a higher incidence of posterior dislocation in snowboarders.

Anterior hip dislocations occur infrequently (about 10% of all hip dislocations) and usually result in anteroinferior dislocation. Forcible abduction, the primary factor in anterior dislocation, presses the femoral neck or trochanter against the rim of the acetabulum and leverages the head of the femur out of its socket. Abduction combined with simultaneous hip flexion and external rotation result in obturator-type luxation. When combined with extension, abduction causes pubic- or iliac-type luxation.

As with most injuries, there are reports of unusual mechanisms of hip injury, usually in the form of case studies. One such study reported traumatic asymmetrical bilateral hip dislocation in an 18-year-old man who was the driver of a vehicle involved in a head-on collision (Lam et al. 2001). After the initial impact, his car spun 90° and was then hit by a second vehicle going in the opposite direction. The authors reported anteroinferior dislocation of the left hip (involving abduction and external rotation) and posterior dislocation of the right hip (with adduction and internal rotation).

Interestingly, there appears to be a relation between femoral structure and the likelihood of hip dislocation. Patients suffering dislocations have significantly less anteversion than a control group; thus, it seems that patients exhibiting relative retroversion may be predisposed to hip dislocations (Upadhyay et al. 1985). Given the anatomical stability of the normal hip and the rare occurrence of hip dislocation, these observations suggest that people who experience recurrent hip dislocations have structural abnormalities (Levin and Browner 1991).

Although most hip dislocations result from trauma, there is a class of injury in young infants, known as congenital dislocation, in which the hip spontaneously dislocates. These occurrences depend

Bo Jackson

On January 13, 1991, Bo Jackson, arguably one of the greatest all-around athletes of all time, dislocated his hip while being tackled during an NFL playoff game. He reportedly said that he popped his femur back into place (i.e., self-reduction), though some doubt the report. Nonetheless, the dislocation and accompanying acetabular fracture resulted in compromised blood flow and an eventual diagnosis of avascular necrosis in Jackson's injured hip. The injury ended Jackson's professional football career and threatened to end his professional baseball career as well. He did return to play pro baseball following a hip arthroplasty, hitting a home run in his first at-bat upon returning to the Chicago White Sox in 1993. Bo was back—but only for two seasons. Jackson retired from baseball following the 1994 season. If current surgical and treatment techniques, such as hip resurfacing arthroplasty (Morse et al. 2021), had been available in 1991, Bo Jackson might have extended his professional sports career.

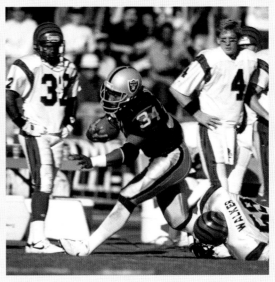

AP Photo / Al Messerschmidt

on joint position: Hamstrings acting on a flexed hip and extended knee are associated with posterior dislocation, and iliopsoas acting on an extended hip is associated with anterior dislocation.

Hip Osteoarthritis

As described in the previous chapter, osteoarthritis (OA) is the most common form of arthritis and is a disabling condition worldwide. OA of the hip, in particular, is a major cause of disability, especially in older persons. The high mechanical loads placed on this major load-bearing joint put it at risk for OA.

Hip OA affects an estimated 10 million Americans. Age is the greatest risk factor for hip OA. The exact mechanism responsible for the strong relation between OA and age remains speculative. One possible explanation implicates a molecular mechanism involving the accumulation of advanced glycation end products (AGEs) in the cartilage collagen. AGE cross-linking increases stiffness of the collagen network and may play a role in the network's decreased ability to resist damage (Verzijl et al. 2002; Verzijl et al. 2003). Other risk factors include the following:

- *Bone mineral density.* Persons with hip OA have higher bone mineral density (BMD) than age-matched controls.

- *Developmental deformities.* Childhood hip disorders can directly cause premature hip OA.

- *Sex.* There is conflicting evidence; some studies show equal prevalence in men and women, whereas other studies (e.g., Quintana et al. 2008) report slightly higher rates in women (possibly attributable to estrogen-related effects).

- *Genetic predisposition.* There is strong evidence of a genetic predisposition for OA, believed to be attributable to collagen structural defects or altered bone or cartilage metabolism linked to gene abnormalities.

- *Joint overload.* Repetitive joint overload may be a predictive risk factor for hip OA. Participation in heavy physical activity and in high joint-loading sports at an elite level is related to consequent hip OA. Farming, in particular, and occupations involving heavy lifting also are implicated. Some have hypothesized that drivers of vehicles with high levels of whole-body vibration are at higher risk of hip OA. One recent study, however, did not find evidence to support that hypothesis (Jarvholm et al. 2004).

- *Nutrition.* Limited literature is available relating hip OA to nutritional status. High intake of dietary antioxidants and anti-inflammatories may provide some protection.

• *Obesity or body mass index (BMI)*. Obesity and BMI are often cited as risk factors for osteoarthritis. Evidence of a relation between obesity and knee OA is clear. The evidence associating obesity with hip OA is less clear and remains controversial. An evaluation of nine research studies concluded that there was moderate evidence for a positive association between obesity and hip OA (Lievense et al. 2002).

• *Smoking*. Evidence is mixed, but some research (e.g., Cooper et al. 1998; Lee 2019) reports a negative association between smoking and OA (i.e., smoking associated with lower incidence of hip OA). Roux et al. (2021) found no association between cigarette smoking and joint function, pain, or need for arthroplasty, but did report fewer osteophytes in the smoking group.

• *Trauma and injury*. Hip injury is associated with unilateral OA, likely attributable to injury-induced alterations in mechanical function and resultant abnormal joint loading.

• *Comorbid conditions*. Persons with heart disease, diabetes, and obesity have higher rates of OA (Barbour et al. 2017).

Thigh Injuries

The thigh region spans the hip and knee joints and consists of the longitudinally aligned femur surrounded by three muscular compartments (anterior, medial, posterior), which are defined by their location and muscular actions (figure 6.3). The anterior compartment includes the iliopsoas (iliacus and psoas major), tensor fasciae latae, pectineus, sartorius, and quadriceps group (vastus lateralis, vastus medialis, vastus intermedius, and rectus femoris). Included in the medial compartment are the three adductor muscles (adductor longus, adductor magnus, and adductor brevis) and gracilis. The posterior compartment contains three muscles (semitendinosus, semimembranosus, biceps femoris), collectively termed the *hamstrings*.

Quadriceps Contusion

Contusions are among the most common thigh injuries, especially in contact sports such as soccer, American football, and rugby. The anterolateral aspect of the thigh is frequently involved, with resultant injury to the quadriceps muscle group. The predominant injury mechanism is compression

from a nonpenetrating blunt force, most commonly in the form of an impactor's knee, helmet, or shoulder. The resulting capillary rupture, edema, inflammation, infiltrative bleeding, and muscle crush can lead to pain, swelling, and decreased knee range of motion. Injury severity depends on impact site, level of muscle activation, age, and degree of fatigue (Beiner and Jokl 2001). Most quadriceps contusions are mild or moderate but in rare instances may be severe and accompanied by compartment syndrome (Diaz et al. 2003; Joglekar and Rehman 2009).

Despite extensive description of the symptoms, treatment, and sequelae of quadriceps contusion, little is known about the underlying pathophysiological mechanisms of tissue injury. Crisco and colleagues (1994) examined selected biomechanical, physiological, and histological aspects of contusion injuries using a reproducible, single-impact model on the gastrocnemius muscle complex of anesthetized rats. Despite some limitations and the speculative nature of extrapolating the results of animal studies to human clinical observations, the results proved enlightening. Gross observation of the muscle surface within 2 hours of injury showed muscle disruption at the center of the impact site with extensive surrounding intramuscular–interstitial hematoma but no damage at either the proximal or distal myotendinous junction. An observed increase of 11% in muscle weight was attributed to hemorrhage and edema. Acute injury also resulted in a 38% decrease in maximal tetanic tension compared with uninjured contralateral controls.

The course of acute injury, degeneration, regeneration, and normalization also was examined microscopically. At day 0, injury to the gastrocnemius was localized near the site of impact and extended deep into the muscle complex. Intracellular vacuolation of intact myofibers was present, along with gross disruption of myofibers. Two days after injury, the muscle exhibited a marked inflammatory response, with evidence of macrophages, polymorphonucleocytes, and degenerating contractile proteins. By day 7, extensive cellular proliferation of myoblasts and fibroblasts was evident. Within 24 days the injured specimens were essentially indistinguishable from control muscles.

The study by Crisco and colleagues (1994) also provided the following instructive observations with respect to impact mechanics and tissue responses:

1. Impact pressures on the skin produce stress to the underlying muscle tissue. When these

stresses exceed some critical value, damage results. The authors hypothesized that this is the mechanism of contusion injury.

2. Mass and velocity (see equation 3.24) of the impacting object alone are not sufficient to describe the event; the size and shape of the impacting object need to be considered as well.

3. Assuming that passive failure (i.e., inactive muscle loaded to failure) is indicative of tissue strength, contusion injuries may be more susceptible to subsequent strain injuries at the site of injury until fully healed.

Myositis Ossificans

Myositis ossificans (MO) is described as a "benign, solitary, frequently self-limiting, ossifying soft-tissue mass typically occurring within skeletal muscle" (Kransdorf et al. 1991, p. 1243) (figure 6.6). The most common form of MO, *myositis ossificans traumatica*, results from severe acute or repeated blunt force trauma to a muscle. The calcified mass formation within the muscle typically develops several weeks after the initial injury (e.g., Rosset-

tini et al. 2018). The most common sites for myositis ossificans are the anterior upper arm (biceps brachii) and the anterior thigh (quadriceps group) (Leadbetter 2001), and often are sport-related (e.g., soccer, American football, rugby).

Although data are limited, studies have reported the presence of calcification in 9% to 17% of patients with quadriceps contusion (Hierton 1983; Norman and Dorfman 1970; Rothwell 1982). Myositis ossificans is most commonly seen in young adults and is seen only rarely in children (Gindele et al. 2000). The advent of improved padding has limited the incidence of myositis ossificans in some sports (e.g., American football) but not in other sports (e.g., rugby) whose players wear limited protective gear (Beiner and Jokl 2002).

This pathogenic bone may form contiguously with normal bone (periosteal) or free of any connection with bone within the muscle belly. The periosteal type may appear as flat new bone formation immediately adjacent to the diaphysis or as a mushroom-shaped formation attached to the bone (King 1998).

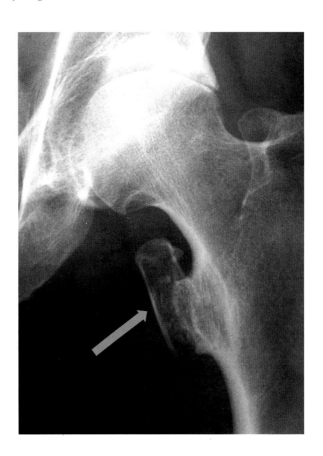

FIGURE 6.6 Myositis ossificans.
Dr P. Marazzi/Science Source

The precise mechanism of myositis ossificans remains poorly understood, but it has been theorized that the condition results from ossification of proliferating fascial connective tissue, via an inflammatory cascade and its sequelae (Walczak et al. 2015). Medici and Olsen (2012) describe the process more fully as involving endothelial–mesenchymal transition, in which vascular endothelial cells differentiate into skeletal cells (osteoblasts) that induce heterotopic (i.e., formed in an abnormal place) bone formation. Myositis ossificans typically self-resolves in a period of weeks or months, but in rare cases that do not naturally resolve, surgical excision may be indicated (Orava et al. 2017).

Femoral Fracture

Although femoral neck fractures (discussed earlier) present one of the most urgent health concerns of older people, fracture to other regions of the femur is also consequential. For example, the incidence of femoral shaft fractures in the United States is about 1:10,000 (DeCoster and Swenson 2002; Weiss et al. 2009), which translates into more than 30,000 cases annually. Most fractures of the femoral diaphysis (shaft) result from high-energy trauma and can thus be both life-threatening and a source of severe disability. A study of 520 femoral fractures, for example, reported that nearly 78% resulted from automobile, motorcycle, or automobile–pedestrian collisions (Winquist et al. 1984).

Fracture patterns typically are classified by the fracture's location, level of comminution or fragmentation, and configuration (e.g., spiral, oblique, or transverse; see figure 5.5). A long-standing system by Winquist and Hansen (1980) classifies femoral fractures by the degree of segmental lesion and comminution (figure 6.7).

- Type 0: No comminution
- Type I: Small butterfly fragment less than 25% of bone width
- Type II: Butterfly fragment 25%-50% of bone width
- Type III: Comminuted with a butterfly fragment greater than 50% of bone width
- Type IV: Severe comminution of an entire section of bone

A more current classification system, adopted by the Orthopaedic Trauma Association (OTA), classifies fractures according to the bone (e.g., tibia), location (e.g., proximal, diaphyseal, distal), fracture type (e.g., simple or multifragmented), fracture group (e.g., spiral, oblique, transverse, wedge), and subgroup (as defined for each specific bone). With this system, the OTA guidelines identify more than 100 femoral fracture classifications.

Femoral fractures in adolescents require special consideration, especially when the fracture occurs near joints or through the epiphyses. There is

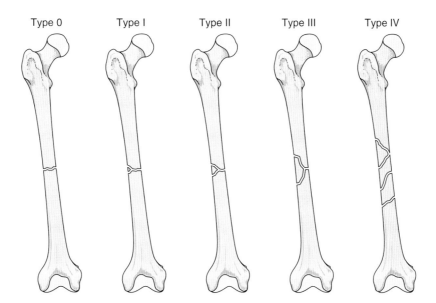

Type 0   Type I   Type II   Type III   Type IV

FIGURE 6.7   Winquist–Hansen classification of femoral fractures.

potential for long-term problems associated with abnormal growth and development following injury and the possibility of subsequent osteoarthritis.

Gunshot, or ballistic, wounds provide a unique example of injury mechanisms. Obviously bullets can strike anywhere in the body, but we restrict our attention here to those that strike the femur. Gunshot fracture patterns depend on numerous factors, including bullet diameter (caliber), velocity, weight, shape, and tumbling characteristics (Brien et al. 1995). Low-velocity bullets (<600 m/s), typical of small-caliber handguns, tend to cause splintering of the femoral diaphysis. In one study, the vast majority (93%) of low-velocity gunshot-related fractures were classified as grade III or IV (Wiss et al. 1991). In addition to causing severe bone fracture, high-velocity bullets (>600 m/s) from rifles and close-range shotgun blasts cause more extensive soft tissue damage and considerable cavitation.

Long and colleagues (2003) classified gunshot injuries (grades 1-3) based on evidence of deep soft-tissue necrosis: These authors described grade 1 injuries as having small entry and exit wounds (<2 cm) and an absence of high-energy injury characteristics, grade 2 as having small wounds (<5 cm) with evidence of high-energy injury, and grade 3 as causing muscle tissue necrosis at the fracture site.

A final example of femoral fracture mechanisms can be seen in skiing injuries. Femoral fractures, like other skiing injuries, depend on skier ability, snow conditions, level of physical conditioning, age, and mechanism of injury. Sterett and Krissoff (1994) examined 85 cases of femoral fractures in alpine skiing, focusing on the mechanisms of injury as a function of skier age. These authors reported that in the youngest age group (3-18 years), femoral fracture tended to result from torsional loading of the femoral shaft, usually while skiers were moving at high speed and catching the ski in wet or heavy snow. In older skiers, such torsional loading would more likely result in soft tissue injury at the knee. Fractures in young adults (18-45 years) occurred mostly from high-energy, direct-impact collisions with an object (e.g., rock or tree) and not surprisingly resulted in high-grade comminuted fractures. In older skiers (>45 years), the majority of fractures were localized in the hip area (femoral neck and peritrochanteric) and were caused by low-energy impact falls on firm snow.

Overall, expert skiers are less likely to sustain injuries than novices. Femoral fracture, however, is one of the few injuries more prevalent in advanced skiers than in beginners. This is attributable largely to the high energy levels required for femoral fracture. Advanced skiers typically ski at higher speeds and over more difficult terrain than novices. The greater speeds result in higher kinetic energy (see equation 3.20), which on impact is transferred to musculoskeletal tissues, including the femur.

Hamstring Strain

Muscle strain (see previous discussion of strains in chapter 5) involves injury to a musculotendinous complex. Strain is classified as an indirect injury because it results from excessive tension loads and not from direct trauma.

Injury typically occurs during forced lengthening or eccentric muscle action used to control or decelerate high-velocity movements (e.g., sprinting or throwing). Hamstring strains are common. In a study of strain injuries in Australian football from 1992 to 1999, 69% involved the hamstring group, followed by the quadriceps (17%) and calf (14%) muscle groups (Orchard 2001). Hamstring strains range from mild (slight pain, no muscle tearing) to severe (complete muscle rupture, usually resulting from an explosive movement) (Peterson and Renström 2017).

At the muscle level, animal studies implicate excessive sarcomere mechanical strain as the primary cause of injury (Lieber and Friden 2002). These authors hypothesize that excessive mechanical strain allows extracellular or intracellular membrane disruption that may permit hydrolysis of structural proteins. This leads to myofibrillar disruption and local inflammation that further degrade and weaken the muscle tissue.

The significance of active versus passive muscle as related to muscle strain has been well documented. As discussed in the previous chapter, Garrett et al. (1987) reported that force generated at failure was only 15% higher in stimulated rabbit extensor digitorum longus muscles compared with unstimulated ones, whereas the energy absorbed was approximately 100% higher at failure in the activated muscles. This suggests that any compromise in a muscle's contractile capacity (e.g., fatigue) may reduce its ability to absorb energy and increase injury risk.

In addition to fatigue, many other risk factors for muscle strain have been identified. These include muscle strength imbalances, lack of flexibility, insufficient warm-up, age, history of injury, muscle weakness, poor training, use of inappropriate drugs, presence of scar tissue, and incomplete or overly aggressive rehabilitation (Croisier et al. 2002; Opar et al. 2012; Verrall et al. 2003; Worrell 1994).

Certain muscles seem more prone to strain injury than others. Muscles in the hamstring group (semitendinosus, semimembranosus, biceps femoris), in particular, are susceptible to muscle strain. These muscles, with the exception of the short head of the biceps femoris, have biarticular function. This structural arrangement dictates that muscle length is determined by the conjoint action of the hip and knee joints. Hip flexion and knee extension each lengthen the semitendinosus, semimembranosus, and biceps femoris (long head). Simultaneous hip flexion and knee extension place the hamstrings in a lengthened state that contributes to the muscles' susceptibility to injury (figure 6.8).

The circumstances of hamstring strain in sprinters and hurdlers illustrate a common injury mechanism. Strain injury usually occurs late in the swing phase or early in the stance phase. During late swing, the hamstrings work eccentrically to decelerate both the thigh and lower leg in preparation for ground contact. Early in stance, the hamstrings act concentrically to extend the hip. Kinetic analyses have shown that peak torques at the hip and knee occur during these phases. An additional suggested contributing factor is the relatively high proportion of fast-twitch (type II) muscle fibers found in hamstring muscles, which would allow for higher levels of intrinsic force production, though one study (Evangelidis et al. 2017) failed to find support for this hypothesis. The combination of these factors places the hamstrings at elevated risk of injury in high-velocity movements.

Locating the precise injury site often proves difficult. Which of the hamstring muscles, for example, is most likely to sustain injury? Computed tomography (CT) used to localize hamstring muscle strain showed that injuries tended to be proximal and lateral within the hamstring group, most often in the long head of the biceps femoris (Garrett et al. 1989). More recent studies have confirmed that the biceps femoris is the most likely hamstring muscle to be injured. Koulouris and Connell (2003), for example, reported that 80% of 154 hamstring injuries involved the biceps femoris. The semimembranosus (14%) and semitendinosus (6%) were rarely implicated. Thelen and colleagues (2005) hypothesized that the high propensity for biceps femoris injury may be attributable, at least in part, to intermuscle differences in hamstring moment arms about the hip and knee joints.

Strain injury in the muscle–tendon unit occurs most often at the myotendinous junction (MTJ). The MTJ's microscopic structure makes it a likely site for focused mechanical loading (stress riser). The MTJ has structural features that aim to reduce the stress riser effect. First, the structural folding of the junctional membrane (figure 6.9) increases the surface area by at least 10 times and thus reduces stress. Second, the folding configuration aligns the membrane so that it experiences primarily shear forces rather than tensile forces. Third, the folding may increase the adhesive strength of the muscle cell to the tendon. Fourth, the sarcomeres near the junction are stiffer than those distant from the junction and thus have limited extensibility (Noonan

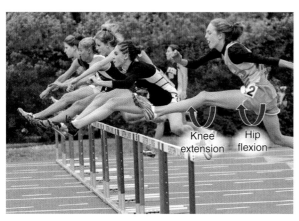

FIGURE 6.8 Simultaneous hip flexion and knee extension place the hamstring muscle group in an elongated position and increase the risk of strain injury.

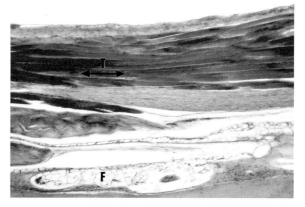

FIGURE 6.9 Electron micrograph of myotendinous junction. The muscle cell appears to interdigitate with the tendon (arrowheads). The tendon contains fibroblasts (F) and dense collagen fibers (T). (Inset bar = 3.0 μm.)

Kateryna Kon/Dreamstime.com

and Garrett 1992). Despite these structural characteristics, however, the MTJ remains a likely site of musculotendinous injury.

Recurrent hamstring strains are quite common. Among the reasons for injury recurrence are premature return to action, weakened tissues, strength deficits, and altered mechanical characteristics. Evidence suggests that previously injured hamstring muscles reach their peak torque at significantly shorter lengths than do uninjured muscles (Brockett et al. 2004; Proske et al. 2004). This shift in torque-length profile may predispose the hamstring muscles to further injury and help account for the high rate of reinjury.

Although recurrent hamstring strains are common, there is evidence suggesting that appropriate prevention programs can reduce injury risk. An effective injury prevention program may include eccentric overload (Askling et al. 2003), strength training (Croisier et al. 2002), mild eccentric exercise (Proske et al. 2004), stretching while fatigued, sport-specific training drills, high-intensity anaero-

bic interval training (Verrall et al. 2005), and combined eccentric strength and flexibility training (Arnason et al. 2008).

In summary, the hamstrings' gross and microscopic anatomical structure, biarticular arrangement, and involvement in controlling high-velocity movement all contribute to this muscle group's particular risk for strain injury. This risk can be reduced, but not eliminated, by appropriate prevention, treatment, and rehabilitation protocols.

Knee Injuries

The knee joint contains three articulating surfaces: between the patella and the femur (patellofemoral joint) (figure 6.10a) and between the medial and lateral condyles of the femur and tibia (tibiofemoral joint) (figure 6.10c). Although often classified as a hinge joint (which implies uniplanar movement), the knee is more correctly classified as double condyloid, because it has movement potential in both flexion–extension and rotation (when the knee is

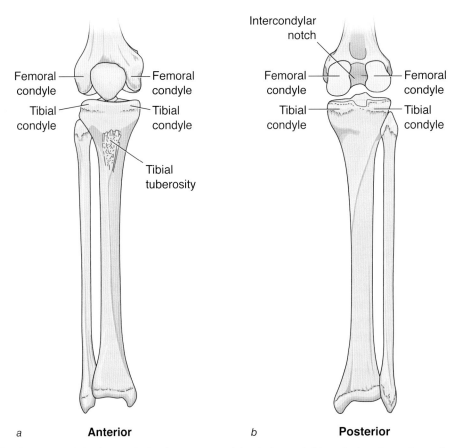

FIGURE 6.10 Anatomy of the knee: skeletal structures, *(a)* anterior and *(b)* posterior views; knee ligaments, *(c and d)* anterior and *(e)* posterior views.

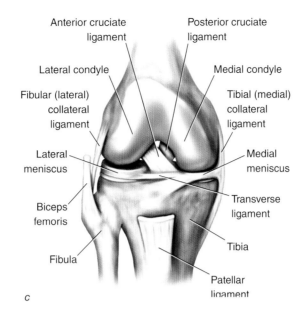

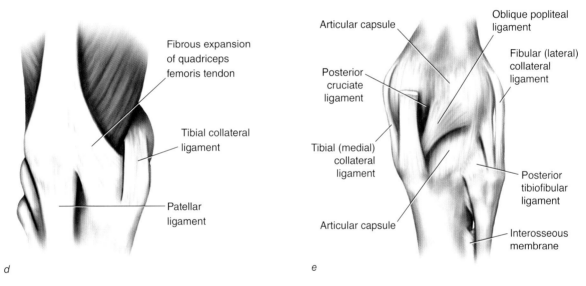

FIGURE 6.10 *(continued)*

flexed). The muscles acting about the knee joint are depicted in figure 6.3 and summarized in table 6.2.

Knee joint movement is among the most complex of all joint movements in the human body. Although its primary movement is flexion–extension, the joint's structure dictates a non-hingelike motion characterized by a variable instantaneous axis of rotation and combined rotational, sliding, and rolling movements (figures 3.19b and 3.20). In addition to serving predominant flexion and extension functions, the tibiofemoral joint also has rotational capability when the joint is flexed as well as limited varus–valgus movement.

One unique feature of the tibiofemoral joint is the so-called **screw-home mechanism** (Hallén and Lindahl 1965; Hallén and Lindahl 1966). During the final 20° to 30° of knee extension, a relative rotation (~10°) between the tibia and femur locks the joint in place at full extension by rotationally "screwing" the bones together. If the tibia is fixed, the femur rotates internally (medially) at extension. Conversely, if the femur is fixed, the tibia experiences a relative lateral rotation into place. At the initiation of flexion, the tibiofemoral joint unscrews, reversing the relative tibial and femoral rotations.

TABLE 6.2 Muscles of the Knee

Muscle	Action
Gracilis	Flexes the leg
Sartorius	Flexes the leg
Quadriceps femoris group Rectus femoris Vastus intermedius Vastus lateralis Vastus medialis	Extends the leg
Hamstring group Biceps femoris Semimembranosus Semitendinosus	Flexes the leg

As a synovial joint, the knee has a strong fibrous capsule that attaches superiorly to the femur and inferiorly to the articular margin of the tibia. Given its relatively poor bony fit, the knee relies on ligaments (along with muscles and tendons) for much of its structural strength and integrity. Among the most important—and most often injured—are the collateral ligaments and the cruciate ligaments (figure 6.10c and d). The collateral ligaments span the medial and lateral aspects of the knee and resist valgus and varus loading. *Valgus* loading at the knee results in an inward curvature of the leg at the knee (i.e., knock-kneed). *Varus* loading results in an outward curvature of the leg at the knee (i.e., bowlegged).

The lateral (fibular) collateral ligament (LCL) is extracapsular and extends from the lateral epicondyle of the femur to the lateral surface of the fibular head. The medial (tibial) collateral ligament (MCL) spans from the medial femoral epicondyle to the superomedial surface of the tibia. Unlike the LCL, the MCL is a capsular ligament that connects directly to the capsule and the medial meniscus. This structural arrangement, as discussed later, has important implications for the MCL's susceptibility to injury. Reference to the MCL as a singular ligament understates its anatomical complexity. The MCL has superficial and deep components that act synergistically to restrict knee joint movements. The posterior oblique ligament is a capsular thickening just posterior to the superficial MCL (Peterson and Renström 2017). Some authors also include the posterior oblique ligament as part of the MCL complex.

The two cruciate ligaments (figure 6.11), named for their oblique or X-shaped orientation to one

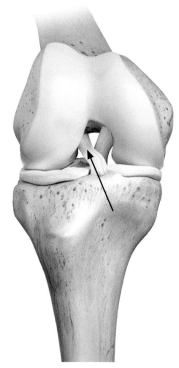

FIGURE 6.11 Anterior cruciate ligament.
SCIEPRO/SCIENCE PHOTO LIBRARY/Getty Images

another, extend between the femur and tibia. The weaker of the two, the anterior cruciate ligament (ACL), attaches proximally on the posteromedial aspect of the lateral condyle of the femur and distally on the anterior portion of the intercondylar surface of the tibia. The ACL is composed of two major bundles: the anteromedial bundle, which is tight in flexion and relatively lax in extension, and the posterolateral bundle, which is tight in extension and lax in flexion. The likelihood of injury to a bundle obviously depends on the degree of knee flexion at the time of injury. The ACL's primary function is to restrict anterior movement of the tibia relative to the femur (or, conversely, to limit posterior movement of the femur relative to the tibia) and secondarily to provide resistance to valgus, varus, hyperextension, and tibial rotation.

The stronger posterior cruciate ligament (PCL) attaches proximally on the anteromedial aspect of the medial condyle of the femur, passes medial to the ACL, and secures distally to the posterior portion of the intercondylar area of the tibia. The PCL also consists of two bundles (Anderson et al. 2012). The larger anterolateral bundle (ALB) tightens in flexion and is relatively lax in extension, and the smaller

Varus, Valgus, Vexation!

Confusing terminology is nothing new. In 1980, Houston and Swischuk published a paper, "Varus and Valgus—No Wonder They Are Confused," in the *New England Journal of Medicine,* taking issue with the use of the terms **varus** and **valgus**. Excerpts from their notes highlight the confusion caused by the use of these terms in the medical literature.

"In lecturing on pediatric bone disease to medical students, we have become painfully aware that the terms varus and valgus cause great confusion. Every year, when shown a radiograph of coxa valga and asked for the appropriate diagnosis, about a third of the students vote for coxa vara, a third for coxa valga, and a third admit that they do not know.

"Since radiologists, orthopedic surgeons, and pediatricians use varus and valgus regularly in their conversation and in their reports, we have attributed the ignorance of medical students to their inexperience, coupled with the unfortunate omission of high-school Latin as a prerequisite for entrance to medical school. This year one of us criticized the incorrect usage of the term varus in reviewing a book written by the other. This led to consultation with current and early dictionaries and to a survey of major orthopedic textbooks.

"To our surprise, we learned that the original Latin meaning of varus was knock-kneed, and of valgus bowlegged, exactly opposite to current pediatric and radiological usage.

"To show that current usage is consistently opposite to the derivation and the definitions of most dictionaries through the years, one of us checked 24 current orthopedic textbooks. . . . To our surprise, we could find a definition of the terms in only two of these texts. W.A. Crabb's *Orthopedics for the Undergraduate* (1969) provided this definition of varus: 'Deviation of a limb towards the midline of the body.' Robert B. Salter's *Textbook of Disorders and Injuries of the Musculoskeletal System* (1970) gave detailed and helpful definitions and was the only one of the 24 to mention the historical discrepancy. Under the heading, 'Varus and Valgus,' Salter stated, 'This particular pair of terms has caused more confusion than any other pair, partly because the original Latin terms had the opposite meaning to that which is now universally accepted.' All 24 texts referred to bowlegs as genu varum, even though the knee in this condition is away from the midline of the body. Thus, varus is now used to indicate a tilt toward the midline of the bone beyond the joint, regardless of whether the prefix is the name of the joint or the bone beyond it. This obviously is confusing.

"Since confusion is universal, since current usage is directly contrary to derivation, and since use of these terms in the directional sense is at the least misleading and at the most dangerous, we suggest that the simple English words bowlegged and knock-kneed are far superior to genu valgum and genu varum.

"In summary, it would seem best to avoid the terms varus and valgus altogether. Anyone who persists in using them should follow the lead of Crabbe and Salter and define them clearly. Furthermore, dictionaries should point out, in unambiguous fashion, not only the derivation of these terms, but the opposite way in which they are used in modern orthopedic literature" (pp. 471–472).

Houston and Swischuk's recommendation that use of *varus* and *valgus* be avoided has not found favor in the scientific and medical communities. Both terms still are widely used and continue to create confusion. We are tempted not to use these terms, but given their continued prevalence in the literature, we will use the terms *varus* and *valgus* in the following chapters. In so doing, however, we provide precise definitions for each term.

Adapted by permission from C.S. Houston and L.E. Swischuk, "Varus and Valgus: No Wonder They Are Confused," *The New England Journal of Medicine*, 302 (1980): 471–472. © 1980 Massachusetts Medical Society. Reprinted with permission from Massachusetts Medical Society.

posteromedial bundle (PMB) is tightest in extension and relatively lax in flexion (figure 6.12). The PCL limits posterior movement of the tibia relative to the femur (or, conversely, restricts anterior movement of the femur relative to the tibia). In addition, the PCL limits hyperflexion of the knee and assists in stabilizing the femur when a flexed knee is bearing weight.

In addition to receiving capsular and ligamentous support, the knee contains two menisci. Each meniscus is a wedge-shaped fibrocartilage pad with peripheral attachment to the joint capsule. The menisci project centrally and move freely in non-weight-bearing flexion. Both menisci have a characteristic crescent shape (figure 6.13).

The medial meniscus has a larger radius of curvature than the lateral meniscus and a semilunar shape. It averages about 10 mm in width in the posterior horn and is narrower in the middle and anterior zones. Several structural characteristics of the medial meniscus increase its risk of injury. These include its tight connection with the joint capsule and MCL and its frequent connection with the ACL.

The lateral meniscus exhibits a tighter curvature and forms a nearly closed curve. Its posterior horn is wider than the corresponding region of the medial meniscus. The lateral meniscus attaches posteriorly to the femoral intercondylar fossa and has only a loose attachment to the joint capsule and no direct connection with the LCL. The nature of these attachments allows more mobility for the lateral meniscus than for the medial meniscus in both unloaded (figure 6.14) and loaded conditions.

The patella, located between the **quadriceps tendon** and its attachment on the tibial tuberosity (via the **patellar tendon**, also known as the **patellar ligament**), increases the mechanical advantage of the knee extensor mechanism. The articulation of

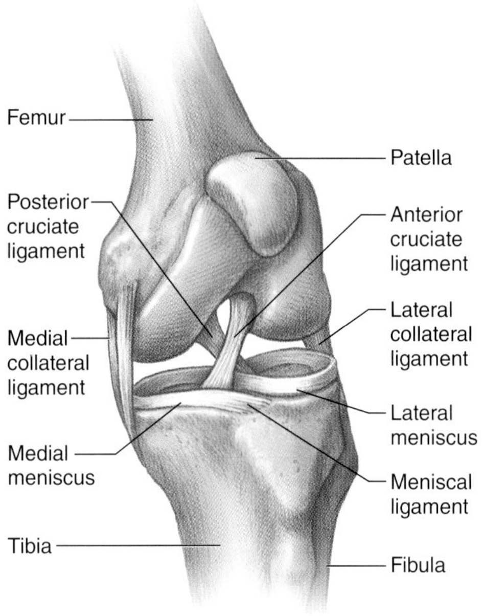

FIGURE 6.12 Posterior cruciate ligament.

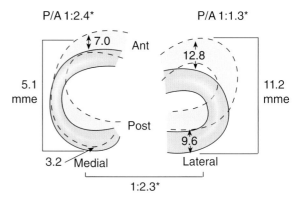

FIGURE 6.14 Diagram of mean meniscal excursion (MME) along the tibial plateau. Ant, anterior; Post, posterior; P/A, ratio of posterior to anterior meniscal translation during flexion. Values other than ratios are given in millimeters. *$p < .05$ by student's *t*-test analysis.

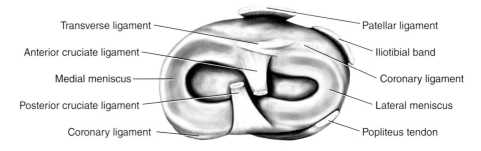

FIGURE 6.13 Menisci of the knee.

the patella with the femur forms the patellofemoral joint (PFJ). The PFJ experiences large loads when the knee is in a flexed position (figure 6.15) and thus is predisposed to certain injuries.

Posterior Cruciate Ligament Injury

Considerable literature on cruciate ligament injury has accumulated since the first description of ACL rupture in the mid-19th century and initial attempts at surgical reconstruction early in the 20th century. Growing participation in exercise and sports in recent years has presaged an increased incidence of cruciate injuries, especially in girls and women.

The prevalence of PCL injury is much lower than that of ACL injury. In fact, the PCL was once thought to be rarely injured, although advances in diagnostic techniques, along with knowledge gained from recent anatomical and biomechanical studies, have improved our understanding of PCL injury (Arthur et al. 2020; Kannus et al. 1991; LaPrade et al. 2015; van Kuijk et al. 2019; Wind et al. 2004). Of PCL injuries, fewer than half are isolated (PCL only), with the remainder (60%) involving other ligaments and knee structures (e.g., menisci) (Fanelli and Edson 1995). Combined injury to the PCL and ACL, in particular (along with potential medial and lateral ligament involvement), presents

an especially complex situation and requires careful evaluation and surgical treatment, including recognition of surgery-related considerations (e.g., graft selection and fixation methods, tunnel crowding, vascular status, surgery timing) (Duethman et al. 2020; Fanelli and Edson 2020; Stannard et al. 2020).

About half of PCL injuries are attributable to trauma resulting from motor vehicle crashes. Most of the remaining cases happen during sporting activities (40%) and industrial accidents (10%). Motor vehicle crashes and industrial accidents typically involve high-energy dynamics, whereas sport-related injuries involve relatively low-energy dynamics.

There are many mechanisms of PCL failure. Some are quite common; others are relatively rare. Five of these mechanisms are illustrated in figure 6.16. Most commonly, PCL injury occurs in vehicular crashes when an unrestrained occupant is thrown into the dashboard. With the knee flexed 90°, the PCL is taut, and the posterior capsule is lax. The impact force drives the tibia posteriorly and causes PCL rupture (figure 6.16*a*). In a fall onto a flexed knee with a plantarflexed foot, the impact occurs on the tibial tuberosity. The proximal tibia is again driven posteriorly (figure 6.16*b*). Forced knee flexion with the foot either plantarflexed or dorsiflexed can result in PCL injury (figure 6.16*c*). Sudden and violent hyperextension of the knee can cause PCL rupture, often with accompanying ACL damage (figure 6.16*d*). Rapidly shifting weight from one foot to another while rotating the body quickly on a minimally flexed knee causes internal rotation and anterior translation of the femur and resulting PCL damage (figure 6.16*e*) (Andrews et al. 1994).

Most PCL injuries involve some level of posteriorly directed tibial force. The amount of this posterior tibial force transmitted to the PCL is highly sensitive to knee flexion angle. Greater knee flexion angles increase the proportion of posterior tibial force seen in the PCL (Markolf et al. 1997). Addition of a valgus moment to the posterior tibial force greatly increases PCL forces and increases the likelihood of injury.

PCL injury can occur in the absence of posterior tibial forces, although this is relatively rare. Markolf and colleagues (1996) reported highest PCL forces with combined internal tibial torque and a varus moment at 90° of knee flexion (in the absence of posterior tibial force). As in this case, combined loading frequently increases injury risk.

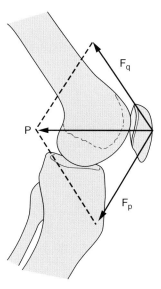

FIGURE 6.15 Patellofemoral joint reaction force (*P*). Vector *P* is formed by the vector sum of the force vector of the quadriceps tendon (F_q) and the force vector of the patellar tendon (F_p).

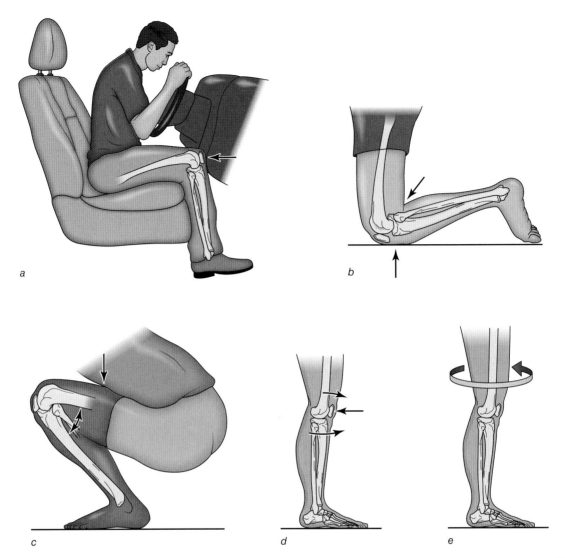

FIGURE 6.16 Mechanisms of posterior cruciate ligament injury. *(a)* Motor vehicle collision in which impact with the dashboard forces the tibia posteriorly relative to the femur. *(b)* Fall on a flexed knee pushing the tibia posteriorly. *(c)* Forced knee flexion. *(d)* Forced knee hyperextension. *(e)* Cutting (changing direction) on a minimally flexed knee.

Anterior Cruciate Ligament Injury: A Closer Look

Few injuries, if any, have received more clinical and research attention than those of the anterior cruciate ligament (ACL). Over the last 40 years, more than 15,000 research and clinical articles related to the ACL have been published. This is not at all surprising given the important role the ACL plays in knee joint function and the high economic toll associated with ACL injury. Although there is no doubt about the functional importance of the ACL, controversy persists with respect to its injury diagnosis, treatment, and rehabilitation. Because of the frequency of injury and the extensive research available, we present a more detailed review of ACL injuries than of other injuries in this chapter.

Epidemiology

Estimates of the incidence of ACL injuries varies, with reported annual rates of 1:3,000 in the United States (Miyasaka et al. 1991) and 1:5,000 in the United Kingdom (Dandy 2002). Estimates of ACL pathology in the United States vary considerably, ranging from 80,000 to 200,000 (or more) tears annually (Gornitzky et al. 2015; Griffin et al. 2000; Hubbell and Schwartz 2005; Kaeding et al. 2016; Singh 2018; Vavken and Murray 2013). Many ACL injuries are sports related, with the highest incidence seen in

15- to 25-year-olds participating in sports that involve cutting and pivoting (Griffin et al. 2000).

In light of the multifactorial nature of ACL pathology, ACL injury rates are, not surprisingly, sport and sex specific (e.g., Agel et al. 2016; Bjordal et al. 1997; Bradley et al. 2002; Montalvo et al. 2019).

Tissue Structure and Function

The ACL is a complex ligament that connects the femur and tibia (figures 6.10 and 6.11). Proximally, the ACL attaches to the medial surface of the lateral femoral condyle. The ACL attaches distally to the anterior surface of the midtibial plateau. The ACL presents through its midsubstance as a band of regularly oriented connective tissue; at its attachment sites the ACL fans out to create a broader attachment area.

The ACL consists of two bands or bundles: anteromedial (AM) and posterolateral (PL). Each band plays a unique role in stabilizing the tibiofemoral articulation. In knee flexion, the AM band is taut whereas the PL band is relatively lax. With knee extension, the PL band becomes taut and the AM band remains taut, but less so than the PL band (Dienst et al. 2002). The role of each band was confirmed in an in situ cadaver study that reported higher PL band forces than AM band forces at knee flexion angles less than 15° in response to a 110 N anterior tibial load (Allen et al. 1999).

The ACL acts as the primary restraint to anterior tibial translation (ATT). In this role, the ACL limits ATT relative to a fixed femur or, conversely, restricts posterior movement of the femur on a fixed tibia. As the primary restraint to ATT, the ACL accepts 75% of anterior forces at full knee extension and 85% at 90° of flexion (Peterson and Renström 2017).

The ACL acts as a secondary restraint to internal tibial rotation. The ACL's role as a secondary restraint to varus–valgus angulation and external rotation is less clear, although generally accepted. The ACL also works in concert with the posterior cruciate ligament (PCL) to limit knee hyperextension and hyperflexion.

Tissue Mechanics

Woo and colleagues (1991) tested paired femur–ACL–tibia complexes to assess the effect of load orientation and age on ACL mechanical properties. These authors performed tensile tests under two conditions: (1) tensile loading along the preserved anatomical axis of the ACL (anatomical orientation) and (2) tensile loading along the long axis of the tibia (tibial orientation). The researchers reported

that young specimens (22-35 years) tested in anatomical orientation had significantly higher ultimate loads (2160 N or 485 lb) than those tested in tibial orientation (1602 N or 360 lb). Specimens tested in anatomical orientation also were stiffer (242 N/mm) than those in tibial orientation (218 N/mm). The authors explained these results by noting that in anatomical orientation, more of the ACL's fibers are aligned to accept tensile loads. The authors also reported significant decreases in ultimate load and stiffness with age, regardless of load orientation.

The ACL's complex structure makes it extremely difficult to load all ligament fibers uniformly while using the entire complex. Investigators therefore have also tested each of the ACL's bands separately to assess their individual mechanical properties. For example, in tests of seven cadaveric ACL–bone units, the anterior bundles developed significantly higher moduli, maximal stresses, and strain energy densities compared with the posterior bundles (Butler et al. 1992).

Injury Mechanisms

Anterior cruciate ligament rupture can result from a variety of mechanisms (Yu and Garrett 2007). ACL injury happens most often in response to valgus loading in combination with external tibial rotation or to hyperextension with internal tibial rotation. Combined loading conditions place the ACL at great risk of injury (Markolf et al. 1995).

The first mechanism (valgus rotation) typically happens in what is termed a *noncontact injury* in which the foot is planted on the ground, the tibia is externally rotated, the knee is near full extension, and the knee collapses into valgus (Myer et al. 2005). The collapse into valgus appears to be a critical element. Evidence using biomechanical models suggests that sagittal plane knee joint forces cannot rupture the ACL during sidestep cutting maneuvers and that valgus loading is a more likely mechanism (McLean et al. 2004).

The situation is exacerbated if a force is applied to the knee while the foot is in contact with the ground (contact injury). This is common in contact sports such as American football, rugby, and soccer when another player impacts the lateral aspect of the knee, accentuating the valgus loading and rotation. Loaded knee valgus combined with external tibial rotation severely stresses the ACL. Although contact injuries are much less common than noncontact injuries (Boden et al. 2000), the added force of impact in contact injuries greatly increases the likelihood of injury occurrence and severity.

A second mechanism involves knee hyperextension with internal tibial rotation. Although a less common mechanism overall, hyperextension may be the predominant mechanism in certain populations such as basketball players or gymnasts, whose injuries often occur as they land following a jump and violently hyperextend their knee (figure 6.17a). Identification of the injury mechanism is important, because jumping-related injuries are associated with a higher incidence of meniscus tears and possible predisposition to subsequent degenerative changes (Paul et al. 2003). In rare instances, ACL rupture can be caused by excessive varus loading.

One approach to determine mechanisms of ACL injury uses magnetic resonance imaging (MRI) to assess the bone lesions associated with these injuries. Valgus loading, as previously described, results in compressive forces between the lateral femoral condyle and the lateral tibial plateau. Speer and colleagues (1992) identified an injury pattern they termed the "MRI triad"—consisting of ACL rupture, terminal sulcus osseous lesion, and bone or soft tissue injury (or both) at the posterolateral corner—and proposed several mechanisms consistent with this pattern of lesions. These mechanisms include valgus loading with subsequent lateral joint compression and hyperextension. The authors were prudent in their conclusions by making a statement that holds true for many injuries: "The great difficulty in resolving the injury into a single mechanism may be that the issue is not resolvable; that is, both mechanisms may come into

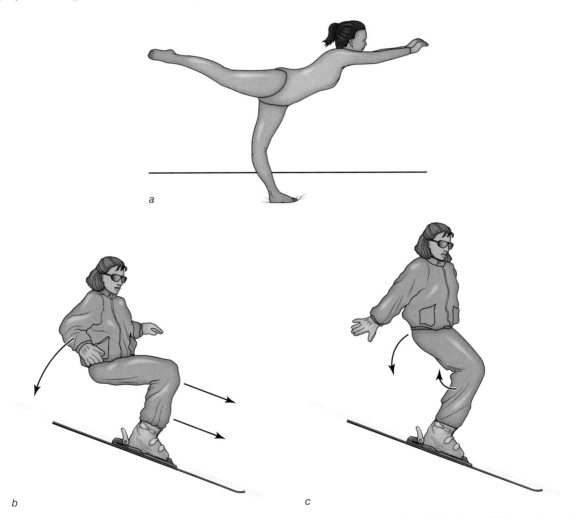

FIGURE 6.17 Mechanisms of anterior cruciate ligament injury. *(a)* Hyperextension of the knee. *(b)* Anterior cruciate ligament (ACL) injury caused by a backward fall. This mechanism forcibly pushes the tibia anteriorly relative to the femur and stresses the ACL. *(c)* Anterior cruciate ligament injury caused by the phantom foot provided by the section of ski posterior to the boot.

play depending on the nature of applied extrinsic and intrinsic forces" (Speer et al. 1992, p. 387).

A similar approach has been taken to investigate the hypothesis that for downhill skiers, various mechanisms may be involved in ACL injury. Bone bruise patterns suggest that there is less valgus loading in skiers, as evidenced by greater variety of presentation of injury across the posterior tibial rim (Speer et al. 1995). These data are consistent with observations that ACL injury in skiers is often associated with a backward fall. In such a fall, the skis and boots accelerate forward relative to the body and, because of modern boot design, take the tibia along. This creates an **anterior drawer mechanism** (i.e., anterior tibial translation) that is consistent with ACL failure in what is termed a *boot-induced* ACL injury.

A second mechanism of ACL injury unique to skiing has been described as the *phantom foot*, referring to the lever formed by the rear section of the ski that effectively forms another "foot" in the posterior direction. In a backward fall, this phantom foot levers the flexed knee into internal rotation of the tibia relative to the femur and amplifies stress in the ACL. Research has indicated that a change in ski binding design may help reduce the incidence of ACL injury resulting from the phantom foot mechanism (St-Onge et al. 2004).

Injury to either cruciate ligament may be an isolated injury or may occur in concert with damage to other structures. An example of a combination injury is one known variously as O'Donoghue's triad, or the **unhappy triad**, in which the ACL, medial collateral ligament (MCL), and medial meniscus sustain damage. This injury typically involves the valgus rotation mechanism described earlier.

Conservative Treatment

Following ACL rupture, the decision whether to pursue conservative treatment or surgical repair is difficult. In a review of studies comparing conservative versus surgical outcomes, Linko and colleagues (2005) concluded that there is insufficient evidence to determine which approach is best overall. Many factors are involved in the decision-making process, including patient age, physical condition, related injuries, and anticipated postsurgery activities. Conservative treatment usually is best suited for very young and very old patients.

The decision for surgical repair may be easier for younger persons who want to return to an active lifestyle involving sport activities. In older persons, however, the decision is more difficult, because ACL deficiency may not compromise performance of low-load activities such as walking. Pursuit of conservative (i.e., nonsurgical) treatment is not without risk, however, because ACL-deficient knees have been associated with knee instability, secondary injury to other structures (e.g., menisci, articular cartilage), and premature onset of osteoarthritis (Woo et al. 2001).

Conservative treatment initially involves control of swelling and pain management and may also include use of a brace for support, **cryotherapy**, and anti-inflammatory medications. Exercises to increase range of motion and strengthen muscles are added progressively, as are noncutting exercises such as swimming, cycling, and sagittal-plane walking and light jogging.

Surgical Repair

Surgical ACL reconstruction is indicated in many cases, especially in patients who plan to resume an active lifestyle that includes cutting or pivoting movements (e.g., tennis or basketball). The number of ACL reconstructions has increased in recent years (Dodwell et al. 2014; Lyman et al. 2009).

Once the decision in favor of surgery is made, the next critical question involves the source of the replacement tissue, or **graft**. The choices include tissue taken from the patient (**autologous graft**, or **autograft**), tissue from a cadaver (**allograft**), or artificial synthetic grafts. Although each choice has its advantages and limitations, the vast majority of ACL replacement surgeries use autografts involving either a bone–patellar tendon–bone (BPTB) graft or a hamstring (e.g., semitendinosus or gracilis) tendon (HT) graft.

A primary advantage of the BPTB approach is the presence of bone plugs at each end of the donor graft (figure 6.18). These plugs provide good fixation of the graft within the femoral and tibial attachment sites and provide initial stability. A limitation of the BPTB procedure is the morbidity seen at the graft excision site.

Proponents of the HT procedure cite the advantages of lower donor site morbidity and comparable graft strength and stiffness (using current techniques). The absence of bone plugs in the HT graft, however, reduces the initial integrity of attachment site fixation.

Debate continues as to which graft source is superior; each has its proponents. A meta-analysis of 11 reports comparing BPTB and HT found no

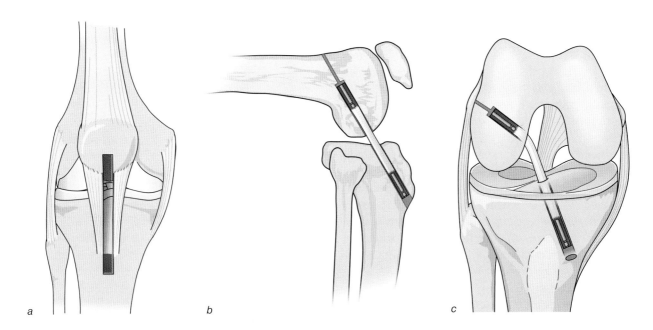

FIGURE 6.18 Surgical ACL repair with bone–patellar tendon–bone (BPTB) graft. *(a)* The graft is excised from the middle of the patellar tendon. *(b)* The graft, with bone plugs on the undersurface of each end, is threaded through an osseous tunnel created by drilling from the posterior aspect of the tibia into the inferior aspect of the femur. *(c)* The graft is fixed using screws.

significant difference between the two grafts in the incidence of instability and concluded that graft choice should be based on patient needs and the surgeon's preference and experience; before the decision is made, the patient and surgeon should consider the benefits and risks of each approach (Goldblatt et al. 2005).

Rehabilitation

Although protocols for rehabilitation after ACL reconstructive surgery must be individualized, general rehabilitative guidelines apply. These guidelines include restoration of knee joint range of motion, reduction of muscle inhibition, control of pain and swelling, muscle strengthening, and progressive return to normal activity. The time line of rehabilitation varies. Older and less conditioned patients may require longer rehabilitation than younger athletes who want to return to their sport as quickly as possible. The appropriate level of rehabilitation aggressiveness, especially for athletes, is controversial (Cascio et al. 2004).

Filbay and Grindem (2019) note that in recent decades, rehabilitation has transitioned from a time-based approach to individualized and criteria-based content and progression. They provide an exemplar framework for ACL rehabilitation with a set of recommended phases and goals for evidence-based ACL rupture rehabilitation (table 6.3).

Providing details of specific rehabilitation programs is beyond the scope of this book. The interested reader is referred to the sources listed at the end of the chapter.

Prevention

Numerous studies have noted an alarming increase in the incidence of ACL injuries in female athletes, disproportionate to those seen in men. Female intercollegiate soccer players, for example, are three times more likely to sustain ACL lesions than their male counterparts in the same sport. In basketball, the difference jumps to 3.6 times (Agel et al. 2005). Similar differences have also been reported for female competitive alpine ski racers, who are 3.1 times more likely to suffer ACL injury than males (Stevenson et al. 1998).

The reasons for these differences in ACL injury rates are unclear, and consensus now points to the multifactorial nature of the problem (Ireland 2002). Among the suggested predisposing factors have been a woman's wider pelvis, greater flexibility, less-developed musculature, hypoplastic vastus medialis obliquus, femoral notch geometry, genu valgum, and external tibial torsion. Body movement in sport, muscular strength and coordination, shoe-surface

TABLE 6.3 Evidence-Based ACL Rupture Rehabilitation Recommendations

Phase	Main goals
Preoperative phase	No knee joint effusion, full active and passive range of motion, 90% quadriceps strength symmetry
Acute phase (immediately following surgery)	No knee joint effusion, full active and passive range of motion, straight-leg raise without lag
Intermediate phase	Control of terminal knee extension in weight-bearing positions, 80% quadriceps strength symmetry, 80% hop test symmetry with adequate movement quality
Late phase	90% quadriceps strength symmetry, 90% hop test symmetry with adequate movement quality, maintain and build athletic confidence, progress sport-specific skills from closed skills with internal focus to open skills with external focus
Continued injury prevention phase	Maintain muscle strength and dynamic knee stability, manage load

Adapted from S.R. Filbay and H. Grindem, "Evidence-based Recommendations for the Management of Anterior Cruciate Ligament (ACL) Rupture," *Best Practice & Research Clinical Rheumatology* 33, no. 1 (2019): 33-47. Distributed under the terms of the Creative Commons Attribution 4.0 International License (http://creativecommons.org/licenses/by/4.0/).

characteristics, level of conditioning, joint laxity, limb alignment, and ligament size must also be considered (Arendt and Dick 1995; Ireland and Ott 2001). In addition, hormones (Dragoo et al. 2003), knee shape (van Kuijk et al. 2021), and menstrual cycle (Arendt et al. 2002; Wojtys et al. 2002) may play a role. The exact combination of factors responsible for the sex discrepancies in ACL injury remains elusive and is a subject of intense clinical debate.

Video analysis of actual ACL injuries implicates a "position of no return" that typically is seen in rapid yet awkward stops or landings (Ireland 2002). This position of no return involves loss of hip and pelvis control, internal femoral rotation, knee valgus, forward trunk lean, and external tibial rotation on a pronated foot. Avoiding the position of no return may dramatically reduce ACL injury risk.

One element of this position, knee valgus, has been studied extensively. McLean and colleagues (2005), for example, found that female intercollegiate athletes had significantly larger peak valgus moments, initial hip flexion, and internal rotation in a sidestepping task compared with male athletes. The authors concluded that a training program to reduce knee valgus loading may help prevent ACL injury, especially in females.

Emerging evidence strongly suggests that the incidence of ACL injury can be dramatically reduced through training programs targeting specific movements and neuromuscular control strategies (Hewett et al. 2005). Positive results have been reported in female athletes in soccer (Mandelbaum et al. 2005) and team handball (Myklebust et al. 2003; Petersen et al. 2005), and across sexes in skiing (Urabe et al. 2002).

One early study (Mandelbaum et al. 2005), involving a 2-year follow-up of female soccer players aged 14 to 18 who received a sport-specific training intervention, reported a 74% to 88% decrease in ACL injuries. The intervention included education, stretching, strengthening, plyometric training, and sport-specific agility drills. These elements replaced the traditional warm-up. The authors concluded that a neuromuscular training program may directly reduce the number of ACL injuries in female soccer players.

More recently, numerous studies and meta-analyses have confirmed the effectiveness of neuromuscular training (NMT) programs in reducing ACL injury risk (e.g., Myer et al. 2013; Noyes and Barber-Westin 2018; Petushek et al. 2019; Ramirez et al. 2014).

In summary, Ireland (2002) concludes,

Multiple factors are responsible for ACL tears. The key factor in the [sex] discrepancy appears to be dynamic, not static, and proximal, not distal. The factors involved in evaluating the female ACL are multiple. However, it is the dynamic movement patterns of hip and knee position with increased flexion and a coordinated proximal muscle firing pattern to keep the body in a safe landing position that are the most critical factors. An ACL injury at an early age is a life-changing event. We can very successfully reconstruct and rehabilitate an ACL, but we cannot stop there. We must now go into the prevention arena. (pp. 648-649)

Meniscus Injury

The menisci are fibrocartilaginous discs located on the medial and lateral tibial plateaus (figure 6.13).

The menisci once were believed to be useless remnants of intra-articular attachments. We now know, however, that the menisci play an essential role in maintaining normal knee function. Compression of the menisci facilitates the distribution of nutrients to adjacent structures. Of greater interest in our discussion of injury mechanisms are the mechanical functions of the menisci, specifically weight bearing, shock absorption, stabilization, and rotational facilitation. Emerging evidence shows that the mechanobiologic response of meniscal cells are critical to the physiologic, pathologic, and repair response of the meniscus, and that mechanical factors are essential to degeneration, regeneration, and health maintenance (McNulty and Guilak 2015).

The menisci transmit varying percentages of forces across the knee joint depending on knee position. In full extension the menisci accommodate 45% to 50% of the load, whereas in 90° of flexion they accept 85% of the load (Ahmed and Burke 1983; Ahmed et al. 1983). The load distribution between the medial and lateral menisci differs. Medially, the meniscus and articular cartilage share the load equally. Laterally, the meniscus assumes 70% of the load transmission (Seedhom and Wright 1974; Walker and Erkman 1975). A recent finite-element simulation study showed that longitudinal tears of the meniscal horns lead to increased magnitude and altered distribution of stress on the menisci, particularly on the posterior horn of the medial meniscus (Zhang et al. 2019) (figure 6.19).

The tibiofemoral (knee) joint experiences a combination of compressive, tensile, and shearing forces that vary according to both the individual and the task. Most obvious is the compressive force created by the ground reaction forces of contact (e.g., at foot strike in walking or running). These compressive loads are typically accommodated through a circumferential **hoop effect** in which the forces are directed

peripherally along the lines of greatest collagen fiber stiffness. Tensile forces are seen in the structures resisting **distraction** between the tibia and femur. Shear forces arise from the rotational loads in movements involving rapid change of direction.

Because meniscal injury often is caused by high rates of force application, the biphasic (i.e., solid and fluid) character of the meniscus plays a fundamental role in determining the mechanical response. Even though circumferential stresses dominate the tissue's response (attributable to the hoop effect), circumferential strains are relatively small, and the fluid phase carries a significant part of the applied load (Spilker et al. 1992).

In broad terms, meniscal injury is either traumatic or degenerative. Traumatic injuries arise from acute insult to the meniscus and are usually seen in young, active individuals. Degenerative meniscal tears are chronic injuries, usually found in older persons, and typically result from simple movements, such as deep knee bends, that load the weakened meniscal tissue. Degenerative, transverse (radial), and horizontal tears (figure 6.20a) are all more common in adults (Stanitski 2002).

The combination of complex joint movement and continuously varying loading patterns creates a formidable puzzle in terms of identifying specific meniscal injury mechanisms. Nonetheless, certain mechanisms are implicated. Damage usually occurs when the meniscus is subjected to a combination of flexion and rotation, or extension and rotation, during weight bearing and resultant shear between the tibial and femoral condyles (Sibley et al. 2012; Siliski 2003). For example, when an athlete whose foot is planted on the ground attempts a rapid change of direction, internal femoral rotation on a fixed tibia causes posterior displacement of the medial meniscus. The meniscal attachment to the joint capsule and MCL resists this movement and places the meniscus under tensile loading.

Because of structural considerations (e.g., medial meniscus attachment to other medial structures) and movement characteristics (e.g., valgus rotation loading during cutting movements), the medial meniscus is five times more likely to be injured than its lateral counterpart. External rotation of the foot and lower leg (relative to the femur) predispose the medial meniscus to injury. In contrast, internal rotation of the foot and leg makes the lateral meniscus more vulnerable.

Rapid extension of the knee generates forces sufficient to cause a longitudinal tear of the medial

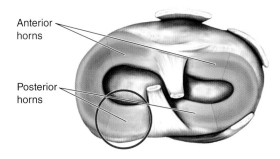

FIGURE 6.19 Posterior horns of the medial meniscus.

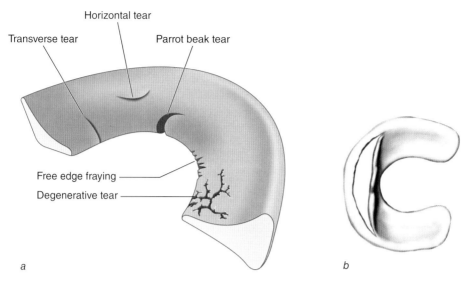

FIGURE 6.20 Types of meniscal tears: *(a)* Transverse, horizontal, parrot beak, and degenerative tears; free edge fraying. *(b)* Bucket-handle tear.

meniscus. On occasion the loading is large enough to cause a vertical longitudinal tear that extends into the anterior horn, an injury termed a **bucket-handle tear**. The bucket-handle pattern more typically arises from repeated insult to a partial tear that progresses to span a large portion of the meniscus (figure 6.20*b*). Bucket-handle tears happen predominantly in skeletally immature persons.

Predisposition to meniscal injury is activity dependent; that is, certain sports are associated with high incidence of meniscal injury. Leading the list is soccer, in which players experience frequent collisions with opponents and often change direction and body position while their cleats are embedded in the turf. Meniscal injury also is common in track and field (e.g., knee torsion in the shot put or discus) and skiing (e.g., ski slippage or catching that imparts a sudden twist to the knee). Occupations involving sustained or repeated squatting (e.g., mining, carpet laying, or gardening) are also implicated in meniscus injury, often attributable to the degenerative processes that accompany prolonged knee flexion and its attendant structural loads.

Collateral Ligament Injury

Injury to the medial collateral ligament (MCL) complex is quite common, with involvement of the lateral collateral ligament (LCL) much less frequent. Both injuries result from sudden and violent loading. Proper physical examination, in conjunction with

MRI evaluation, is required for treatment and rehabilitation of both MCL and LCL injuries (Quarles and Hosey 2004).

Medial Collateral Ligament

The medial collateral ligament (MCL) is a primary knee stabilizer, and is the most commonly injured of the knee's ligaments (Andrews et al. 2017). Impact on the lateral side of the knee causes knee valgus and tensile loading of the medial aspect (figure 6.21*a*), a mechanism that can produce MCL injury. The MCL is most effective in resisting valgus loading when the knee is flexed 25° to 30° (Swenson and Harner 1995). Other structures play a relatively greater role when the knee is at full extension than when the knee is partially flexed. Each part of the MCL is differentially loaded at varying angles of knee flexion. At 5° of knee flexion, the superficial MCL accounts for 57% of medial stability, with the deep MCL at 8% and the posterior oblique ligament at 18%. When the knee is further flexed to 25°, the superficial MCL increases to 78% while the deep MCL and posterior oblique each drop to 4% (Peterson and Renström 2001).

The role of the MCL in resisting valgus loading has been demonstrated experimentally (Grood et al. 1981; Piziali et al. 1980; Seering et al. 1980). Research suggests that the MCL is the primary valgus restraint, with only secondary involvement provided by the cruciate ligaments. In cases of

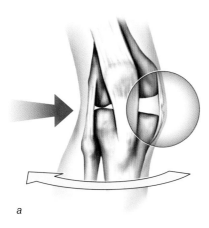

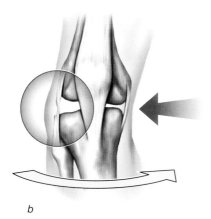

FIGURE 6.21 Collateral ligament injury at the knee. *(a)* Valgus loading of the medial collateral ligament. *(b)* Varus loading of the lateral collateral ligament.

isolated MCL failure, however, residual structures, particularly the ACL, are able to resist varus–valgus moments (Inoue et al. 1987). Although most MCL injuries are acute and traumatic, overuse syndromes also have been implicated, specifically associated with the whip-kick technique used by swimmers performing the breaststroke.

Lateral Collateral Ligament

LCL injury usually results from varus loading, often in combination with hyperextension. Varus loading happens when an impact is applied to the knee's medial aspect while the foot is planted on the ground (figure 6.21*b*). The varus loading creates tensile forces in the lateral knee structures. Given its extracapsular structure, the LCL is more likely than the MCL to sustain isolated injury. Nonetheless, combined injury to the LCL and one of the cruciate ligaments is not uncommon.

The degree of impact affects the progression of injury. Moderate impact results in isolated LCL rupture. Violent impact causes LCL rupture in concert with ACL failure. Extremely violent impacts rupture the LCL, ACL, and PCL (Peterson and Renström 2017).

Knee Extensor Disorders

The knee joint complex forms the critical middle link in the kinetic chain of the lower extremity, and its loading and motion characteristics dictate effective limb function. Aberrations in any of the many functional components of the knee joint complex increase injury risk. Arguably the most important component is the so-called **knee extensor mechanism**, which consists of the quadriceps muscle group, the patellofemoral joint, and the tendon group (quadriceps tendon and patellar tendon) connecting these elements.

The patella serves as the central structure in the knee extensor mechanism. In that role it acts as a fulcrum, or pivot, to enhance the mechanical advantage of the quadriceps during knee flexion and extension. The patella effectively displaces the tendon line of action away from the instantaneous joint center (axis) and thus increases the moment arm (figure 6.22). A given force then produces a greater moment of force or torque.

Force created by the quadriceps is transmitted through the quadriceps tendon and patellar tendon (also called *patellar ligament*) to the tibial tuberosity. Past researchers erroneously assumed that the force in the quadriceps tendon (F_Q) was the same as that in the patellar tendon (F_P). However, this has been disproven by research showing that F_Q and F_P are not equal (e.g., Ahmed et al. 1987; Huberti et al. 1984). The actual forces in each tendon depend on the knee joint angle (figure 6.23). Tendofemoral contact in positions of extreme flexion (e.g., in a deep squat) carries a significant portion of the contact force, thus reducing the load on the patella. In addition, across the range of knee motion (0°-60°), the F_P/F_Q ratio was significantly greater for axial loading than for multiplane loading, suggesting that loading orientation affects the transfer of forces from the quadriceps tendon to the patellar tendon (Powers et al. 2010).

Patellofemoral Disorders

Patellofemoral pain (PFP) is one of the most common lower-extremity pathologies. Despite its prevalence, controversy persists regarding its cause, evaluation,

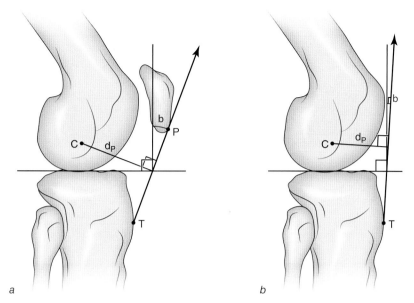

a   b

FIGURE 6.22 Effect of the patella in increasing the mechanical advantage of the knee extensor mechanism. *(a)* The patella effectively moves the tendon line of action away from the knee joint instantaneous center (axis of rotation, *C*), increasing the moment arm (d_p) of the quadriceps group and thus enhancing its mechanical advantage. *(b)* Without a patella, the moment arm (d_p) is shorter, the angle of pull (β) is smaller, and the mechanical advantage is reduced. *T* is the patellar tendon attachment site at the tibial tuberosity.

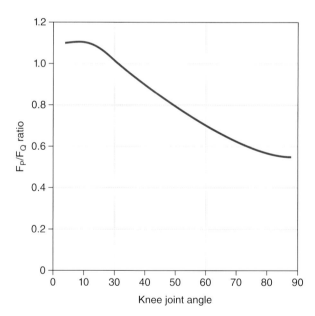

Knee joint angle

FIGURE 6.23 Ratio of patellar tendon force (F_P) to quadriceps tendon force (F_Q) as a function of knee flexion angle. Generally, in early flexion (0°-30°), the F_P/F_Q ratio is slightly above 1.0, indicating that $F_P > F_Q$. Beyond about 30° of knee flexion, the ratio drops below 1.0 (i.e., $F_Q > F_P$).

and treatment, and much remains to be done to identify the mechanisms involved. Powers (2003) suggested that comprehensive evaluation of PFP should include consideration of hip–pelvic motion and foot–ankle motion and should not focus solely on structures of the knee or events involving the knee.

As forces are transmitted through the knee extensor mechanism, a component of the force is directed through the patella toward the joint center and pushes the patella against the femur. Near full extension, the patella rides high on the femur. As the knee flexes, the patella slides into the intercondylar groove. This movement of the patella along the femur is referred to as **patellar tracking**.

Effective patellar tracking depends on congruence between the patella and femur. This congruence is typically measured by congruence angle, lateral patellofemoral angle, and patellar tilt angle (figure 6.24). Caution is warranted in interpreting these measures based on osseous landmarks, because the surface geometry of the cartilage may not match the osseous morphology (Staubli et al. 1999).

Proper tracking also depends on a complex interaction of muscle forces (i.e., vector sum of the individual force vectors of the vastus medialis, vastus lateralis, vastus intermedius, and rectus femoris), **patella alta** (patella positioned abnormally high on the femur), geometry of the intercondylar groove, and other forces (e.g., retinacula) and structural considerations (e.g., **Q angle**; figure 6.25). As the patella moves, contact pressures develop between

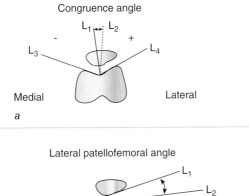

Congruence angle

Medial

Lateral

a

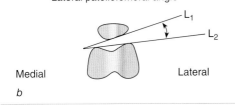

Lateral patellofemoral angle

Medial

Lateral

b

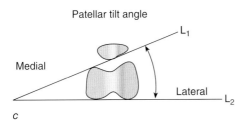

Patellar tilt angle

Medial

Lateral

c

FIGURE 6.24 Patellofemoral angle measures. *(a)* Congruence angle (between lines L_1 and L_2). *(b)* Lateral patellofemoral angle. *(c)* Patellar tilt angle.

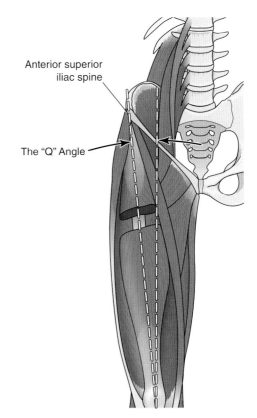

Anterior superior iliac spine

The "Q" Angle

FIGURE 6.25 Quadriceps (Q) angle, measured as the angle formed by a line drawn from the anterior superior iliac spine to the midpatella and a line drawn from the midpatella to the tibial tuberosity.

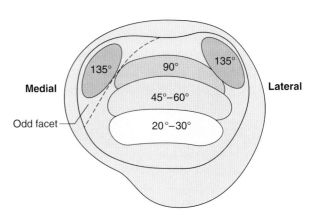

FIGURE 6.26 Patellofemoral contact areas as a function of change in degree of knee flexion. As the knee is flexed from full extension (0°) through 90°, the contact area migrates from the inferior retropatellar surface to the superior region. At 135° of flexion, the contact area is on both the superolateral surface and the medial odd facet.

the patella and femur. These pressures, as well as the contact area and contact force, vary with the degree of knee flexion. In one of the earliest studies of patellofemoral dynamics, Huberti and Hayes (1984) reported increases in contact area, contact pressure, and contact force as the knee flexes from 20° to 90°.

Patellar movement simultaneously changes the location of the patellofemoral joint reaction force and the moment arm about the instantaneous knee joint axis. As the patella slides down within the groove, the retropatellar contact area changes (figure 6.26). Brechter and colleagues (2003) established the efficacy of using MRI to quantify patellofemoral joint contact area. MRI has also been used to confirm the results of earlier studies (e.g., Hungerford and Barry 1979) reporting that as the knee flexes, patellofemoral joint contact area increases and migrates superiorly on the retropatellar surface as the patella glides deeper into the intercondylar groove (Salsich et al. 2003). Most of the increase in contact area happens in the first 45° to 60° of flexion (Salsich et al. 2003). The increase

in contact area permits wider distribution of the escalating contact forces and thus helps moderate the patellofemoral joint pressure (and stress). At knee angles greater than 60°, contact area levels off and may actually decrease with extreme knee flexion at 120° under certain loading conditions (Huberti and Hayes 1984).

Patellofemoral joint stress and contact area have important clinical ramifications, as demonstrated in the following studies:

- Brechter and Powers (2002) reported significantly higher patellofemoral joint stress (attributable to smaller contact area) in subjects with PFP compared with subjects without pain.

- Studies of the influence of patella alta on patellofemoral joint stress have shown that subjects with patella alta had significantly less contact area and greater patellofemoral stress compared with controls (Ward and Powers 2004; Ward et al. 2007).

- Salem and Powers (2001) studied collegiate female athletes performing squats to three depths (70°, 90°, 110° of knee flexion) using 85% of their one repetition maximum (1RM). The results suggested that peak patellofemoral joint reaction force and patellofemoral joint stress do not vary significantly between 70° and 110°. Thus, the authors concluded that deep squats are no more challenging to the patellofemoral joint than shallow squats.

- Besier et al. (2005) reported that in weight-bearing conditions, patellofemoral contact areas increased by 24%, and concluded patellofemoral contact area varies across sex, knee flexion postures, and physiologic loading conditions.

- Studies using MRI have reported changes in articular cartilage thickness and deformation (e.g., Freedman et al. 2015; Lange et al. 2019) and joint congruence (e.g., Clark et al. 2019) throughout ranges of knee flexion.

- Multiplane loading of the knee extensor mechanism overestimates contact pressure at 0° of knee flexion (i.e., full extension) and underestimates contact pressure at 90° of knee flexion when compared to axial loading, and loading of individual vasti muscles affects patellar kinematics (Powers et al. 1998).

As stated, controversy still exists regarding the causes of patellofemoral pain. Powers (2003, p. 639) suggested that "abnormal motion(s) of the tibia and femur in the transverse and frontal planes are believed to have an effect on patellofemoral joint mechanics and therefore PFP." Thomeé and colleagues (1995, p. 237) suggested that "chronic overloading and temporary overuse of the patello-femoral joint, rather than malalignment, contribute to patellofemoral pain."

Dye (2004) took issue with the malalignment theory for PFP, asking,

———

If the presence of malalignment is crucial in the genesis of anterior knee pain, why does one find patients with bilateral radiographically determined patellofemoral malalignment (i.e., patellar tilts) with only unilateral symptoms? Why do more than 90% of patients with patellofemoral pain who have a diagnosis of malalignment as the cause have a successful response to conservative therapy, even though there has been no "correction" or restoration of the supposed underlying indicators of malalignment (e.g., a high Q angle or a shallow trochlea)? . . . One can logically assume that the perception of patellofemoral pain, in most instances, is a function of nociceptive neurological output of any combination of innervated patellar and peripatellar tissues. (pp. 5-7)

In summary, the integrity of patellofemoral movement is dictated by the neuromechanical synergy between patellofemoral tracking, patellofemoral contact pressures, and neuromotor control of patellofemoral agonists. The precise relation between patellofemoral movement and patellofemoral pain remains unclear. Given the multifactorial nature of PFP, controversy about its source will persist (e.g., Powers et al. 2017; Crossley et al. 2019).

Disturbance of patellofemoral integrity often leads to injuries. Injuries to the knee extensor mechanism result from direct trauma, indirect trauma, or chronic overuse. Whatever the cause, there is little doubt that the injuries are both myriad and prevalent.

In chapter 5, we cautioned against the use of nonspecific injury descriptors. Two such terms commonly used to referring to patellofemoral pathologies are *jumper's knee* and *chondromalacia patella*. The former term refers to tendon pain of the knee extensor mechanism developed through repeated jumping. We suggest the use of more clinically useful terms that identify the location and condition of the involved tissue (e.g., *quadriceps tendinitis, patellar tendinitis, apophysitis of the tibial tuberosity,* or *Osgood–Schlatter disease*).

The second term, chondromalacia patella, has evolved into an all-too-common descriptor for generalized patellar pain; however, the term is best reserved to specifically describe the degeneration of retropatellar articular cartilage. Once believed to be a primary condition of unknown etiology, **chondromalacia patella** is now thought to most often occur secondary to other mechanisms, including both traumatic (e.g., patellar fracture) and chronic (e.g., patellar malalignment, chronic subluxation, pathological patellar tracking) events.

Quadriceps Tendon and Patellar Tendon Ruptures

Extreme forces or continued mechanical insult to an already weakened knee extensor mechanism may lead to tendon rupture (see Case Study: Patellar Tendon Rupture). Quadriceps tendon rupture typically occurs in people over age 40 and is localized at the osteotendinous junction of the superior patellar pole. Calcification at the rupture site suggests that quadriceps tendon rupture tends to occur in areas of previous microtrauma. In contrast, patellar tendon ruptures tend to afflict those younger than 40, most often tearing at the inferior patellar pole.

The injury mechanism typically involves a violent quadriceps contraction against resistance at the knee and requires substantial loads to induce rupture. Although rare, several cases of bilateral patellar tendon ruptures have also been reported in the literature (e.g., Divani et al. 2013; Foley et al. 2019; Kellersmann et al. 2005; Rose and Frassica 2001; Sibley et al. 2012; Tarazi et al. 2016). Some of these injuries have identifiable mechanisms (e.g., jumping, tripping, or specific athletic tasks) and predisposing risk factors (e.g., systemic disease or steroid use), whereas others appear as idiopathic events in otherwise healthy individuals.

Osgood–Schlatter Disease

Osgood–Schlatter disease (OSD)—named after physicians Robert Bayley Osgood and Carl Schlatter, who in 1903 simultaneously and independently identified the disorder (Nowinski and Mehlman 1998)—is a **traction apophysitis** of the tibial tuberosity. Commonly found in adolescent athletes, OSD is characterized by inflammation of the bone where the patellar tendon attaches to the tibial tuberosity (figure 6.27). OSD is distinguished from patellar tendinitis, which manifests as inflammation of the patellar tendon near its attachment at the tibial tuberosity.

The injury mechanism most associated with OSD is repetitive high-load quadriceps action in adolescents during periods of rapid growth (Peterson and Renström 2017). Sports involving jumping and running (e.g., basketball and volleyball) are commonly implicated. In addition to activity, anatomical structure, body weight, muscle tightness and

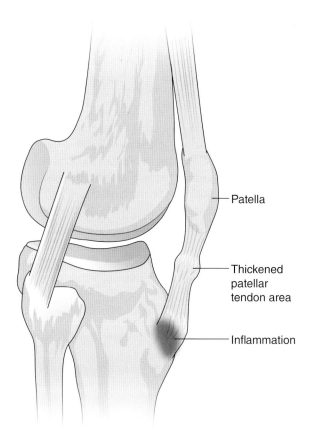

FIGURE 6.27 Knee with Osgood–Schlatter disease.

weakness, and hamstring tightness may play a role in the risk of OSD. Demirag and colleagues (2004) concluded that OSD may be caused, at least in part, by a patellar tendon that attaches more proximally and across a broader area of the tibia.

Magnetic resonance imaging has been used to describe the progression of OSD: swelling (edema) and inflammation at the tibial tuberosity, followed by tears at the secondary ossification center and ossicle formation from a partially avulsed portion of the tuberosity (Hirano et al. 2002).

OSD most commonly happens in boys between the ages of 10 and 16 and usually disappears when the adolescent reaches full maturity. However, this sex difference may be decreasing as female participation in high-impact sports (e.g., basketball, volleyball) increases (Ladenhauf et al. 2020). Although most studies report that OSD is self-limiting, one study suggested that persons with a history of OSD may experience a higher level of knee disability in later years than those with no history of OSD (Ross and Villard 2003).

Iliotibial Band Syndrome

The iliotibial band (ITB) is a thickened band of fascial tissue spanning from the iliac crest (with partial insertion from the tensor fasciae latae) to the lateral tibial condyle (at Gerdy's tubercle) (figure 6.28). In full extension (0° of flexion), the ITB lies anterior to the lateral femoral epicondyle. As the knee flexes through about 30°, the ITB passes over the lateral femoral epicondyle to a position posterior to the epicondyle (figure 6.28). The area where the ITB rubs on the lateral epicondyle is sometimes referred to as the *impingement zone* (Farrell et al. 2003).

When the ITB passes over the lateral femoral epicondyle, friction is created between the ITB and the lateral epicondylar surface, and with repeated flexion–extension cycles, the ITB can become irritated, resulting in a painful inflammatory condition called **iliotibial band syndrome** (ITBS), also termed *iliotibial band friction syndrome* (ITBFS). However, some dispute the role of friction as the causal factor in ITBS, and instead implicate fat compression beneath the tendon tract as a more likely cause (e.g., Fairclough et al. 2006).

ITBS is commonly found in runners, cyclists, and military personnel (Kirk et al. 2000), whose knees experience repeated flexion–extension through limited range of motion. In a study of military recruits, ITBS was associated with running and abrupt increases in training volume and was second only to ankle sprains as the most frequent injury diagnosis (Almeida et al. 1999).

In cycling, the knee moves through the 30° flexion range with each pedaling cycle. Farrell and colleagues (2003) found that foot–pedal forces at the impinge-ment zone during cycling were only 18% of those found at the foot–ground interface in running, and these researchers concluded that repetition appears to be more important than force levels in hastening the onset of ITBS. The authors also noted that ITBS may be aggravated by improper cycle seat height, anatomical differences, and training errors.

Excessive foot pronation has been associated with ITBS (Peterson and Renström 2017), but some (e.g., Khaund and Flynn 2005) contend that research support for this theory is lacking. Other potential risk factors include ITB tightness; high running mileage; interval training; muscle weakness in the knee extensors, knee flexors, and hip abductors; genu varum (bowleggedness); tibial rotation; and leg-length discrepancy (Khaund and Flynn 2005; Peterson and Renström 2017). In addition, Louw and Deary (2014) identify decreased rear foot eversion, tibial internal rotation and hip adduction angles at the knee, and decreased hip abduction and adduction ranges of motion as potential factors associated with ITBS. Evidence for the role of hip abductor weakness as a factor in ITBS is limited or conflicting (van der Worp et al. 2012).

Lower-Leg Injuries

The lower leg (also called *leg* or *shank*) spans the knee and ankle joints and contains two longitudinally aligned bones, the tibia (medial) and fibula (lateral). Four muscle compartments (anterior, lateral, superficial posterior, deep posterior) surround these bones, with tight fascia enclosing each compartment. The anterior compartment contains the

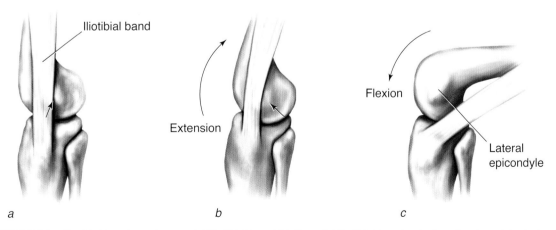

FIGURE 6.28 Iliotibial band syndrome. *(a)* Iliotibial band friction. *(b)* Iliotibial band anterior of epicondyle during knee extension. *(c)* Iliotibial band rubs over epicondyle and moves posterior to the epicondyle when knee is flexed more than 30°.

Case Study: Patellar Tendon Rupture

Musculoskeletal injuries typically do not happen under conditions that permit quantitative assessment of the injury dynamics. In most cases, clinicians and researchers are limited to qualitative evaluation. On rare occasions, however, circumstances do allow for quantitative examination. One such case occurred when a weightlifter's patellar tendon ruptured during a national weightlifting competition that was being filmed for biomechanical analysis (Zernicke et al. 1977).

The world-class light heavyweight lifter was attempting to complete the second phase of a clean-and-jerk movement using 175 kg (385 lbs) when his right patellar tendon ruptured. The tendon was torn completely, with evidence of damage at the distal pole of the patella and at the patellar tendon insertion on the tibia. Using a multilink, rigid-body model, Zernicke and colleagues (1977) were able to estimate the tensile force in the tendon at the instant of rupture. The force was approximately 14.5 kN, or more than 17.5 times the lifter's body weight.

This exceptional example highlights the complex dynamics of injury and provides evidence of the high stresses applied to and tolerated by biological tissues and the importance of loading rate on tissue response to mechanical loading.

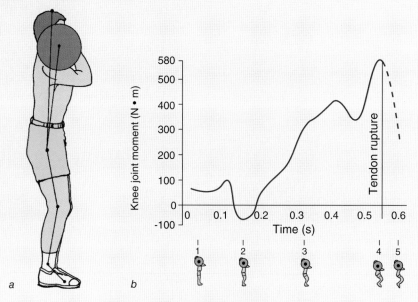

Patellar tendon rupture. *(a)* Five-segment, rigid-body model of weightlifter. *(b)* Mean resultant knee joint moments from the beginning of the jerk movement until after tendon failure.

(a) Adapted by permission from R.F. Zernicke, J. Garhammer and F.W. Jove, "Human Patellar-Tendon Rupture," *The Journal of Bone and Joint Surgery* 59, no. 2 (1977): 180. *(b)* Adapted by permission from R.F. Zernicke, J. Garhammer and F.W. Jove, "Human Patellar-Tendon Rupture," *The Journal of Bone and Joint Surgery* 59, no. 2 (1977): 181

tibialis anterior, extensor hallucis longus, extensor digitorum longus, and peroneus tertius. The lateral compartment contains the peroneus longus and peroneus brevis. The largest compartment in terms of muscle mass is the superficial posterior compartment, which contains the gastrocnemius and soleus (together termed the *triceps surae*) and plantaris. The deep posterior compartment houses the flexor hallucis longus, flexor digitorum longus, and tibialis posterior (figure 6.29). The actions of

the foot and ankle muscles are summarized in table 6.4.

Compartment Syndrome

Acute injury or chronic exertion often increases fluid accumulation within muscle compartments of the arms, feet, and legs. The excess fluid may be attributable to hemorrhage, edema, or both. Given the relative inextensibility of the surrounding fascia, the fluid increase results in greater compartmental

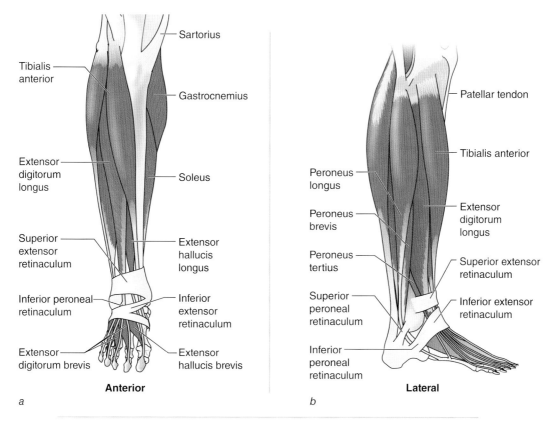

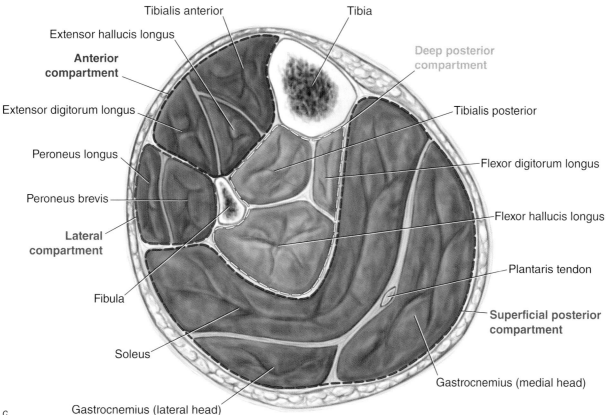

FIGURE 6.29 Muscles of the lower leg. *(a)* Anterior view. *(b)* Lateral view. *(c)* Four compartments of the lower leg.

TABLE 6.4 Muscles of the Lower Leg and Ankle

Muscle	Action
Anterior compartment	
Tibialis anterior	Dorsiflexes the ankle and inverts the foot
Extensor hallucis longus	Dorsiflexes the ankle and inverts the foot
Extensor digitorum longus	Dorsiflexes the ankle and everts the foot
Peroneus tertius	Dorsiflexes the ankle and everts the foot
Lateral compartment	
Peroneus longus	Plantarflexes the ankle and everts the foot
Peroneus brevis	Plantarflexes the ankle and everts the foot
Superficial posterior compartment	
Gastrocnemius	Plantarflexes the ankle and flexes the leg
Soleus	Plantarflexes the ankle
Plantaris	Plantarflexes the ankle and flexes the leg
Deep posterior compartment	
Popliteus	No action at ankle or foot; flexes and medially rotates the leg
Flexor hallucis longus	Plantarflexes the ankle and inverts the foot
Flexor digitorum longus	Plantarflexes the ankle and inverts the foot
Tibialis posterior	Plantarflexes the ankle and inverts the foot

pressure. This creates a **compartment syndrome** (CS), defined as "a pathologic condition of skeletal muscle characterized by increased interstitial pressure within an anatomically confined muscle compartment that interferes with the circulation and function of the muscle and neurovascular components of the compartment" (Garrett 1995, p. 48).

From a mechanical perspective, compartment syndromes are a consequence of the relations among mass, volume, and pressure (see chapter 5). Increasing the mass within a fixed volume increases the internal pressure. This is the essence of a compartment syndrome.

The mechanism of CS may be either chronic (*chronic compartment syndrome*, also *chronic exertional compartment syndrome*) (e.g., Buerba et al. 2019) or acute (*acute compartment syndrome*, also *traumatic compartment syndrome*) (e.g., Schmidt 2017). Many conditions can lead to a compartment syndrome, including soft tissue contusion, crush, tibial fracture, bleeding disorders, venous obstruction, arterial occlusion, burn, prolonged compression after drug overdose, surgery, apparel (e.g., medical antishock trousers), and excessive exercise.

In the lower leg, any of the four muscle compartments (anterior, lateral, superficial posterior, deep posterior) may be affected. Most commonly,

the anterior compartment is involved (Schepsis et al. 2005), with all muscles in the compartment affected. In rare instances, an isolated muscle (e.g., tibialis anterior) is involved (Church and Radford 2001).

Increased compartmental pressure compromises vascular and neural function and sets the stage for ischemia and a self-perpetuating cycle of fluid accumulation and restricted flow. The situation is exacerbated by the mechanical properties of the fascia, which has been shown to increase in thickness and stiffness in response to chronic compartment syndrome (Hurschler et al. 1994). The situation is also worsened by a decrease in compartment volume, as might be caused by compression wraps or tight clothing.

Sufficiently large compartment pressures result in vessel closure and potentially catastrophic physiological consequences. Venous collapse severely reduces blood return and leads to capillary congestion and decreased tissue perfusion. Local tissues then suffer the consequences of hypoperfusion (e.g., ischemia and eventual necrosis), necessitating eventual amputation.

Transient increases in compartment pressures are normally seen in response to exertion. In people without chronic compartment syndrome (CCS), resting pressures vary, ranging from 0 to 20 mmHg (Dayton and Bouche 1994). During exertion, pressures may exceed 70 mmHg but quickly return to resting levels within minutes of exercise cessation. A person with CCS, in contrast, may exhibit resting pressures of 15 mmHg that climb to more than 100 mmHg during exercise, with prolonged postexercise decline (figure 6.30).

Relief from CCS is achieved surgically by fascial incision (fasciotomy) to release the compartment and effectively increase its volume and reduce internal pressure. Some controversy exists over the threshold pressure above which fasciotomy is indicated. Suggested values range from 30 to 45 mmHg. However, many other factors should be considered as well:

- Intracompartmental pressures do not measure neuromuscular ischemia. Ischemic development depends on both the magnitude and duration of the elevated pressure.
- Patient tolerance to ischemia may vary.
- Injured muscle may be less tolerant of ischemia and elevated pressure than uninjured muscle (Gulli and Templeman 1994).

Medial Tibial Stress Syndrome

Medial tibial stress syndrome (MTSS) is described as exercise-induced pain along the posteromedial

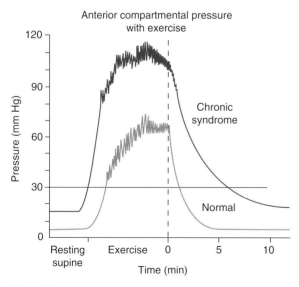

FIGURE 6.30 Anterior compartment pressures recorded in a patient with chronic anterior compartment syndrome and in a normal subject.

Reprinted by permission from S.J. Mubarak, *Compartment Syndromes and Volkmann's Contracture* (Philadelphia, PA: W.B. Saunders Company, 1981), 218.

tibial border, with recognizable pain upon palpation of the posteromedial tibial border over a length of more than 5 cm (Moen et al. 2009; Yates and White 2004). The underlying pathology for MTSS remains equivocal (Winters 2020). Early evidence suggested that MTSS may be associated with fasciopathy (Johnell et al. 1982), but more recent reports have implicated bone overload and lower regional bone mineral density (Magnusson et al. 2001), as well as tibial bending during chronic weight-bearing activities (Beck 1998).

MTSS results from excessive tensile forces applied to the fascia by the eccentric action of musculotendinous units, most often the soleus and flexor digitorum longus. Controversy exists over whether the tibialis posterior may be involved. The condition initially manifests as fasciitis and with continued loading may progress to periostitis and ultimately to diminished bone mineral density in the affected area (Magnusson et al. 2001).

MTSS often is seen in runners, dancers, and military personnel, and is the most common source of exercise-induced lower-leg pain. Yates and White (2004) reported a MTSS incidence of 35% in a group of 124 naval recruits undergoing a 10-week basic training program. Women recruits were more likely than men (53% vs. 28%) to develop MTSS.

MTSS was diagnosed in 16% of persons with running-related injuries (Mulvad et al. 2018). It is a multifactorial overuse syndrome related to the runner's anatomical structure, training program, flexibility, muscle strength, footwear, and running mechanics. Changes in any of these variables may lead to a MTSS-related injury. Despite the prevalence of MTSS, its diagnosis is problematic in light of differential diagnoses of stress reaction and stress fracture (discussed in the following section), tendinitis, musculotendinous strain, and chronic compartment syndromes.

MTSS treatment begins with conservative management (e.g., rest and ice) but may require surgical treatment if conservative measures fail. The surgery involves a deep posterior compartment **fasciotomy** to relieve pressure in the affected area. Surgical outcomes are mixed. In a study of surgical treatment of MTSS, Yates and colleagues (2003) reported excellent (35%), good (34%), fair (22%), and poor (9%) results in 78 patients. Although surgery may relieve pain in a majority of patients, return to full activity may be precluded for many. Yates and colleagues reported significant pain reduction in 72% of patients, but only 41% were able to fully return to their presymptom activity level.

Tibial Stress Reaction and Stress Fracture

Bone responds to repetitive loading by adapting its structure according to Wolff's law (see chapter 4). This process includes resorption where the loading conditions render bone unnecessary and depositing bone in regions needed to sustain the new mechanical loads. If, however, the magnitude and frequency of loading exceed the bone's ability to adapt, injury occurs. The most recognizable form of injury is bone fracture. As discussed in the previous chapter, fracture may occur acutely (traumatic fracture) or in response to chronic loading (**stress fracture**). Chronic loading fractures are most often associated with a sudden increase in activity (e.g., athletes, military recruits) and are termed **fatigue fractures**. Less recognized are chronic fractures found in persons with no increase in activity but with decreased bone density. These stress fractures are called **insufficiency fractures**.

The term *stress fracture* itself suffers from overuse, or perhaps misuse, because it is often used to describe bone with no clear evidence of discontinuity or line of fracture. The term **stress reaction** describes bone with evidence of remodeling but with an absence of radiological evidence of fracture. Such stress reactions are quite common and are detectable using a combination of radiographs, bone scans, and magnetic resonance imaging scans (figure 6.31).

Actual fractures occur much less frequently than pure mechanical loading (i.e., material fatigue failure) alone would predict, suggesting that the process leading to stress reaction and subsequent stress fracture involves physiological processes of bone adaptation to mechanical loading. This is not to discount completely the role of mechanical fatigue, however, because microfractures have been detected at remodeling sites.

Verifiable stress fractures most frequently happen in the tibia, accounting for up to 50% of all stress fractures. Most long-bone stress fractures are oriented transversely to the longitudinal axis of the bone; longitudinally directed stress fractures are uncommon and usually found on the anterior cortex of the distal tibia (Tearse et al. 2002).

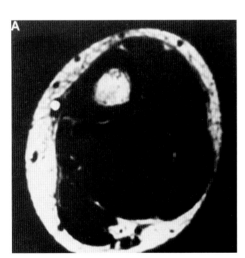
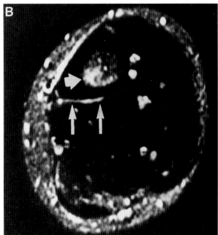
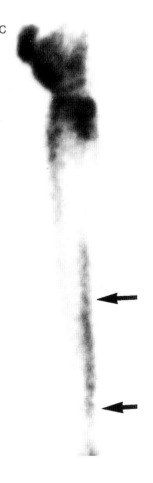

FIGURE 6.31 Stress reaction in the lower left leg of an 18-year-old female varsity runner. Axial T1-weighted magnetic resonance image *(a)* shows no detectable abnormality, but the T2-weighted image *(b)* shows moderate periosteal edema (long arrows) along the posterior and medial aspect of the tibia. There is also marrow edema (short arrow) in the adjacent part of the tibia. The bone scintigraphy *(c)* shows increased activity along the distal half of the tibial diaphysis (arrows).

Reprinted by permission from M. Fredericson et al., "Tibial Stress Reaction in Runners: Correlation of Clinical Symptoms and Scintigraphy with a New Magnetic Resonance Imaging Grading System," *The American Journal of Sports Medicine* 23, no. 4 (1995): 472–481, reprinted by permission of SAGE Publications.

Shin Splints

Of the many catch-all terms in the medical literature, perhaps none can match *shin splints* when it comes to nonspecificity, lack of consensus on meaning, and continuing misunderstanding and confusion. Although current literature seems to associate the term *shin splints* most often with medial tibial stress syndrome (MTSS), we present a few of the various past and current descriptions of the term.

- "Diffuse areas of increased tenderness over the anterior or posterior bony attachments of the tibialis anterior muscles to the tibia. . . . This relatively mild condition must be distinguished from its two more disabling cousins, tibial stress fracture and chronic exertional compartment syndrome" (Kibler and Chandler 1994, p. 549).

- "Medial tibial stress syndrome (MTSS), commonly referred to as shin splints, describes the pain on the medial side of the shin bones experienced by many athletes as a result of microtrauma on the tibia" (Hammad et al. 2018, p. 1).

- "Pain in the shin may be related to overuse or stress of the muscles within the extensor or flexor groups, stress fracture, or induced ischemia within muscular compartments leading to compartment syndrome" (Ciullo and Shapiro 1994, p. 661).

- "Painful injury to and inflammation of the tibial and toe extensor muscles or their fasciae that is caused by repeated minimal traumas (as by running on a hard surface)" (Merriam-Webster 2005, p. 758).

- "A nondescript pain in the anterior, posterior, or posterolateral compartment of the tibia. It usually follows strenuous or repetitive exercise and is often related to faulty foot mechanics such as pes planus or pes cavus. The cause may be ischemia of the muscles in the compartment, minute tears in the tissues, or partial avulsion from the periosteum of the tibial of peroneal muscles" (Venes 2005, p. 1987).

- A "painful condition of the front lower leg, associated with tendinitis, stress fractures, or muscle strain, often occurring as a result of running or other strenuous athletic activity, especially on a nonresilient surface" (Dictionary.com 2021).

And among the most confusing of all, from *Stedman's* (2005):

- *Shin-splints* (hyphenated)—"Tenderness and pain with induration and swelling in the anterior tibial compartment, particularly following athletic overexertion by the untrained."

- *Shin splints* (two words, nonhyphenated)—"A collective term for various injuries to the leg including acute and chronic exertional compartment syndrome, medial tibial stress syndrome, and periostitis."

O'Donoghue (1984, p. 591) astutely noted, "As with many names in common use, there is considerable and often heated argument as to what is actually meant by the term. As is usual in these circumstances, the term 'shin splints' is a wastebasket one including many different conditions. The authors of various articles on the subject are inclined to state very definitely that it is caused by one particular thing to the exclusion of all others, which causes great confusion."

As we urged in chapter 5, the term *shin splints* should be relegated to O'Donoghue's wastebasket, and we instead recommend using terms that are clinically correct, specific, and useful. We echo the sentiment of Batt (1995, p. 53) that "the term shin splint be recognized as generic, rather than diagnostic, and that specific conditions that currently exist under this term be differentiated."

Stress fracture location depends somewhat on activity. The mechanical demands of specific movements appear to play a prominent role in determining the fracture site. Runners, the most common victims of tibial stress fracture, exhibit fractures focused between the middle and distal thirds of the tibia. Athletes in jumping sports (e.g., basketball and volleyball) tend to experience proximal fractures. Dancers, in contrast, sustain more midshaft fractures.

Traumatic Fractures of the Tibia and Fibula

Mechanical insult to the lower leg may result in traumatic fracture of the tibia, fibula, or both. The sources of the applied force vary but most commonly involve vehicle–pedestrian collisions and sports-related movements. Other causes include slip-and-fall accidents, falls from a height, direct blows, crushing, gunshot, and overuse (Court-Brown and McBirnie 1995).

Causal mechanisms can be classified as either low energy (e.g., slip and fall, sports-related injury) or high energy (e.g., direct blows, motor vehicle crashes). Low-energy fractures often involve torsion or bending of the tibia with minimal soft tissue involvement. Torsional loading occurs when the lower leg is twisted about its long axis (see chapter 5), such as when a ski provides an extended moment arm for applying torques to the skier's tibial shaft. Bending loads are created when parallel and oppositely directed forces are applied simultaneously to the bone. The classic boot-top fracture (shown in figure 3.35c) illustrates this bending mechanism.

High-energy injuries, in contrast, involve direct impact or high bending forces and result in transverse fractures and considerable fragmentation or comminution (Watson 2002) (figure 6.32). Motor vehicle crashes account for the majority of direct impact, or crushing, fractures.

One study identified baseball bats as a causal agent in tibial fractures. The fractures did not occur during athletic competition but rather resulted from the bats being used as weapons. Levy and colleagues (1994) reported 47 such bat-induced fractures during a 1-year period at an urban trauma center. Eleven of these fractures were to the tibia, and many involved extensive comminution and complications (e.g., delayed union or compartment syndrome).

Case Study: Bilateral Spiral Fracture

Many thousands of skiing-related injuries happen every year, sometimes because of excessively tight bindings or binding release malfunctions (Hull and Mote 1980). Zernicke (1981) reported the case of an injury in which a skier, on his first run of the day on the beginner's slope, unintentionally began to "snowplow" uncontrollably, forcing both legs into extreme internal rotation. Failure of the bindings to release resulted in spiral fractures in both tibias. Subsequent testing of the skis, boots, and bindings using a biomechanical model (see figure) provided quantitative estimates of the torques transmitted to the lower leg as lateral forces were applied to the skis. The data showed that the bindings placed the skier at high risk of injury, because "for nearly all applications of lateral loads to the ski, this skier's bindings would not have released prior to exceeding the torsional elastic threshold of the tibia" (Zernicke 1981, p. 243).

Fortunately, poor bindings such as the ones in this case are no longer in use. This example nonetheless demonstrates the potential for injury in skiing and points to the importance of proper equipment selection and maintenance in reducing the risk of musculoskeletal injury.

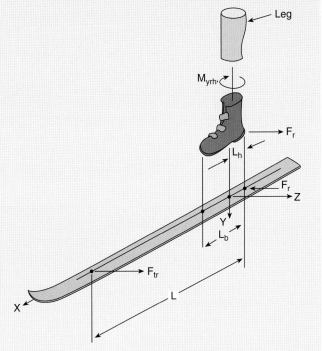

Schematic diagram of leg–boot–ski binding system. M_{yrh} = torque transmitted to skier's lower leg; F_r = lateral release force applied to heel; L_h = distance from vertical axis of the tibia to the heel point; L_b = distance from the heel to the toe pivot point (i.e., length of the boot); F_{tr} = lateral force applied to the ski at a distance (L) in front of the heel-release point; Z = z-coordinate axis; Y = y-coordinate axis; X = x-coordinate axis.

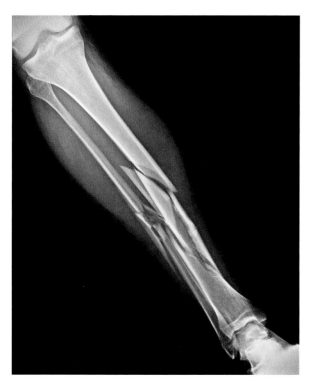

FIGURE 6.32 Tibial and fibular fractures.
thesleepless1/iStock/Getty Images

Whatever the mechanism, tibiofibular fracture is a serious injury because of the injured bone's compromised ability to carry loads in its role as a critical link in the lower extremity's kinetic chain.

Ankle and Foot Injuries

Given their numerous bones, ligaments, and articulations, the foot and ankle are arguably the human body's most complex region. The ankle joint is formed by articulation of the tibia, fibula, and talus. The tibia and fibula create a deep socket, or mortise, that houses the talus. In a dorsiflexed position, the talus fits snugly within the mortise and is quite stable. As the ankle plantarflexes, the narrower posterior section of the talus rotates into the area between the malleoli. This looser fit compromises joint stability, resulting in a relatively unstable ankle in the plantarflexed position (figure 6.33).

Many ligaments reinforce the ankle. Medially, the strong deltoid ligament complex provides resistance to forceful eversion. On the lateral aspect, three ligaments are primarily responsible for restricting inversion. The weakest of the three, the anterior talofibular ligament (ATFL), extends anteromedially from the fibular malleolus to the neck of the talus. The calca-

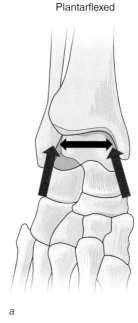

Plantarflexed

a

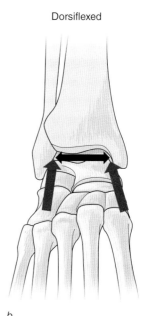

Dorsiflexed

b

FIGURE 6.33 Ankle joint in *(a)* plantarflexion, and *(b)* dorsiflexion. The narrow talar width between the tibial and fibular malleoli (*a*, black arrow) results in the looser bony fit (*a*, red arrows). This puts the ankle at greater risk of injury when compared to the wider talar width and tighter bony fit in the dorsiflexed position (*b*).

neofibular ligament (CFL) passes posteroinferiorly from the tip of the fibular malleolus to the lateral surface of the calcaneus. The posterior talofibular ligament (PTFL) connects the fibular malleolar fossa to the lateral tubercle of the talus (figure 6.34).

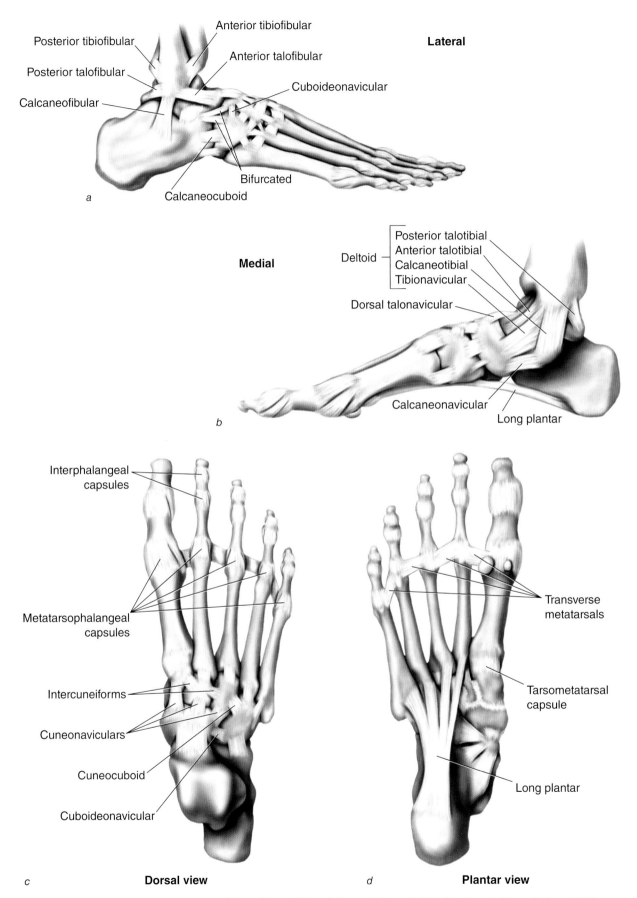

FIGURE 6.34 Tendons and ligaments of the ankle and foot. *(a)* Lateral view. *(b)* Medial view. *(c)* Dorsal view. *(d)* Plantar view.

Each foot contains 26 bones (figure 6.35). The largest of these, the calcaneus, serves as the attachment for the calcaneal (Achilles) tendon, which transmits the force of the triceps surae muscles in plantarflexing the ankle. The articulation of the calcaneus with the talus forms the subtalar (talocalcaneal) joint, an articulation essential to proper function of the foot and ankle complex during load bearing. The subtalar joint axis runs obliquely, as shown in figure 6.36.

The bones of the foot form two primary arches: the longitudinal arch, running from the calcaneus to the distal ends of the metatarsals, and the transverse arch, which extends from side to side across the foot (figure 6.37). The longitudinal arch is divided into a medial portion that includes the calcaneus, the talus, the navicular, three cuneiforms, and the three most medial metatarsals. The lateral portion is much flatter and is in contact with the ground during

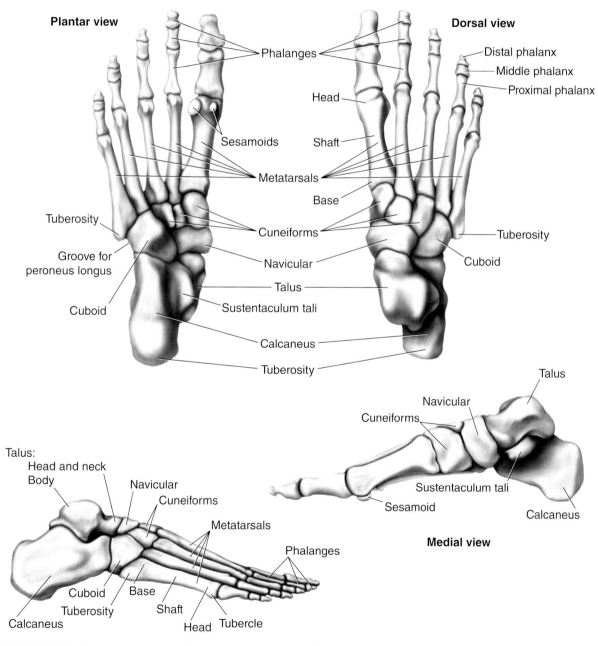

FIGURE 6.35 Bones of the foot: Plantar, dorsal, lateral, and medial views.

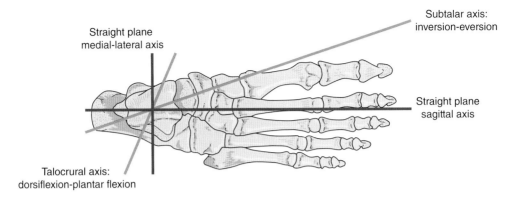

FIGURE 6.36   Anatomy of the subtalar joint axis.

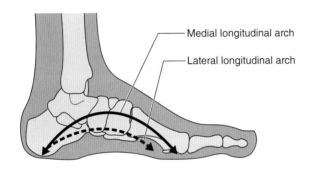

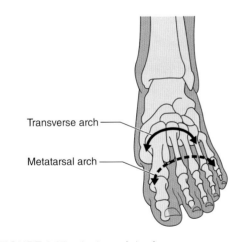

FIGURE 6.37   Arches of the foot.

Reprinted by permission from W.C. Whiting, *Dynamic Human Anatomy*, 2nd ed. (Champaign, IL: Human Kinetics, 2019).

standing. The transverse arch is formed by the cuboid, cuneiforms, and bases of the metatarsals.

During weight-bearing activities, the arches compress to absorb and distribute the load. Several ligaments assist in this force distribution. These include the plantar calcaneonavicular ligament (spring ligament), the short plantar ligament, and the long plantar ligament. The integrity of the arches

and their ability to absorb loads are maintained by the tight-fitting articulations between foot bones, the action of intrinsic foot musculature, the strength of the plantar ligaments, and the plantar aponeurosis (plantar fascia).

Ankle Sprain

As a result of its relative anatomical instability and supportive function, the ankle joint (figure 6.38) frequently suffers injury. In certain sports (e.g., basketball, volleyball), ankle sprains are the most common injury. Despite their prevalence, ankle sprains continue to present clinicians with diagnostic and therapeutic challenges (Safran et al. 1999).

To present a meaningful discussion of ankle injury mechanisms, we must review several anatomical structures and their functional characteristics. As briefly described earlier, the ankle joint is formed by articulation of the tibia, fibula, and talus. The talar body is wedge-shaped, with its anterior portion being wider than its posterior. This irregularity contributes directly to the joint's positional stability. In dorsiflexion, the wider part wedges between the malleoli, lending stability to the joint. The narrow portion of the talus, however, moves between the malleoli in plantarflexion, permits talar translation and tilt, and results in lateral instability. The juxtaposition of the tibia and fibula is maintained by a tibiofibular syndesmosis, which consists of an interosseous ligament (thickening of the interosseous membrane), an anterior inferior tibiofibular ligament, a posterior inferior tibiofibular ligament, and an inferior transverse tibiofibular ligament (Carr 2003).

Ankle sprain is somewhat of a misnomer because the injury typically involves both the ankle and subtalar joints. These two joints move in concert to execute what should be correctly viewed as com-

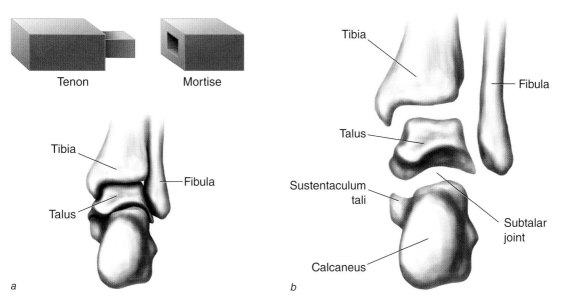

FIGURE 6.38   Skeletal anatomy of the ankle joint. *(a)* The talocrural joint as a mortise-(tibia and fibula) and-tenon (talus) joint. *(b)* Posterior view of the ankle, showing the subtalar joint.

bined ankle–foot movement. Our movement conventions are described and illustrated in figure 6.39.

The determining factors in ankle injury, as in most injuries, are the joint position at the time of injury; the magnitude, direction, and rate of applied forces; and the resistance provided by joint structures. The joint motions commonly involved in ankle–foot injuries are precipitated by walking on uneven surfaces, stepping in holes, rolling the ankle during a cutting maneuver, or landing on another player's foot when descending from a jump in sporting events (figure 6.40). Resulting injuries range from fracture–dislocation to ligamentous damage (sprain). Ankle sprains are more common in women than men, in children than adults, and in court and indoor sports (Doherty et al. 2014).

The vast majority (85%-90%) of ankle sprains are termed **inversion sprains**. According to our nomenclature, the mechanism is supination (i.e., a combination of ankle plantarflexion, subtalar inversion, and internal rotation of the foot in which the longitudinal midline of the foot deviates, or rotates, medially). The term *inversion sprain* is so entrenched in the literature, however, that its extinction seems unlikely. An alternative term, **lateral ankle sprain**, may be more appropriate.

In most cases there is an orderly sequence of ligament failure (figure 6.41). The anterior talofibular ligament (ATFL) fails first because of its orientation

at the instant of loading and its inherent weakness (Siegler et al. 1988). When the ankle assumes a plantarflexed position (as it does in ankle–foot supination), the ATFL aligns with the fibula and functions as a collateral ligament (Carr 2003). This alignment, taken together with the ATFL's relative weakness, predisposes the ATFL to injury. About 65% to 70% of ligament injuries at the ankle involve isolated ATFL damage.

The calcaneofibular ligament (CFL) is next injured, followed by rare failure of the posterior talofibular ligament (PTFL). When the ankle is dorsiflexed, the CFL aligns with the fibula and provides collateral reinforcement. Isolated CFL injuries are rare; the CFL is most often injured in combination with the ATFL (20%).

An interesting structural relation between the ATFL and CFL was described more than four decades ago by Inman (1976). He described considerable variation (70°-140°) in the angle between the ATFL and CFL (figure 6.42). Inman hypothesized that a larger angle may be associated with lateral ankle joint laxity and possibly a greater injury risk.

Occasionally, the anterior portion of the deltoid ligament is injured during an inversion injury. At first glance, this may appear incongruous. Why would a medial structure incur damage from forcible inversion? The answer lies in the complexity of joint action, specifically that the anterior portion of

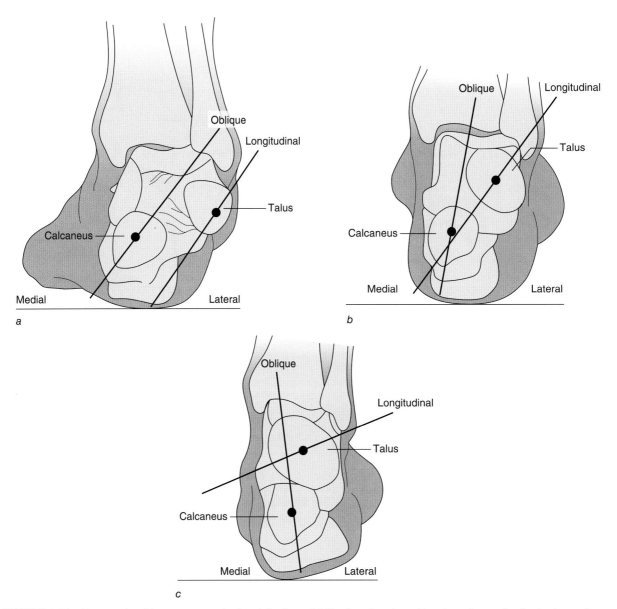

FIGURE 6.39 Foot and ankle movement in the right foot. *(a)* **Supination** (combined motions of subtalar inversion, ankle plantarflexion, and foot internal rotation). *(b)* Neutral position. *(c)* **Pronation** (combined motions of subtalar eversion, ankle dorsiflexion, and foot external rotation).

the deltoid ligament is taut in ankle plantarflexion. Because the ankle is plantarflexed at the time of injury, the anterior portion of the deltoid ligament becomes a candidate for injury. As an inherently strong ligament, however, the deltoid ligament is rarely injured in so-called inversion sprains. The opposite movement pattern creates **eversion sprain** (pronation by our definition); the injury mechanism involves ankle dorsiflexion, subtalar eversion, and lateral rotation of the foot. An alternative term, **medial ankle sprain**, may be more appropriate.

Given the inherent strength of the medial collateral (deltoid) ligament group, injuries resulting from this mechanism are both less frequent (about 5%) and less severe. In this mechanism the talus is forced against the lateral malleolus. Because the lateral malleolus is longer and thinner than the medial malleolus, the talus cannot rotate over the lateral malleolus. This may result in malleolar fracture. Rupture of the deltoid ligament may occur, although this is rare and is always seen in conjunction with other ligament tears.

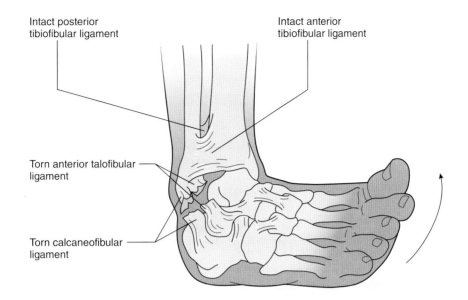

FIGURE 6.40 Common mechanism of ankle injury.

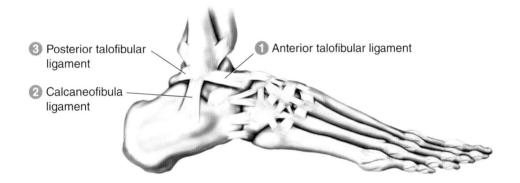

FIGURE 6.41 Sequential failure pattern of the lateral ankle ligaments. Typically the ATFL (1) fails first, followed by the CFL (2) and rarely the PTFL (3).

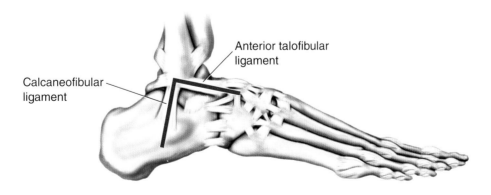

FIGURE 6.42 Angle between the ATFL and CFL.

In some cases applied loads separate the distal fibula from the tibia with sufficient force to tear the syndesmosis (interosseous membrane and tibiofibular ligaments) in what is termed a **high ankle sprain** (figure 6.43). Ligament damage can be seen in the anterior tibiofibular ligament, the posterior tibiofibular ligament, or both, along with possible fracture (Hunt et al. 2015). Likely mechanisms for a high ankle sprain include talar torsion, forced ankle dorsiflexion, and traumatic impact. The highest incidence of high ankle sprains are reported in American football, wrestling, and ice hockey (Mauntel et al. 2017). Unrecognized and untreated syndesmotic injuries may lead to chronic instability and ankle arthrosis.

In general, ankle sprains that go undiagnosed and untreated can result in residual physical disability, including chronic ankle instability (Herzog et al. 2019).

Calcaneal Tendon Pathologies

Ever since the Greek warrior Achilles was felled by an arrow judiciously aimed at his unprotected heel, the calcaneal region has been associated with susceptibility to injury.

The calcaneal (Achilles) tendon, the largest and strongest tendon in the body, is formed by merging of the distal tendons of the gastrocnemius and soleus about 5 to 6 cm proximal to its insertion site on the posterior surface of calcaneus. At the insertion site, tendon width varies from 1.2 to 2.5 cm. Approximately 12 to 15 cm proximal to the insertion, the calcaneal tendon begins to spiral, twisting about 90° as it approaches its calcaneal insertion (Schepsis et al. 2002).

Frequent and repeated loading of the calcaneal tendon predisposes it to overuse pathologies, most commonly peritenonitis (inflammation of the peri-

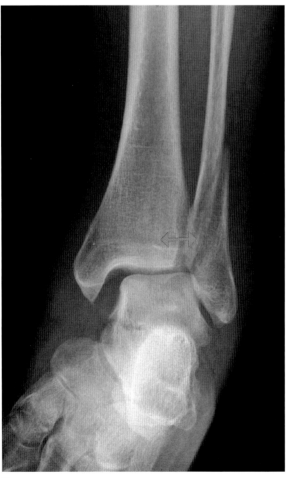

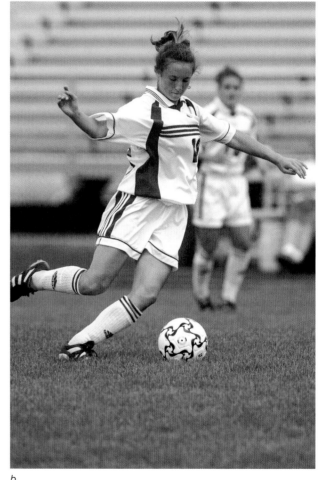

a   *b*

FIGURE 6.43   High ankle sprain. *(a)* Tibia and fibula pried apart by talar rotation. *(b)* Left foot rotation with ankle dorsiflexed.

(a) Steven Needell/Science Source

tenon), insertional disturbances (e.g., bursitis or insertion tendinitis), myotendinous junction injury, or tendinopathies (Kvist 1994).

The calcaneal tendon transmits substantial loads from the triceps surae muscle group (gastrocnemius and soleus) to its attachment on the posterior calcaneus. A sample of studies confirms the high loads transmitted by the calcaneal tendon:

- Burdett (1982), using a biomechanical model, estimated peak calcaneal tendon forces ranging from 5.3 to 10.0 times body weight during the stance phase of running.

- Fukashiro and colleagues (1995), using an implanted tendon force transducer, reported peak calcaneal tendon force of 2233 N (502 lb) in the squat jump, 1895 N (426 lb) in the countermovement jump, and 3786 N (851 lb) in hopping.

- Giddings and colleagues (2000), using experimental data and a quantitative model, predicted maximal calcaneal tendon force 3.9 times body weight for walking and 7.7 times body weight for running, with the peak loads at 70% of the stance phase for walking and 60% of stance for running.

- Bogey and colleagues (2005), using an electromyograph-to-force processing technique, estimated peak calcaneal tendon force of 2.9 kN (652 lb) during gait.

- Pourcelot and colleagues (2005), using a noninvasive ultrasonic technique, found peak calcaneal tendon forces of about 850 N (191 lb) during the stance phase of walking.

- Revak and colleagues (2017), using kinematic and force plate measures, reported lower calcaneal tendon loading in bilateral and seated heel-raising and -lowering exercises when compared to unilateral and standing conditions.

- Gheidi and colleagues (2018) using a musculoskeletal model, compared calcaneal tendon loading during weight-bearing exercises, with highest peak force (6.68 times body weight) in a unilateral jump landing, and lowest peak force (0.77 times body weight) in a squat exercise.

Although the calcaneal tendon clearly is subjected to high magnitude loads across a spectrum of activities, Komi and colleagues (1992) suggested that the loading rate may be more clinically relevant than the loading magnitude.

Four primary mechanisms have been implicated in calcaneal tendon rupture (Mahan and Carter 1992; figure 6.44): (1) sudden dorsiflexion of a plantarflexed foot (e.g., a lacrosse player in the act of throwing), (2) pushing off the weight-bearing foot while extending the ipsilateral knee joint (e.g., a basketball player executing a rapid change of direction), (3) sudden excess tension on an already taut tendon (e.g., catching a heavy weight), and (4) a taut tendon struck by a blunt object (e.g., softball bat). These mechanisms suggest, and epidemiological evidence confirms, that most calcaneal tendon ruptures are unilateral. Although rare, bilateral calcaneal tendon ruptures have been reported (Garneti et al. 2005).

The cause of calcaneal tendinopathies is multifactorial; contributing factors include training errors, running terrain, malalignments (e.g., combined flat foot and excessive pronation) and biomechanical faults, improper footwear, trauma, age, sex (men are at 5-6 times greater risk of rupture than women), anthropometrics, environment, and psychomotor factors. The tendon also may be weakened, and thus put at even greater risk, by systemic diseases, steroids, and fluoroquinolone antibiotics (Casparian et al. 2000; Maffulli and Wong 2003; Vanek et al. 2003). Nonuniform tendon stresses attributable to individual muscle contributions may also contribute to injury risk (Arndt et al. 1998).

Tendon degeneration may eventually lead to complete tendon rupture. Calcaneal tendon ruptures typically happen in sedentary, 30- to 40-year-old men who suddenly exert themselves in a sporting task that involves running, jumping, or rapid change of direction (Järvinen et al. 2001; Schepsis et al. 2002; Yinger et al. 2002). In many instances these spontaneous tendon ruptures seem to "just happen." Postinjury assessment, however, shows evidence of degeneration in the ruptured tendon. Tendon rupture thus often occurs secondary to degenerative processes rather than as a spontaneous primary injury.

Calcaneal tendon rupture usually occurs about 2 to 6 cm proximal to the calcaneal insertion in a region known to be **hypovascular**. This fact, combined with decreased blood flow associated with age, helps explain the frequency of rupture in middle-aged people. The calcaneal tendon has a poor blood supply that previously was thought not to vary along its length (Ahmed et al. 1998). A study

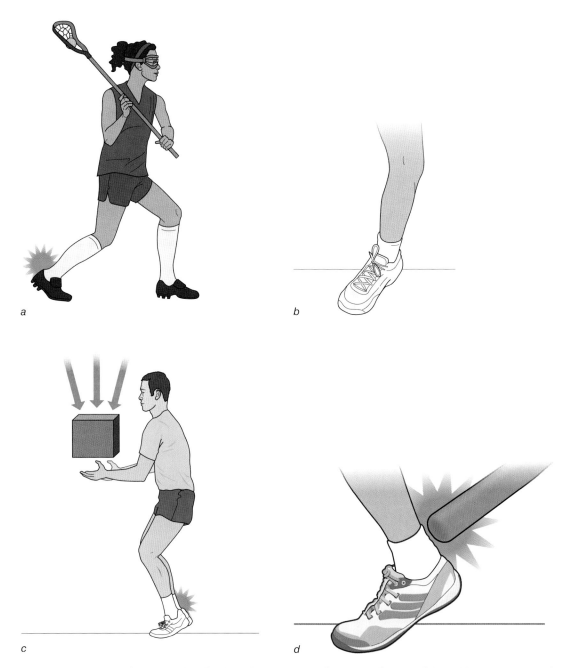

FIGURE 6.44 Mechanisms of calcaneal (Achilles) tendon rupture. *(a)* Rapid dorsiflexion of the ankle by a lacrosse player. *(b)* Cutting maneuver with rapid change of direction. *(c)* Catching a falling weight. *(d)* Blunt trauma to a taut tendon.

using a novel method, however, reported an avascular region close to the calcaneal insertion site and regional differences in vascular density along the tendon length (Zantop et al. 2003). The middle part of the calcaneal tendon had a much lower vascular density (28.2 vessels/cm^2) than either the proximal part (73.4 vessels/cm^2) or the distal part (56.6 vessels/cm^2). The authors identified this reduced vascularization (and resulting **hypoxia**) as a predisposing factor for calcaneal tendon degeneration and

eventual rupture. In addition, the distal portion of the Achilles tendon is at greater risk of rupture due to its smaller cross-sectional area distally compared to proximally (Reeves and Cooper 2017).

As a side note of interest, there may be a relation between blood type and increased incidence of tendon rupture. Persons with type O blood seem to be more likely to suffer from tendon rupture in general (Józsa et al. 1989) and calcaneal tendon rupture in particular (Kujala et al. 1992) compared with people who have other blood types, suggesting a genetic link between one's ABO blood group and the molecular structure of tendon tissue. Another study, however, found no significant relation between the proportions of ABO blood groups and Achilles tendon rupture (Maffulli et al. 2000). Maffulli and colleagues concluded that the association between blood group and tendon rupture may be attributable to differences in blood group distribution in genetically segregated populations. Genetic factors also play a role in predisposition to calcaneal tendon rupture (Ribbans and Collins 2013).

Predisposition to rupture also may be affected by collagen type. Eriksen and colleagues (2002) found type III collagen accumulation at the rupture site, likely attributable to microtrauma and healing events. Similar results of higher type III collagen at calcaneal tendon rupture sites have been reported (Pajala et al. 2009). Increased type III collagen content may contribute to lower tendon tensile strength and enhanced rupture risk.

In summary, the theoretical explanations for Achilles tendon ruptures and other chronic pathology suggest a sequence of events that is initiated with an intrinsic tendon pathology associated with disuse, age-related tendon change, and hypovascularity, resulting in localized degeneration and tendon weakening. This decreases the tendon's threshold to rupture. The precise proprioceptive and pathomechanical position and load that causes the injury remains obscure. It is probably a complex equation of neuromuscular control and endocrine factors that result in the Achilles tendon rupture. (Yinger et al. 2002, p. 234)

Plantar Fasciitis

Plantar fasciitis (PF) has been described as an inflammatory condition of the plantar fascia in the midfoot or at its insertion on the medial tuberosity of the calcaneus that involves microtears or partial rupture of fascial fibers. *Plantar fasciitis* is yet another catch-all term that has become entrenched in the literature as a general descriptor of pain in the plantar area of the posterior foot. A more appropriate nonspecific designation is *plantar heel pain* or *heel pain syndrome*, with *plantar fasciitis* reserved for inflammation specifically to the plantar fascia. Given the reported presence of noninflammatory evidence (e.g., myxoid degeneration with fragmentation of the plantar fascia) in the plantar fascia of patients undergoing fascial release surgery (La Porta and La Fata 2005), some have suggested *plantar*

fasciosis (Thomas et al. 2010) or *plantar fasciopathy* (Trojian and Tucker 2019) as a more accurate descriptor for this condition. In a 2018 consensus paper, the American College of Foot and Ankle Surgeons wrote, "Finally, fasciopathy has historically been used as a general term that includes both short-term inflammation (fasciitis) and long-term degeneration (fasciosis). In an attempt to simplify the terminology for the purposes of the present CCS, only the term 'fasciitis' has been used in this document" (Schneider et al. 2018, p. 372).

Differential diagnoses of plantar fasciitis include tarsal tunnel syndrome, acute calcaneal fracture, bone tumor, calcaneal apophysitis, Achilles tendinitis, plantar fascia rupture, and retrocalcaneal bursitis (Goff and Crawford 2011; Thomas et al. 2010).

In most cases, PF develops in response to repeated loading (e.g., running) in which compressive forces flatten the longitudinal arch of the foot. Forces in the plantar fascia during running have been estimated to be 1.3 to 2.9 times body weight (Scott and Winter 1990). This flattening of the arches stretches the fascia and absorbs the load in much the same way a leaf spring bends to accommodate heavy weights, in what is termed a **truss mechanism** (figure 6.45*a*). Extension of the toes puts added stress on the structures by way of a **windlass mechanism**, as depicted in figure 6.45*b*.

Plantar fasciitis is hastened or worsened by lack of flexibility. Tightness of the calcaneal tendon, for example, limits ankle dorsiflexion and results in greater plantar fascial stress. Ankle strength and flexibility deficits have been observed in the symptomatic limbs compared with the unaffected limbs and with an asymptomatic control group (Kibler et al. 1991).

In addition to strength and flexibility, other factors are associated with PF, including overtraining, leg length discrepancies, fatigue, fascial inextensibility, and poor movement mechanics. Excessive pronation during running provides a good example of how a pathological movement pattern contributes to PF. During pronation the subtalar joint everts, causing plantar fascial elongation and increased tissue stress. Repetition of this pathological loading leads to microdamage and attendant inflammation. Although overpronation has been associated with PF, there is not a clear link between PF and **pes cavus** (high foot arch) or **pes planus** (flat foot) (Peterson and Renström 2001). The cause of plantar fasciitis remains unclear.

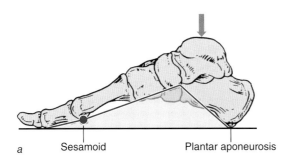 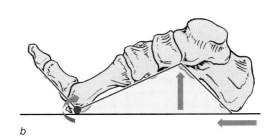

a   Sesamoid   Plantar aponeurosis   b

FIGURE 6.45   *(a)* Truss mechanism in which body weight compresses the longitudinal arch. *(b)* Windlass mechanism (first proposed by Hicks 1954) in which hyperextension of the toes increases tension in the plantar structures.

Toe Injuries

Jacques Lisfranc, a field surgeon in Napoleon's army, described amputation through the tarsometatarsal joint of a gangrenous foot (Vuori and Aro 1993). Although his description did not include reference to fracture–dislocation of the joint, his name is now given to these injuries to the tarsometatarsal region (see figure 6.46). Lisfranc fracture–dislocations involve the tarsometatarsal, intermetatarsal, and anterior intertarsal joints (Lau et al. 2017).

The circumstances of Lisfranc joint injury vary and include both low-energy injuries (e.g., tripping or stumbling) and high-energy trauma (e.g., fall from a height, direct crush, vehicular crash). Several mechanisms have been suggested to explain Lis-

franc fracture–dislocations. One relatively uncommon mechanism is direct force, as when a heavy object is dropped on the foot. Direct force applied to the metatarsal pushes the bone down and causes plantar dislocation and possible accompanying fracture. Force applied proximal to the tarsometatarsal joint results in dorsal dislocation.

A second mechanism involves axial loading of the region when indirect forces (e.g., ground reaction force) are applied to a foot in extreme plantarflexion. This occurs when a person is in a tiptoe position at the instant of load application. A similar loading may occur in dorsiflexion as well. In both cases the metatarsal is forcibly pushed out of joint. Such an injury is typically accompanied by capsular rupture and metatarsal fracture.

Violent abduction, induced by a twisting mechanism, is another cause of Lisfranc injury. This is classically illustrated by an equestrian injury in which the rider's foot is fixed in the stirrup while the rider falls, pushing the metatarsals into extreme abduction.

Although Lisfranc fracture–dislocations have instructive value in demonstrating mechanisms of injury, their incidence is quite low. A review of nearly 700 cases of metatarsal fracture found that less than 10% involved Lisfranc joint injuries (Vuori and Aro 1993). More recently, Stødle et al. (2020) reported a Lisfranc injury incidence of 14:100,000 person-years and an incidence of unstable injuries, meaning injuries with detectable displacement of the tarsometatarsal joints, of 6:100,000 person-years.

Other foot and toe injuries are more prevalent. Among these is **turf toe**, an injury involving damage

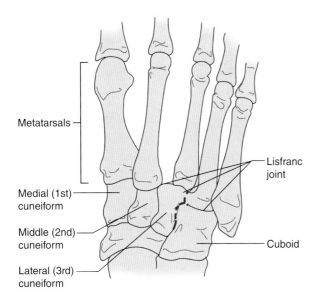

Metatarsals

Lisfranc joint

Medial (1st) cuneiform

Middle (2nd) cuneiform

Cuboid

Lateral (3rd) cuneiform

FIGURE 6.46   Lisfranc fracture–dislocation.

to the capsuloligamentous structures of the first metatarsophalangeal (MP) joint. Multiple mechanisms have been implicated in turf toe injuries, most commonly hyperextension of the toe while the ankle is plantarflexed (Allen et al. 2004; Poppe et al. 2019). This injury typically occurs when the foot is planted on the ground with the first MP joint in extension. A load, such as another player falling on the foot, forces the joint into hyperextension and damages joint structures (figure 6.47). Much less frequently, turf toe results from a hyperflexion mechanism. Turf toe also may happen secondarily in response to excessive valgus and varus loading of the first MP joint. Although once thought to be a relatively minor injury, turf toe is now recognized as a condition with significant short-term effects and potentially serious long-term consequences (Seow et al. 2020).

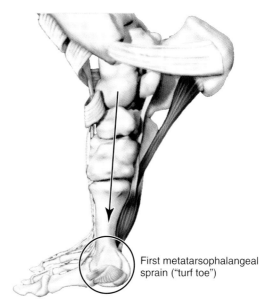

First metatarsophalangeal sprain ("turf toe")

FIGURE 6.47 Turf toe injury caused by hyperextension of the hallux (big toe) with simultaneous compressive loading.

Copyright Primal Pictures Ltd.

Chapter Review

Key Points

- Lower-extremity injuries are common and affect posture, walking, running, and other load-bearing tasks.
- Increased participation in competitive and recreational sports in recent decades, especially by girls and women, has contributed to the increased incidence of lower-extremity injuries.
- Lower-extremity injury risk is multifactorial.
- Demographic and sociological changes logically predict future increases in certain lower-extremity injuries (e.g., hip fractures in older persons).
- Injury prevention programs have proven effective in reducing the incidence of certain injuries (e.g., ACL ruptures).

Questions to Consider

1. This chapter's *A Closer Look* examined anterior cruciate ligament injury in detail. Select another injury presented in the chapter and write your own *A Closer Look* for that injury.
2. Explain, using specific examples, how lower-extremity injuries may affect posture, walking, running, and other load-bearing tasks.
3. Select a lower-extremity injury described in the text and explain how and why it might be considered a multifactorial problem.
4. The text describes how predicted demographic changes will likely increase the incidence of hip fracture. Select another injury and explain how demographic changes may predict future increases (or decreases) in risk for the injury you have selected.

Suggested Readings

Browner, B.D., J. Jupiter, C. Krettek, and P.A. Anderson, eds. 2019. *Skeletal Trauma: Basic Science, Management, and Reconstruction* (6th ed.). Philadelphia: Elsevier.

Bulstrode, C., J. Wilson-MacDonald, D.M. Eastwood, J. McMaster, J. Fairbank, P.J. Singh, S. Bawa, P.D. Gikas, T. Bunker, G. Giddins, M. Blyth, D. Stanley, P.H. Cooke, R. Carrington, P. Calder, P. Wordsworth, and T. Briggs, eds. 2011. *Oxford Textbook of Trauma and Orthopaedics* (2nd ed.). New York: Oxford University Press.

Canata, G.L., P. d'Hooghe, K.J. Hunt, G.M.M.J. Kerkhoffs, and U.G. Longo, eds. 2019. *Sports Injuries of the Foot and Ankle: A Focus on Advanced Surgical Techniques*. New York: Springer.

Diermeier, T., B.B. Rothrauff, L. Engebretsen, A.D. Lynch, O.R. Ayeni, M.V. Paterno, . . . S.J. Meredith. 2020. Treatment after anterior cruciate ligament injury: Panther Symposium ACL Treatment Consensus Group. *Knee Surgery, Sports Traumatology, Arthroscopy* 28: 2390-2402.

Fanelli, G.C., ed. 2015. *Posterior Cruciate Ligament Injuries: A Practical Guide to Management* (2nd ed.). New York: Springer.

Feliciano, D., K. Mattox, and E. Moore, eds. 2020. *Trauma* (9th ed.). New York: McGraw-Hill.

Filbay, S.R., and H. Grindem. 2019. Evidence-based recommendations for the management of anterior cruciate ligament (ACL) rupture. *Best Practice & Research Clinical Rheumatology* 33: 33-47.

Griffin, B.L.Y., M.J. Albohm, E.A. Arendt, et al. 2006. Understanding and preventing noncontact anterior cruciate ligament Injuries: A Review of the Hunt Valley II Meeting. *The American Journal of Sports Medicine* 34: 1512-1532.

Kruse, L.M., B. Gray, and R.W. Wright. 2012. Rehabilitation after anterior cruciate ligament reconstruction: A systematic review. *Journal of Bone & Joint Surgery* 94(19): 1737-1748.

Noyes, F.R., and S. Barber-Westin, eds. 2018. *ACL Injuries in the Female Athlete: Causes, Impacts, and Conditioning Programs* (2nd ed.). New York: Springer.

Noyes, F.R., and S. Barber-Westin, eds. 2019. *Return to Sport after ACL Reconstruction and Other Knee Operations: Limiting the Risk of Reinjury and Maximizing Athletic Performance*. New York: Springer.

Porter, D.A., and L.C. Schon, eds. 2020. *Baxter's the Foot and Ankle in Sport* (3rd ed.). Philadelphia: Elsevier.

Richie, D.H. 2021. *Pathomechanics of Common Foot Disorders*. New York: Springer.

Rodríguez-Merchán, E.C., and A.D. Liddle, eds. 2019. *Disorders of the Patellofemoral Joint: Diagnosis and Management*. New York: Springer.

Tornetta, P., III, W. Ricci, C.M. Court-Brown, M.M. McQueen, and M. McKee, eds. 2019. *Rockwood and Green's Fractures in Adults* (9th ed.). Philadelphia: Lippincott Williams & Wilkins.

van Melick, N.E., R.E.H. van Cingel, M.P.W. Tijssen, and M.W.G.N van der Sanden. 2016. Assessment of functional performance after anterior cruciate ligament reconstruction: A systematic review of measurement procedures. *Knee Surgery, Sports Traumatology, Arthroscopy* 21(4): 869-879.

Upper-Extremity Injuries

Healing is a matter of time, but sometimes also a matter of opportunity.

Hippocrates (460-375 BC)

OBJECTIVES

- To describe the relevant upper-extremity anatomy involved in musculoskeletal injury
- To identify and explain the mechanisms involved in musculoskeletal injuries to the major joints (shoulder, elbow, wrist, and fingers) and segments (upper arm, forearm, and hand) of the upper extremities

A day rarely passes without media reports of some notable musculoskeletal injury. Headlines such as "Child Severely Injures Hand in Fireworks Accident" or "High Incidence of Carpal Tunnel Syndrome Found in Factory Workers" or "Star Basketball Player Suffers Torn Rotator Cuff" are all too common. Upper-extremity injuries are of special concern because they impair one's ability to manipulate the environment. Even simple tasks such as opening a jar or putting a key in a lock become difficult for a person with impaired dexterity. Significant injury to the shoulder, elbow, wrist, or fingers can end a career, necessitate a change of occupation, or hinder participation in recreation.

Effective diagnosis, treatment, and rehabilitation of upper-extremity injuries depend on a sound understanding of injury mechanisms. Only when the causal relations between applied forces and resultant injury are established and understood can appropriate programs of intervention and prevention be designed and implemented.

As was done for ACL injuries in chapter 6, this chapter includes a detailed exploration of glenohumeral impingement and rotator cuff injuries in

Rotator Cuff Pathologies: A Closer Look. In that section we expand our discussion beyond the mechanisms of injury to include detailed descriptions of shoulder complex structure and tissue mechanics and discussion of clinical evaluation, treatment, and rehabilitation of rotator cuff pathologies.

Shoulder Injuries

The shoulder (or pectoral) girdle contains two bones: the scapula and clavicle. The clavicle attaches medially to the sternal manubrium (sternoclavicular joint) and laterally to the acromion process of the scapula (acromioclavicular joint) (figure 7.1). The acromioclavicular (AC) joint is a plane (gliding) synovial joint with articular surfaces separated by an articular disc. The acromioclavicular ligament supports the AC joint superiorly, with inferior support provided by the coracoclavicular ligament.

The humerus of the upper arm articulates with the scapula at the glenohumeral (GH) joint (also called *shoulder joint*), the body's most mobile joint, where the humeral head fits loosely into the shallow glenoid fossa of the scapula. The fibrocarti-

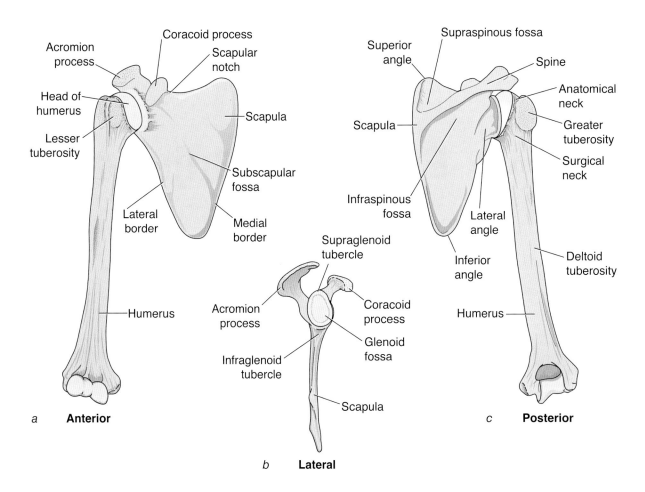

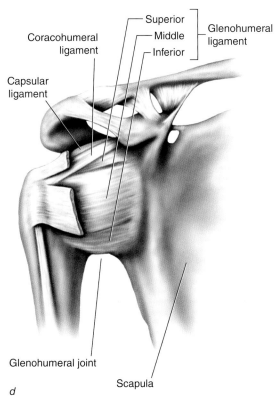

FIGURE 7.1 Bones of the shoulder girdle: *(a)* Anterior view, *(b)* lateral view, and *(c)* posterior view. *(d)* Shoulder ligaments.

laginous glenoid labrum attaches to the rim of the glenoid fossa and improves the joint's bony fit. Two ligaments strengthen the GH joint: the glenohumeral ligament (a thickening of the anterior joint capsule) and the coracohumeral ligament, which anchors the humerus to the coracoid process of the scapula.

The GH joint's ball-and-socket structure permits triplanar motions referred to as *flexion–extension* (sagittal plane), *abduction–adduction* (frontal plane), and *internal–external rotation* (transverse plane). The muscles responsible for producing and controlling movements at the GH joint are shown in figure 7.2 and summarized in table 7.1. Among the

most important (and often injured) GH muscles are the four muscles of the rotator cuff group (subscapularis, supraspinatus, infraspinatus, and teres minor). These muscles assist in stabilizing the GH joint by forming a cuff around the humeral head and pulling the humerus into the glenoid fossa.

Significant injuries to the shoulder include acromioclavicular sprain, glenohumeral instability and dislocation, biceps tendinitis, impingement syndrome, rotator cuff rupture, and labral pathologies. These injuries often are associated with specific sports (table 7.2) and often are position dependent (Perry and Higgins 2001). For example, shoulder injuries are more common in

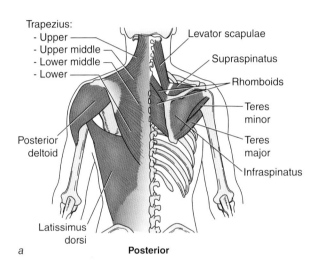

a **Posterior**

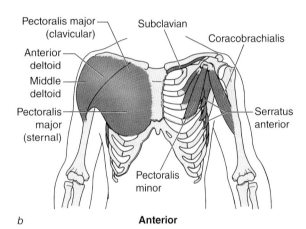

b **Anterior**

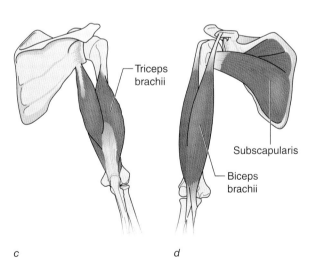

c　　　　*d*

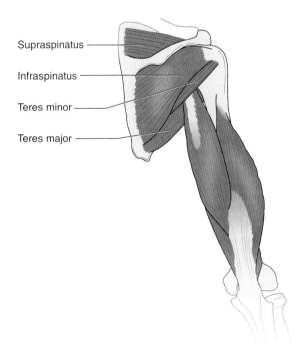

e

FIGURE 7.2　Musculature of the shoulder: *(a)* Posterior muscles. *(b)* Anterior muscles. *(c)* Triceps brachii. *(d)* Biceps brachii and subscapularis. *(e)* Posterior view of supraspinatus, infraspinatus, teres minor, and teres major.

TABLE 7.1   **Muscles of the Shoulder**

Muscle	Action
Biceps brachii	Flexes the arm
Coracobrachialis	Flexes and adducts the arm
Deltoid	Abducts the arm; posterior fibers extend and externally (laterally) rotate the arm; anterior fibers flex and internally (medially) rotate the arm
Infraspinatus*	Externally rotates and slightly adducts the arm
Latissimus dorsi	Adducts, extends, and internally rotates the arm
Pectoralis major	Adducts, flexes, and internally rotates the arm
Subscapularis*	Internally rotates the arm
Supraspinatus*	Abducts the arm
Teres major	Adducts, extends, and internally rotates the arm
Teres minor*	Externally rotates, slightly adducts, and extends the arm
Triceps brachii (long head)	Extends the arm

*Muscles included in the rotator cuff group.

TABLE 7.2   **Injury Rate of Sport-Specific Shoulder Injuries in High School Athletes**

Sport	Sex	Overall	Competition	Practice
Soccer	Female	0.39	0.88	0.19
	Male	0.57	1.19	0.30
Basketball	Female	0.45	0.76	0.32
	Male	0.47	0.90	0.30
Softball	Female	1.10	1.46	0.91
Baseball	Male	1.90	2.38	1.64
American football	Male	5.09	16.2	2.72
Volleyball	Female	1.07	0.72	1.26
Overall	Female	0.72	0.94	0.61
	Male	3.05	6.64	1.85
	Combined	2.27	4.41	1.46

Injury rates (per 10,000 athlete-exposures), 2005-06 and 2006-07 school years, National High School Sports-Related Injury Surveillance Study.

Adapted from J.E. Bonza, S.K. Fields, E.E. Yard, et al., *Journal of Athletic Training* 44, no.1 (2009): 76-83; https://doi.org/10.4085/1062-6050-44.1.76.

baseball pitchers and swimmers competing in the butterfly and freestyle events than in baseball players at other positions and swimmers competing in other events. Acute sports-related shoulder injuries account for nearly one-third of all shoulder injuries (Enger et al. 2019).

Acromioclavicular Sprain

Acromioclavicular (AC) sprain results from applied forces that tend to displace the scapular acromion process from the distal end of the clavicle. This injury commonly is referred to as **shoulder separation** and should not be confused with a shoulder dislocation (see next section). The synovial AC joint is classified as a plane-type joint and contains an intra-articular disc that normally degenerates with age (Hatta et al. 2013; Horvath and Kery 1984). Superior and inferior AC ligaments provide horizontal stability, with vertical stability provided by the coracoclavicular ligaments.

Acromioclavicular injury results from either direct or indirect forces. Direct force applied to the point of the shoulder with the arm in an adducted position is the most common cause of AC injury (Buss and Watts 2003). This mechanism is seen when a person collides with a solid object or surface, and the impact force drives the acromion inferiorly relative to the clavicle (figure 7.3*a*). In the absence of fracture, increasing force levels cause AC injury progression as follows: (1) mild sprain of the AC ligament, (2) moderate AC ligament sprain with coracoclavicular ligament involvement, and (3) complete AC dislocation, with tearing of clavicular attachments of the deltoid and trapezius muscles and complete rupture of the coracoclavicular ligament.

Less frequently, AC injuries result from indirect forces, as when a person falls on an outstretched hand or arm (figure 7.3*b*). In this mechanism, contact forces are transmitted up the arm, through the humerus, to the acromion. These superiorly directed loads force separation of the acromion and clavicle. On rare occasions, extreme traction forces applied to the arm may separate the acromion from its clavicular attachment (Edgar 2019).

Classically, AC injury classification identifies six types of AC sprain and dislocation (Williams et al. 1989). The mechanism and resulting injuries for each of the six types are illustrated in figure 7.4. The first three types (types I-III), originally described by Tossy and colleagues (1963) and Allman (1967), are most common, accounting for nearly 98% of all AC injuries (Lambert and Hertel 2002). Types IV through VI are rare.

The six types of AC injury are characterized as follows (Peterson and Renström 2001):

- Type I: Isolated sprain of the AC ligament, with pain over the AC joint; minimal pain with shoulder motion; mild tenderness
- Type II: Widening of the AC joint with elevation of the distal end of the clavicle with disruption of AC ligament; moderate to severe pain; limited shoulder motion

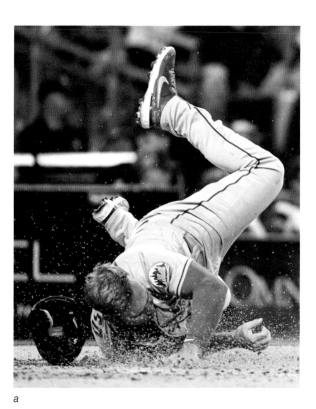

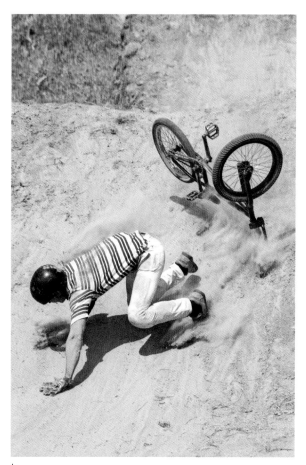

a

b

FIGURE 7.3 Mechanisms of acromioclavicular sprain (separated shoulder). *(a)* Collision with an object or surface. *(b)* Falling on an outstretched hand or arm.

(a) Denis Poroy/Getty Images *(b)* Sergey Lavrentev/fotolia.com

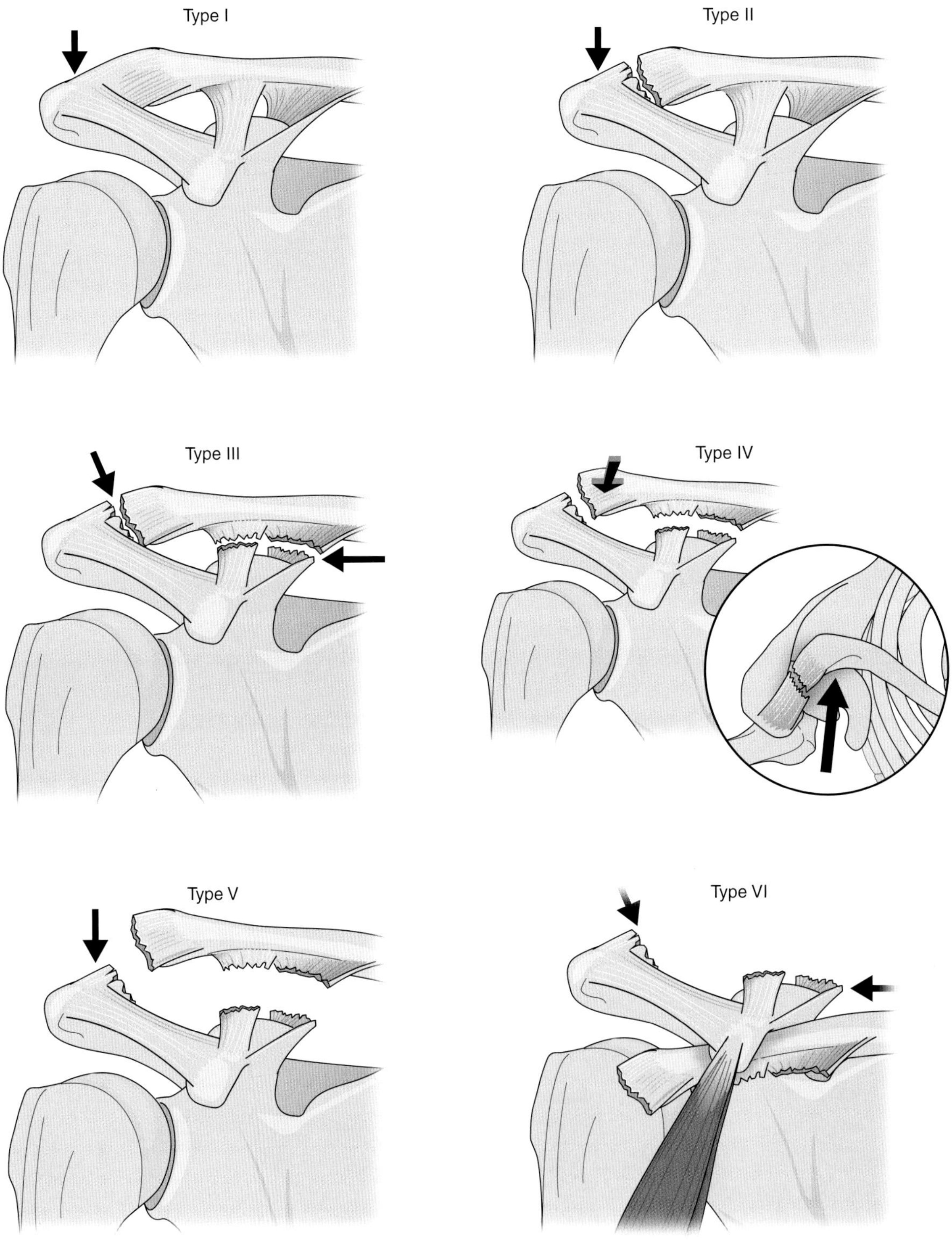

FIGURE 7.4 Types of acromioclavicular joint injury (I-VI).

- Type III: Dislocation of AC joint with superior displacement of clavicle; disruption of coraco-clavicular ligaments; widened coracoclavicular space; moderate to severe pain; upper extremity depressed with possible free-floating clavicle

- Type IV: Dislocated AC joint, with posterior displacement of clavicle into or through trapezius muscle; complete disruption of coracoclavicular ligament; clinically similar to type III but with greater pain and posterior clavicular displacement

- Type V: Disruption of acromioclavicular and coracoclavicular ligaments; gross displacement of AC joint; clinically similar to type III but with more pain and displacement

- Type VI: Disruption of acromioclavicular and coracoclavicular ligaments; inferior displacement of clavicle into subacromial or subcoracoid position

Glenohumeral Instability and Dislocation

The ability of any joint to resist dislocation is directly related to its inherent stability. What the shoulder gains in mobility, it sacrifices in stability. As discussed in chapter 6, joints such as the hip, with good bony fit and extensive surrounding musculature, rarely dislocate. The glenohumeral joint, in contrast, is prone to dislocation (luxation) because of its poor bony fit and limited supporting musculature. The shallowness of the glenoid fossa and limited contact area between the fossa and the humeral head contribute to the joint's instability.

The glenoid labrum improves the joint fit to a limited extent by increasing surface area and deepening the fossa, but nonetheless the glenohumeral joint is arguably the least stable articulation in the body—a dubious distinction substantiated by its frequent dislocation. The factors contributing to its stability, therefore, must be understood to discuss

---

Frozen Shoulder

In 1872, French physician E.S. Duplay described a "peri-arthritis" characterized by shoulder stiffness and limited joint movement. Sixty-two years later, E.A. Codman (1934) coined the term *frozen shoulder* to describe the same condition and its attendant pain and reduced external rotation and abduction.

Neviaser (1945) identified the condition as **adhesive capsulitis,** a term still sometimes used to describe the condition. Frozen shoulder is an idiopathic condition involving shoulder stiffness and pain affecting the anterior joint capsule and the rotator cuff interval (between the subscapularis and supraspinatus). Magnetic resonance arthrographic assessment points to a thickening of the coracohumeral ligament in the rotator cuff interval (Mengiardi et al. 2004).

The three primary symptoms of frozen shoulder are insidious shoulder stiffness, severe pain, and loss of both passive and active external rotation (Cho et al. 2019; Dias et al. 2005; Robinson et al. 2012). Frozen shoulder most commonly afflicts persons 40 to 70 years of age and is more common in women than men.

Although the cause of frozen shoulder is unknown, several factors have been associated with the condition. These include rotator cuff pathology, diabetes, thyroid and autoimmune disease, cervical spine disease, trauma, chest disease, or hyperlipidemia (Clasper 2002).

Frozen shoulder typically resolves in 1 to 3 years but not always completely. Three clinical stages have been described (Chan et al. 2017; Clasper 2002; Dias et al. 2005):

- *Stage 1.* Painful (freezing) stage—gradual pain onset, especially at night. Stiffness results in less arm use.

- *Stage 2.* Stiffening (adhesive) stage—pain reduction with residual stiffness. Reduced joint movements, especially shoulder external rotation.

- *Stage 3.* Thawing (resolution) stage—improved joint range of motion.

Despite progress in the diagnosis and treatment of frozen shoulder, much of what Codman said in 1934 still holds true: "This is a class of cases that I find difficult to define, difficult to treat, and difficult to explain from the point of view of pathology" (Codman 1934, p. 216).

adequately the mechanisms of glenohumeral dislocation.

Stabilizing factors are classified as active (dynamic) or passive (static). **Active stabilization** is provided by muscles surrounding and acting at the glenohumeral joint. These include the deltoid, trapezius, latissimus dorsi, pectoralis major, and muscles of the rotator cuff group (subscapularis, supraspinatus, infraspinatus, and teres minor). In midrange positions, shoulder muscles act as powerful glenohumeral stabilizers. At end-range positions, however, certain muscles (e.g., deltoid and pectoralis major) may contribute to glenohumeral instability (Labriola et al. 2005).

Passive stabilization is provided by the joint capsule and supporting ligaments. At the extremes of joint movement, tension in the capsuloligamentous structures provides resistance to dislocation. The laxity in these structures necessary for the exceptional movements at the glenohumeral joint precludes their involvement as stabilizers throughout normal ranges of motion. During normal ranges of motion, other stabilizing mechanisms are necessary. These include the combined effects of negative intracapsular pressure and the mechanisms of concavity compression and scapulohumeral balance.

In a normal (i.e., undamaged capsule) glenohumeral joint, a small negative intracapsular pressure helps stabilize the joint (Speer 1995). Although not especially large, this force (90-140 N) nonetheless contributes to maintaining glenohumeral stability throughout its range of motion.

The mechanisms of concavity compression and scapulohumeral balance also contribute significantly to joint stabilization. **Concavity compression** refers to the stability created when a convex object is pressed into a concave surface (Lippitt and Matsen 1993). When the surfaces are pressed together, there is greater resistance to translational movement between the surfaces. At the surface between the humeral head and the glenoid fossa, numerous muscle forces increase the articular pressure and stabilize the joint. Translational resistance at the glenohumeral articulation is greater in the superior–inferior direction than in the anterior–posterior direction and increases with greater compressive loads. Despite the resistance, translation occurs with combined abduction, extension, and external rotation of the glenohumeral joint.

Using a three-dimensional position sensor and force and torque transducers, Harryman and colleagues (1990) reported translation of the humeral head with passive glenohumeral motion. They found significant anterior translation during glenohumeral flexion and cross-body movement and posterior translation with extension and external rotation. Their results have clinical relevance because they indicate that the glenohumeral joint does not function purely as a ball-and-socket mechanism and that even passive manipulation of the joint causes significant translation of the humeral head across the glenoid fossa.

More recently, Klemt et al. (2018) reported compressive and shear forces during activities of daily life (ADLs) and emphasized the importance of glenohumeral loading in designing implants, surgical procedures, and rehabilitation protocols. Exemplar glenohumeral loads are presented in table 7.3.

Scapulohumeral balance refers to the coordinated muscle action that maintains the net joint reaction force within the fossa. As seen in figure 7.5, when the reaction–force line of action is directed into the glenoid, the joint is stable. The joint becomes unstable as the line of action moves away from the geometric center of the glenoid and beyond the surface boundary. Responsibility for maintaining appropriate glenohumeral congruity lies most immediately with the rotator cuff muscles and secondarily with the deltoid, trapezius, serratus anterior, rhomboids, latissimus dorsi, and levator scapulae. Fatigue in any of these muscles (e.g., from repeated throwing) compromises the compensatory capability of the musculoskeletal complex at the shoulder and predictably increases the potential for injuries such as tendinitis, impingement, rotator cuff pathology, joint instability, and glenohumeral luxation.

Individuals with congenitally lax shoulders may experience atraumatic dislocations caused by minimal forces. Most cases of shoulder dislocation, however, arise from traumatic insult to the glenohumeral complex. In the vast majority of these cases (>90%), dislocation occurs anteriorly. Anterior dislocation occurs most often from indirect forces when axial loads are applied to an abducted, extended, and externally rotated arm (figure 7.3b). Less frequently, anterior dislocation results from direct forces applied to the posterior aspect of the humerus (figure 7.6a).

Though rare, several cases of bilateral glenohumeral dislocations have been reported. In one unique case, a young man experienced bilateral anterior glenohumeral dislocation while he was performing a bench press. The lifter became fatigued,

TABLE 7.3 GLENOHUMERAL LOADS DURING ACTIVITIES OF DAILY LIVING

Activity	Glenohumeral (GH) contact force (% body weight)	Ratio of GH shear force (superior [+], inferior [–]) to compression force	Ratio of GH shear force (posterior [+], anterior [–]) to compression force
Reach back of head	33	0.13	–0.24
Clean back	39	–0.57	–0.16
Eat with spoon	32	0.09	–0.16
Lift shopping bag from floor	53	–0.32	–0.21
Sit to stand	164	0.41	–0.50
Pull	38	–0.77	–0.14
Push	38	–0.81	–0.19
Abduction (slow)	58	0.28	–0.23
Abduction (fast)	54	0.30	–0.18
Flexion (slow)	54	0.13	–0.19
Flexion (fast)	51	0.14	–0.14

Adapted by permission from C. Klemt et al., "Analysis of Shoulder Compressive and Shear Forces During Functional Activities of Daily Life," *Clinical Biomechanics* 54, (2018): 34–41. Distributed under the terms of the Creative Commons Attribution 4.0 International License (http://creativecommons .org/licenses/by/4.0/).

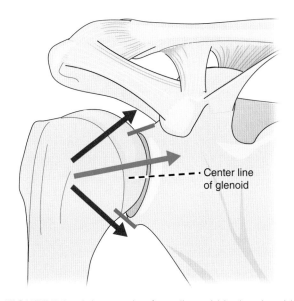

Center line of glenoid

FIGURE 7.5 Joint reaction force line within the glenoid (green arrow, stable) and outside of the glenoid (red arrows, unstable). The joint reaction force line of action can move outside the glenoid boundaries (blue lines) through movement of the humerus, reorientation of the glenoid, or a combination of both.

causing the weight of the bar to force his arms into hyperextension while in a midabducted position. His humeral shafts pivoted on the bench and forced the humeral heads to dislocate anteriorly (Cresswell and Smith 1998). Other bilateral dislocations have

resulted from seizures (Rudy and Hennrikus 2017; Taneja et al. 2013), falls (Agrahari et al. 2020; Khedr et al. 2017; Silva et al. 2015), and horseback riding (Turhan and Demirel 2008).

Approximately 25% of anterior shoulder dislocations are complicated by concomitant fracture. Risk factors for fracture–dislocations are age (≥40 years), first episode of dislocation, and mechanism (e.g., fall from heights, fight or assault, or motor vehicle crash) (Emond et al. 2004).

Posterior glenohumeral dislocations are relatively rare, largely due to static stabilizers (posterior labrum, joint capsule, posterior-inferior glenohumeral ligament) and dynamic stabilization from the subscapularis (Doehrmann and Frush 2021). Mechanisms of posterior dislocation essentially reverse those just described for anterior dislocation. Indirect forces transmitted through a flexed, adducted, and internally rotated shoulder drive the humerus posteriorly (figure 7.6*b*). Posterior dislocation also results from direct trauma to the anterior aspect of the humerus (figure 7.6*c*) or to an arm subjected to forceful internal rotation and adduction (Samilson and Prieto 1983).

Cases have been reported in which violent muscle contractions during electrical shock or seizures have caused posterior dislocations. In such cases, the substantial forces of fully activated internal rotators (subscapularis, latissimus dorsi, and pectoralis

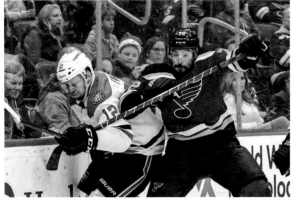

a

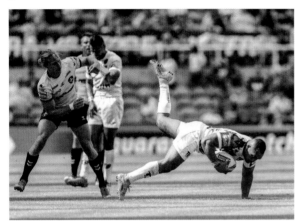

b

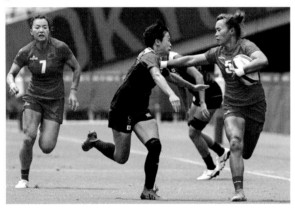

c

FIGURE 7.6 Mechanisms of glenohumeral dislocation (luxation). *(a)* Anterior glenohumeral dislocation from direct force applied to the posterior aspect of the shoulder. *(b)* Posterior glenohumeral dislocation from indirect force applied through the arm in a flexed, adducted, and internally rotated position. *(c)* Posterior glenohumeral dislocation from direct force applied to the anterior aspect of the shoulder.

(a) Rick Ulreich/Icon Sportswire via Getty Images *(b)* Lee Parker - CameraSport via Getty Images *(c)* GREG BAKER/AFP via Getty Images

major) overwhelm the external rotators (infraspinatus and teres minor) and leverage the humeral head from the glenoid fossa. Occasional inferior dislocations occur from a hyperabduction mechanism that creates a fulcrum between the humeral neck and the acromion process and levers the head out inferiorly.

Rotator Cuff Pathologies: A Closer Look

 Rotator cuff problems are a common source of pain and dysfunction in persons who use overhead movements in their work or play. Because of the prevalence of rotator cuff pathologies and the resultant potential for disability, we present in this section a detailed review of glenohumeral impingement and rotator cuff injury.

Tissue Structure and Function

The morphology of the rotator cuff musculotendinous unit and surrounding structures dictates glenohumeral motion and the joint's susceptibility to impingement syndrome and rotator cuff lesions. Table 7.4 summarizes the structural and functional characteristics of the muscles of the rotator cuff group.

The rotator cuff muscles receive their vascular supply from a number of arteries. A critical zone of hypovascular tissue has been demonstrated in the distal 1.0 to 1.5 cm of the supraspinatus and infraspinatus tendons. The hypovascularity in this area has been suggested by some as a predisposing factor in rotator cuff pathology, but "the existence and extent of a true critical zone, and its significance relative to the pathological changes occurring with the rotator cuff, remains in question" (Malcarney and Murrell 2003, p. 995).

Healthy rotator cuff tendons contain predominantly water and type I collagen fibers (with trace quantities of type III collagen). Type I collagen fibers present in a parallel orientation. Type III fibers, in contrast, tend to orient in a more random pattern, are smaller, and have a lower tensile strength than type I fibers. Greater amounts of type III collagen are found in tendons undergoing repair and those that are aging and degenerating. From a structural perspective, it is not surprising that damaged and aging rotator cuff tendons are more susceptible to injury.

We stress the importance of recognizing the integral relations among glenohumeral impingement, joint instability, and rotator cuff lesions. Rotator cuff ruptures often are rooted in prior impingement syndromes, with a continuum of causality progressing from mild impingement to complete rotator cuff

TABLE 7.4   Structural and Functional Characteristics of the Rotator Cuff Muscles

	Subscapularis	**Supraspinatus**	**Infraspinatus**	**Teres minor**
Origin	Ventral scapula	Superior scapula	Dorsal scapula	Dorsolateral scapula
Insertion (on humerus)	Lesser tuberosity	Greater tuberosity	Greater tuberosity	Greater tuberosity
Innervation	Subscapular nerve (C5-C8)	Suprascapular nerve (C4-C6)	Suprascapular nerve (C4-C6)	Axillary nerve (C5-C6)
Movement function (at glenohumeral joint)	Internal rotator	Abductor	External rotator	External rotator

rupture. Thus, separating the discussion of these two types of injury is, to some extent, arbitrary. A comprehensive discussion of shoulder pathology should not involve either one of these conditions at the exclusion of the other.

Glenohumeral Impingement

An **impingement** syndrome occurs when increased pressure within a confined anatomical space deleteriously affects the enclosed tissues. With respect to the glenohumeral joint, impingement syndrome is an ill-defined term and can refer to either of two major glenohumeral impingement types: subacromial impingement and internal impingement.

Types of Impingement   **Subacromial impingement** refers to shoulder abduction that results in suprahumeral structures (most notably the distal supraspinatus tendon, subacromial bursae, and proximal tendon of the long head of the biceps brachii) being forcibly pressed against the anterior surface of the acromion and the coracoacromial ligament (which together form the **coracoacromial arch**) (figure 7.7). In addition to affecting suprahumeral structures, subacromial impingement may result in glenohumeral articular cartilage lesions (Guntern et al. 2003).

Subacromial contact pressures are elevated in patients with impingement syndrome; maximal contact pressure develops with the arm in a hyperabducted position or with the arm adducted across the patient's chest with the arm internally rotated (Nordt et al. 1999). **Acromioplasty** has proved effective in reducing subacromial contact pressure by cutting or shaving bone to flatten the acromion.

Walch and colleagues (1992) described another form of impingement (**internal impingement**), in which the supraspinatus tendon contacts the posterior–superior rim of the glenoid fossa and the posterior labrum. This mechanism may be signifi-

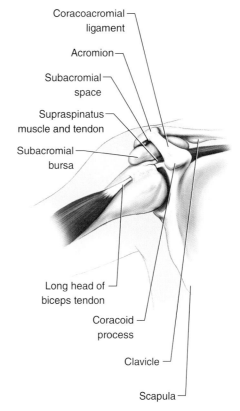

FIGURE 7.7   Abducting the arm elevates the humeral head, impinging the subacromical bursa, distal tendon of the supraspinatus, and proximal tendon of the biceps brachii (long head) against the coracoacromial arch.

cant in the development of rotator cuff pathologies (Edelson and Teitz 2000). Internal impingement often happens in throwing, when the shoulder is abducted and externally rotated (e.g., cocking phase in an overhead throw), but is not limited to throwers (McFarland et al. 1999). Internal impingement may involve undersurface (articular-sided) tears of the supraspinatus or infraspinatus tendons, posterosuperior labral fraying, anterior labral fraying, and osteochondral lesions (Giaroli et al. 2005;

Paley et al. 2000). Caution is warranted in attributing all undersurface rotator cuff lesions to internal impingement, because other mechanisms may be responsible (Budoff et al. 2003).

In their review of subtypes of anterior impingement (e.g., subcoracoid impingement, anterosuperior impingement, "chondral print," frayed upper subscapularis with impingement [FUSSI] lesion), Cunningham and Lädermann (2018) concluded, "Although advances in biomechanical research and arthroscopic technologies have helped to better understand these entities, current scientific literature is still riddled with conflicting theories and results" (p. 359).

Etiology Impingement pathologies fall into two broad age-based categories. Impingement in those younger than 35 years usually happens to participants in sports (e.g., swimming, water polo, baseball, or American football) or occupations (e.g., carpenter or painter) involving extensive overhead movements. Overhead-throwing athletes are at particular risk for internal impingement (Corpus et al. 2016; Lin et al. 2018). Older individuals are more likely to suffer from the effects of degenerative processes that lead to bone spur formation, capsular thinning, decreased tissue perfusion, and muscular atrophy, all of which can contribute to age-related degenerative rotator cuff tears (Keener et al. 2019).

Jobe and Pink (1993) proposed an injury classification based on age-related differences. Group I injuries are characterized by isolated impingement with no joint instability and are usually found in older (>35 years) recreational athletes. Group II injuries result from overuse, typically in young (18-35 years) overhead athletes, and present primarily as glenohumeral instability with secondary impingement. Group III injuries also are common to young overhead athletes and are closely associated with group II. They are differentiated from group II by the presence of generalized ligamentous laxity at the elbow, knee, and fingers.

Repeated abduction places large stresses on the musculotendinous and capsuloligamentous structures and eventually leads to tissue microtrauma. Continued mechanical loading further weakens the tissues and hastens their failure. Tissue failure, in turn, contributes to glenohumeral instability and greater joint movement. This increases the chance of humeral subluxation, which further aggravates the impingement condition. Thus, the person is trapped in an unfortunate loop of joint deterioration and compromised function.

A well-established association exists between (1) rotator cuff muscle weakness and subacromial impingement (e.g., Reddy et al. 2000) and (2) altered glenohumeral and scapulothoracic kinematics (e.g., Halder et al. 2001; Yamaguchi et al. 2000). The question of whether rotator cuff weakness hastens the impingement, or whether the impingement ultimately weakens the muscles, remains unresolved.

Acromial structure also is cited as a factor in glenohumeral impingement. The most commonly used system for classifying acromial morphology, first presented by Bigliani et al. (1986), specifies three shapes, as shown in figure 7.8. Farley et al. (1994) also suggested a fourth acromion type (inferiorly convex).

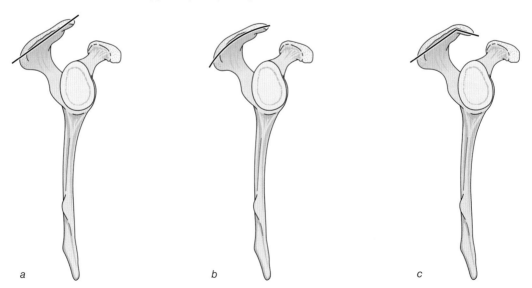

a   b   c

FIGURE 7.8 Variation in acromion shapes (lateral view). *(a)* Type I, flat. *(b)* Type II, curved. *(c)* Type III, hooked.

Other morphological features have been implicated in impingement and rotator cuff lesions. These include thickening of the coracoacromial ligament (Farley et al. 1994; Ogata and Uhthoff 1990; Soslowsky et al. 1996), anterior tilt of the acromion (Prato et al. 1998), age-related changes in acromial morphology (Wang and Shapiro 1997), and **os acromiale** (Hutchinson and Veenstra 1993). McLean and Taylor (2019) provide a recent review of acromial classifications and measures.

Research using alternative methods of classifying acromial morphology has found a stronger relation between arch geometry and shoulder dysfunction (Prato et al. 1998; Tuite et al. 1995; Vaz et al. 2000). Kaur et al. (2019) reported a higher prevalence of impingement and rotator cuff tears associated with low lateral acromial angle, larger critical shoulder angle, and lower acromiohumeral distance, but no relation between acromial type and cuff lesions. In summary, the exact relation between acromial shape and rotator cuff pathology remains equivocal.

In light of the evidence, there is likely no single mechanism of impingement injury, but rather a variety of factors specific to each individual's morphological characteristics and history of joint loading.

Risk factors for glenohumeral impingement syndrome are the same as those associated with other cumulative trauma disorders of the shoulder (e.g., bicipital tendinitis, subacromial bursitis, or **thoracic outlet syndrome**). These factors include awkward or static postures, heavy work, direct load bearing, repetitive arm movements, working with hands above shoulder height, and fatigue resulting from lack of rest.

Impingement syndrome affects special populations as well. Wheelchair athletes, for example, suffer a high incidence of rotator cuff impingement, with muscle imbalance suggested as a causal mechanism. The typical pattern of imbalance in wheelchair athletes differs from that seen in overhead athletes such as baseball pitchers, swimmers, and water polo players. Muscle imbalance in the overhead athlete appears as a relative weakness in the abductors and external rotators. Wheelchair athletes, in contrast, typically exhibit relative weakness in the adductors and overall rotator strength deficiency. The resulting abductor dominance exaggerates superior movement of the humeral head and leads to impingement in the subacromial space (Burnham et al. 1993). In addition to wheelchair athletes, individuals with spinal cord injury (SCI) using manual wheelchairs are at risk for glenohumeral impingement during

scapular plane elevation and propulsion (Mozingo et al. 2020).

The mechanisms underlying rotator cuff impingement are the subject of ongoing debate. In a broad sense, the mechanisms can be intrinsic (inflammatory changes within the cuff), extrinsic (forces acting outside the rotator cuff), or both.

Rotator Cuff Rupture

Rupture of musculotendinous structures in the rotator cuff typically results from a chain of events that begins with minor inflammation and progresses (with continued overuse) to advanced inflammation, microtearing of tissue, and eventual partial or complete cuff rupture. Compromised tissue integrity and muscle fatigue contribute to altered movement mechanics, and these modified movements further stress the involved tissues and hasten their eventual failure. The supraspinatus is the most commonly injured muscle in the rotator cuff group (Goldberg et al. 2001) (figure 7.9). Supraspinatus injury, in particular, is associated with repeated, and often violent, overhead movement patterns (e.g., throwing, striking, hammering, or painting). Less frequently, other cuff muscles suffer damage.

Many of the complex movements at the shoulder stress the muscles of the rotator cuff group. The throwing motion, in particular, places exceptional loads on the shoulder. As a result of these loads, the rotator cuff is especially susceptible to injury. The entire rotator cuff synergistically resists distraction

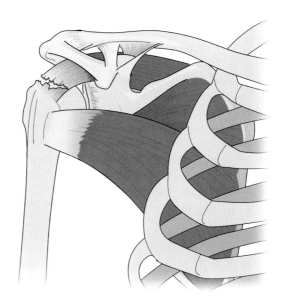

FIGURE 7.9 Rotator cuff tear (distal tendon of supraspinatus).

forces that tend to pull the humeral head from the glenoid. Injury or fatigue to any of these muscles leads to altered throwing mechanics and increases the chance of additional tissue damage.

Intrinsic mechanisms have long been implicated as a cause of impingement-related rotator cuff lesions, suggesting that the degenerative process is inherent to the supraspinatus itself. This is largely attributable to compromised blood flow resulting from impingement pressures and regions of relative avascularity in the supraspinatus near its humeral attachment. Convincing evidence supports this concept. First, rotator cuff lesions are often seen in the absence of any extrinsic involvement. Second, studies have shown that degeneration first occurs on the articular surface of the tendon rather than on the bursal side. Support for the role of hypovascularity in impingement pathologies, however, is not universal.

The extrinsic approach, originally suggested by Neer (1972), implicates external factors such as compression of the rotator cuff tendon by external structures. Other extrinsic factors that may hasten glenohumeral impingement and resultant rotator cuff tears include faulty posture, capsular tightness, altered joint kinematics and structural pathologies in the coracoacromial arch (Michener et al. 2003), and osteophytes (bone spurs) in the joint spaces that serve as stress risers, focusing forces on the supraspinatus tendon and producing a functionally smaller supraspinatus outlet.

Kinematic Patterns and Cuff Lesions The specific muscles with pathological involvement depend on the shoulder movement pattern. In a classic study, Burkhart (1993) identified four distinct patterns of rotator cuff kinematics associated with specific cuff lesions. All of the patterns involve injury to the supraspinatus. Burkhart (1993) reported that type I (stable fulcrum kinematics) lesions showed tears of the supraspinatus and part of the infraspinatus but not to a level that disrupted essential force couples. Patients had normal motion and near-normal strength levels.

Patients with type II lesions (unstable fulcrum kinematics, posterior cuff tear pattern) exhibited massive tears of the superior and posterior portions of the rotator cuff, which resulted in an uncoupling of the essential force couples and led to an unstable fulcrum for glenohumeral motion. Type II patients could perform little more than a shoulder shrug.

Type III (captured fulcrum kinematics) and type IV (unstable fulcrum kinematics, subscapularis tear pattern) lesions both involved tears of the subscapularis. The less severe type III patterns had partial subscapularis tears (accompanying superior and posterior damage). Muscle damage in type III patients prevented the humeral head from centering in the glenoid fossa, and the humerus subluxated superiorly and formed a captured acromiohumeral fulcrum that restricted humeral elevation. Type IV lesions involved tears of the supraspinatus and subscapularis, with the posterior cuff muscles remaining intact. This was a reversal of the type II pattern in which an unstable glenohumeral fulcrum attributable to the force couple imbalances was created by the muscle tears. Shoulder elevation in the type IV patients was poor (Burkhart 1993). The type IV category included injuries resulting from a traumatic event such as a fall. Macrotrauma may be associated with contact sports (Blevins 1997) such as American professional football, where the most common mechanism for full-thickness rotator cuff tears is a fall onto the shoulder (Foulk et al. 2002).

Acromion Types and Cuff Tears Evidence of an association between acromion type and rotator cuff lesions is inconsistent. A hooked (type III) acromion (figure 7.8c) has been associated with higher incidence of rotator cuff tears; however, evidence of this association is mixed. Some studies have reported a positive relation between acromial type and rotator cuff lesions (Blake et al. 2013; Bigliani and Levine 1997; Toivonen et al. 1995), whereas others have failed to find a significant relation (Banas et al. 1995; Chalmers et al. 2020; Farley et al. 1994). The primary difficulty with finding a significant relation may be the fair-to-poor interobserver reliability in determining acromion type (Bright et al. 1997; Haygood et al. 1994; Jacobson et al. 1995; Zuckerman et al. 1997).

Treatment of Rotator Cuff Pathologies

Proper treatment of rotator cuff pathologies is essential to restoring upper-extremity function. Conservative (i.e., nonsurgical) treatment typically is the first course of action and often proves effective. In more severe cases, surgical intervention may be indicated.

Conservative Treatment The choice of treatment for subacromial impingement syndrome and other rotator cuff pathologies is difficult because of the multifactorial nature of the condition (Michener et al. 2003). Conservative (nonoperative) treatment of impingement and rotator cuff pathology begins with avoidance of aggravating activities and includes use of stretching to increase range of motion, nonsteroidal medications to control inflammation, occasional corticosteroid injections, and physical modalities. These treatments continue until pain is reduced. As pain decreases, a progressive strength training program can begin. Such a treatment program results in patient satisfaction about 50% of the time (Ruotolo and Nottage 2002).

Several factors have been identified that predict a poor prognosis for conservative treatment. These include rotator cuff tears greater than 1 cm, severe muscle weakness, and a history of symptoms lasting more than 1 year (Bartolozzi et al. 1994). Itoi and Tabata (1992) also found a 12-month history of symptoms to be a significantly poor prognostic indicator. Hawkins and Dunlop (1995) reported sleep-interrupting pain as a poor prognostic factor for conservative treatment.

There is ongoing debate about conservative versus surgical treatment for degenerative (i.e., nontraumatic) rotator cuff tears. Some studies have reported similar outcomes when comparing conservative and surgical approaches (Kukkonen et al. 2014; Kukkonen et al. 2015). Others have found mixed results. For example, Lambers Heerspink et al. (2015), using a randomized control study, compared conservative versus surgical treatment of full-thickness rotator cuff tears. Using the Constant-Murley score, a 100-point scale composed of individual parameters (pain, activities of daily living, strength, range of motion) they found no differences in functional outcomes, but significant differences in pain and disabilities that favored surgical treatment. Still other studies have reported improved outcomes for surgical (versus conservative) treatment (Piper et al. 2018; Schemitsch et al. 2019).

Studies with short follow-up periods have shown no or smaller differences than longer-term studies. Moosmayer et al. (2019) reported that differences in outcome between surgery and physiotherapy for small and medium-sized rotator cuff tears were greater 10 years after treatment compared to shorter follow-ups in the same patients. The longer-term differences favored surgical repair.

Surgical Treatment   More than a century ago, Codman (1911) reported his surgical repair of a completely ruptured supraspinatus tendon. Since that time, remarkable progress has been made in our understanding of rotator cuff morphology, shoulder pathomechanics, and treatment techniques.

In terms of pain relief and return of muscle strength, surgical repair of traumatic rotator cuff tears typically has a higher success rate than conservative approaches (Ruotolo and Nottage 2002; Wittenberg et al. 2001). Surgical treatment of a rotator cuff tear is indicated for four groups:

- An active 20- to 30-year-old patient with an acute cuff tear, accompanied by serious functional deficit
- A 30- to 50-year-old patient with an acute tear secondary to a particular event
- A high-level competitive athlete, especially one who participates in overhead or throwing activities
- A patient who does not respond to conservative treatment

Although a detailed account of the many surgical techniques used to repair rotator cuff tears is beyond the scope of our discussion, mention is warranted of the pioneering work of Charles Neer, whose recognition of the anterior acromion's role in the pathogenesis of rotator cuff lesions laid the foundation for all subsequent surgical techniques. The goals of Neer's approach to cuff repair were to close the cuff defect, eliminate impingement, preserve the deltoid, and prevent stiffness (Neer 1990). "His surgical technique of an open superior approach, acromioplasty, coracoacromial ligament excision, tendon mobilization, and tendon repair to bone remains the 'gold standard' to which all contemporary methods of surgical treatment of rotator cuff tears must be compared" (Williams et al. 2004, p. 2765).

Whatever the surgical technique used, one must be mindful of the biomechanical aspects of surgical repair. As Burkhart (2000, p. 89) noted, "Much of the history of rotator cuff repair has been checkered by ill-advised attempts to simply cover the hole in the cuff. By ignoring shoulder mechanics, many of these methods can actually make the shoulder worse. . . . Meticulous attention to detail at every step is critical. A loose suture or a poorly placed anchor can mean loss of integrity of the entire construct. In orthopaedic surgery as in structural engineering, structural integrity is built one step at a time."

Among the important issues requiring consideration are indications for and timing of surgical repair, surgical method (i.e., open, mini-open, or arthroscopic), the need for acromioplasty or coracoacromial ligament excision, and management of irreparable cuff tears (Williams et al. 2004).

All surgical methods have proved successful. Open rotator cuff repair has a long history of success. More recently, mini-open and arthroscopic surgical techniques have also gained favor, often with comparable or better results (Buess et al. 2005; Rebuzzi et al. 2005). Most studies have found little or no difference in results between arthroscopic and mini-open rotator cuff repair in terms of long-term outcomes (Sauerbrey et al. 2005; Warner et al. 2005; Youm et al. 2005), but the arthroscopic group has shown less pain and greater shoulder flexion immediately after surgery (Karakoc and Atalay 2020; Kelly et al. 2019; Liu et al. 2017). In summary, "The effects of arthroscopic compared to mini-open rotator cuff repair, on function, pain and range of motion are too small to be clinically important at 3-, 6-, and 12-month follow ups" (Nazari et al. 2019, p. 2).

One of the key factors in successful cuff repair is early operative intervention when tears are smaller, tendon degeneration is minimized, and the risk of re-rupture is reduced (Williams et al. 2004). Early diagnosis and repair of rotator cuff tears may also limit deterioration of the biceps tendon (Chen et al. 2005).

In cases of massive rotator cuff tears (MRCT), also termed *functionally irreparable rotator cuff tears* (FIRCT), a decision must be made about the surgical approach. Procedures to be considered include **debridement**, acromioplasty, biceps tendon splitting or tenodesis, superior capsule reconstruction, graft interposition, and balloon implantation (Burnier et al. 2019).

The most common option for MRCT and its attendant deficits, however, is muscle–tendon transfer (Kany 2020). Muscle–tendon transfer procedures have traditionally involved use of the pectoralis major for anterosuperior lesions (e.g., Wirth and Rockwood 1997) or the latissimus dorsi or teres major for posterosuperior cuff tears (e.g., Warner and Parsons 2001). More recently, lower trapezius tendon transfer with incorporated calcaneal tendon allografts has proved effective in dealing with MRCT (Stoll and Codding 2019). Transfer of the latissimus dorsi to the lesser tuberosity of the humerus is currently being considered as an alternative to pectoralis major transfer for massive subscapularis tears (Burnier et al. 2019).

Tendon transfers usually are limited to younger individuals (Lädermann et al. 2015). Older persons with chronic MRCT may have good clinical outcomes from a reverse total shoulder arthroplasty (Thorsness and Romeo 2016).

In cases where surgery is not feasible or successful, tissue engineering and regenerative medicine (TERM) solutions hold promise. Early studies by Funakoshi and colleagues (2005, 2006), for example, demonstrated the feasibility of rotator cuff regeneration using tissue engineering techniques, using a nonwoven chitin fabric as an acellular matrix for rotator cuff regeneration (type III collagen) in rabbits.

Currently, various technologies are being explored and developed for rotator cuff augmentation and repair. These technologies include extracellular tendon patches, scaffolds created by electrospinning (Hong et al. 2019; Stace et al. 2018), stem cells, growth factors, platelet-rich plasma, and chitosan–glycerol phosphate/blood implants for cartilage repair (Després-Tremblay et al. 2016).

Postoperative Care and Rehabilitation Following surgery, a well-designed rehabilitation program is essential for full recovery and return to normal activities. Each rehabilitation program should be individualized. Elements of a sound rehabilitation program include the following. Initially, the rotator cuff repair must be protected for 5 to 6 weeks. Immediately postsurgery, the patient begins exercises aimed at maintaining active elbow, wrist, and hand movements. Shoulder shrugs and scapular adduction exercises are included early on, along with pendulum exercises and gentle isometric exercises with a neutrally positioned arm. Three to four weeks postsurgery, passive mobilization can be added. Active assisted elevation can be added at 6 weeks, with other progressive resistance exercises added as allowed. Three months postsurgery, patients can return to most typical daily activities but no strenuous movements (e.g., lifting heavy objects or ballistic movements). Although tendon healing may be nearly complete by 3 months, return to full strength may take up to 1 year (Millstein and Snyder 2003).

The American Society of Shoulder and Elbow Therapists outlined time line components for rehabilitation following arthroscopic rotator cuff repair (Thigpen et al. 2016). These include the following:

- Phase 1 (0-6 weeks): Patient education; modalities (e.g., cryotherapy); passive range of motion (PROM) exercises

- Phase 2 (6-12 weeks): Near-full PROM; introduce active assisted range of motion (AAROM) and active range of motion (AROM) exercises; light strengthening when pain is well controlled; begin active arm elevation exercises

- Phase 3 (12-20 weeks): Emphasize muscle and tendon strengthening consistent with range of motion (ROM) milestones and goals; keep electromyographical (EMG) activity levels in the 30% to 49% of maximum range; overhead strengthening only for patients who demonstrate adequate tolerance of resisted elevation in the scapular plane

- Phase 4 (20-26 weeks): Continued and advanced strengthening as tolerated; exercises ≥50% EMG

Rotator Cuff Pathology Prevention

Given the prevalence of both symptomatic and asymptomatic impingement and rotator cuff lesions, prevention is a primary issue, especially for those at risk. A sound prevention program should include two elements: (1) a physical conditioning program, and (2) recognition and modification of any underlying pathomechanics. Any injury prevention approach focused solely on improving physical condition may ultimately prove ineffective if underlying pathomechanics (e.g., improper movement mechanics) are not addressed as well. Moreover, these preventive steps must be supplemented with early recognition and intervention strategies.

The physical conditioning program should involve muscles that stabilize and move the glenohumeral and scapulothoracic joints, with emphasis on improving the strength and endurance of the rotator cuff muscles. Special attention should be given to strengthening the subscapularis. Range of motion improvement also is indicated at both the glenohumeral joint (taking care not to overstretch the anterior joint capsule) and scapulothoracic joint. Activity should also be monitored to reduce movements that might aggravate the condition. Technique correction may help prevent injury (Jobe 1997).

Labral Pathologies

The glenohumeral labrum is a fibrocartilage rim that encircles the articular surface of the scapular glenoid fossa. Inferiorly, the labrum appears as a rounded fibrous structure continuous with the hyaline articular cartilage. Superiorly, the labrum is more meniscus-like with loose attachment to the glenoid (Nam and Snyder 2003). The labrum's vascular supply arises from capsular or periosteal vessels and is more pronounced peripherally than centrally. Compared with other labral areas, the superior and anterosuperior portions have reduced vascularity (Cooper et al. 1992). Overall, blood supply to the labrum is adequate to enable its reattachment following injury (Alashkham et al. 2017).

Age-Related Rotator Cuff Pathologies: Normal or Not?

In older persons, the rotator cuff can degenerate with accompanying osteophyte formation, thinning of the joint capsule, decreased blood perfusion, muscular atrophy, and eventual muscle tears. These pathologies may result in significant pain and loss of function. More than half of persons in their 80s present with rotator cuff tears (Tashjian 2012).

Studies also have found rotator cuff tear pathologies in asymptomatic individuals. Templehof and colleagues (1999) reported evidence of rotator cuff tears in 23% of 411 asymptomatic adults (≥50 years old), with a clear pattern of more tears with increasing age. In the oldest group (age >80 years), 51% of patients had cuff tears in the absence of symptoms. Other studies have reported similar results (Milgrom et al. 1995; Sher et al. 1995; Worland et al. 2003). In a cadaveric population, Lehman and colleagues (1995) found an increase in full thickness rotator cuff tears with increasing age; 30% of cadavers more than 60 years of age showed evidence of rotator cuff tears. More recently, others have confirmed the high prevalence of asymptomatic rotator cuff tears in older adults (Keener et al. 2015; Minagawa et al. 2013).

These studies show that rotator cuff tears "must to a certain extent be regarded as 'normal' degenerative attrition, not necessarily causing pain and functional impairment" (Tempelhof et al. 1999, p. 296). In summary, initially, asymptomatic rotator cuff tears (1) are prevalent in the general population, but especially so in older persons, (2) are likely to become symptomatic over time, and (3) eventually result in decreased function, strength, and range of motion (Lawrence et al. 2019).

Labral injuries can happen acutely or chronically, and are caused by a variety of mechanisms, including compression attributable to falls, traction (tension) from lifting, throwing in overhead sports, and glenohumeral dislocation–subluxation.

Anterior dislocation can cause an avulsion of the anteroinferior glenoid labrum at the attachment site of the inferior glenohumeral ligament complex (IGHL) in what is termed a **Bankart lesion** (figure 7.10*a*). The Bankart lesion, first described by British orthopedist Arthur Bankart (1923), is invariably accompanied by joint capsule disruption and

IGHL stretching. IGHL compromise contributes to recurrent anterior glenohumeral instability.

In 1990, Snyder and colleagues coined the term **SLAP lesion** (superior labrum anterior–posterior) to describe superior labral injuries. These investigators identified four types of SLAP lesions:

- Type I: Fraying of the superior labrum with no detachment at the biceps insertion (figure 7.10*b*)
- Type II: Detachment of the superior labrum and biceps tendon (figure 7.10*c*)

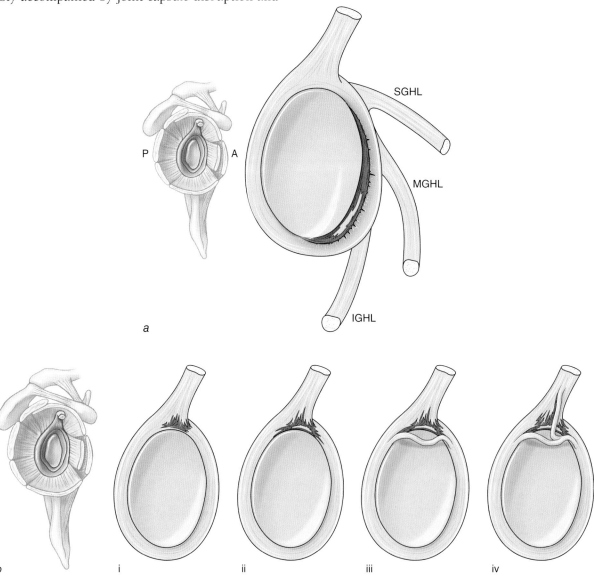

FIGURE 7.10 Labral injuries. *(a)* Bankart lesion involving an avulsion of the anteroinferior glenoid labrum at the attachment site of the inferior glenohumeral ligament (IGHL) complex. A = anterior; MGHL = middle glenohumeral ligament; P = posterior; SGHL = superior glenohumeral ligament. *(b)* Types of superior labrum anterior–posterior (SLAP) lesions. *(i)* Type I: Fraying of the superior labrum with no detachment at the biceps insertion. *(ii)* Type II: Detachment of the superior labrum and biceps tendon. *(iii)* Type III: Bucket-handle tear of the superior labrum with an intact biceps. *(iv)* Type IV: Bucket-handle tear of the superior labrum with tearing of the biceps tendon.

- Type III: Bucket-handle tear of the superior labrum with an intact biceps (figure 7.10*d*)
- Type IV: Bucket-handle tear of the superior labrum with tearing of the biceps tendon (figure 7.10*e*)

The prevalence of lesion type varies considerably among studies. For example, the prevalence of type I lesions in three studies ranged from 9.5% to 74%, whereas prevalence of type II lesions ranged from 21% to 55% (Handelberg et al. 1998; Kim et al. 2003; Snyder et al. 1995).

Morgan and colleagues (1998) subdivided type II SLAP lesions into three subtypes according to the location of the labral–biceps tendon detachment: anterior, posterior, and combined anterior–posterior. Type II SLAP lesions have been associated with the so-called *dead arm syndrome*, which limits a thrower's velocity and control, largely attributable to the pain and uneasiness associated with labral injury (Burkhart and Morgan 2001; Burkhart et al. 2000).

Andrews and colleagues (1985) first described superior labral tears near the origin of the long head of the biceps brachii in a population of overhead throwing athletes. The authors postulated that tension in the biceps tendon during throwing pulled the labrum from its attachment.

Several mechanisms have been suggested for SLAP lesions. Andrews and colleagues (1985) theorized a traction (tension) mechanism. Snyder and colleagues (1990, 1995) promoted a compression mechanism as seen in a fall or collision. Maffet and colleagues (1995) suggested a traction or pulling mechanism. Others (Jobe 1995; Walch et al. 1992) implicated contact with the rotator cuff muscles (e.g., supraspinatus) when the throwing arm is in a cocked position. Burkhart and Morgan (1998) and Morgan and colleagues (1998) described a mecha-

nism involving "peel-back" of the superior labrum when the biceps attachment is twisted during abduction and external rotation. Age-related degenerative SLAP lesion tears can also happen secondary to general wear and tear patterns associated with advancing age (Varacallo et al. 2021).

The reported frequency of SLAP lesion mechanisms varies, likely due to differences in the populations being assessed, including their age, physical condition, activity patterns, and associated injuries (e.g., rotator cuff pathology). Available information suggests that compression is likely the most common mechanism (table 7.5).

Upper-Arm Injuries

The upper arm (also called simply the *arm*) spans the shoulder and elbow joints and contains the humerus, which is surrounded by two muscle compartments. The anterior compartment contains the biceps brachii, brachialis, and coracobrachialis; the posterior compartment houses only the triceps brachii, a muscle complex with three heads: the long head, medial head, and lateral head (see figure 7.2). The humerus articulates proximally with the scapula and distally with the radius and ulna at the elbow joint.

Humeral Fracture

Fractures of the humerus account for about 5% to 8% of all fractures, with fracture risk increasing considerably with advancing age (Court-Brown and Caesar 2006; Ekholm et al. 2006; Praemer et al. 1999; Updegrove et al. 2018). Fracture location differs depending on age and sex, with younger males suffering more distal humeral fractures and older females more proximal fractures, usually resulting from falls and related to osteoporosis (Court-Brown and Caesar 2006; Kim et al. 2012). If current trends continue, an estimated 500,000 humeral fractures

TABLE 7.5 Mechanisms of SLAP Lesion Injuries

	Snyder et al. (1995) (N = 140)	Handelberg et al. (1998) (N = 32)
Compression (fall or compression)	43 (31)	9 (28)
Traction (lifting weight)	23 (16)	7 (22)
Dislocation–subluxation	27 (19)	7 (22)
Throwing (overhead sports)	16 (12)	8 (25)
Nonspecific onset	31 (22)	1 (3)

Values are n (%).

will happen in the United States in 2030 (Kim et al. 2012).

Humeral fractures result from either direct or indirect trauma. Direct injuries typically are high energy and exhibit extensive comminution (i.e., bone fragmentation) and soft tissue disruption, whereas indirect trauma involves less energy and minimal bony displacement.

The pattern of bone fracture varies: Compressive forces lead to proximal and distal end disruption, bending results in transverse shaft fracture, torsional loads create spiral fractures, and combined torsion and bending can cause oblique fracture or butterfly fragmentation. A commonly used classification system for humeral shaft fractures is presented in figure 7.11.

Humeral fractures typically result from direct trauma (e.g., fall on an outstretched hand or arm, motor vehicle crash). Fractures also occur, although rarely, in response to violent muscular contractions, as first reported by Wilkinson (1895).

The pattern of fracture depends on the magnitude, location, and direction of applied forces, with segment movement determined by the action of muscles in the area. For example, when fracture occurs proximal to the pectoralis major attachment site, the distal segment is displaced medially by the pectoralis major, whereas the proximal segment is abducted and internally rotated by the rotator cuff (figure 7.12a). If the fracture site is between the attachments of the pectoralis major and the deltoid, the distal segment is

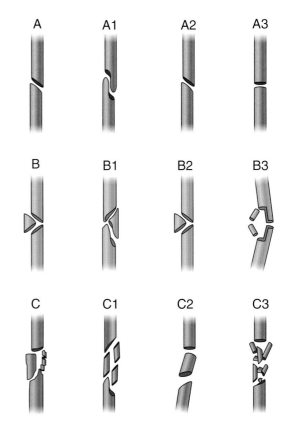

FIGURE 7.11 Classification system for humeral shaft fractures: A = simple fractures, B = wedge (butterfly) fractures, and C = complex (comminuted) fractures.

Reprinted from by permission from B.D. Browner et al., *Skeletal Trauma*, 3rd ed. (Philadelphia: Saunders, Ltd, 2003): 1485, with permission from Elsevier.

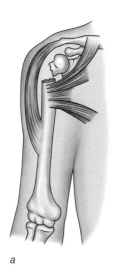
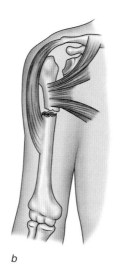
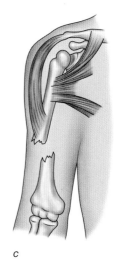

| a | b | c |

FIGURE 7.12 *(a)* Fracture proximal to the pectoralis major insertion. *(b)* Fracture distal to the pectoralis major insertion and proximal to the deltoid insertion. *(c)* Fracture distal to the deltoid insertion.

abducted through action of the deltoid, whereas the proximal segment is pulled medially by the pectoralis major, latissimus dorsi, and teres major (figure 7.12*b*). In fractures distal to the deltoid attachment, the proximal segment is abducted and flexed, with the distal segment displaced superiorly (figure 7.12*c*).

In most injuries, age plays a prominent role in determining the nature and extent of tissue damage, and the same is true of humeral fractures. Humeral fractures in older persons most commonly result from falls (Kim et al. 2012; Tytherleigh-Strong et al. 1998), whereas in young people the usual culprits are direct impact or vigorous throwing. Humeral fractures have been documented as a result of throwing objects as varied as baseballs, javelins, and hand grenades (e.g., Callaghan et al. 2004; Kaplan et al. 1998). Various theories have been proposed to explain throwing-related fractures, including factors of antagonistic muscle action, violent uncoordinated muscle action, poor throwing mechanics, excessive torsional forces, and fatigue.

A report on a series of 12 spontaneous humeral fractures in baseball players who played regularly in an over-30 league noted that the injured players had been inactive for years before joining the league. The prolonged layoff period may have contributed to disuse atrophy in the humerus and may have predisposed the athletes to both sudden and stress fractures. Four risk factors for fracture were identified: age (average age of the injured players was 36), prolonged absence from pitching activity, lack of regular exercise, and prodromal (precursory) arm pain (Branch et al. 1992). With fracture, as with many injuries, a person's condition and activity pattern play an important role in determining their susceptibility to injury.

Biceps Tendon Injuries

The proximal tendon of the long head of the biceps brachii (LHBB) has attachments at both the supraglenoid tubercle (or **biceps anchor**) and the superior rim of the glenoid labrum. The biceps anchor provides primary restraint for the LHBB tendon, with secondary restraint given by the labral attachment (Healey et al. 2001). From this attachment the biceps tendon courses through the rotator cuff interval in the bicipital groove of the humerus. Distally, the biceps brachii attaches to the radial tuberosity.

The primary action of the biceps brachii is to flex the elbow (with lesser involvement as a glenohumeral flexor). The proximal biceps tendon is predisposed to injury because of its intimate involvement with the action of the rotator cuff and

its attachment at the superior labrum. Injuries to the biceps tendon include chronic tenosynovitis and acute subluxation, dislocation, and rupture.

The cause of biceps injury is unclear, in large part because of the complex interaction of impingement and instability pathologies and considerable anatomical variability. Biceps tenosynovitis commonly is associated with repeated overhead tasks such as throwing. Acutely, tenosynovitis manifests as swelling and inflammation. With repeated insult, chronic tenosynovitis progresses to include tendon fraying, synovial proliferation, fibrosis, and eventual tendon rupture or dislocation (Ptasznik and Hennessy 1995).

The biceps tendon typically dislocates medially, often in conjunction with rotator cuff lesions and acute trauma. The mechanisms of biceps dislocation include abduction with external rotation, falls onto an outstretched hand, direct lateral impact, hyperextension, and anterior glenohumeral dislocation. Anatomical features, most notably the depth and angulation of the bicipital groove, have been implicated as predisposing factors in biceps tendon dislocation. The tendon is more likely to dislodge from a shallow or low-angled groove.

Given the integral relation between rotator cuff and biceps tendon pathologies, the mechanisms that encourage cuff lesions (e.g., impingement) also are strongly associated with biceps tendon degeneration. Rupture of the biceps tendon is a logical consequence of progressive tissue degradation. Biceps tendon rupture has been associated with distal traction and active biceps contraction, as when a person is actively pulling and their arm is suddenly jerked distally.

The structural congruity of the glenoid labrum and proximal biceps tendon often results in combined injuries at the bicipital–labral junction (e.g., SLAP lesion). Although the exact mechanism of injury is unresolved, both biceps tendon traction and humeral head traction may be involved.

Elbow Injuries

The elbow joint is structurally classified as a synovial hinge joint formed by dual articulations of the capitulum of the humerus (figure 7.13*a*) with the head of the radius (figure 7.13*c*) and the trochlea of the humerus (figure 7.13*a* and *b*) with the trochlear notch of the ulna (figure 7.13*c*). The radius and ulna articulate at the proximal radioulnar joint (figure 7.13*c* and *d*). Normal elbow motion is confined to uniplanar flexion–extension, with forearm

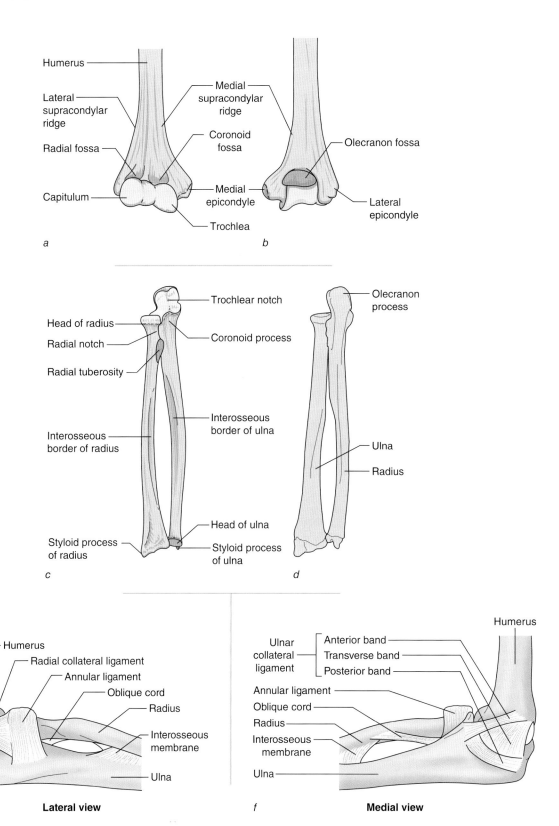

FIGURE 7.13 *(a-d)* Bones and *(e and f)* ligaments of the elbow joint.

pronation–supination produced by the combined rotations of the proximal and distal radioulnar joints. As a synovial joint, the elbow is surrounded by a thin fibrous capsule that runs from its proximal humeral attachment to become continuous distally with the synovial capsule of the proximal radioulnar joint.

The elbow is reinforced by the radial collateral ligament (RCL) complex, which extends from the lateral epicondyle of the humerus to the annular ligament of the radius (figure 7.13e). The elbow also is reinforced by the ulnar collateral ligament (UCL) (also called the medial collateral ligament [MCL]) complex (figure 7.13f), which connects the medial epicondyle with the coronoid process and olecranon of the ulna (figure 7.13c-f). The RCL complex consists of three ligaments (radial collateral ligament, annular ligament, and lateral ulnohumeral ligament) and provides primary restraint against varus loading (i.e., laterally directed force on the medial aspect of the elbow). The UCL contains three distinct bundles (anterior, posterior, transverse). The anterior and posterior bundles resist valgus loading (i.e., medially directed force on the lateral aspect of the elbow), whereas the transverse bundle plays a minimal role in joint stabilization. Muscles controlling elbow motion are shown in figure 7.2 and summarized in table 7.6.

Before considering specific injuries, we need to address several pervasive wastebasket terms used to describe elbow injuries. The most common of these is the ubiquitous *tennis elbow*, a term with varied meanings, ranging from a general descriptor of any pain in and around the elbow to a specific diagnosis of lateral epicondylitis (see next section). In the latter case, *tennis elbow* can be triply confusing because it can be interpreted to mean that tennis is solely responsible for epicondylitis, that epicondylitis is the only elbow injury seen in tennis players, or that all tennis players suffer from the condition. None of these suppositions is correct. For these reasons, we refrain from using the colloquial *tennis elbow* and its cousins, *Little League elbow*, *golfer's elbow*, and *climber's elbow* and instead focus on specific clinical descriptors.

Significant injuries to the elbow include epicondylitis, tendinitis, myotendinous strain, **osteochondritis dissecans**, **osteochondrosis**, dislocation, bursitis, ligamentous sprain, and fractures of the humerus, ulna, and radius. Many of these injuries are common among athletes and are specific to athletic tasks (table 7.7).

TABLE 7.6 Muscles of the Elbow

Muscle	Action
Anconeus	Extends the forearm
Biceps brachii	Flexes the forearm; also supinates the forearm and flexes the arm
Brachialis	Flexes the forearm
Brachioradialis	Flexes the forearm
Triceps brachii	Extends the forearm; long head also extends the arm

TABLE 7.7 Sport-Specific Elbow Injuries

Sport	Injuries and mechanisms
Baseball/Softball	Medial epicondylitis, ulnar collateral ligament (UCL) sprain and rupture, valgus extension overload, ulnar neuritis (cubital tunnel syndrome), flexor tendinitis
Basketball	Tendinitis, bursitis, lateral epicondylitis, dislocation, fracture
Golf	Medial and lateral epicondylitis, tendinitis
Gymnastics	Hyperextension, dislocation, fracture, UCL rupture, osteochondritis dissecans, medial epicondylitis
Tennis	Lateral epicondylitis (backhand), medial epicondylitis (forehand and serving)
Volleyball	Medial epicondylitis, valgus extension overload (spiking)

Epicondylitis

Most elbow injuries are overuse conditions characterized by progressive tissue degeneration. As with most chronic injuries, repeated loading produces tissue microtrauma before the condition becomes symptomatic. Even in asymptomatic individuals, evidence of intracytoplasmic calcification, collagen fiber splitting and kinking, and abnormal fiber cross-links has been reported (Kannus and Józsa 1991). The causes of these histopathologies have not been clearly established but may be mechanical or vascular in nature.

Continued loading worsens the microscopic damage and eventually leads to symptomatic tissue involvement in the form of initial inflammation, inflexibility, and tissue weakness. At the elbow, these events often manifest as epicondylitis, involving soft tissue attachments on humeral epicondyles. Task specificity determines whether the medial or lateral epicondyle is involved.

Nirschl (1988) described four stages in the progression of epicondylitis:

- Stage 1: Inflammation not associated with pathologic tissue alterations

- Stage 2: Pathologic tissue alterations characterized by disrupted collagen architecture in the form of a fibroblastic and immature vascular response (tendinosis) in the relative absence of inflammatory cells

- Stage 3: Tendinosis with tissue structural failure (e.g., microtearing)

- Stage 4: Continued structural failure with fibrosis or calcification

The term *epicondylitis* may be misleading, because there is scant evidence of inflammatory markers present at the affected site, and there is significant disagreement about several other aspects of the disorder (Ciccotti and Charlton 2001, p. 77; Nirschl and Ashman 2003). Alternative designations for epicondylitis have been suggested, including *tendinosis* (Kraushaar and Nirschl 1999), *angiofibroblastic tendinosis* (Nirschl and Ashman 2003), and *epicondralgia* (Hotchkiss 2000). Nonetheless, the term *epicondylitis* is so embedded in the literature that its extinction seems unlikely. Whatever name is used, Whaley and Baker remind us that "the disease itself is not an inflammatory process, but rather a degenerative process" (2004, p. 688).

Lateral Epicondylitis

Lateral epicondylitis is characterized by pain on the lateral aspect of the elbow and is most often attributed to pathology at the proximal attachment of the extensor carpi radialis brevis (ECRB) (Abrams et al. 2012; Nirschl and Pettrone 1979). Lateral epicondylitis arises from repetitive occupational or athletic activities, specifically those involving wrist extension and radioulnar supination (Tosti et al. 2013).

Lateral epicondylitis is prevalent in tennis players, with between 40% and 50% of players experiencing this injury at some time during their years of playing. The injury is most common in players between 30 and 50 years old. The suspected causal mechanisms include faulty stroke mechanics, off-center ball contact, grip tightness, and racket vibration. Repeated impact of the racket and ball stresses the muscles that stabilize and control movement of the wrist. These stresses can result from both concentric and eccentric muscle actions.

The mechanics of the backhand stroke in particular have been associated with the incidence of lateral epicondylitis (Priest et al. 1980). Electromyographic studies have shown high levels of wrist extensor activity, especially in the ECRB, during the backhand stroke (Giangarra et al. 1993; Morris et al. 1989). When a player (usually a novice) leads with the elbow, greater forces are generated in the wrist extensors. These loads are transferred through the active and stiffened musculature to the proximal attachment on the lateral humerus.

Despite scant support in the literature, use of a two-handed backhand stroke has been associated by some with a lower incidence of lateral epicondylitis because the simplified and coordinated action of trunk rotation and arm movement imposes fewer mechanical demands on the musculoskeletal system. Giangarra et al. (1993), for example, concluded that "The decreased occurrence of lateral epicondylitis in players using a double-handed backhand may not be caused by decreased extensor activity, but rather by factors associated with flawed stroke mechanics more often seen in the single-handed technique" (p. 394).

Lateral epicondylitis is not exclusive to tennis players. Other striking sports such as racquetball and golf are implicated, as are occupations and manual job tasks involving repetitive motions of the wrist and elbow (Haahr and Andersen 2003; van Rijn et al. 2009). Specifically, research has shown that pinching and grasping with the fingers and hand always produce flexor moments at the wrist and that extensor moments are generated to maintain equilibrium. Overuse of the extensor mechanism in repeated pinching and grasping, such as in chronic work with hand tools or writing, increases the susceptibility to lateral epicondylitis (Snijders et al. 1987).

Medial Epicondylitis

Medial epicondylitis occurs infrequently compared with lateral epicondylitis (Barco and Antuña 2017). The actual numbers vary, with Leach and Miller (1987) reporting lateral epicondylitis to be 7 to 10 times more common than medial epicondylitis, and Shiri et al. (2006) more recently finding it 3.25 times more common.

Many cases of medial epicondylitis are sport related. In tennis, for example, medial epicondylitis results from excessive loading during the forehand and service strokes. These motions, especially by advanced players, involve forcible extension of the wrist. The eccentric action of the wrist flexor muscles in controlling wrist extension places considerable stress on these muscles and their attachment on the medial aspect of the humerus.

Medial epicondylitis occurs more often in throwers whose movement patterns include a high-velocity valgus extension mechanism (e.g., baseball or javelin) (Wilson et al. 1983). Valgus loading during throwing, especially during the late-cocking and acceleration phases, produces high tensile forces on the elbow's medial aspect. Repeated valgus loading can presage medial epicondylitis (Grana 2001). Repetitive valgus loading also can cause other injuries, including damage to the ulnar collateral ligament (UCL), the flexor–pronator musculotendinous unit, and the ulnar nerve (Safran 2004).

Valgus-Extension Loading Injuries

Numerous studies have examined the kinematics, kinetics, and muscle involvement at the elbow during the overhead throwing motion. The throwing motion typically is divided into five phases: wind-up, cocking, acceleration, deceleration, and follow-through. A sixth phase, stride, sometimes is included between wind-up and cocking.

Several studies (e.g., Fleisig et al. 1995) have quantified elbow kinetics during throwing and reported large and potentially injurious forces and moments. Near the end of the cocking phase when the elbow is approaching terminal extension, the elbow experiences valgus loading that is resisted by a varus torque produced by musculotendinous and periarticular tissues (figure 7.14). Varus torques at this point have been estimated as ranging from 64 to 120 N·m, with predicted joint force between the radius and humerus of approximately 500 N (Fleisig et al. 1995; Werner et al. 1993).

The coupling of valgus torque and elbow extension produces a so-called **valgus-extension overload mechanism** that can lead to medial elbow injuries, including epicondylitis, ulnar collateral ligament rupture, avulsion fracture, and nerve damage. In addition, the valgus stress in extension causes impingement of the medial aspect of the olecranon on the olecranon fossa and radial head impingement on the capitulum. Repeated impingement may lead to inflammation, chondromalacia, osteophyte formation, and olecranon stress fracture (Ahmad and ElAttrache 2004).

In throwing, as in other dynamic movements, the largest loads are developed during eccentric actions that resist and control high-velocity motion. Repeated application of these high loads may lead to progressive degeneration and eventual tissue failure. Although this process is common, it is not inevitable. Some athletes and workers are able to load their tissues repeatedly with minimal, if any, symptomatic response. Why does a particular loading history cause injury in one person but not in another? The answer likely lies in the fact that injury is a multifactorial puzzle and that some people are more susceptible to injury than others. To define this susceptibility, Meeuwisse (1994) proposed a model that incorporates

---

Not-So-Funny Bone

The so-called *funny bone* is neither a bone nor particularly funny. The name derives from the transient sensation of numbness and tingling experienced when the posteromedial aspect of the elbow is struck. In this area, the ulnar nerve passes by the posterior aspect of the humeral epicondyle on its way from the shoulder to the forearm and hand. Violent compression on the ulnar nerve against the humerus causes a temporary blockage of nerve impulses. This creates the "funny" sensation when this nerve is struck.

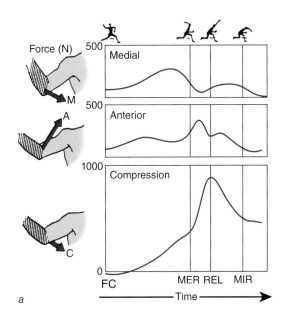

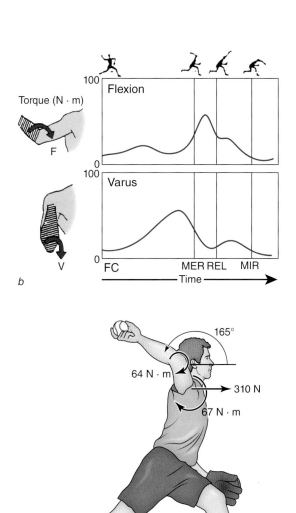

FIGURE 7.14 Kinetics of baseball pitching. *(a)* Force applied to the forearm at the elbow in the medial (M), anterior (A), and compression (C) directions. The instants of front foot contact (FC), maximum external rotation (MER), ball release (REL), and maximum internal rotation (MIR) torque are shown. *(b)* Torques applied to the forearm at the elbow in the flexion (F) and varus (V) directions. *(c)* Shortly before maximum external rotation, the arm was externally rotated 165° and the elbow was flexed 95°. At this instant there were 67 N·m of internal rotation torque, 310 N of anterior force at the shoulder, and 64 N·m of varus torque at the elbow.

Adapted by permission from G.S. Fleisig et al., "Kinetics of Baseball Pitching with Implications About Injury Mechanisms," *The American Journal of Sports Medicine* 23, no. 2 (1995): 236–268. Reprinted by permission of SAGE Publications.

both intrinsic (e.g., age, strength, flexibility, previous injury) and extrinsic (e.g., biomechanics of movement skills, equipment, environmental conditions, schedule, inherent demands) factors.

Throwing, by its repetitive nature, provides an instructive example of chronic injury development and the interactive nature of these intrinsic and extrinsic factors. Kibler (1995) characterized progressive degeneration as a negative feedback cycle in which the following five complexes interact to create a downward spiral, leading to tissue failure:

1. Tissue overload
2. Clinical symptoms
3. Tissue injury
4. Functional biomechanical deficit
5. Subclinical adaptation

Applying this model to the overhead throwing motion, for example, we see how the complexes interactively contribute to elbow injury. During the late cocking phase, the valgus extension mechanism causes *tissue overload* on the medial aspect of the elbow in the form of asymptomatic microtrauma. Repeated mechanical insults lead to *clinical symptoms* of point tenderness over the medial epicondyle and *tissue injury* to flexor–pronator group attachments and ulnar collateral ligaments. The elbow then suffers *functional biomechanical deficits* in the form of flexor–pronator inflexibility and weakness, coupled with elbow inflexibility and muscle imbalance. The thrower then alters their technique (*subclinical adaptation*) in an attempt to compensate for the deficits. These compensations further overload the tissues, and the insidious cycle continues until

Tendon Transplantation Surgery

In 1974, holding a 13-3 record, Los Angeles Dodgers pitcher Tommy John was en route to one of his best seasons ever. Then John ruptured the ulnar collateral ligament (UCL) in his pitching arm, and his career appeared to be over. He reportedly asked team physician Frank Jobe to "make up something" to salvage his pitching arm—and Dr. Jobe did just that. In what has become known as *Tommy John surgery*, Dr. Jobe reconstructed John's UCL using a free tendon (palmaris longus) graft from John's nonpitching arm.

At the time, no one knew what the outcome would be. John missed the 1975 baseball season and returned in 1976 to test his repaired arm. He passed the test with flying colors. Postsurgery, Tommy John pitched for an additional 13 years and amassed 164 wins. These wins, combined with 124 preinjury victories, left John with 288 career triumphs when he finally retired in 1989. Postinjury, John was a three-time All-Star (1978, 1979, 1980) and finished second in the Cy Young Award voting in 1977 and 1979.

Dr. Jobe continued to perform and refine his UCL reconstruction techniques (Jobe et al. 1986) and share his procedure with other professional colleagues. Jobe and colleagues reported good to excellent results in 80% of patients (Conway et al. 1992). The most notable result, however, remains that of Tommy John. John's 288 career wins may be forgotten, but his name will not. The name Tommy John will always be associated with the pioneering surgery that saved his pitching career. As John said, "I'd never have been able to win 288 games without the surgery. We're going to be linked forever."

As for John's perspective of the surgery and his baseball career, he said, "You know what I'm most proud of? . . . I pitched 13 years after the procedure and I never missed a start. I had not one iota of trouble. I'd like people to remember that about me, too."

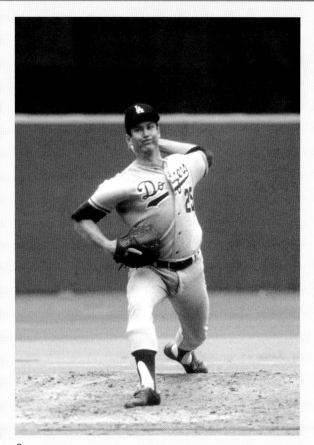

a

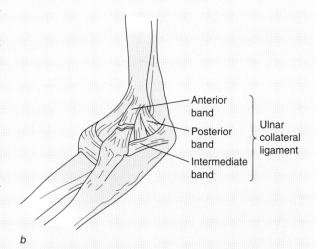

b

(a) Tommy John pitching after his groundbreaking surgical repair. *(b)* Ulnar collateral ligament consisting of three bands: anterior, intermediate, posterior. Anterior band shown with complete tear.
(a) Focus on Sport/Getty Images

ultimate tissue failure. Appropriate rehabilitation must address all five complexes to break the negative feedback cycle.

Elbow Dislocation

Given its relative stability, it is not surprising that the elbow is more than three times less likely than the shoulder to become dislocated (Praemer et al. 1999). Elbow dislocation, nonetheless, is not uncommon. Because joint luxations are rarely isolated—they are often accompanied by extensive soft tissue damage as the bones are forcibly displaced—elbow dislocations typically involve complete rupture or avulsion of both the ulnar and radial collateral ligaments. Elbow dislocation is most prevalent in young individuals and in conjunction with sport activities.

The elbow's bony configuration provides exceptional resistance to anterior dislocation. As such, the vast majority of dislocations happen posteriorly (Rettig 2002) and can be directed straight–posterior, posteromedial, or posterolateral (figure 7.15). Dislocation tends to be posterolateral (Nestor et al. 1992; O'Driscoll et al. 1991) to allow the coronoid to pass inferiorly to the trochlea (O'Driscoll 2000). The propensity for posterior dislocation is also seen in children. In one study (Rasool 2004) of 33 elbow dislocations in children (all caused by falls), 91% were posterior.

The most common mechanism for elbow dislocation involves axial force applied to an extended or hyperextended elbow. This force effectively levers the ulna out of the trochlea and causes capsular and ligament rupture that then allows joint dislocation (Hotchkiss 1996). During the forcible hyperextension, the joint's alignment also creates valgus stresses that can lead to rupture of the ulnar collateral ligament and sometimes rupture at the origin of the flexor–pronator group on the medial aspect of the humerus.

O'Driscoll and colleagues (1991, 1992) described posterolateral rotatory instability (PLRI), which results from combined axial compression, valgus instability, and supination. PLRI involves injury to the radial collateral ligament (RCL) complex (Anakwenze et al. 2014). According to O'Driscoll et al., PLRI progresses through four stages of severity:

- Stage I: Disruption of the ulnar portion of the RCL complex with resultant posterolateral subluxation and spontaneous reduction
- Stage II: Continued disruption anteriorly and posteriorly with accompanying subluxation
- Stage IIIA: Disruption of all soft tissues except for the anterior bundle of the ulnar collateral ligament; complete posterior dislocation
- Stage IIIB: Complete rupture of the ulnar collateral complex with gross valgus and varus instability

Elbow Fractures

Fractures can occur to any of the three bones (humerus, ulna, or radius) of the elbow. The involvement of each depends on the nature, magnitude, location, and direction of the applied forces.

- Humeral fractures can involve various areas of the distal humerus, including the supracondylar, intercondylar (Y and T fractures), condylar, epicondylar, and articular regions (figure 7.16a).
- Ulnar fractures commonly involve the olecranon and result either directly from violent impact to the posterior aspect of the elbow or indirectly from falls that load the elbow joint (figure 7.16b).
- Coronoid fractures happen during joint dislocation when the trochlea shears off the tip of the coronoid process of the ulna (figure 7.16c). Coronoid fracture in conjunction with radial head fracture especially compromises elbow joint stability (Cohen 2004).
- Radial head fractures most often result from either longitudinal loading of the radius as a result of a fall or accompanying elbow dislocation (figure 7.16d). Radioulnar fractures are more fully described in the following section.

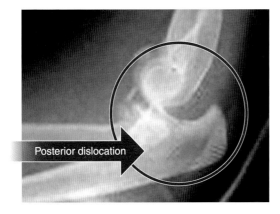

FIGURE 7.15 X-ray of posterior elbow dislocation, caused by falling on an outstretched hand (FOOSH).

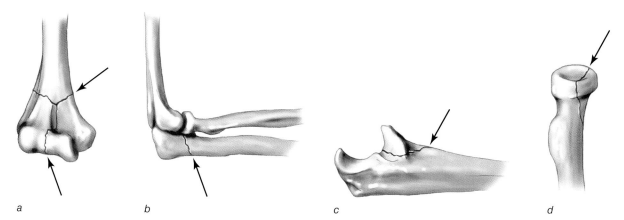

a   b   c   d

FIGURE 7.16 Elbow fractures. *(a)* Fracture of the distal humerus. *(b)* Ulnar fracture. *(c)* Coronoid fracture. *(d)* Radial head fracture.

Forearm Injuries

The forearm spans the elbow and wrist joints and consists of two longitudinally aligned bones, the radius (lateral) and ulna (medial), which are surrounded by numerous muscles that function at the elbow, radioulnar, and wrist joints and whose distal tendons continue to the hand to control finger movements (figure 7.17*a*). The forearm muscles are divided into two major groups: the flexor–pronator group and extensor–supinator group. Specific muscles in each of these groups are presented in table 7.8.

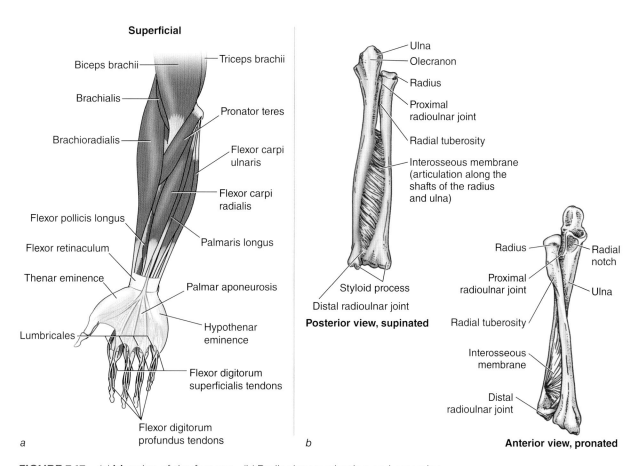

FIGURE 7.17 *(a)* Muscles of the forearm. *(b)* Radioulnar supination and pronation.

TABLE 7.8   Muscles of the Forearm

FLEXOR–PRONATOR GROUP	
Superficial group	Pronator teres
	Flexor carpi radialis
	Palmaris longus
	Flexor carpi ulnaris
	Flexor digitorum superficialis
Deep group	Flexor digitorum profundus
	Flexor pollicis longus
	Pronator quadrates
EXTENSOR–SUPINATOR GROUP	
Extensors, abductors, and adductors of the wrist	Extensor carpi radialis longus
	Extensor carpi radialis brevis
	Extensor carpi ulnaris
Extensors of the four medial digits	Extensor digitorum
	Extensor indicis
	Extensor digiti minimi
Extensors and abductors of the thumb	Abductor pollicis longus
	Extensor pollicis brevis
	Extensor pollicis longus

The radius and ulna articulate with one another at the proximal radioulnar joint, which is a synovial pivot joint between the head of the radius and the radial notch of the ulna, and at the distal radioulnar joint, which is a synovial pivot joint between the head of the ulna and the ulnar notch of the radius. Coordinated action of these two joints creates the forearm motions of pronation and supination. In pronation, the radius rolls over a relatively fixed ulna. The reverse occurs in supination, when the radius returns to its anatomical position (figure 7.17b).

Diaphyseal Fractures of the Radius and Ulna

Fractures of the radius and ulna can occur in isolation or combination, with numerous suggested injury mechanisms. Identification of the injury mechanism is important because it suggests the location and type of fracture. Combined injury to both the radius and ulna typically involves direct, high-energy trauma, such as motor vehicle crashes or gunshot wounds, or the lower-energy impact of a fall.

Isolated fractures of the upper two-thirds of the radius (proximal fractures) are rare because of the protection offered by the overlying musculature. Forces sufficient to cause radial fracture in this region most often fracture the ulnar shaft as well. Fracture at the junction between the middle and distal thirds of the radius is more common and often is associated with injury to the distal radioulnar joint. Fractures of the distal third of the radius are termed **Galeazzi fractures** (Galeazzi 1934) and result most often from a direct blow on the dorsolateral side of the wrist or a fall on an outstretched arm that axially loads a hyperpronated forearm (Jupiter and Kellam 2003).

Isolated fracture of the ulna arises from various mechanisms. Injury from direct trauma is colloquially termed a **nightstick fracture**, referring to the situation in which a person, in response to an impending overhead blow, raises their arm and exposes the medial surface to impact.

Another mechanism of isolated ulnar fracture involves dislocation of the radial epiphysis. This mechanism was originally suggested in 1814 by Giovanni Monteggia, who described fracture of the proximal ulna associated with anterior dislocation of the radial head.

Bado (1967) proposed the term **Monteggia lesion** and enlarged the scope of the injury to include all ulnar fractures resulting from radial epiphyseal luxation. Bado suggested a classification system consisting of four types (I-IV) of injury, as depicted in figure 7.18.

• *Type I (anterior dislocation).* These Monteggia fractures are the most common, accounting for about 70% of Monteggia lesions (Wilkins 2002). Several

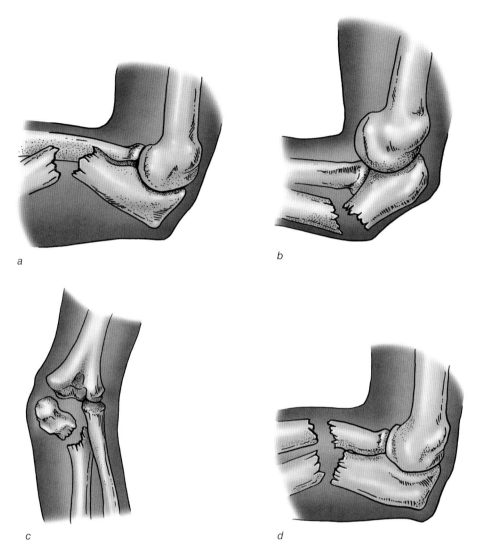

FIGURE 7.18 Classification of Monteggia fractures. *(a)* Type I, anterior dislocation of radial head and fracture of ulnar diaphysis with anterior angulation. *(b)* Type II, posterior or posterolateral dislocation of radial head and fracture of ulnar diaphysis with posterior angulation. *(c)* Type III, lateral or anterolateral dislocation of radial head and fracture of ulnar metaphysis. *(d)* Type IV, anterior dislocation of radial head and fracture of proximal third of radius and ulna.

mechanisms have been proposed for type I injuries. In the 1940s, Smith (1947) and Speed and Boyd (1940) suggested that a direct blow to the posterior forearm caused a fracture in the ulnar diaphysis, followed by forcing of the radial head into anterior dislocation. In 1949, Evans described a hyperpronation mechanism from forced pronation that causes ulnar fracture and eventual anterior displacement of the radial head. The current, most accepted mechanism is the hyperextension mechanism proposed by Tompkins (1971). In this case, falling on an outstretched arm hyperextends the elbow. The biceps brachii strongly resists the hyperextension and dislocates the radial head. The compressive load is then transferred to the ulnar diaphysis,

which fails in tension in the form of a complete oblique or greenstick fracture (Wilkins 2002).

- *Type II (posterior dislocation).* Type II Monteggia fractures result from posterior elbow dislocation in which the ulnar shaft fractures before ulnar collateral ligament failure. In this mechanism, a longitudinal force is directed up the forearm with the elbow flexed. This results in failure of the posterior ulnar cortex and posterior radial head dislocation (Penrose 1951). Four subtypes of type II injuries have been identified based on the location and loading mechanism (bending, shearing, or compression) of the ulnar fracture (Jupiter et al. 1991).

- *Type III (lateral dislocation).* Type III lesions are the second most common type, accounting for nearly 25% of Monteggia lesions. Wright (1963) described a varus load applied to an extended elbow that results in ulnar failure followed by lateral or anterolateral radial head displacement.

- *Type IV (anterior dislocation with radial head fracture).* Type IV lesions are rare, accounting for about 1% of all Monteggia lesions. Type IV injuries have a similar mechanism to type I, with the added presence of radial head fracture.

The complexity of Monteggia lesions is increased by comminution of the proximal ulna, level of radial head fragmentation, reduction of the radial head, and humeroulnar instability (Kim and London 2020). Given the importance of the forearm in mediating movement between the elbow and fingers, clinicians must accurately assess injury mechanisms, make an informed diagnosis, and plan appropriate treatment.

Fracture of the Distal Radius

Fractures of the distal radius are common, accounting for up to one-sixth of all fractures. The most common mechanism is falling on an outstretched arm (Rettig and Raskin 2000). Young males and elderly females greatly outnumber their opposite-gender counterparts in the incidence of fracture.

The literature is replete with eponyms for fractures of the distal radius. These include *Colles'*, *Smith's*, and *Barton's fractures*, each with their own distinguishing characteristics. Here, we use the clinical descriptions with parenthetical reference to corresponding eponymic designations.

Many classification systems have been proposed to describe distal radial fractures. One useful system groups these fractures according to their mechanisms of injury rather than by radiological characteristics (Fernandez and Jupiter 1996). Five types are included (figure 7.19):

- Type I: Bending fractures
- Type II: Shearing fractures of the joint surface
- Type III: Compression fractures of the joint surface
- Type IV: Avulsion fractures
- Type V: Combined fractures

Type I bending fractures result from landing on an outstretched arm. Axial compressive loads cause bending of the radius with a fracture pattern (Colles'

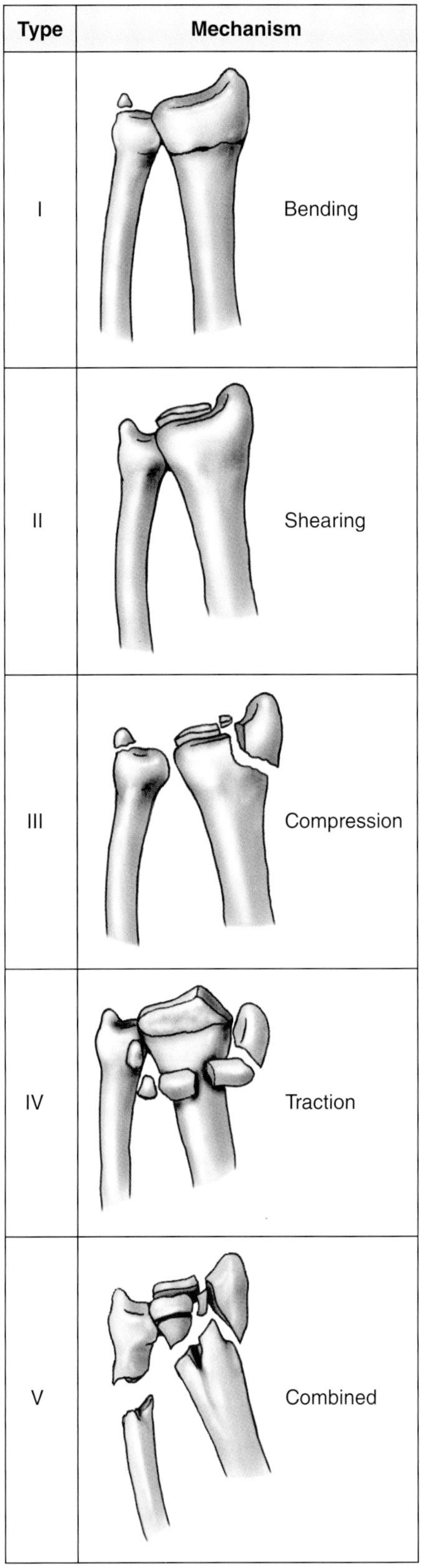

Type	Mechanism
I	Bending
II	Shearing
III	Compression
IV	Traction
V	Combined

FIGURE 7.19 Fractures of the distal radius as characterized by injury mechanism.

fracture, figure 7.20*a*) showing volar (anterior or palmar) metaphyseal cortex failure in tension and varying degrees of comminution on the dorsal (posterior) surface. These type I injuries constitute the majority of distal radial fractures. An opposite bending results from a fall on either a flexed wrist or an outstretched and supinated arm. The compressive loading then results in tensile failure (**Smith's fracture**, figure 7.20*b*) on the dorsal (posterior) aspect of the metaphysis and compressive comminution on the volar aspect. This fracture pattern also is seen when a slightly flexed clenched fist hits a rigid surface.

High-energy loading, particularly in young individuals, produces type II shearing fracture (**Barton's fracture**, figure 7.20*c*) in which the volar lip of the radial articular surface is sheared off. In type III fractures, high compressive loads (such as those generated in landing from a high fall) cause intra-articular fractures of the joint surface with disruption of the subchondral and cancellous bone.

Mechanical loading that creates high stresses on the osteoligamentous attachments, as in exaggerated torsion, produces avulsion (type IV) fractures. The most complex mechanism of distal radial fracture is type V, or combined fracture, which usually results from high-energy injuries including combinations of bending, compression, shearing, or avulsion mechanisms.

Dorsal

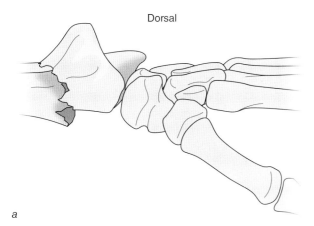

a

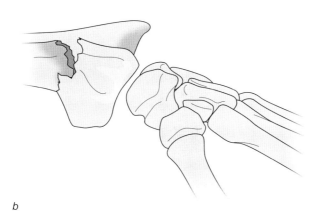

b

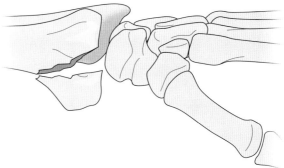

c

FIGURE 7.20 Fractures of the distal radius. *(a)* Colles' fracture. *(b)* Smith's fracture. *(c)* Barton's fracture.

Ulnar Variance

The relative lengths of the ulna and radius play an important role in forearm and wrist mechanics. This length difference is referred to as **ulnar variance (UV)**. (Note: *ulnar variance* should not be confused with *ulnar deviation*, which describes frontal plane wrist–hand movement toward the ulnar side of the forearm.)

If the radius and ulna are the same length, UV is zero. When the ulna is longer than the radius, there exists a **positive ulnar variance**. Conversely, a **negative ulnar variance** exists when radial length exceeds ulnar length. Measures of UV vary, with reported means ranging from −0.84 mm to 0.2 mm (Kristensen et al. 1986; Nakamura et al. 1991). Recently, Sayit et al. (2018) found a median UV of 0.65 mm (across 600 wrist measurements), and reported a significant difference between males (median: 0.4, minimum: −3.8, maximum: 5.1) and females (median: 0.85, minimum: −4.8, maximum: 5.7).

Caution is warranted in interpreting mean values because UV varies by age, ethnicity, and sex. In addition, UV is determined by genetics, elbow pathology, and loading history (De Smet 1994). Loading history is most relevant to our discussion of injury mechanisms. Although the wrist is not designed to function as a load-bearing joint, certain activities (e.g., gymnastics) expose the wrist to considerable loads. These compressive loads are transmitted through the carpals to the radius and ulna, with the radius accepting approximately 80% of the load. In cases of repetitive compressive loading in the skeletally immature individual, this loading differential may dictate premature closure of the radial growth plate. Continued growth of the ulna then would create an acquired ulnar variance.

Gymnasts are especially prone to UV. The dual risk factors of early onset (beginning training at a relatively young age) and repetitive upper-extremity load bearing account for the prevalence of wrist lesions in this population. Age-matched elite gymnasts had a positive UV of 0.46 mm (De Smet et al. 1994) compared with −1.1 mm in nonelite gymnasts (DiFiori et al. 1997) and −2.3 mm in non-gymnasts (Hafner et al. 1989). This disproportionately positive UV in gymnasts suggests that the high loads placed on gymnasts' wrists may inhibit growth of the distal radius, stimulate growth of the ulna, or both (DiFiori et al. 1997). Despite the plausibility of inhibited distal radial growth, conclusive evidence remains elusive (Caine et al. 1997).

Certain gymnastics skills place the athlete's wrist at particular risk. The back handspring, for example, loads the wrist with forces up to 2.4 times body weight, and the radius accepts most of the load (Koh et al. 1992). For men, the pommel horse is the main culprit. Joint forces of up to 2 times body weight and loading rates of up to 219 times body weight per second have been reported (Markolf et al. 1990). The gymnast's wrist assumes a load-bearing role for which it is ill designed. The consequences manifest in an ulnar impaction syndrome, characterized by progressive degeneration of the triangular fibrocartilage complex and the ulnar carpus.

How much joint loading is too much? Because of the multifactorial nature of the problem, the question remains unresolved. Some guidance is provided by a study that examined factors associated with wrist pain in young gymnasts. Training intensity, relative to the age of the participant and the age when training began, seems to be a critical determinant of wrist pain development (DiFiori et al. 1996). Although wrist pain is common in gymnasts, radiographic evidence suggests that UV is not associated with wrist pain or injury of the distal radial physis (DiFiori et al. 2002).

Wrist and Hand Injuries

The wrist is not a single joint but rather a group of articulations that include the distal radioulnar, radiocarpal, and intercarpal joints. The hand contains numerous articulations, namely the carpometacarpal (CM), metacarpophalangeal (MP), and interphalangeal (IP) joints (figure 7.21). All of these are synovial joints. Structurally, the MP joints are condyloid, whereas the

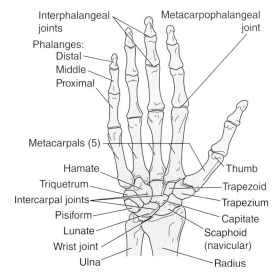

FIGURE 7.21 Bones and articulations of the wrist and hand.

IP joints are hinge joints. Both MP and IP joints are strengthened by palmar and collateral ligaments.

Muscles in the forearm primarily control wrist and finger motion, with assistance from intrinsic muscles of the hand. The distal tendons of most flexor muscles in the forearm pass along the ventral aspect of the wrist, where they are held firmly in place by the flexor retinaculum, a thick and relatively inextensible fascial sheath. These tendons, along with neurovascular structures, pass through the so-called carpal tunnel formed by the carpal bones and the flexor retinaculum (figure 7.22). The distal tendons of the extensors are secured similarly between the carpal bones and the extensor retinaculum.

Carpal Tunnel Syndrome

Injuries resulting from repeated tissue stress are collectively known as *cumulative trauma disorders* (CTDs), also called *repetitive strain injury*, *chronic microtrauma*, *overuse syndrome*, and *cumulative trauma syndrome*. These chronic injuries have been increasing at an alarming rate, especially in occupational settings, and account for a majority of all new nonfatal occupational illnesses. CTDs are prevalent in many occupations and prove costly in both economic and human terms.

One of the most debilitating chronic disorders is **carpal tunnel syndrome** (CTS), a condition first reported by Paget in 1854 (Lo et al. 2002), which is characterized by swelling within the carpal tunnel that creates a compressive neuropathy affecting the median nerve (figure 7.22) (Padua et al. 2016). Like other entrapment syndromes, CTS involves increased pressure within a confined space. The inextensible borders formed by the carpal bones and the flexor retinaculum (also called the *transverse carpal ligament*) preclude an increase in tunnel size. Inflammation and edema in response to repeated loading compress neurovascular tissues and compromise their function. Of greatest consequence is compression of the median nerve, which results in sensory symptoms of numbness, tingling, burning, and pain in the wrist and radial 3-1/2 fingers. Sensory deficits from CTS are more pronounced than reductions in motor function.

Symptoms of CTS are associated with specific movement patterns (e.g., wrist flexion–extension) and tasks (e.g., assembly work, typing, playing a musical instrument, polishing, sanding, scrubbing, or hammering). Carpal tunnel syndrome has also been documented in workers across a diverse range of jobs, including keyboard operators, sheet metal workers, supermarket checkers, sheep shearers, fish-processing workers, and sign language interpreters. Making a causal connection in all cases warrants caution, however, because discrimination can be tenuous between work-related and non-work-related cases of CTS. Estimated prevalence of CTS in the general population varies in the 1% to 5% range, with Atroshi et al. (1999) reporting 3.8% prevalence. Historically, CTS has been reported as more common among women than men in a ratio of about 2:1 (Phalen 1966; Praemer et al. 1999).

The etiology of CTS is complex, because many mechanisms and risk factors play a contributing

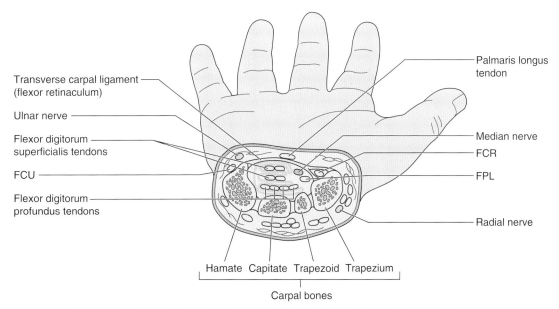

FIGURE 7.22 Structure of the carpal tunnel. Neurovascular structures, including the median nerve, pass through the carpal tunnel bounded by the flexor retinaculum and the carpal bones.

role. Fundamentally, the pathophysiology of CTS involves a combination of ischemia and mechanical trauma (Viikari-Juntura and Silverstein 1999; Werner and Andary 2002).

Accurate diagnosis of CTS can be difficult initially because repetitive stress is implicated in other hand and wrist pathologies, such as tendinitis. Once diagnosed, CTS remains mechanically problematic because there are multiple risk factors, including forceful exertions, repetitive or prolonged activities, awkward postures, localized contact stresses, vibration, and cold temperatures.

Silverstein and colleagues (1987) evaluated 652 workers to assess the role of force and repetition on the prevalence of CTS in workers. These authors found the lowest prevalence (0.6%) in workers with low-force, low-repetition jobs and the highest occurrence (5.6%) in workers in high-force, highly repetitive jobs. Silverstein and colleagues concluded that of the two factors, high repetitiveness appeared to be a greater risk factor than high force. Although studies such as this shed some light on the relations among CTS risk factors, unraveling the interrelations and relative contributions of all risk factors remains a challenge.

Carpal Fractures

Wrist fractures encompass osseous injury to the radius and ulna (discussed previously) and fractures to any of the eight carpal bones. The most common mechanism of injury is a compressive load applied to a hyperextended (dorsiflexed) wrist (figure 7.23). Other, less

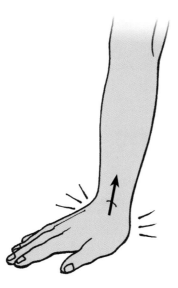

FIGURE 7.23 Mechanism of injury attributable to compressive load applied to a hyperextended wrist at impact.

common mechanisms have been implicated in carpal fracture. These mechanisms include hyperflexion and rotational loading against a fixed object or surface.

The vast majority of carpal fractures occur when axial loads are transmitted through a hyperextended wrist. With the wrist in this position, compressive forces are transmitted through the carpals to the distal radioulnar complex. Predictably, certain carpals are more likely to suffer injury than others. Mitigating influences include the degree of radial or ulnar deviation, amount of energy absorbed, point of application and direction of the applied forces, and relative strength of the bones and ligaments.

Given the 80:20 load distribution between the radius and ulna, respectively, the scaphoid and lunate are most likely to be fractured because of their articulations with the radius. Scaphoid fractures are most common (Fowler and Hughes 2015; Sabbagh et al. 2019) and account for 60% to 70% of all carpal fractures (Botte and Gelberman 1987). Scaphoid fractures are most likely to occur when the wrist is hyperextended past 95° and the radial portion of the palm accepts most of the load (Dias 2002; Weber and Chao 1978). Typically, the palmar aspect of the scaphoid then fails in tension, with the dorsal aspect failing in compression (Ruby and Cassidy 2003). Less commonly, scaphoid fracture can result from a compressive force applied to a neutral or slightly flexed wrist, colloquially referred to as *puncher's fracture* (Horii et al. 1994). Other carpal fractures (triquetrum, trapezium, capitate, pisiform, trapezoid, lunate, and hamate) each account for a small percentage of overall carpal fractures (Hey and Chong 2011; Suh et al. 2014), with injury mechanisms ranging from a direct blow to impingement caused by hyperflexion or hyperextension of the wrist.

Thumb Injuries

Because the thumb is essential to our prehensile abilities, injury to the thumb can severely impair a person's manual dexterity. We describe common thumb injuries (sprain, fracture, and neural lesion) to illustrate injury mechanisms that can significantly impair thumb function.

The most common sprain in the hand damages the ulnar collateral ligament of the first metacarpophalangeal joint (figure 7.24). This injury, colloquially referred to as *gamekeeper's thumb* or *skier's thumb*, can involve chronic tensile loading (stretching) of the ligament or acute loading that result in any level of sprain, including complete rupture. This

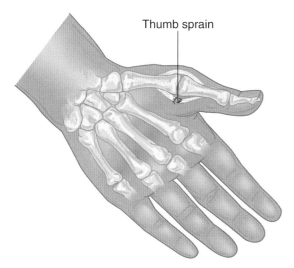

Thumb sprain

FIGURE 7.24 Abductor mechanism causing rupture of the ulnar collateral ligament of the thumb.

injury most commonly occurs when a skier falls onto an outstretched hand with the thumb in an abducted position. The ski pole handle effectively holds the thumb in abduction as the compressive load of the fall is accepted by the hand. The forceful abduction places excessive tensile loads on the ulnar collateral ligament and hastens its failure.

Ulnar collateral sprain can also result from hyperextension of the first metacarpophalangeal joint, such as when a collision occurs between two athletes. A softball player tagging an opponent who is sliding into second base may have her thumb forcibly hyperextended by the contact force between her thumb and the foot or leg of the incoming base runner.

Fracture subluxation of the trapeziometacarpal joint (**Bennett's fracture**) is an intra-articular fracture of the first metacarpal (thumb) resulting from axial force applied when the metacarpal bone is in flexion. Many circumstances can cause this injury, but it is classically observed as a result of a poorly delivered punch in a boxing match or fist fight.

A neural lesion characterized by perineural fibrosis of the ulnar digital nerve of the thumb, known as *bowler's thumb*, most commonly involves symptoms of **paresthesia** (tingling) and, to a lesser extent, tenderness and **hyperesthesia** (pathological sensitivity). The injury mechanism is repeated blunt trauma to the thumb's ulnar digital nerve (e.g., caused by the gripping and release of a bowling ball). This condition can be treated conservatively or prevented by redrilling the bowling ball or modifying the grip mechanics to lessen the repetitive trauma to the nerve.

Metacarpal and Phalangeal Conditions

Metacarpal and phalangeal fractures are common injuries, particularly among athletes (Cotterell and Richard 2015; Wahl and Richard 2020). The pattern of fracture and dislocation involving the metacarpals and phalanges directly depends on the circumstances of injury (direct impact, crushing, indirect trauma) and the nature of the force application (e.g., magnitude, location, direction). Among the implicated injury mechanisms are direct trauma caused by an implement or fall, forcible hyperextension or hyperflexion, twisting forces, violent distraction, forced leverage, crushing, or a combination of these mechanisms.

Chapter Review

Key Points

- Impairment to any structural component of the upper limb compromises our ability to effectively manipulate or propel objects.

- The upper extremity is designed for mobility, and loss of dexterity can have profound effects on our ability to efficiently perform grasping or manipulative tasks.

- Cumulative trauma and repetitive strain injuries are major burdens for today's workplace and the health care system.

- Acute or chronic injuries to any of the upper-extremity joints can significantly affect activities of daily living, work, and recreation and ultimately reduce a person's quality of life.

Questions to Consider

1. This chapter's *A Closer Look* examined rotator cuff pathologies in detail. Select another injury presented in the chapter and write your own *A Closer Look* for that injury.

2. Explain, using specific examples, how upper-extremity injuries may compromise our ability to effectively manipulate or propel objects.

3. Chapter 3 discussed a mobility–stability continuum, which states that greater joint stability (i.e., resistance to dislocation) usually is associated with lesser mobility, and conversely that greater joint mobility is associated with lesser stability. Upper-extremity joints are among the most mobile joints in the body and hence are relatively unstable. Describe, using specific examples, how this lack of stability may increase injury risk.

4. The text presents carpal tunnel syndrome as an example of a cumulative trauma disorder (CTD). Describe in detail other examples of CTD in the upper extremity.

Suggested Readings

Andrews, J.R., K.E. Wilk, and M.M. Reinold, eds. 2008. *The Athlete's Shoulder* (2nd ed.). New York: Churchill Livingstone.

Bauer, A.S., and D.S. Bae, eds. 2019. *Upper Extremity Injuries in Young Athletes (Contemporary Pediatric and Adolescent Sports Medicine)*. New York: Springer.

Browner, B.D., J. Jupiter, C. Krettek, P.A. Anderson, eds. 2019. *Skeletal Trauma: Basic Science, Management, and Reconstruction* (6th ed.). Philadelphia: Elsevier.

Bulstrode, C., J. Wilson-MacDonald, D.M. Eastwood, J. McMaster, J. Fairbank, P.J. Singh, S. Bawa, P.D. Gikas, T. Bunker, G. Giddins, M. Blyth, D. Stanley, P.H. Cooke, R. Carrington, P. Calder, P. Wordsworth, and T. Briggs, eds. 2011. *Oxford Textbook of Trauma and Orthopaedics* (2nd ed.). New York: Oxford University Press.

Feliciano, D.V., K. Mattox, and E. Moore, eds. 2020. *Trauma* (9th ed.). New York: McGraw-Hill.

Fu, F.H., and D.A. Stone. 2001. *Sports Injuries: Mechanisms, Prevention, Treatment* (2nd ed.). Philadelphia: Lippincott Williams & Wilkins.

Gomes, N.S., L. Kovačič, F. Martetschläger, and G. Milano, eds. 2020. *Massive and Irreparable Rotator Cuff Tears: From Basic Science to Advanced Treatments*. New York: Springer.

Kibler, W.B., and A.D. Sciascia. 2019. *Mechanics, Pathomechanics and Injury in the Overhead Athlete: A Case-Based Approach to Evaluation, Diagnosis and Management*. New York: Springer.

Morrey, B.F., J.S. Sotelo, and M.E. Morrey, eds. 2017. *The Elbow and Its Disorders* (5th ed.). Philadelphia: Elsevier.

Provencher, M.T., B.J. Cole, A.A. Romeo, P. Boileau, and N. Verma, eds. 2019. *Disorders of the Rotator Cuff and Biceps Tendon: The Surgeon's Guide to Comprehensive Management*. Philadelphia: Elsevier.

Slutsky, D. 2014. *Operative Orthopedics of the Upper Extremity*. New York: McGraw-Hill.

Tornetta, P., III, W. Ricci, C.M. Court-Brown, M.M. McQueen, and M. McKee, eds. 2019. *Rockwood and Green's Fracture in Adults* (9th ed.). Philadelphia: Lippincott Williams & Wilkins.

Waters, P.M., D.L. Skaggs, and J.M. Flynn, eds. 2020. *Rockwood and Green's Fracture in Children* (9th ed.). Philadelphia: Wolters Kluwer.

Head, Neck, and Trunk Injuries

You only get one brain.

Dr. Ann McKee (Director of Neuropathology, Department of Veterans Affairs)

OBJECTIVES

- To describe the relevant head, neck, and trunk anatomy involved in musculoskeletal injury
- To identify and explain the mechanisms involved in musculoskeletal and neurological injuries to the head, neck, and spine

Of all the body's regions, the head, neck, and trunk are of paramount importance in controlling life-sustaining functions. Trauma to structures in these regions (e.g., brain, spinal cord, heart) poses the greatest danger to our physical well-being. In the preceding chapters we discussed injuries to the extremities that may result in varying degrees of disability but are rarely fatal. Injuries to the head, neck, and trunk, in contrast, have real and immediate potential to be life threatening. Understanding the mechanisms responsible for these injuries can assist with their proper diagnosis, treatment, and prevention.

This chapter includes a detailed exploration of concussive injuries in *Concussion: A Closer Look*. In that section we expand our discussion beyond the mechanisms of injury to include detailed descriptions of neural tissue structure and mechanics and explanations of clinical evaluation, treatment, and rehabilitation for concussive injuries.

Anatomy

The head includes the skull, which encapsulates the brain, meninges, cranial nerves and the origins of the spinal cord. Structures in the head are protected by an intricate collection of 28 bones. The cranial bones, those that compose the vault holding the brain, include the frontal, occipital, ethmoid, and sphenoid bones, and paired temporal and parietal bones (figure 8.1). Anterior and anterolateral to the cranial bones are the 14 facial bones: paired nasal, maxillae (upper jaw), zygomatic (cheek), lacrimal, palatine, and inferior nasal conchae bones and singular mandible (lower jaw) and vomer bones. The six of the remaining bones are housed within the ear and referred to as the auditory ossicles (paired incus, stapes, and malleus bones). The hyoid, suspended from the styloid process of the temporal bone by ligaments and muscles, lies outside of the cranial structure, but is sometimes included among the bony structures of the head.

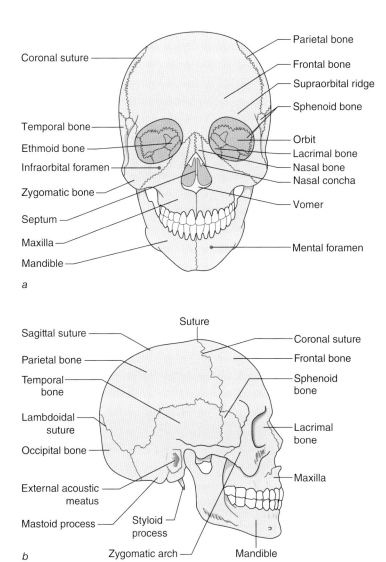

FIGURE 8.1 Bones of the skull from *(a)* frontal and *(b)* lateral views.

The brain and its protective meningeal covering are housed in a cranial vault. The brain is composed of three primary structures: the cerebrum, the cerebellum, and the brain stem (figure 8.2). The cerebrum, the largest and most superior of the brain structures, comprises the right and left hemispheres, which are joined by a band of fibers called the **corpus callosum**. Each hemisphere is divided into lobes (frontal, parietal, temporal, occipital), each with unique and complementary roles in thought and sensorimotor processing.

The second largest brain structure, the cerebellum, is located inferior to the cerebrum and posterior to the brain stem. Among its functions are coordination of the subconscious movements of skeletal muscles, movement error detection, maintenance of equilibrium and posture, and prediction of the future position of the body during a particular movement. The cerebellum also plays a role in emotional development by modulating sensations of pleasure and anger.

Lastly, the brain stem sits inferior to the cerebrum, functions as the link between the cerebrum and the spinal cord, and comprises the medulla oblongata, pons, midbrain, and hypothalamus. The brain stem largely serves as a pathway for most sensory and motor information passing between the cerebrum and spinal cord while also housing numerous vital reflex centers essential for life-supporting functions, such as heart rate, respiration, blood pres-

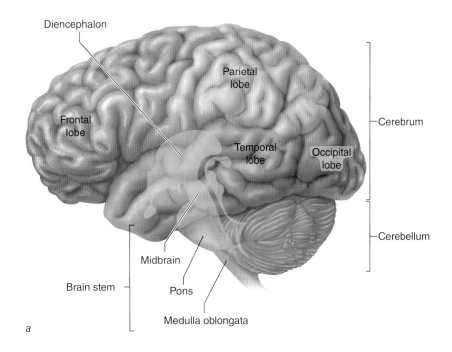

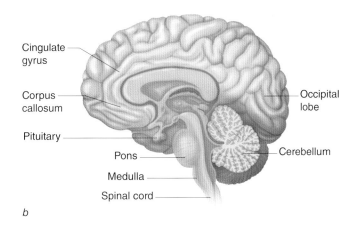

FIGURE 8.2 Anatomy of the brain. *(a)* Lateral view. *(b)* Sagittal section.

sure, and levels of consciousness. The brain stem also contains the nuclei for most of the 12 cranial nerves (table 8.1).

The cerebrum, brain stem, and spinal cord are covered by three layers of protective tissue known as **meninges**: the dura mater, the arachnoid mater, and the pia mater. The outermost layer is the **dura mater** (Latin for "tough mother"), a tough connective tissue comprised of two layers. The outer of the two layers (called the periosteal or endosteal) adheres tightly to the inner surface of the cranial cavity and does not extend beyond the foramen magnum, where the brain stem transitions to become the spinal cord. The inner layer of the dura mater is called the meningeal layer and lies just below the periosteal layer and extends outside of the cranial cavity to encapsulate the spinal cord. The middle meningeal layer, the **arachnoid**, appears as a web-like membrane. The **pia mater** (Latin for "tender mother") is the thinnest and most delicate of the meninges and adheres closely to the contours of the brain. **Cerebrospinal fluid (CSF)** flows in the space between the arachnoid and pia mater (i.e., **subarachnoid space**) and circulates around the brain

TABLE 8.1 Cranial Nerves

Nerve	Name	Sensory functions	Motor functions
I	Olfactory	Smell	None
II	Optic	Vision	None
III	Oculomotor	None	Eyeball movement, upper eyelid, pupil constriction
IV	Trochlear	None	Eyeball movement
V	Trigeminal	Sensation of the teeth and face	Mastication
VI	Abducens	None	Eyeball movement
VII	Facial	Taste	Facial expression, saliva and tear secretion
VIII	Vestibulocochlear	Balance, hearing	None
IX	Glossopharyngeal	Taste and gag reflex	Saliva secretion, swallowing, phonation
X	Vagus	Sensations from many organs	Swallowing, involuntary actions of the heart, lungs, and digestive tract
XI	Accessory	None	Head turn, shoulder shrug, some phonation
XII	Hypoglossal	None	Tongue movement during speech and swallowing

and spinal cord and provides supportive, protective, and nutritive functions.

Head Injuries

Head injuries have the potential to range from mild to life threatening, with both immediate and long-term consequences. The term *head injury* is encompassing of all injuries related to the bony structure and soft tissue of the head, including the skull, brain, and skin, among others. Injury severity depends, in part, on several principles, including the magnitude of the insult, the anatomical structures involved, age, and several others. We introduce several terms and discuss principles of head injuries here before exploring specific head injuries in detail.

Head injuries can result from a number of mechanisms, with mechanical injuries characterized as direct or indirect. Direct (contact) loading results from impact (e.g., helmet-to-helmet contact on the football field). Indirect (inertial) loading occurs when forces are transmitted to the head through adjacent structures such as the neck (e.g., whiplash mechanism). Whether direct or indirect, the applied force either accelerates or decelerates the head. Forces applied to a stationary head will tend to accelerate its mass, typified by a forceful blow, whereas forces acting in opposition to the head's motion will decelerate it, such as when the

head's motion is abruptly stopped by an unyielding surface (figure 8.3).

Numerous interrelated factors combine to determine the exact mechanism of injury depending on the type of force and its magnitude, location, direction, duration, and rate. Less understood are blast-related injuries that result from overpressure, but these can have the same structural and clinical outcomes on the brain as an acceleration injury resulting from a mechanical force (Bryden et al. 2019).

Subsequent to a force applied to the head is the motion that occurs in response to loading. Forces directed through the head's center of mass cause linear translation of the head (figure 8.4a), whereas forces acting eccentrically (off center) from the center of mass result in rotation of the head in any or all of the three primary planes (figure 8.4b). Because the skull is attached to the cervical spinal column, pure linear or rotational acceleration cannot occur, thus the applied forces cause combined translational and rotational, or general, motion of the skull and its contents.

The mechanical properties of the head's constituent tissues play an important role in determining the location and severity of injury. The skull forms a stiff, yet slightly compressible container housing the brain and its covering structures. The brain, in contrast, is more compliant, with the consistency of gelatin. When describing potential injury mechanisms, we must consider the different mechanical responses and relative mobility of these tissues. When a load is applied to the head, the stress–strain profiles of each structural component dictate a complex (and not completely understood) response.

The brain and other intracranial tissues develop internal stresses in response to loading. Each of the three principal stresses (compression, tension, shear) can be present and result in tissue deformation and strain. Injury occurs when the capacity of the tissue to withstand the applied load is exceeded. Dependent on the location of the structural damage, the injury is categorized either as a closed head injury or penetrating injury. Closed head injuries (e.g., concussion, cerebral edema, diffuse axonal injury) result in an injury to the brain or its covering structures but with no exposure to the external environment. Penetrating injuries, in contrast, occur when an object (e.g., bullet, javelin, arrow) directly penetrates the skull and its neurovascular contents.

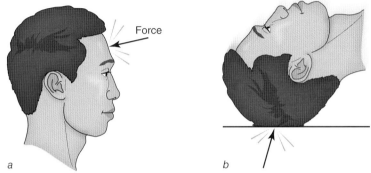

FIGURE 8.3 *(a)* Force applied to a stationary head. *(b)* Impact force created by contact of a moving head with an unyielding surface.

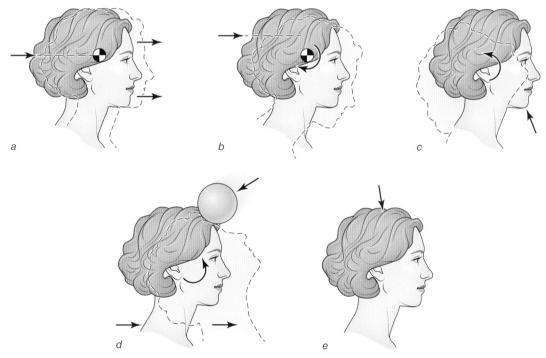

FIGURE 8.4 Effect of forces applied to the head (solid line = original position; dashed line = position following force application). *(a)* Force applied through the head's center of mass causes linear translation of the head. *(b)* Force applied eccentrically (off center) causes rotation of the head. *(c)* Force applied to the chin causes rotation of the head. *(d)* Simultaneous impact by a ball to the head and contact force to the back produce both rotation of the head and translation of the body. This combination accentuates the hyperextension mechanism in the cervical spine. *(e)* Blunt trauma to the superior aspect of the head causes a depressed skull fracture.

The factors just described do not necessarily occur in isolation; rather two or more of them may be used to characterize any given injury. For example, the unfortunate recipient of an upper-cut punch in boxing might experience an acceleration injury that creates violent hyperextension (figure 8.4*c*). In another example, a soccer player who, while heading the ball, is simultaneously contacted in the back by an opponent (figure 8.4*d*) would experience the combined effects of forward linear translation of the trunk and hyperextension of the neck.

We offer two final observations before considering specific head injuries:

- Head injuries often are insidious, in that evidence at the time of primary injury may provide little or no indication of associated secondary injuries that will subsequently develop.

- Injury to superficial structures does not necessarily and invariably result in intracranial damage to the brain and its coverings. Evidence of extensive superficial damage (e.g., copious bleeding), for example, does not always predict cerebral injury. Conversely, extensive brain injury can occur in the absence of superficial damage. In most cases, the overall severity of a head injury is best judged by the degree of internal damage to neural structures because these are responsible for effective cognitive, sensory, and motor function. Indeed, some brain injuries may be slow to develop (e.g., subdural hematoma) and may require advanced medical imaging to diagnose. For these reasons, the continued monitoring of head injury patients is strongly advised.

Skull Fracture

The study of skull fracture biomechanics has a long history, with the majority of injuries resulting from blunt trauma as the head hits a surface or object (e.g., as a result of falls or motor vehicle collisions) or from a direct blow to the head by an object (e.g., a baseball bat). Pioneering work by Gurdjian and colleagues in the 1940 and 1950s (e.g., Gurdjian and Webster 1946; Gurdjian et al. 1947, 1949, 1953) and Hodgson and colleagues in the 1960 and 1970s (e.g., Hodgson 1967; Hodgson and Thomas 1971, 1972, 1973) provided valuable information on skull strength and fracture characteristics.

More recent research has added to our understanding of skull mechanics. Yoganandan and col-

leagues (1995), for example, tested cadaver skulls and reported failure loads ranging from 4.5 to 14.1 kN (1,011-3,168 lb). The skulls had higher mean failure loads (11.9 kN or 2,674 lb) when loaded dynamically than when loaded quasistatically (6.4 kN or 1,438 lb). Skull strength varies regionally, with highest strength in the occipital (posterior) region, followed by the lateral (side) regions and the frontal region (Yoganandan and Pintar 2004).

Skull fractures can occur along the convexity, or vault, of the skull or through the skull base and are commonly categorized as linear, depressed, or compound. **Linear fractures** result from low-velocity blunt trauma, generating cracks in the cranial bone with no depression or displacement. The deleterious consequences of linear fractures are typically minimal. Higher magnitude blunt trauma can cause a **depressed skull fracture** (figure 8.4*e*), which presents as an indentation in the bone and can potentially cause cerebral contusion and intracranial bleeding involving the protective layers (meninges) of the brain. **Compound fractures** are the most serious, with disruption to the overlying skin and penetration of the meningeal layers that exposes the brain tissue. Fractures occurring at the base of the skull are called **basilar skull fractures** and are commonly caused by high-velocity acceleration and deceleration (e.g., motor vehicle collision). Basilar skull fractures have the added risk of damage to the spinal cord and blood vessels that pass through the foramen magnum. The location of the cranial nerves, on the ventral surface of the brain, also puts them at risk for injury.

Second to fracture may be injury to underlying intracranial structures. These injuries include cerebral contusions, intracranial hemorrhage, and, in cases of exposure to contaminants (as with scalp laceration or exposure to the nasal cavity and para-nasal sinuses), infection of the cerebrospinal fluid (**meningitis** or **cerebritis**). The extensive meningeal vasculature increases the likelihood of hemorrhage between the layers, resulting in **epidural**, **subdural**, or **subarachnoid hematoma**:

- *Epidural hematoma.* Rupture of the meningeal artery that bleeds into the space between the dura mater and the skull. Collection of blood in the epidural space compresses the brain, resulting in the rapid onset of headache, alterations in consciousness, and possible impaired pupil and eye function. Surgical intervention includes reliving the pressure through a burr hole or craniotomy.

• *Subdural hematoma.* Blood accumulation from a venous injury in the subdural space between the outer protective layer (dura mater) of the brain and the middle layer (arachnoid). Subdural hematoma is the most common form of intracranial mass lesion. Acute subdural hematoma can result from a traumatic event (e.g., rapid acceleration–deceleration or blunt force trauma), whereas chronic subdural hematoma can occur over an extended period of days or weeks as a result of minor head trauma (more often in older persons).

• *Subarachnoid hematoma.* Blood accumulation in the subarachnoid space between the middle (arachnoid) and inner (pia mater) layers covering the brain. Subarachnoid hematoma typically happens as a result of head trauma but also can result from a cerebral aneurysm.

Skull fracture is strongly predictive of intracranial hemorrhage. The absence of fracture, however, should not be interpreted as precluding brain injury, because approximately 20% of fatal head injuries show no evidence of skull fracture (Gennarelli and Graham 2005).

Blood accumulation caused by any hematoma is serious and, depending on the size, may raise the intracranial pressure (ICP) on the delicate brain tissues. Unchecked increases in ICP can cause permanent brain damage and eventual death.

Facial Fracture

Facial fractures are of particular concern because of the close proximity of the facial bones to vital neural and sensory structures. Facial fractures are most common in those between 20 and 40 years of age (Neuman and Eriksson 2006), and neurological injury associated with facial fractures can be as high as 76% (Haug et al. 1994). The mechanism of injury in the vast majority of cases is forceful blunt trauma, with impact velocity, rather than impact force, correlating most highly with fracture severity (Rhee et al. 2001).

The impacting object takes a variety of forms. Collisions with a part of another person's body (e.g., head, shoulder, elbow), an implement (e.g., hockey stick, baseball bat), a projectile (e.g., cricket ball, baseball, golf ball), or an unyielding surface (e.g., vehicle steering wheel) have all been reported to cause facial fractures. Facial fractures have historically been most commonly the result of automobile crashes. Worldwide, the role of vehicular crashes in facial fracture is a concern. Studies report that crashes account for 45% of facial fractures in Brazil (Brasileiro and Passeri 2006), 70% in Canada (Hogg et al. 2000), 45% in Germany (Kühne et al. 2007), and 56% in Nigeria (Adebayo et al. 2003). However, a recent increase in facial fractures resulting from violent assault suggests a disturbing trend. Lim and colleagues (1993), for example, reported that in Australia assault accounted for 51.2% of 839 facial fractures reviewed. Similarly, Alvi and colleagues (2003) reported that 41% of facial fractures treated at a trauma center in Chicago were caused by assault, followed by automobile collisions at 26.5%.

The shift in facial fracture etiology has been, in part, the result of increased seat belt use in automobiles. At impact, unrestrained drivers are launched chest first into the steering wheel (figure 8.5*a*). In

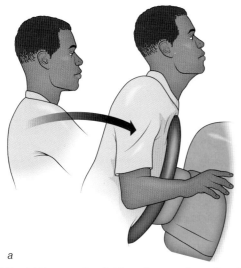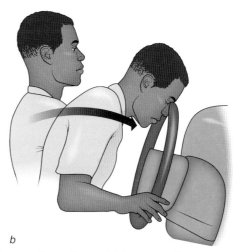

a   *b*

FIGURE 8.5   *(a)* Unrestrained driver thrown chest-first into the steering column. *(b)* The torso of a driver restrained by a lap-only seat belt rotates forward and results in head impact with the steering wheel assembly.

contrast, the driver who is restrained by a lap belt only (no shoulder strap) is more likely to sustain head injury as the cranium is thrown toward the steering wheel (figure 8.5*b*). Drivers who wear shoulder-restraint systems have fewer head injuries than unrestrained drivers, but may have more abdominal injuries because the body is rapidly decelerated by the restraint straps. A higher prevalence of gastrointestinal injury, in particular, has been reported for restrained adults (Wotherspoon et al. 2001) and children (Sokolove et al. 2005).

In addition to seatbelts, airbags have lowered the number of facial fractures. In most cases, airbags can prevent or reduce injury severity, but they will never be 100% effective. Substantial injury can still occur when crash speeds exceed the ability of the airbag to dissipate force or other scenarios (e.g., rollover crash) go beyond the airbag's intended design.

Because facial injury typically results from direct trauma, the risk of fracture depends largely on the strength of the bony tissue at the impact site (figure 8.6). Several researchers have been prominent in reporting facial bone strength. Among these are Hodgson (1967), Nahum and colleagues

(1968), Schneider and Nahum (1972), Hopper and colleagues (1994), and Yoganandan and colleagues (1993). Hampson (1995) summarized craniofacial bone tolerances for the zygoma, zygomatic arch, mandible, maxilla, frontal bone, and nose.

Reaching valid conclusions regarding facial fracture tolerances is difficult because of the limited number of specimens typically used in impact studies, differences in testing protocols, and specimen age. Nonetheless, Allsop and Kennett (2001) identified some trends:

- Fracture characteristics are not significantly affected by bone mineral content.
- Force pulse duration does not substantially affect fracture force.
- Fracture force is not affected by rate of force onset and strain rate.
- Initial fracture may happen at less than maximal force.
- Skull bone thickness significantly affects fracture force.
- Impact area of the testing apparatus significantly affects fracture force.

Isolated facial fractures are typically uncomplicated injuries, particularly when the bone is not displaced. However, given the high level of vasculature, nervous tissue, and other structures of the head, secondary injury is not uncommon. Nerves can be entrapped (i.e., pinched) following fracture and can result in permanent damage if not resolved quickly. Fractures to the orbital socket can result in impingement of the muscles that control the eye. Fractures to the frontal bones may result in crushed sinuses, leading to infection.

Facial fractures are particularly problematic because they often cross disciplinary boundaries. Treatment of injuries associated with facial fractures frequently requires the combined expertise of orthopedists, neurologists, dentists, ophthalmologists, and other medical specialists.

Penetrating Injuries

Penetrating injuries result from impact forces that exceed the tensile strength of the skull, resulting in exposure of the intracranial space to the external environment. The term is sometimes used in this broad sense to describe injuries from any cause, including motor vehicle collisions, occupational and sports injuries, and an object penetrating the skull.

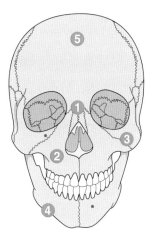

Area	MFTL	PT
1	25-75	342-450*
2	140-445	668-1801
3	200-450	489-2401
4	425-925	402-1607
5	800-1600	1000-6494

FIGURE 8.6 Force and pressure tolerances for facial bones. 1 = nasal arch, 2 = maxilla, 3 = zygoma, 4 = mandible, 5 = frontal bone. MFTL = minimal fracture tolerance level (lbs), PT = pressure tolerance (N). *In this case, there is a 50% risk of fracture from an applied force of 450 to 850 N. (Cormier, 2010).

Data from Hampson (1995), Cormier et al (2010), Pappachan and Alexander (2012), and Weisenbach et al. (2020).

The Curious Case of Phineas Gage

Most of today's head-penetration injuries result from gunshot wounds. In contrast to these all-too-common contemporary tragedies stands the peculiar case of Phineas Gage, a 25-year-old railroad construction foreman in mid-19th century Vermont. Gage was working late one hot summer afternoon placing explosives to blast stone from the planned path of the Rutland & Burlington Railroad when the explosive powder, which had been placed in a hole drilled in the stone, detonated prematurely and launched the iron rod Gage was using to tamp the powder into the hole (Damasio 1994). The rod, which weighed more than 13 lb (5.9 kg) and measured 1-1/4 inches (3.2 cm) in diameter and more than 3-1/2 feet (1.1 m) in length, penetrated Gage's head. As graphically described by Damasio (p. 4), "The explosion is so brutal. . . .

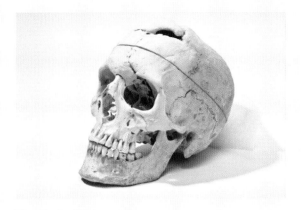

The skull of Phineas Gage.
Used with permission of Warren Anatomical Museum collection, Center for the History of Medicine in the Francis A. Countway Library of Medicine, Harvard University.

The bang is unusual, and the rock is intact. The iron enters Gage's left cheek, pierces the base of the skull, traverses the front of his brain, and exits at high speed through the top of the head. The rod has landed more than a hundred feet away, covered in blood and brains. Phineas Gage has been thrown to the ground. He is stunned, in the afternoon glow, silent but awake." Miraculously, Gage survived and was "able to talk and walk and remain coherent immediately afterward" (p. 5).

Gage was pronounced fully cured (at least physically) within two months of the accident and had no difficulty walking, touching, hearing, or speaking. It seems that the areas and networks of his brain responsible for language, perception, and motor function had survived the accident relatively unaffected. Gage, however, suffered from devastating and progressive alterations in his personality; his social reasoning skills were forever changed.

The implications of Gage's response to injury are profound. "Gage's story hinted at an amazing fact: Somehow, there were systems in the human brain dedicated more to reasoning than to anything else, and in particular to the personal and social dimensions of reasoning. The observance of previously acquired social convention and ethical rules could be lost as a result of brain damage, even when neither basic intellect nor language seemed compromised" (Damasio 1994, p. 10).

More commonly, penetrating injuries are limited to those in which an object pierces the cranium, exposing the contents of the cranial vault. These injuries are typically the result of high-velocity missiles (e.g. bullet), with secondary injury to the cerebral tissue resulting from the shock wave propagating through the tissue; or low-velocity missiles (e.g. knife) that fractures the thinner sections of bone, but with lower secondary shock-wave propagation. One remarkable and infamous case of a penetrating injury is described in the following sidebar.

The majority of penetrating head injuries are the result of gunshots. **Ballistics** is the science dealing with the motion of projectiles or missiles. **Wound ballistics** deals with the interaction of penetrating projectiles and living body tissues (Fackler 1998). In the case of bullets or shrapnel fragments, ballistic principles govern the path and mechanical characteristics that set the stage for head injury upon penetration. With respect to ballistic injuries, projectile flight can be divided into three phases (Volgas et al. 2005):

- **Internal ballistics** concern the effect of bullet and weapon design and materials on the projectile while in the barrel of the weapon.

- **External ballistics** concern the effect of external factors (e.g., wind, velocity, drag, gravity) on projectile flight from the barrel to the target.

• **Terminal ballistics** concern the behavior of projectiles in tissues.

Internal and external ballistics determine the initial conditions for terminal ballistics (i.e., speed, angle, and spin of a bullet). The entering projectile can cause tissue damage via three mechanisms: direct cutting or tearing of tissues, creation of a permanent cavity, and creation of a temporary cavity (Volgas et al. 2005). The permanent cavity is the path along which the projectile moves through the tissue, and in the absence of fragmentation, the cavity is usually small. A temporary cavity may form from the impulse waves emanating perpendicularly from the projectile's path. The amount of temporary cavitation depends on projectile speed, tissue density, and whether the projectile tumbles or fragments. The temporary cavity creates a vacuum that draws tissue and other material into the cavity space. This is followed by tissue rebound, which creates a second temporary cavity as tissues collide and rebound off each other in the vacuum space (Volgas et al. 2005). Cavitation is shown in figure 8.7.

Projectiles, by virtue of their motion, possess kinetic energy as described in equation 3.20:

$$E_k = \frac{1}{2} \cdot m \cdot v^2$$

where m = mass and v = linear velocity. The destructive potential of a bullet is determined, in part, by the magnitude of its kinetic energy at the moment of impact. The magnitude of injury is therefore partly determined by the mass and velocity of the projectile. The squared value placed on velocity indicates the greater influence it has on overall kinetic energy. Doubling a bullet's mass, for example, will double its kinetic energy—but doubling its velocity quadruples its kinetic energy.

In mechanical terms, the energy absorbed (E_a) by the tissues of the head (or elsewhere) is the amount of kinetic energy lost between bullet impact and exit:

$$E_k = E_i - E_e = \frac{1}{2} \cdot m \cdot \left(v_i^2 - v_e^2 \right) \tag{8.1}$$

where E_i = kinetic energy at impact, E_e = kinetic energy at exit, m = mass, v_i = impact velocity, and v_e = exit velocity. In cases where the bullet does not exit the skull, all the kinetic energy is absorbed intracranially. When the bullet has sufficient energy to traverse the brain but not enough to pierce the skull a second time and exit the cranium, the bullet may ricochet off the interior surface of skull, transferring additional energy to the brain and causing additional damage as it burrows back into the tissue.

Because energy dissipation alone does not entirely determine the type and extent of tissue disruption, velocity and energy measures only indicate the potential for injury and are not predictive of the nature and extent of injury (Santucci and Chang 2004). Two projectiles with the same kinetic energy on entry can therefore cause vastly different injury patterns (Fackler 1996). In addition to velocity and energy, the characteristics of tissue disruption are determined by the following factors (Bartlett 2003):

• Projectile stability and entrance profile (e.g., spin, pitch, and yaw).

• Caliber, construction, construction materials, configuration, and shape of the projectile.

• Distance and path of the projectile in the body.

• Biologic characteristics of the tissues (e.g., strength, elasticity, density). Denser tissues, for example, provide greater retarding resistance and contribute to greater energy loss. A bullet penetrating the skull would lose more energy in the brain tissue than would a bullet penetrating an air-filled lung.

• Mechanism of tissue damage (e.g., stretching, crushing, tearing).

• Projectile deformation and fragmentation. Bullets designed and constructed to deform or fragment after impact enhance kinetic energy loss and increase the severity of tissue damage.

All of the foregoing factors interact to determine the complex energy transfer profile as energy dis-

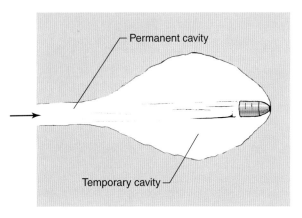

FIGURE 8.7 Cavitation caused by a projectile penetrating tissue.

sipates from the missile and is absorbed by the tissue surrounding the missile's path. The regrettable trend of firearm design toward more powerful, faster, and more deformable bullets portends an increase in destructive potential and inevitably greater levels of injury and catastrophic death.

Traumatic Brain Injury

Traumatic brain injury (TBI) is broadly defined as an injury to the brain brought about by direct or indirect force application to the head. TBI is a

major public health issue with nearly 3 million occurrences in the United States each year, mostly the result of falls (52%), followed by motor vehicle collisions (20%), and being struck by or against an object (17%) (CDC 2019). Because TBIs commonly lack a visible injury, they have been characterized by the U.S. Centers for Disease Control and Prevention (CDC) as a "silent epidemic" (Langlois et al. 2004).

The severity of injury largely depends on impact magnitude. Various scales have been devised to measure the degree of neural dysfunction from TBI

Football Risks

No other sport in the 21st century has come under scrutiny as intensely as football. Among the most popular sports in the United States, football is played by those from all walks of life and is deeply intertwined with American culture. Although the risk of orthopedic injury has long been known and accepted, increased scrutiny has more recently been placed on both the short- and long-term risk of concussion and repeated head impacts that have long been considered a routine part of the game.

From a physical perspective, football raises many interesting issues. Football athletes participate in perhaps the most vigorous of all sports, one that requires an efficient combination of power, speed, agility, coordination, and stamina. To a greater degree than most other athletes, football athletes subject themselves to substantial physical abuse that comes with participating in a heavy-contact sport. Football-related injuries range from minor cuts and abrasions to more severe damage, such as head and neck trauma. Ligament injuries to the upper and lower extremity occur most frequently, with the knee being the most commonly injured joint. Concussion accounts for less than 10% of football-related injuries, but the risk of concussion in football is among the highest of all sports (Van Pelt 2021).

In their most severe form, football injuries can lead to sudden death. In 2019, 20 athletes across all levels of play died as a direct or indirect result of football participation—one death per every 250,000 participants (Kucera et al. 2020).

Second to these acute injuries is the potential for cumulative neurological injuries that develop after repeated mechanical insult. Commonly referenced as **chronic traumatic encephalopathy (CTE)**, the deleterious effect of repeated head impacts with and without concussion on neurological function have been in the medical literature for more than 100 years. Harrison Martland's (1928) seminal work identified 23 boxers as "punch drunk" as a result of repeated head impacts. Numerous other investigators evaluated the effects of concussion and head impacts on boxers and animal models throughout the 20th century, but CTE was not linked to American football until 2005, when Bennet Omalu published a case study on former Pittsburgh Steelers player Mike Webster (Omalu et al. 2005).

Scientists are in the early stages of understanding the nuance of CTE, and prospective longitudinal studies are need to fully quantify risk. Clearly, an athlete participating in a noncontact sport (e.g., swimming) who never sustains a concussion has no increased risk. Similarly, there are currently no data to suggest that athletes who sustain a single concussion that is rapidly identified and managed appropriately is at risk for long-term deleterious outcomes (Giza et al. 2013). Intuition would tell us that increased exposure to concussion or repeated head impacts would increase the chances of a poor outcome, but only a small percentage of former football athletes have been diagnosed with CTE. Diagnosis rates among those participating in other heavy-contact sports (e.g., ice hockey) are lower. Yet, intrinsic (e.g., genetic) and extrinsic (e.g., diet, exercise, environment) factors are likely to modify the risk among those with the highest exposure to concussion and head impacts.

Despite a lack of comprehensive evidence, some have called for banning football outright, whereas others believe nothing should change. Between these two extremes have been changes to medical guidelines (McCrory et al. 2017), helmets (Rowson et al. 2014), and practices and competitions that have made the game safer for athletes (Wiebe et al. 2018).

as mild (concussion), moderate, or severe based clinical features. Historically, the most commonly used system has been the **Glasgow Coma Scale (GCS)**, which measures a patient's auditory, motor, and visual response to stimulation and determines the level of brain dysfunction on a 13-point scale ranging from 3 to 15 (table 8.2). A summed GCS score of 13 to 15 indicates mild injury, 9 to 12 moderate injury, and 3 to 8 severe injury. Mild injuries, which involve a functional change in the neural tissue, may also be referred to as *concussions*.

Moderate and severe injuries commonly involve structural changes to the neural tissue in addition to the functional changes. Tissue damage following impact may be restricted to a limited area (**focal injury**) or may pervade a large region of neural tissue (**diffuse injury**). Both diffuse and focal injuries can occur simultaneously.

Cerebral Contusion

Because the skull and brain are only loosely connected, acceleration or deceleration of the skull from an impact results in a lag motion from the brain. When the impact and resultant motion is large enough, the brain may collide with the inner surface of the cranial cavity, injuring the brain directly beneath the site of skull impact (**coup lesion**) or opposite the location of skull impact (**contrecoup lesion**) (figure 8.8). Either mechanism may result in a bruising of the cerebral tissue known as a **cerebral contusion**.

Not every head impact will produce a coup–contrecoup injury. As Valsamis (1994) noted,

> the rates of acceleration and deceleration will determine whether contact will be made at the initiation or cessation of skull movement. Thus, fast acceleration and relatively slow deceleration will result in a coup lesion. Relatively slow acceleration coupled with rapid deceleration will result in a contrecoup lesion. If both the components are rapid, a "coup–contrecoup" lesion will be produced, and, if both components are relatively slow, no contusion will result. (pp. 176-177)

The importance of head rotation, rather than translation, in the development of shearing loads in cerebral tissue has been appreciated for many decades. Holbourn (1943), for example, noted that

TABLE 8.2   Glasgow Coma Scale

EYE OPENING	
Spontaneous	4
To speech	3
To pain	2
None	1
BEST MOTOR RESPONSE	
Obeys	6
Localizes	5
Withdraws	4
Abnormal flexion	3
Extends	2
None	1
VERBAL RESPONSE	
Oriented	5
Confused conversation	4
Inappropriate words	3
Incomprehensible sounds	2
None	1

Scoring based on the modified GCS ranking: Severe: 3–8; moderate: 9–12; mild: 13–15.

Adapted from "Glasgow Coma Scale," Center for Disease Control, accessed June 30, 2022, https://www.cdc.gov/masstrauma/resources/gcs.pdf.

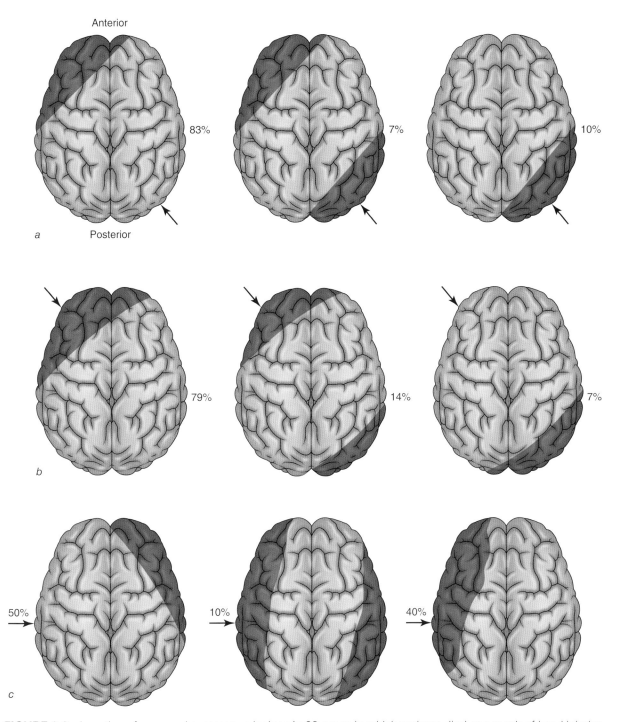

FIGURE 8.8 Location of coup and contrecoup lesions in 63 cases in which patients died as a result of head injuries. (Arrows indicate location of impact force. Shaded areas indicate areas of cerebral lesions.) *(a)* Occipital impacts. *(b)* Frontal impacts. *(c)* Lateral impacts.

Adapted by permission from K. Sano et al., "Mechanisms and Dynamics of Closed Head Injuries (preliminary report)," *Neurologia Medico-Chirurgica* 9, no. 22 (1967).

the shear strains produced by linear acceleration of the head are small compared with those developed in response to rotational accelerations. This fact was experimentally verified by Ommaya and

colleagues (1971, p. 515), who discounted the role of linear motion ("pure head translation has never been demonstrated as an injury producing factor for the brain") and submitted that "skull distortion and head rotation . . . explains a greater number of observations on coup and contrecoup injuries." Although much has been learned about the mechanisms of coup and contrecoup lesions, many questions remain regarding this complex set of cerebral contusion injuries.

Brain Swelling

Contusions and other traumatic brain lesions are often accompanied secondarily by brain swelling (edema), a serious and potentially fatal condition in which the contents of the cranial vault increase in volume. The increased fluid within the cerebral tissue causes an overall increase in brain size and ICP. Depending on the degree of swelling, the result can be compromised neurovascular function, cerebral ischemia, or herniation into adjacent intracranial spaces.

Brain swelling may be attributable to cerebral **hyperemia** (increased blood volume) or **cerebral edema**, a specialized condition characterized by increased tissue fluid content. Five types of cerebral edema have been identified (Miller 1993):

- Vasogenic: Caused by vascular injury (e.g., contusion) that damages the blood–brain barrier and allows for additional fluid to leak into the brain space
- Hydrostatic: Caused by increased arterial pressure
- Cytoxic: Caused by compromised energy supplies to the brain (e.g., ischemia), resulting in a buildup of sodium ions and associated fluids
- Osmotic: Caused by additional fluid moving from the blood into the brain because of very low sodium levels in the circulatory system (e.g., hyponatremia)
- Interstitial: Caused by unregulated production of cerebrospinal fluid

Concussion: A Closer Look

Medical recognition of concussion dates back to the 5th century BC as "commotion of the brain" resulting in loss of speech, hearing, and sight (McCrory and Berkovic 2001). Since that time, over 101 definitions have been proposed in the scientific literature (Kristman et al. 2014). Although they vary somewhat in their exact wording, they contain the elements of the classic characterization as "traumatic paralysis of neural function in the absence of lesions" (Denny-Brown and Russell 1941, p. 159). The most widely accepted definition of **concussion**, or sport-related concussion (SRC), created by the Concussion in Sport Group and updated in 2016 (McCrory et al. 2017) includes several common features:

Sport related concussion is a traumatic brain injury induced by biomechanical forces. Several common features that may be utilised in clinically defining the nature of a concussive head injury include:

- SRC may be caused either by a direct blow to the head, face, neck or elsewhere on the body with an impulsive force transmitted to the head.
- SRC typically results in the rapid onset of short-lived impairment of neurological function that resolves spontaneously. However, in some cases, signs and symptoms evolve over a number of minutes to hours.
- SRC may result in neuropathological changes, but the acute clinical signs and symptoms largely reflect a functional disturbance rather than a structural injury and, as such, no abnormality is seen on standard structural neuroimaging studies.
- SRC results in a range of clinical signs and symptoms that may or may not involve loss of consciousness. Resolution of the clinical and cognitive features typically follows a sequential course. However, in some cases symptoms may be prolonged.

This definition concludes that "The clinical signs and symptoms cannot be explained by drug, alcohol, or medication use, other injuries (such as cervical injuries, peripheral vestibular dysfunction, etc.) or other comorbidities (e.g., psychological factors or coexisting medical conditions)" (McCrory et al. 2017).

Whether concussion is its own unique entity or can be used interchangeably with *mild traumatic brain injury* (MTBI) is up for debate. Traditional thought would suggest MTBI implies some form of structural brain injury, whereas concussion is usually described as involving neural dysfunction without structural brain damage. However, modern scientific techniques (e.g., diffusion tensor imaging) are able to show alterations in white matter tract integrity following injury that would suggest structural damage at the microscopic level.

Definition and Grading   Concussion has been historically graded based on the presence or absence of unconsciousness and its duration. By 2001 there were no fewer than nine concussion grading scales available, many of which ranked the injury as 1, 2, or 3 to represent increasing severity, although some had as many as six levels (Cantu 2001). In 2004, the

Concussion in Sport Group suggested a dichotomous grading system of "simple" or "complex" injuries (McCrory et al. 2005). Since that time, the majority of medical organizations and the Concussion in Sport Group have recommended concussion severity grading be abandoned altogether (Broglio et al. 2014; Harmon et al. 2019; McCrory et al. 2017).

Concussion has been defined as a heterogenous injury, with no two injuries presenting the same both within and between people. Symptoms of concussion may include headache, dizziness, nausea, visual disturbances, **tinnitus**, confusion, "not feeling right," and others. Physical manifestations of concussion may include loss of consciousness, confusion, amnesia, compromised balance and coordination, unsteady gait, slowness in answering questions or following directions, poor concentration, display of inappropriate emotions, vomiting, vacant stare, slurred speech, personality changes, and inappropriate playing behavior (McCrory et al. 2005). Although the symptoms are transient by definition, the time course of recovery varies considerably, ranging from several seconds to months. Approximately 50% of concussed individuals will recover within two weeks of their injury and 90% within a month (McCrea et al. 2013). A small number of individuals will continue to report symptoms beyond that point, but those reporting symptoms longer than three months may be suffering from post-concussive syndrome (American Psychiatric Association 2013).

The medical management of concussion has changed dramatically since the turn of the century. Prior to that point, an athlete continuing to play while concussed was often seen as a point of pride or ignored altogether. Since the early 2000s, however, the understanding of concussion, educational efforts, and state laws have all led to higher reporting rates and more treatment.

Epidemiology Accurate estimates of concussion incidence are elusive, attributable in part to underreporting and difficulty with definitive diagnosis (McCrea et al. 2004). Bazarian and colleagues (2005) estimated an annual concussion incidence of 127.8 in 100,000 based on emergency department cases. These data do not, however, include concussions seen in nonemergency venues (e.g., personal physician's office) or possible concussions for which no medical attention is sought. Some have an estimated the annual incidence of concussion resulting from sport and recreation, including unreported injuries, to range from 1.6 to 3.8 million (Langlois et al. 2006).

The primary causes of concussion are predictable: falls, motor vehicle trauma, accidental head impact, assault, and sport and recreational activities. Arguably, the best estimates of concussion incidence come from sport settings, which offer controlled environments that are typically monitored by medical professionals (i.e., athletic trainers or physicians). Concussion risk varies across sports, with contact and collision sports among the highest. A meta-analytic review of concussion risk reported rugby as having the highest overall risk (28.23 per 10,000 athletic exposures), followed by American football (8.72 per 10,000) and ice hockey (7.87 per 10,000) (Van Pelt et al. 2021).

It is clear, however, that when looking across a number of sports, women have a higher injury risk in sex-comparable sports (e.g., soccer; see Van Pelt et al. 2021). Scientists are not entirely sure why this is, but some evidence suggests women have smaller neck musculature relative to head mass (see Tierney et al. 2005) and may be more susceptible to injury at certain points in the menstrual cycle. Women are also more likely to report their injury to a medical provider (Wunderle et al. 2014).

Tissue Structure and Function Nearly every concussion definition describes the injury as a neural dysfunction in the absence of structural damage at the macro level. The force transmitted to the brain, be it direct or indirect, is thought to stretch the neural tissue, mechanically opening the voltage-gated channels and causing the indiscriminate flux of ions across the membrane (Giza and Hovda 2014). Because the body will constantly seek to maintain homeostasis, the sodium–potassium ion pumps are upregulated to restore ion balance, at the cost of additional energy use. The state of **hyperglycolysis** is concurrent with increased intracellular calcium and extracellular potassium and reduced cerebral blood flow. The brain will eventually return to its natural state over time, with most individuals returning to preinjury levels of functioning within 4 weeks (McCrea et al. 2013).

Brain tissue, because of its incompressibility, handles compressive loads well but is much less resistant to shearing loads caused by head rotation. Research attempting to quantify the magnitude at which concussion occurs has been conducted at all levels of sport, with surprising consistency (Broglio et al. 2010; Guskiewicz et al. 2007; Pellman et al. 2003). Although there is significant individual variability both within and between athletes, a mean linear acceleration near 100 g and rotational acceleration of 4500 rad/s^2 are commonly reported. Interestingly, the estimated rotational acceleration needed to produce concussion is lower for adults (4500 rad/s^2) than for infants (10,000 rad/s^2). This contrast points to differences in mechanical response between an adult skull and brain and those of a developing child. These differences are attributable to contrasting constitutive material properties, structural geometries, age-dependent physiological responses to mechanical stress, overall mass, and structural properties of the head (Ommaya et al. 2002). Brains of various sizes have dissimilar injury thresholds and age-related mechanical properties (Goldsmith and Plunkett 2004).

Mechanisms of Injury Concussion results from a change in momentum of the head and thus most often involves direct impact or acceleration–deceleration mechanisms. In the vast majority of cases, direct impact to the head is implicated, although rapid acceleration–deceleration without direct impact also can cause concussion. Proposed concussion mechanisms include shear strains caused by rotation (Holbourn 1943), coup–contrecoup cavitation caused by displacement between the skull and brain (Gross 1958), linear acceleration causing shear stress or distortion in the brain stem (Gurdjian et al. 1955), and sequential centripetal disruption beginning at the brain surface and extending inward to deeper brain structures (Ommaya and Gennarelli 1974). The importance of rotational acceleration as a mechanism of concussive injury was originally suggested by Holbourn (1943) and has been reiterated by many researchers, notably Ommaya and Gennarelli (1974), who suggested that rotational accelerations to the head cause diffuse and widespread injury, whereas translational accelerations mainly cause focal injuries. Despite extensive research over the past half-century, controversy remains over the exact mechanisms causing concussion (Zhang et al. 2001).

Treatment, Rehabilitation, and Prevention A number of medical and international groups have outlined the appropriate treatment, rehabilitation, and prevention for concussion that are specific to the medical provider (Broglio et al. 2014; Harmon et al. 2019; McCrory et al. 2017). Although differences exist among these documents, all agree that any athlete suspected of sustaining a concussion should immediately be removed from play and not allowed to return until cleared by a medical provider trained in concussion identification and management. Following removal from play, the injured individual should rest for 24 to 48 hours, followed by a return to activities of daily living and then a slow progression back to their regular physical activities. If the individual is a student, the process of returning to the classroom and athletics can occur in parallel,

but a complete return to learning should take place before a complete return to play. Although the vast majority of individuals will recover from their injury within a month and have no discernable long-term consequences, approximately 10% of concussed individuals will continue to experience concussion-related symptoms beyond the 1-month mark, at which point specialized care may be necessary.

Although concussions cannot be eliminated, a focus on prevention can help reduce the risk of injury and its physical, financial, and emotional costs. Concussion prevention has primarily focused on sport and recreational activities, particularly through advances in protective equipment design. Helmets are at the center of this conversation: A helmet's hard outer shell spreads impact forces over a large area to protect against focal injuries (e.g., scalp lacerations); the inner lining helps dissipate kinetic energy via an energy-absorptive mechanism (Bailes and Cantu 2001). Modern football helmet design has been shown to reduce concussion risk relative to older models (Rowson et al. 2014), with the most recent technologies aimed at mitigating postimpact rotational acceleration. The influence of mouth guards on reducing concussion risk is less clear, with mixed findings in the research. A review of literature suggests no effect of mouth guards on concussion risk (Mihalik et al. 2007), although larger epidemiological studies suggest otherwise (Chisholm et al. 2020). Regardless of the ability to mitigate concussion risk, mouth guards are highly effective at reducing dental injuries.

Implementation and enforcement of rules aimed at reducing injuries can also help mitigate risk. For example, limiting contact practice sessions in American football reduces head impact exposure (Broglio et al. 2016), and adjusting the kickoff placement reduces concussion risk (Wiebe et al. 2018). Rules instituted in the 1970s that banned spearing (i.e., using the helmet as a battering device) resulted in a precipitous decrease in cervical spine injuries and concussions (Swartz et al. 2005).

Diffuse Axonal Injury

One of the distinguishing characteristics of concussion is an absence of detectable pathology. As impact forces increase, the likelihood of structural damage increases as well. In cases of more severe injury, neural structures sustain damage that is apparent through imaging (e.g., CT scans). These lesions may be in the form of contusion, laceration, hemorrhage, or axonal damage. Axonal lesions have been described as diffuse degeneration of the white matter,

Second Impact Syndrome

On rare occasions following a concussion, a subsequent blow that directly impacts or indirectly moves the head can result in dramatic escalation of concussive symptoms. Called **second impact syndrome (SIS)**, this injury "occurs when an athlete who has sustained an initial head injury, most often a concussion, sustains a second head injury before symptoms associated with the first have fully cleared" (Cantu 1998, p. 37). SIS can result in cerebrovascular dysregulation, vascular congestion, pupil dilation, increased ICP, cerebral edema, respiratory failure, and possible death.

Children and adolescents are at particular risk for SIS. Many reported cases of SIS involve high school athletes. Age, type of sport, and prior history of concussion are potent risk factors for SIS (Cobb and Battin 2004). Given its rarity, however, clinical evidence for SIS is largely anecdotal. Some researchers have questioned whether SIS exists. McCrory (2001), for example, contends that the evidence for SIS is not compelling and that observed neurovascular declines are likely attributable to diffuse cerebral swelling. Despite the controversy, prudence dictates that individuals with a concussion be restricted from activities in which they might suffer further head impact until concussive symptoms are completely resolved.

---

diffuse white-matter shearing injury, and inner cerebral trauma. Currently, the most common designation is **diffuse axonal injury (DAI)**, a shearing of the axons. However, this term may be a misnomer—DAI is not a diffuse injury to the entire brain, but rather to discrete areas of the brain (Meythaler et al. 2001). Some researchers and clinicians now use the term **traumatic axonal injury (TAI)** or **diffuse traumatic axonal injury (DTAI)** to describe these injuries (Gennarelli and Graham 2005).

DAI results from high-speed impacts, most commonly motor vehicle crashes that involve rapid acceleration and deceleration. DAI has been reported in football, soccer, and ice hockey players (Powell and Barber-Foss 1999; Tegner and Lorentzon 1996), but these are rare. Recent reports have associated DAI with shaken-baby syndrome, in which violent shaking of a baby elicits acceleration and deceleration forces high enough to cause brain trauma (e.g., Case et al. 2001; Duhaime et al. 1998).

Maxwell and colleagues (1993) suggested two mechanisms of injury in nonimpact head injuries: (1) initial axonal shearing and sealing of fragmented axonal membranes, and (2) secondary axonal swelling and disconnection. The mechanical insult brought about by the force of impact may directly disrupt axonal structure, which can result in the secondary mechanism. Delayed and sequential events lead to axonal failure that lead to axonal severance into the distal segments. In these cases, the distal segment predictably experiences Wallerian degeneration (see chapter 5) and becomes deafferented (i.e., separated from its sensory components). Both mechanisms disrupt transmission of the neuronal

signals and, depending on the magnitude of injury, may leave the individual significantly impaired.

Accurate diagnosis of DAI, especially in its mildest forms, remains problematic. Because DAI is an injury at the level of the axon, the mildest cases may not be apparent using CT scans, although it can be identified through careful microscopic examination. In cases where DAI is associated with hemorrhage, which is detectable with CT scan and MRI, DAI is assumed to be present. DAI is thusly graded according to the localization of its lesions (Adams et al. 1989). Grade I DAI is characterized by diffuse axonal injury throughout the brain (e.g. cerebral hemispheres, the corpus callosum, and the brain stem). Grade II injuries add focal lesions in the corpus callosum, whereas grade III DAI lesions show focal lesions in the brain stem.

Cerebral tissue is resistant to compression loads; however, the tissue has limited resistance to shearing loads. Shearing strains arising from angular acceleration of the head are accepted as the cause of most cases of DAI. More specifically, the plane of angular acceleration largely determines the extent of injury. In studies on nonhuman primates, angular acceleration in the sagittal plane resulted in only grade I lesions. Similar levels of angular acceleration in the transverse (horizontal) plane typically caused grade II injuries. The most severe grade III lesions were associated with accelerations in the frontal (coronal) plane. Using a primate model to explore the effect of angular acceleration direction on duration of coma, degree of neurological impairment, and level of DAI, Gennarelli and colleagues (1982) concluded that "axonal damage produced by coronal head acceleration is a major cause of prolonged traumatic coma and its sequelae" (p. 564).

Ommaya's **centripetal theory** is important in explaining lesions after head injury. The collective knowledge of multiple studies "suggested that the distribution of damaging diffuse strains induced by inertial loading would decrease in magnitude from the surface to the center of the approximately spheroidal brain mass" (Ommaya 1995, p. 530). In other words, the higher the impact magnitude, the deeper the injury would be present, along with the associated clinical signs and symptoms. This prediction was in conflict with the long-held view that traumatic unconsciousness was an isolated primary brain stem injury—Ommaya consistently found accompanying peripheral lesions with brain stem injuries.

Our understanding of head injury in general, and DAI in particular, has improved remarkably over the last two decades. Sahuquillo and Poca (2002) first developed the concept that secondary ischemic damage is highly prevalent in the brains of patients suffering fatal head injuries. Efforts to minimize deleterious ischemic effects greatly improve chances of patient survival and recovery. Until as recently as the 1990s, DAI was considered by most to be a primary injury. DAI, however, is not a single event but rather a dynamic physiological process initiated at impact and continuing for a variable time postinjury. Sahuquillo and Poca (2002) conclude, "Experimental evidence has shown beyond any reasonable doubt that DAI is a complex physiopathological entity where primary immediate damage can coexist with a simultaneously evolving secondary process in which axons that initially are structurally intact may progress towards secondary disconnection or axotomy" (pp. 53-54).

Neck Injuries

The neck provides the structural link between the head and trunk and contains components of many of the body's principal systems. Among these are important vascular (common carotid arteries, subclavian arteries and veins, brachiocephalic trunk and veins), respiratory (trachea, larynx), digestive (esophagus), nervous (sympathetic trunk, phrenic nerve, vagus nerve), and endocrine (thyroid and parathyroid glands) structures. The skeletal portion of the neck includes the cervical vertebrae, held in place by a strong system of ligaments (figure 8.9*a*) and musculature. Among the more prominent muscles of the neck are the sternocleidomastoid and trapezius (figure 8.9*b* and *c*).

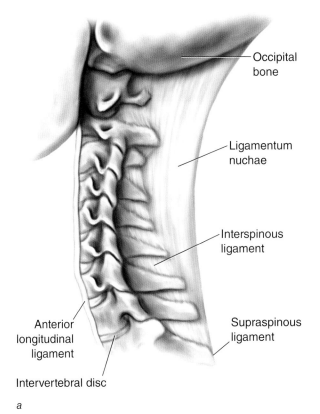

Occipital bone

Ligamentum nuchae

Interspinous ligament

Supraspinous ligament

Intervertebral disc

Anterior longitudinal ligament

a

FIGURE 8.9 *(a)* Cervical vertebrae, with several of their supporting ligaments shown. *(b)* Posterior musculature of the neck. *(c)* Anterior musculature of the neck.

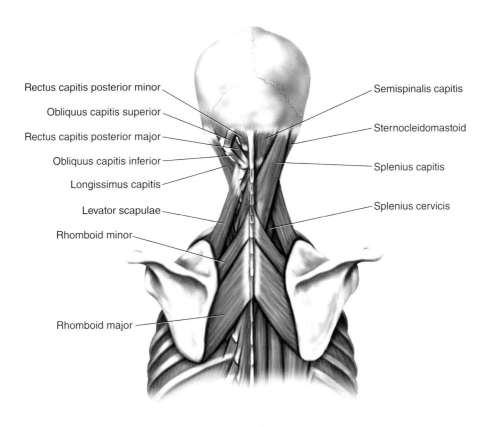

Rectus capitis posterior minor

Obliquus capitis superior

Rectus capitis posterior major

Obliquus capitis inferior

Longissimus capitis

Levator scapulae

Rhomboid minor

Rhomboid major

Semispinalis capitis

Sternocleidomastoid

Splenius capitis

Splenius cervicis

b   **Posterior**

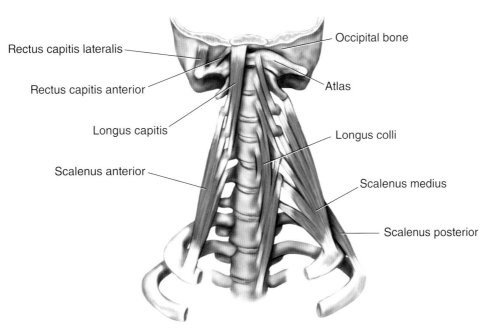

Rectus capitis lateralis

Rectus capitis anterior

Longus capitis

Scalenus anterior

Occipital bone

Atlas

Longus colli

Scalenus medius

Scalenus posterior

c   **Anterior**

FIGURE 8.9   *(continued)*

The vertebral column (spine) is a group of 33 vertebrae extending from the base of the skull to its inferior termination at the coccyx (tailbone). The spine is divided into five regions (figure 8.10): cervical (7 vertebrae), thoracic (12 vertebrae), lumbar (5 vertebrae), sacral (5 fused vertebrae), coccygeal (4 fused vertebrae). Vertebrae in the cervical, thoracic, and lumbar regions are separated by intervertebral discs that are composed of a gelatinous inner mass (nucleus pulposus) surrounded by a layered fibrocartilage network (annulus fibrosus). Each vertebra consists of a body, vertebral arch, and processes projecting laterally (transverse process) and posteriorly (spinous process) from the arch (figure 8.10).

The size and orientation of these structural elements differ between regions (figure 8.11). Just posterior to the vertebral body is an open passage (vertebral foramen) that houses the spinal cord. Other passages (intervertebral foramina) between adjacent vertebrae allow the exit of spinal nerve roots on both sides of the vertebral column. These regional changes in facet orientation play an essential role in determining movement potential between adjacent vertebrae in each region (figure 8.12). Angle values are rough estimates. Actual values vary within regions of the spine and among individuals.

The consequences of spinal cord damage range from mild, as in neurapraxia (transient loss of nerve conduction without structural degeneration), to incomplete or complete bisection. In cases of severe injury, the level of spinal cord involvement is critical in determining the type and extent of sensorimotor deficit. Broadly, injury at a specific level will impair function at the level of the injury and below.

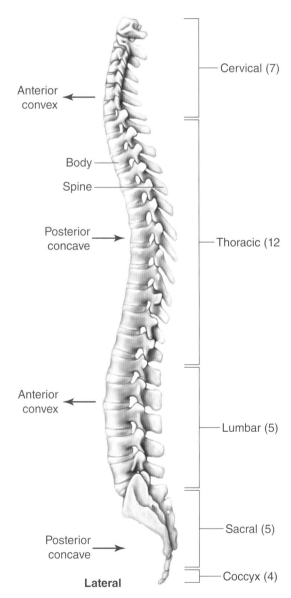

FIGURE 8.10 Skeletal structures of the vertebral (spinal) column.

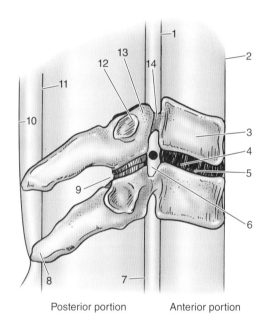

FIGURE 8.11 Sagittal view of a spinal motion segment formed by two adjacent vertebral bodies and the intervening disc. Structures or locations of structures pictured (only the locations of ligaments, and not their structures, are indicated): 1, posterior longitudinal ligament; 2, anterior longitudinal ligament; 3, vertebral body; 4, cartilaginous end plate; 5, intervertebral disc; 6, intervertebral foramen with nerve root; 7, ligamentum flavum; 8, spinous process; 9, intervertebral joint formed by the superior and inferior facets (joint capsules not shown); 10, supraspinous ligament; 11, interspinous ligament; 12, transverse process (intertransverse ligament not shown); 13, vertebral arch; 14, vertebral canal (spinal cord not shown).

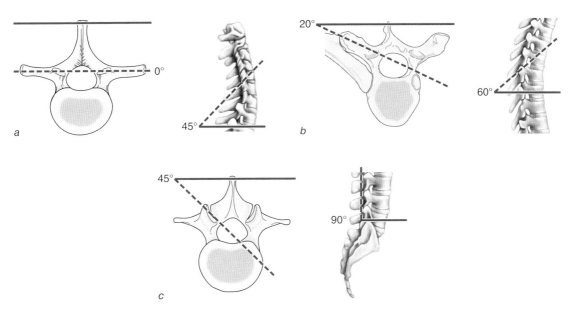

FIGURE 8.12 Orientation of the vertebral facet joints. *(a)* Cervical spine. The vertebral facets in the cervical spine are inclined 45° above the horizontal plane and are parallel with the frontal plane. *(b)* Thoracic spine. The facets in the thoracic region are inclined 60° above the horizontal plane and deviate 20° behind the frontal plane. *(c)* Lumbar spine. Facets in the lumbar spine are inclined 90° above the horizontal plane and deviate 45° behind the frontal plane. These regional changes in facet orientation play an essential role in determining movement potential between adjacent vertebrae in each region. Angle values are rough estimates. Actual values vary within regions of the spine and among individuals.

For example, injury at the C3-C4 level may result in complete paralysis of the trunk and extremities and loss of unassisted respiration. Injury at C5-C6 may allow limited arm movement, whereas lower-level injury at C7-T1 may spare upper-extremity muscle function and limit paralysis to the lower extremities.

Cervical Trauma

The complex structure and intricate motion of the cervical region present unique challenges in identifying and describing mechanisms of cervical injury. The sometimes confusing mixture of engineering and medical terminology used to describe cervical mechanics further complicates the task.

Classification of cervical injury mechanisms requires great care and precision because (1) the overall motion of the head relative to the trunk may not be indicative of local motion between adjacent segments, (2) small deviations (<1 cm) in the point of force application or in head position can change the injury mechanism from compression–flexion to compression–extension, and (3) observed head motions may occur after the instant of injury and thus not reflect the true injury mechanism (McElhaney et al. 2001).

Although various classification systems have been proposed, the system revised by McElhaney et al. (2001) based on the principal loadings of the cervical spine indicates possible injury outcomes (figure 8.13 and table 8.3).

The **compression–flexion mechanism** (or **flexion–compression mechanism**) is the most common injury mechanism for cervical spine injuries. In these cases, the slightly flexed neck aligns the cervical spine axially to eliminate normal lordosis. In this position, the cervical spine becomes a segmented, straightened column that has lost the ability for energy absorption that comes with normal curvature (Cusick and Yoganandan 2002). This position, termed the *stiffest axis*, leaves the cervical structures to absorb all of the loading energy (figure 8.14), placing the spine at greater risk of structural failure (Pintar et al. 1995). When this energy exceeds the capacity of the cervical structures, failure of the intervertebral discs, the body and processes of the vertebrae, or the spinous ligaments may occur. Resulting **wedge fractures** or burst fractures are predictably present. Disruption of supporting structures permits further flexion or rotation of the cervical spine and associated vertebral dislocation. This dislocation carries the risk

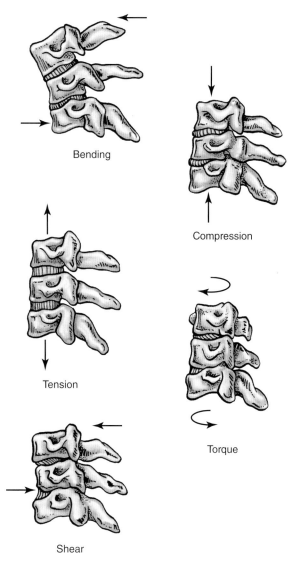

Bending

Compression

Tension

Torque

Shear

FIGURE 8.13 Mechanisms of neck loading.

TABLE 8.3 Cervical Spine Injuries

HYPERFLEXION INJURIES	
Stable	Anterior subluxation Anterior vertebral compression Shoveler's fracture
Unstable	Anterior subluxation (delayed instability) Bilateral facet dislocation Flexion teardrop fracture
FLEXION–ROTATION INJURIES	
Stable	Unilateral facet dislocation
HYPEREXTENSION INJURIES	
Stable	Fracture of posterior arch of atlas Fracture of anterior arch of atlas Laminar fracture Extension teardrop fracture
Unstable	Hangman's fracture Hyperextension dislocation Fracture–dislocation
EXTENSION–ROTATION INJURIES	
Stable	Fracture of articular pillars
VERTICAL COMPRESSION INJURIES	
Stable or unstable	Jefferson fracture C3-C7 burst fracture
COMPLEX OR UNKNOWN MECHANISM	
Unstable	Atlantooccipital dislocation Odontoid fracture

Adapted by permission from Y. Agarwal, P. Gulati, B. Sureka, and N. Kumar, "Radiologic Imaging in Spinal Trauma," in *ISCoS Textbook on Comprehensive Management of Spinal Cord Injuries,* edited by H.S. Chhabra (India: Wolters Kluwer, 2015).

of impinging the spinal cord or spinal nerves. The compression–flexion mechanism is most common in diving and also happens in sports such as football, ice hockey, and surfing.

Cervical injury may also result from a **tension–extension mechanism** in which the head is forcibly hyperextended by posterior impact with forcible resistance applied to the chin (figure 8.15*a*), inertial forces resulting from posterior impact (figure 8.15*b*), or forces applied inferiorly to the posterior aspect of the head (figure 8.15*c*). This mechanism creates tension stresses to the anterior aspect of the cervical structures and can involve disruption of the anterior longitudinal ligament or intervertebral disc or horizontal fracture of the vertebral body. High-energy loading can also result in posterior vertebral displacement and risk of spinal cord injury.

Some cervical injuries result from multiple mechanisms. For example, fracture at the anteroinferior corner of a vertebral body, termed a **teardrop fracture** (figure 8.16), has been attributed to many mechanisms, including axial compression, compression–flexion, tension–extension, and compression–extension loading (McElhaney et al. 2001).

Motor vehicle crashes are the single largest cause of cervical fractures. Multiple factors are at play in understanding the biomechanics of these injuries, but there is agreement on some issues. Yoganandan and colleagues (1989) examined motor vehicle crash–related cervical injuries and concluded the following:

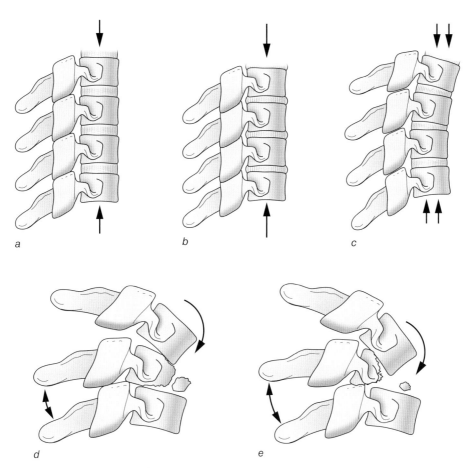

FIGURE 8.14 *(a)* With the neck slightly flexed (approximately 30°), the cervical spine is straightened and functions as a segmented column. *(b)* Axial compressive forces applied to a segmented column initially compress the column. Increased loading causes *(c)* angular deformation, *(d)* buckling, and *(e)* eventual fracture, subluxation, or dislocation.

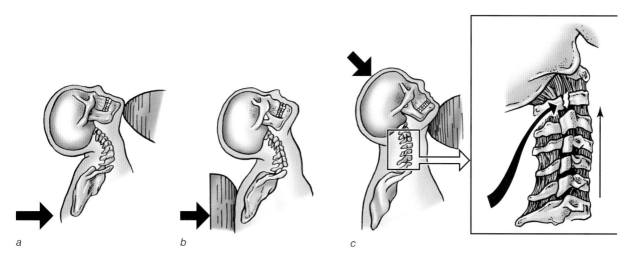

FIGURE 8.15 Tension–extension injury mechanisms. Cervical hyperextension caused by *(a)* posterior impact with forcible resistance on the chin, *(b)* inertial forces from posterior impact, and *(c)* forces applied inferiorly to the posterior aspect of the head with forcible resistance applied to the chin.

Reprinted by permission from R. Levine, *Head and Neck Injury* (Denver, CO and Troy, MI: SAE International, 1994). Permission conveyed through Copyright Clearance Center, Inc.

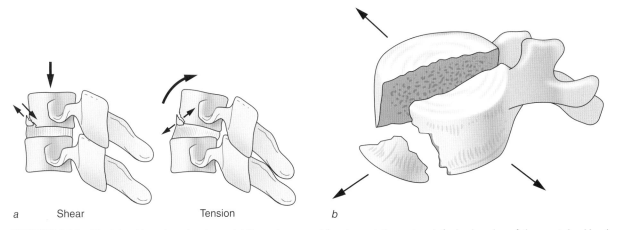

a Shear   Tension   *b*

FIGURE 8.16 Vertebral teardrop fracture. *(a)* Bone fragment fracture at the anteroinferior border of the vertebral body resulting from compressive loading (left) that results in shearing at the fragment interface from spinal extension (right) that creates tensile loading at the fragment interface. *(b)* A three-part, biplanar teardrop fracture with an anteroinferior corner fracture fragment and a sagittal fracture through the vertebral body.

- Cervical injuries focus at the occiput axis and C5-C6 regions of the upper and lower cervical spine, respectively.

- Fatal spinal injury from motor vehicle crashes most commonly happens at the craniocervical junction and upper cervical spine (O-C1-C2).

- Motor vehicle crash survivors tend to have lower cervical spine injury more often than upper cervical involvement.

- Craniofacial injury and cervical spine trauma are closely related, suggesting that occupant restraint systems that limit head and face impact can reduce the incidence of serious cervical spine injury.

Identification of the specific mechanisms of cervical spine injury often is problematic, largely because of the complexity of cervical anatomy, alignment, and loading. Nonetheless, "the influence of cervical alignment and curvature in association with the direction of force application on the potential vertebral component compromise is an important consideration in clarifying the causative forces of specific fracture patterns" (Cusick and Yoganandan 2002, pp. 17-18).

Spinal Cord Injury

Cervical **spinal cord injury (SCI)** can, unfortunately, occur in many activities. The reported incidence of SCI for specific activities varies based on the population, location, and injury circumstances. Car crashes are a commonly cited cause of injury, accounting

for up to half of all SCIs. For example, a nationwide study in Turkey reported motor vehicle crashes as the leading cause of SCI (48.8%), followed by falls (36.5%) (Karacan et al. 2000). Conversely, a study of 20- to 29-year-old patients in the Republic of South Africa identified gunshot wounds as the leading cause of SCI (36%), followed by car crashes (25%) (Hart and Williams 1994). Spinal cord injuries also have been reported attributable to falls from heights, work-related tasks, and sporting and recreational activities. Despite their relative infrequency, sports-related SCIs often achieve notoriety in the media, usually in cases of American football injuries that result in paralysis.

Although rare, spinal cord injury (SCI) can have a catastrophic impact on quality of life. More commonly, cervical injury manifests as a temporary sensorimotor lesion caused by pinching or stretching of cervical nerve roots or the brachial plexus. These so-called *burners* or *stingers* result in burning pain, with numbness and temporary weakness in the affected arm.

Watkins and Watkins (2001) described two mechanisms associated with this injury. The first involves an off-center axial load applied while the neck is extended and laterally flexed. In this position, the spinal canal and foramina narrow and allow the bony borders to impinge on the exiting nerve roots. This mechanism is most commonly seen in American football players during the impacts of blocking, tackling, and ground contact.

In the second mechanism, the shoulder on the involved side is depressed and the head is forcibly pushed away contralaterally. This motion violently stretches the nerve roots and associated brachial plexus and results in transient neurological symptoms. In mild burners, sensorimotor function returns within minutes and recovery is complete within a week or two. More severe injury can result in motor loss to muscles (e.g., biceps brachii, deltoid) that persists for weeks or even months. Subsequent injuries typically result in progressively longer recoveries.

More severe SCI, when the cord itself is damaged, usually results from vertebral fracture, dislocation, or both. Bony fragments can impinge and partially or fully sever the spinal cord. The level of cervical spinal cord injury (C1-C7) is critical in determining the degree of neuromuscular dysfunction and motor deficit (Gardner 2002; Watkins and Watkins 2001). The following summarizes function and deficits according to cervical level:

- *C1-C3.* Limited movement of head and neck. Complete paralysis of trunk and extremities (**quadriplegia**). Patient requires ventilatory support.
- *C3-C4.* Usual head and neck control. C4 may shrug shoulders. Patient requires initial ventilatory assistance.
- *C5.* Head, neck, and shoulder control. Patient can bend elbows and supinate arm to turn palms up.
- *C6.* Head, neck, shoulder, and elbow flexion control. Patient can turn palms up and down and can extend wrist.
- *C7.* Added ability to extend elbow.
- *C8.* Added strength and some finger control, but lack of fine precision hand movements.

Whiplash-Related Injuries

Of all cervical disorders, whiplash-related injuries are among the most common and most misunderstood, because the term is used to describe both an injury mechanism (i.e., cervical acceleration–deceleration) and a clinical syndrome.

Whiplash mechanics are complex and not well understood, but the Quebec Task Force on Whiplash-Associated Disorders defined whiplash as "an acceleration–deceleration mechanism of energy transfer to the neck which may result from rear-end or side impact, predominately in motor vehicle accidents, and from other mishaps. The energy transfer may result in bony or soft tissue injuries (whiplash injury), which may in turn lead to a wide variety of

clinical manifestations (whiplash-associated disorders)" (Cassidy et al. 1995, p. 22).

In recent decades many studies have been conducted to determine the mechanisms of whiplash, which is typically characterized as involving a hyperextension mechanism. Using a motor vehicle crash as an example, the vehicle is violently pushed forward, accelerating the occupant's trunk and shoulders anteriorly. The head remains stable (based on Newton's first law), effectively forcing the neck into hyperextension. Once its inertia is overcome, the head is thrown (whiplashed) forward into flexion.

Modern research efforts have shown the hyperextension model to be too simplistic, inadequately describing the complex motion of the cervical spine during whiplash. "The critical revision brought about by modern research into whiplash is that it is not a cantilever movement that is injurious; i.e., it is not an extension–flexion movement of the head, as was commonly believed previously. Rather, within less than 150 ms after impact, the cervical spine is compressed. During this period the cervical spine buckles; upper cervical segments are flexed while lower segments extend around abnormally located axes of rotation" (Bogduk and Yoganandan 2001, p. 272). The simultaneous upper cervical flexion and lower cervical extension results in an S-shaped neck curvature within 75 ms of impact (figure 8.17), then gives way to a C-shaped hyperextension curvature (Grauer et al. 1997). These motions place both the lower cervical spine and upper cervical spine at risk of injury from the rear-impact mechanism (Panjabi, Pearson et al. 2004).

Although usually viewed as a sagittal plane injury caused by a rear-end impact, whiplash can also result from lateral or frontal forces with their own unique injury pattern. In addition, motion of the neck is not confined to a single plane. If a driver is looking to the side at the moment of impact, for example, the injury mechanism involves a combination of hyperextension and rotation. In this case

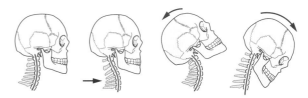

FIGURE 8.17 Neck curvature resulting from simultaneous upper cervical flexion and lower cervical extension.

the pre-impact rotation enhances the effect of the impact as the cervical structures are prestretched, which may enhance the injurious effect of the impact forces.

At first glance, whiplash might appear a simple injury mechanism. However, "in an individual accident there is likely to be a complex interaction between different forces depending upon the speed and direction of impact and the attitude of the head and neck" (Barnsley et al. 1994, p. 288). In addition to the cervical musculature, spinous ligaments, intervertebral discs, vertebral bodies, and facet (zygapophyseal) joints, the brain and even the temporomandibular joint can be involved (e.g., Davis 2000; Ito et al. 2004; Panjabi, Ito et al. 2004; Pearson et al. 2004). Various mechanisms and potential injury sites are shown in figure 8.18. Whiplash-associated disorders can manifest as both clinical and psychosocial symptoms (Eck et al. 2001). Possible symptoms are listed in table 8.4.

From the clinical perspective, whiplash is categorized into five grades (Pastakia and Kumar 2011):

- 0: No neck pain, stiffness, or physical signs
- 1: Complaints of neck pain with stiffness or tenderness but no physical signs noted
- 2: Neck pain and stiffness complaints with decreased range of motion and point tenderness

- 3: Neck pain and stiffness complaints with neurological signs
- 4: Neck pain and stiffness complaints with fracture, dislocation, or spinal cord injury

Cervical Spondylosis

Cervical spondylosis is a term used to describe degenerative changes of the cervical column, typically involving the intervertebral discs and surrounding structures, including osteophytosis of the vertebral bodies, ligamentous instability, and osseous hypertrophy of the laminal arches and facets (Lestini and Wiesel 1989). Cervical spondylosis most often affects the C3-C7 vertebrae (McCormack and Weinstein 1996) and has a markedly different etiology from injuries of an acute onset. Although the onset is less dramatic, chronic injuries nonetheless can cause considerable dysfunction.

As part of the normal aging process, the intervertebral discs lose height and become less flexible over time, in large part due to reduced water content and degradation of the other materials that comprise the disc. Disc degeneration typically leads to increased stresses on articular cartilage, which must take on the abnormal biomechanical loads, and may be accompanied by osteophyte (bony outgrowth) formation. These structural alterations increase the risk of spinal stenosis, a narrowing of the spinal

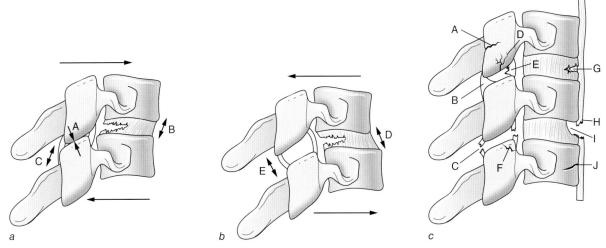

FIGURE 8.18 Potential mechanisms and injury sites for whiplash-related injuries. Shear forces affecting a spinal motion segment. *(a)* Translation of the superior vertebral body anteriorly relative to the inferior body, which stresses the articular surfaces of the zygapophyseal joint (A), the anterior annulus fibrosus (B), and the zygapophyseal joint capsule (C). *(b)* Translation of the superior vertebral body posteriorly relative to the inferior body, which stresses the intervertebral disc (D) and the zygapophyseal joint capsules (E). *(c)* Common lesions affecting the cervical spine following whiplash injury. A, articular pillar fracture; B, hemarthrosis (hemorrhage into a joint) of the zygapophyseal joint; C, rupture or tear of the zygapophyseal joint capsule; D, fracture of the subchondral plate; E, contusion of the intra-articular meniscus of the zygapophyseal joint; F, fracture involving the articular surface; G, tear of the annulus fibrosus; H, tear of the anterior longitudinal ligament; I, end-plate avulsion fracture; J, vertebral body fracture.

TABLE 8.4   Prevalence of Clinical Symptoms Related to Whiplash Injury

Whiplash clinical symptoms	Prevalence
Neck pain	94%
Neck stiffness	96%
Interscapular pain	35%
Headache	44%
Numbness/paresthesia	22%
Vertigo	15%
Vision symptoms	12%
Hearing symptoms	13%
Sleeping problems	35%
Memory problems	15%
Signs of stress	30%

Adapted from B. Rydevik, M. Szpalski, M. Aebi, et al., "Whiplash Injuries and Associated Disorders: New Insights into an Old Problem," *European Spine Journal* 17 (2008): 359-416.

canal, impingement on neural tissue, and impaired blood perfusion of the spinal cord. Symptoms associated with cervical spondylosis occur at the level of the spinal cord and roots that are affected and may include paresthesia, neck and arm pain, weakness, and sensory loss. A good clinical examination can help identify the pathology, but imaging such as magnetic resonance imaging (MRI) will have the best diagnostic accuracy. Considerable debate continues on the value of surgical intervention, but may include a decompression (i.e., removing a section of the intervertebral disc that is impinging the spinal cord) or spinal fusion (i.e., fixing two or more vertebra together when there is excessive movement).

Myelopathy is a neurological deficit related to the spinal cord. Specific to cervical spondylosis, a narrowing of the spinal canal, kyphotic conditions result from cervical flexion, spinal cord compression and related ischemia, and ligamentous ossification. Despite the often insidious onset of cervical spondylosis, its sequelae have significant potential to cause severe neuromuscular dysfunction.

Trunk Injuries

The trunk, sometimes called the *torso*, extends from the base of the neck down to and including the perineum. As the largest body region, the trunk accounts for 45% to 50% of the body's mass and contains a number of vital organs: the heart (and its major vessels), spinal cord, lungs, stomach and intestines, kidneys, liver, and spleen. The thoracic region of the trunk is protected by the sternum and ribs, but offers limited motion, whereas the lumbar region does not have the same level of protection, allowing for increased motion.

The musculature of the trunk serves both movement and protective functions. The principal muscles of the anterior trunk are the pectoralis major, serratus anterior, rectus abdominis, external obliques, internal obliques, and transversus abdominis (figure 8.19a-d). Important posterior trunk muscles include the trapezius, latissimus dorsi, rhomboids (major and minor), and erector spinae (figure 8.19e-f).

Vertebral Fracture

Fractures of the vertebra can result from a number of circumstances, but are commonly associated with osteoporosis or direct trauma. Among postmenopausal women, 25% may suffer from a vertebral fracture, making it a major health concern (Melton 1997). Risk factors associated with vertebral fractures can be classified as *modifiable* or *nonmodifiable*. Among other things, modifiable risk factors include alcohol and tobacco use, osteoporosis, estrogen deficiency, physical frailty, lack of physical activity, fall risk, low body weight, and deficiencies in dietary calcium and vitamin D—all factors associated with overall bone health. Nonmodifiable risk factors include age (advanced), sex (female), early menopause, dementia, race (Caucasian), and adult fracture history (Old and Calvert 2004).

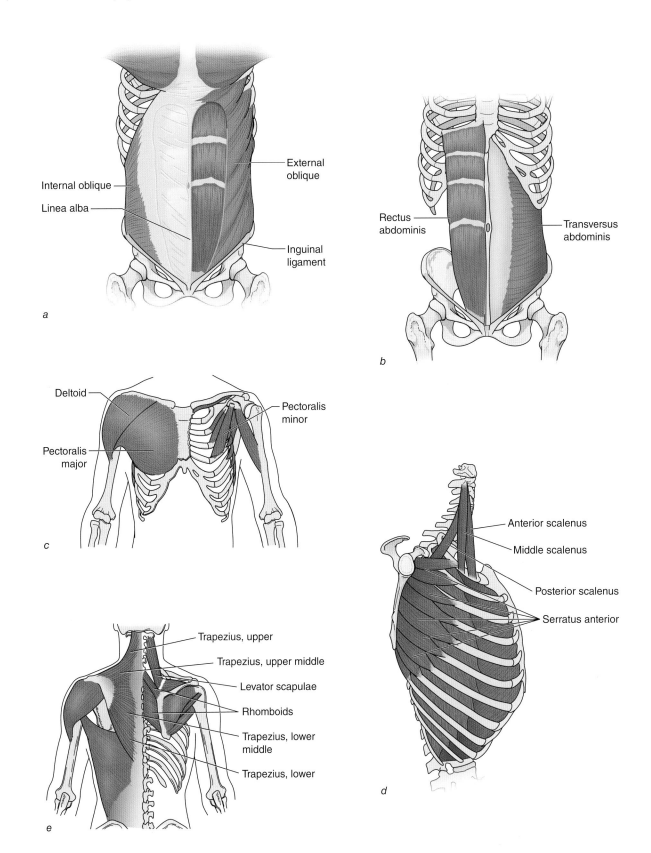

FIGURE 8.19 Musculature of the trunk. *(a-d)* Anterior views. *(e-f)* Posterior views. Deep muscles of the back, including the three subdivisions of the erector spinae group (iliocostalis, spinalis, longissimus) are shown in *(f)*.

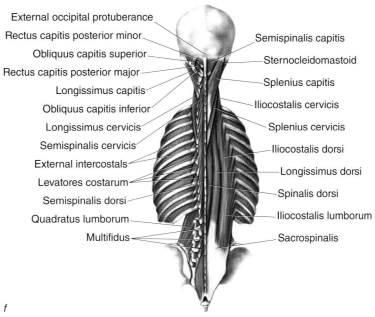

External occipital protuberance

Rectus capitis posterior minor

Obliquus capitis superior

Rectus capitis posterior major

Longissimus capitis

Obliquus capitis inferior

Longissimus cervicis

Semispinalis cervicis

External intercostals

Levatores costarum

Semispinalis dorsi

Quadratus lumborum

Multifidus

Semispinalis capitis

Sternocleidomastoid

Splenius capitis

Iliocostalis cervicis

Splenius cervicis

Iliocostalis dorsi

Longissimus dorsi

Spinalis dorsi

Iliocostalis lumborum

Sacrospinalis

f

FIGURE 8.19   *(continued)*

Rear-End Collisions

Although less than 20% of rear-end collision victims have long-term injury-related symptoms (Radanov et al. 1995), hundreds of research studies over the past half-century have sought to detail injury mechanics to develop better prevention strategies. These studies have involved use of live subjects (in low-speed rear-end impacts), cadaveric simulations, accelerometry, electromyography, and mathematical modeling. As a result of these studies, we have a better understanding of rear-impact dynamics, but cervical dynamics during rear-impact scenarios are complex and still not entirely understood (e.g., Luan et al. 2000).

Pioneering work by Severy (1955) showed that rear-end collisions cause a sequential accel-

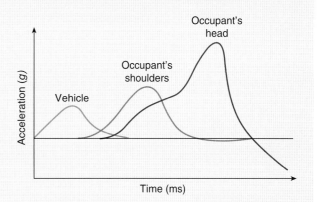

Idealized acceleration curves of an impacted vehicle, an occupant's shoulders, and an occupant's head.
Adapted from L. Barnsley, S. Lord, N. Bogduk, "Whiplash Injury," *Pain* 58, no. 3 (1994): 283-307.

eration of the vehicle, the occupant's trunk and shoulders, and the occupant's head. As the vehicle is impacted from a rear-end collision, it accelerates first, reaching a peak acceleration of almost 5 *g*—that is, five times the acceleration of gravity (A in figure). The vehicle occupant's shoulders reach their peak acceleration of about 7 *g* 100 ms later (B in figure). Finally, the occupant's head reaches its peak acceleration of greater than 12 *g* at 250 ms after initial impact (C in figure). This sequential progression of peak acceleration is evidence of both momentum and energy transfers.

Response of the cervical spine depends on impact awareness, muscle involvement and strength, and direction of impact (Kumar et al. 2005). In an unaware vehicle occupant, muscles are recruited late relative to the impact onset—perhaps 200 to 250 ms after impact, well beyond the point of providing meaningful stability to the head and neck (Bogduk and Yoganandan 2001).

In addition to impact awareness, muscle involvement, and direction of impact, many other factors determine injury risk in rear-end impacts: vehicle mass, velocity, and ability to withstand crashes; road conditions; use of restraint systems; and the occupant's body and head position at impact, neck rotation, gender, history of neck injury, and age.

Axial loading of the spinal column can result in a compressive vertebral fracture, also described by Holdsworth (1970) as a **burst fracture**. When a severe compression force is applied to either cervical or lumbar vertebrae when they are aligned in a straight (noncurved) column, the body of the vertebra can shatter from within (i.e., explode or burst). The applied force results in a fracture to the vertebral body and potentially other vertebral structures. Depending on the magnitude of bony displacement, the spinal cord may be involved. Victims of these injuries commonly suffer from long-term pain, dysfunction, and changes to the spinal curvature.

Loading of the spinal column from the posterior or posterolateral aspects more commonly involve a fracture of the lamina or pedicle and are of particular concern because of their close proximity to the spinal cord. Fractures resulting in displaced spinal fragments can move into the spinal canal and impinge on the cord. This impingement can cause severe neural damage, including paralysis or death, depending on the location. Vertebral fractures usually are caused by axial compressive loads and occur most commonly in the cervical and thoracolumbar regions. Vertebrae in the thoracolumbar region (variably defined to include vertebrae between T11 and L3) are especially susceptible to fracture because of the spine's relatively neutral alignment (minimal curvature) in this region and because this region is a transition zone between the relatively rigid thoracic region and the more flexible lumbar region.

The level of instability created by the fractures is a subject of some controversy, especially in cases with an absence of neurological deficit associated with the fracture. The spinal column is surrounded by significant ligamentous and muscular support, which can often hold bony fragments in place during the healing process. The risk of spinal cord lesion resulting from a displaced bony fragment, however, largely depends on the rate of loading. Fractures that result from high loading rates are more likely to result in encroachment into the spinal canal, whereas low loading rates produce minimal intrusion (Tran et al. 1995). Panjabi and colleagues (1994) found that multiaxial instabilities are commonly present following injuries that involve axial rotation and lateral bending. Their results suggest that treatment of these fractures requires caution and that their fixation and stabilization should be approached conservatively.

Severity of vertebral fractures in the thoracolumbar region are classified based on the type of fracture, associated neurological injury, and any modifiers (Schroeder et al. 2015).

Fracture Morphology
- Type A: Compression injuries
- Type B: Failure of the posterior or anterior ligaments without significant translation
- Type C: Dislocation or displacement in any direction or lack of soft tissue to prevent translation

Neurological Injury
- N0: Neurologically intact
- N1: Transient neurological deficits
- N2: Signs of symptoms of radiculopathy
- N3: Incomplete SCI
- N4: Complete SCI
- NX: Patient cannot be examined

Modifiers
- M1: Indeterminate ligamentous injury
- M2: Patient comorbidities that may affect the treatment

Spinal Deformities

As noted previously, a healthy spinal column curves in an S-shaped pattern from top to bottom. The cervical and lumbar spines curve anteriorly (e.g., lordotic curve), whereas the thoracic and sacral regions have a posterior curve (e.g., kyphotic curve). The curvature allows for shock absorption and stability during upright stance. Injury, disease, and congenital predisposition all can cause abnormalities to the normal structural alignment or alteration of spinal curvatures. Changes or differences in either often result in abnormal force distribution patterns that lead to pathological tissue adaptations and indirectly lead to or exacerbate other musculoskeletal injuries.

Abnormal spinal curvatures are commonly classified into three broad categories: scoliosis, kyphosis, and lordosis (figure 8.20). Each is classified by the magnitude, location, direction, and cause, and they can occur in isolation or in combination. Spinal deformities have long been associated with cardiopulmonary dysfunction. Hippocrates, for example, noted that those with kyphosis had difficulty breathing, and that patients afflicted with scoliosis commonly exhibited **dyspnea** (shortness of breath) (Padman 1995).

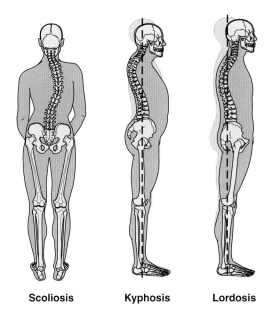

Scoliosis   Kyphosis   Lordosis

FIGURE 8.20 Spinal deformities.

Reprinted by permission from W.C. Whiting, *Dynamic Human Anatomy,* 2nd ed. (Champaign, IL: Human Kinetics, 2019).

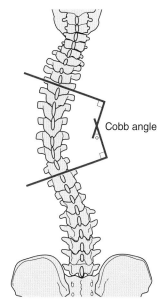

Cobb angle

FIGURE 8.21 Measure of scoliotic spinal curvature: the **Cobb angle**, defined as the angle between the two lines that pass through the upper and lower end vertebrae at each end of the curvature.

Scoliosis

Scoliosis is a lateral (frontal plane) spinal curvature in excess of 10° that is often associated with twisting of the spine (figure 8.21). Mild spinal deviations are well tolerated and usually asymptomatic, but may worsen over time. Severe deformities, in contrast, can markedly compromise breathing and the ability to move. Scoliotic curvatures exceeding 90° greatly increase the risk of cardiorespiratory failure through decreased lung and chest wall compliance, poor blood oxygenation (**hypoxemia**), increased work of breathing, reduced respiratory drive, enlarged heart (**cardiomegaly**), and pulmonary arterial hypertension (Padman 1995).

About 3% of the population suffer from scoliosis, or nearly 10 million people in the United States alone. The vast majority of cases are idiopathic, whereas smaller portions can be attributed to congenital causes (approximately 15%) or occur secondary to neuromuscular disease (10%) (Stehbens 2003). Various mechanisms and theories have been suggested to explain idiopathic scoliosis. Some have suggested idiopathic scoliosis results from genetic factors (e.g., Miller 2000), whereas others have suggested cumulative, repetitive, and asymmetrical biomechanical stresses (e.g., Stehbens 2003). Both are plausible causes, although additional research exploring connective tissue abnormalities, neurological and growth abnormalities, and muscle structure and function is needed. Regardless, "The consensus is that the etiology is multifactorial. With time, continued research will lead to the identification of the various factors involved in the causation of this disorder, which affects so many children and adolescents" (Lowe et al. 2000, p. 1166).

Treatment options for scoliosis largely depend on the magnitude of the curvature and the age and physical maturity of the patient. Among those that have not yet reached full maturation, clinical providers may not intervene so as to not inadvertently alter growth in other parts of the body. This is particularly true when there is no pain or discomfort involved. For mild (<30°) and moderate (30°-45°) cases, electrical stimulation, biofeedback, manipulation, and bracing are the first treatment options. Of these, bracing (figure 8.22*a*) has proved most successful (Parent et al. 2005). A recent review highlights the growing body of evidence that exercise-based approaches can be used to prevent the progression and reverse the signs and symptoms of spinal deformity (Hawes 2003).

For severe scoliotic curvatures (i.e., >45°), operative treatments may be necessary, commonly including rod placement parallel to the spinal column or vertebral fusion of adjacent vertebrae to forestall further progression of the deformity (figure 8.22*b*).

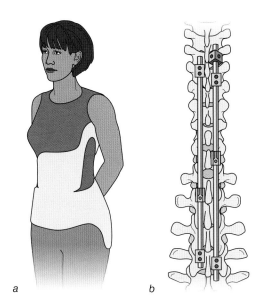

FIGURE 8.22 Methods of treating scoliosis. *(a)* Bracing. *(b)* Surgical implantation of Harrington instrumentation (rods) to stabilize the spine.

Scoliosis is progressive, making the early identification, diagnosis, and intervention important to forestall poor outcomes. Lack of early intervention can result in severe, even life-threatening deformities later in life. Although the causal mechanisms of scoliosis are often unknown, treatment in the form of braces or implanted spinal rods are well established and proven effective.

Kyphosis

Kyphosis is a sagittal-plane spinal deformity characterized by an excessive posterior convex curvature. Although possible in the sacral region of the spine, kyphosis is most common in the thoracic region, producing what is commonly called a "hunchback." Although the thoracic region has a natural kyphotic curvature, a kyphosis deformity is a hyperkyphosis, or exaggerated kyphotic curvature. Clinically, the term *kyphosis* often is used, as here, to describe this hyperkyphotic condition.

The natural kyphotic curve tends to increase with age, albeit more aggressively in women than men. Normal angles among younger individuals range between 20° and 40°. Among older adults, the normal kyphotic angle approaches 45° in men and 50° in women. Kyphosis severity is measured in a manner similar to the Cobb angle (see figure 8.21) or by measuring the horizontal distance between the center of C7 and S1 in the sagittal plane. Those

with osteoporosis are at increased risk of kyphosis (Bradford 1995), but 70% of older adults with kyphosis do not have a bone mineral density issue. Rates of kyphosis are not clearly defined in younger populations, but are thought to occur in 50% of men and 65% of women over the age of 65 (Bartynski et al. 2005).

The best treatment for kyphosis may lie in prevention. Women with satisfactory exercise habits have a significantly lower index of kyphosis, suggesting that physical conditioning programs aimed at proper postural maintenance may delay or prevent the onset of kyphosis associated with aging (Cutler et al. 1993).

Structural kyphosis in children is called **Scheuermann's kyphosis**. Whereas nonstructural kyphosis involves normal bony and intervertebral disc structure, Scheuermann's kyphosis is defined by wedge-shaped discs that are commonly herniated. Conscious postural alignment is not possible, making the condition orthopedically significant because it may be progressive. Pathological progression increases the severity of deformity, which may require bracing or surgery (Wegner and Frick 1999).

Lordosis

Lordosis refers to an excessive posterior concave curvature of the spine, typically in the lumbar region, that produces an anterior tilt of the pelvis, sometimes called a hollow or swayback condition. Similar to kyphosis, the cervical and lumbar regions have a natural lordosis; hyperlordosis (exaggerated inward curve of the spine) is referenced clinically as *lordosis* or *lordotic*.

There is no universally agreed-upon normal angle of the lumbar spine, making defining abnormal curvature difficult. In most people, normal curvature of the lumbar spine ranges from 20° to 60° (Boos and Aebi 2008). As the pelvis tilts anteriorly, the curve of the lumbar region increases. As the lumbosacral (L5-S1) angle increases over its normal orientation (figure 8.23), shear loading on the intervertebral discs and surrounding structures increase, and compressive load on the disc decreases. Lordosis is more common in women and in persons with a higher body mass index (Murrie et al. 2003). Whether lordosis varies with age is unclear. Tuzun and colleagues (1999) reported an increase in lordosis with age; Amonoo-Kuofi (1992) found a tendency for decreased lordosis with age; and Murrie

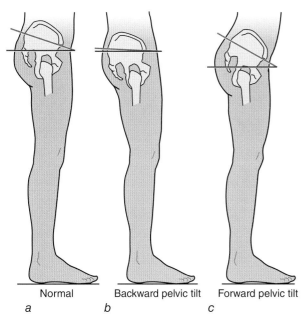

FIGURE 8.23 Effect of pelvic tilting on the lumbosacral (L5-S1) angle. *(a)* Normal standing creates a lumbosacral angle of approximately 30°. *(b)* Tilting the pelvis backward decreases the lumbosacral angle (<30°) and flattens the lumbar spine. *(c)* Tilting the pelvis forward increases the lumbosacral angle (>30°) and exaggerates the lumbar lordosis.

and colleagues (2003) found no change in lordosis in older persons.

Lower-extremity joint pathologies can affect lumbar lordosis. Offierski and MacNab (1983) described a *hip–spine syndrome* in which concurrent pathologies exist at the hip and spine, and they cautioned that failure to recognize the concurrent pathologies may result in misdiagnosis and potential treatment errors. Murata and colleagues (2003) reported what they termed a *knee–spine syndrome*, in which degenerative changes in the knee caused symptoms in the lumbar spine.

Spondylolysis and Spondylolisthesis

Low back pain arises from myriad causes, most commonly related to muscular dysfunction related to overuse or acute strains. In other instances, bony injuries may occur; two such conditions afflicting young and athletic populations are spondylolysis and spondylolisthesis. Typically occurring at the L4-L5 and L5-S1 levels, **spondylolysis** is a defect or stress fracture in the area of the lamina between the superior and inferior articular facets known as the **pars interarticularis** (figure 8.24*a*). Spondylolysis

affects 6% of the adult population across the age span (Herman et al. 2003).

In contrast, **spondylolisthesis** is translational motion, or slippage (typically anterior), between adjacent vertebral bodies (figure 8.24*b*). A recent study using a finite-element model showed that moments created by lateral bending and torsion are associated with the greatest vertebral slippage (Natarajan et al. 2003). The process involved in slippage differs between young and older individuals (typically in women older than 50 years). In older populations, spondylolisthesis occurs most frequently at L4-L5, attributable in part to degenerative lesions associated with arthritis of the facet joints and to relative instability at this level compared with L5-S1. This instability may be caused by a developmental predisposition to more sagittally oriented facet joints at the L4-L5 level (Grobler et al. 1993).

In young athletes, the mechanism allowing spondylolisthesis differs from that observed in adults. In patients between 9 and 18 years old, Ikata and colleagues (1996) found end-plate lesions in all cases of vertebral slip between L5 and S1 exceeding 5%. The implicated mechanism was slippage between the osseous and cartilaginous end plates secondary to spondylolysis. The likelihood of progression (continuing slippage) depends on the type, stability, and degree of slippage and the slip angle (Bradford

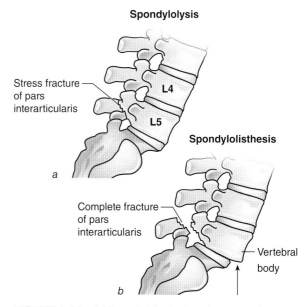

FIGURE 8.24 *(a)* Spondylolysis showing stress fracture of the pars interarticularis with no slippage of the vertebral body. *(b)* Spondylolisthesis exhibiting slippage and complete fracture of the pars interarticularis.

Safe Lifting

Low back injuries resulting from lifting are a significant drain on both industry and the medical system, accounting for as much as 20% of all workplace injuries. The low back is particularly susceptible to injury as a result of its flexibility, which facilitates overall movement. Bending at the waist to pick up an object can be broadly thought of as a lever mechanism, whereby the trunk is the lever arm with the low back serving as the axis.

Torque (i.e., moment of force, see chapter 3) is the amount of force needed to move the lever arm, which is dependent on the length of the lever and the mass of the object being moved. This can be expressed mathematically as $M = F \cdot d$, whereby M is the magnitude of the moment of force, F is the force, and d is the distance from the point of rotation to the end of the lever where the mass is supported.

When bending, the lumbar spine must support the mass of the trunk, in addition to the mass of any object being picked up. Consider the following scenario: While in a weight room, an athlete bends at the waist to pick up a 50 kg dumbbell off the floor, located 0.5 m from the pivot point in the lower back. The mass of her trunk is 32 kg (approximately 53% of total body mass) with a center of mass at 0.3 m from the pivot point.

According to Newton's second law of motion ($F = m \cdot a$), we can rewrite the equation for torque above, and get $M = m \cdot a \cdot d$, which can be applied to our scenario as:
Torque created by the dumbbell (using gravity as the acceleration value):

$$M = 50 \text{ kg} \cdot 9.81 \text{ m/s}^2 \cdot 0.5 \text{ m}$$

$$M = 245.25 \text{ N·m}$$

Torque created by the body mass:

$$M = 32 \text{ kg} \cdot 9.81 \text{ m/s}^2 \cdot 0.3 \text{ m}$$

$$M = 94.176 \text{ N·m}$$

To move the mass, a torque in excess of the total (339.426 N·m) must be generated by the back musculature. If the athlete is unable to generate this amount of torque, forces will be transferred to the static structures (e.g., ligaments), placing them at risk for injury.

To reduce injury risk, the torque must be reduced. This can be accomplished by shortening the moment arm—that is, standing closer to the weight, maintaining a more upright posture and lifting with the legs.

To reduce the risk of low back injury:

- Position the feet at shoulder width or greater to help maintain balance.
- Keep the abdominal muscles engaged to stabilize the lumbar spine and pelvis.
- Lower the body using the knees and not by flexing the spine.
- Keep the spine as vertical as possible.

1995). With continued slippage, the superior vertebra (L5) moves anteriorly relative to the inferior articular surface (S1), the slip angle (figure 8.25) changes, and the degree of slippage (as measured by percentage slip) increases (Stinson 1993). There seems to be considerable slowing of slip progression with each decade (Beutler et al. 2003).

Not surprisingly, the populations most at risk for both spondylolysis and spondylolisthesis are those whose training exposes them to repeated high-force compressive spinal loading, especially in combination with flexion–extension and rotational positions and movements. These include gymnasts, weightlifters, wrestlers, and divers. Spondylolysis is exacerbated by the stresses imposed on the vertebral laminae by the body's lumbar lordosis. Of greatest concern to young athletes is the situation in which repeated loading of the pars region causes microfractures and eventual bone failure.

Spondylolisthesis results from a number of mechanisms, broadly within six categories: dysplastic, isthmic, degenerative, traumatic, pathological, and iatrogenic. The involved anatomical structures and pathogenesis for each type are presented in table 8.5.

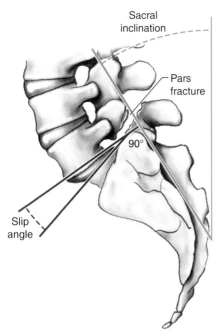

FIGURE 8.25 Schematic of sacral inclination and slip angle.

Approximately 75% of individuals with spondylolisthesis remain asymptomatic. Although as the magnitude of slippage (defined as the percentage translation of the vertebral body) increases, so does the risk for symptoms. With progressing intensity, symptoms may include back pain and tightness as the surrounding musculature braces the deviated vertebra. This in turn may result in altered posture (e.g., increased kyphosis), altered gait, and eventually gluteal dysfunction.

Intervertebral Disc Pathologies

Intervertebral discs are located between the vertebra, resting on the body of the inferior vertebra and supporting the superior vertebra. The intervertebral disc is a viscoelastic structure consisting of two distinct structural elements, the *annulus fibrosus* and *nucleus pulposus*. The disc is separated from the vertebra by a thin layer of hyaline cartilage (cartilaginous end plate). The **nucleus pulposus** is a gelatinous mass consisting of fine fibers embedded in a mucoprotein gel, with water content ranging from 70% to 90%. Water and proteoglycan content are highest in the young and decrease with age. The mechanical consequences of these losses include decreases in disc height, elasticity, energy storage, and load-carrying capacity. The lumbar nucleus pulposus occupies 30% to 50% of the total disc area in cross section and is located slightly posteriorly (rather than centrally) between adjacent vertebral bodies.

The **annulus fibrosus** is composed of fibrocartilage and consists of concentric bands of annular fibers that surround the nucleus pulposus and form the outer boundary of the disc. The collagen fibers of adjacent annular bands run in opposite directions (figure 8.26), creating a crisscrossed orientation that allows the annulus to accommodate multidirectional torsional and bending loads.

Lumbosacral injuries can involve any of the many structures comprising the spinal column and involve three mechanisms: (1) spinal compression or weight bearing; (2) torsional loading, which results in various patterns of shearing in the transverse (horizontal) plane; and (3) tensile stresses resulting from excessive spinal motion (Watkins and Williams 2001). Intervertebral disc pathologies are a good representation of the mechanisms for other lumbosacral injuries.

Normal activities load the intervertebral discs in complex ways. The combined effects of spinal

TABLE 8.5   Classification of Spondylolisthesis

Type	Name	Anatomical involvement	Etiology
I	Dysplastic	Upper facets of S1 and lower facets of L5	Hereditary or congenital facet orientation anomalies
II	Isthmic	Pars interarticularis abnormality	Succession of microfractures; mechanical, hormonal, hereditary causes
III	Degenerative	Facet arthritis and ligamentum flavum weakness	Advanced pan-column degenerative changes
IV	Traumatic	Neural arch	Acute trauma
V	Pathological	Pars and other components	Infection
VI	Iatrogenic	Pars and other components	Surgical complications

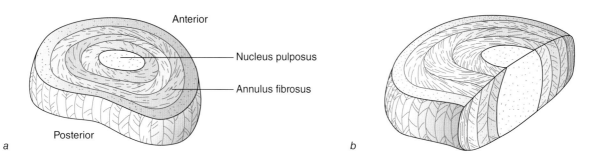

FIGURE 8.26 *(a)* Concentric rings of the annulus fibrosus surrounding the centrally located nucleus pulposus, with alternating fiber angulation. *(b)* Vertical section.

flexion–extension, lateral bending, and rotation exert high forces on the discs and their supporting structures. These forces are highest in the lumbar region, largely attributable to the compressive forces imposed by the weight of superior body segments.

When subjected to compressive loading, the primary disc components respond differently. The nucleus pulposus distributes pressure evenly across the disc and to the lower vertebrae. In an unloaded state, the nucleus pulposus exhibits an intrinsic pressure of 10 N/cm^2 attributable to preloading provided by the longitudinal ligaments and the ligamenta flava. In a loaded state, the nucleus pulposus accepts 1.5 times the externally applied load, whereas the annulus experiences only 0.5 times the compressive load (figure 8.27). Under normal loading conditions, motion of the lumbar spine results in a slight displacement of the nucleus in the opposite direction (e.g., forward flexion of the spine results in posterior translation of the nucleus). Because of the relative incompressibility of the nucleus pulposus, the load is transmitted (see Poisson's effect, described in chapter 3) as a tensile load to the fibers of the annulus fibrosus. These forces radiate circumferentially in what is described as a *hoop effect*. The resulting tensile stresses may be four to five times greater than the externally applied compressive load (Nachemson 1975).

Injuries to the intervertebral discs typically fall into two categories: herniation and degeneration. Herniation involves the protrusion of the nucleus pulposus through the annulus fibrosus. The mechanism for protrusion can vary, but is seen from high-force motions, direct trauma, or gradual deterioration of the annulus. Rotational body movements produce shearing stress in the annular fibers and can lead to circumferential and radial tears. The resulting weakness in the annular layers reduces the ability of the annulus to contain the nucleus pulposus. Compressive loads then squeeze the

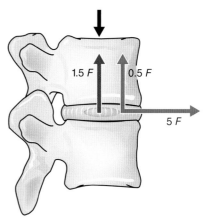

FIGURE 8.27 Uneven stress distribution across the lumbar intervertebral disc. A uniform compressive load (*F*) applied through the vertebral body creates an axial stress of 1.5 *F* (per unit area) in the nucleus pulposus. The annulus fibrosus, in contrast, generates an axial stress of only 0.5 *F*. The orthogonal stress in the annulus (perpendicular to the applied load) can reach levels up to five times the applied force (5 *F*).

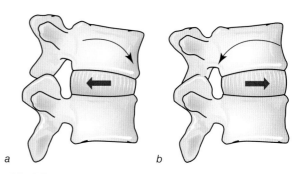

FIGURE 8.28 Intervertebral disc stress in response to bending *(a)* forward and *(b)* back. In bending, one side of the disc experiences compression while the other side undergoes tension. The compressive and tensile stresses are at a maximum at the outer borders of the disc and decrease toward the center of the disc. Forward flexion of the spine tends to squeeze the nucleus pulposus posteriorly.

Low Back Pain

Low back pain will afflict up to 80% of individuals at some time during their lives and is the most common occupation-related disability. For some the pain is merely a temporary annoyance, resolving within 6 weeks. For others, low back pain may last for months, if not years, and be completely debilitating.

Low back pain arises from mechanical dysfunction that results in chemical or mechanical irritation of pain-sensitive nerve endings in structures of the lumbar spine. Chemical irritation is associated with inflammatory diseases or tissue damage. Mechanical irritation, in contrast, can result from stretching of ligaments, periostea, tendons, or joint capsules. Compression of spinal nerves by a herniated intervertebral disc, damage to the disc itself, local muscle spasms, and zygapophyseal joint pathology can also cause low back pain. Whatever its source, low back pain either can be felt locally in the lumbar region or may be referred to the buttocks, lower extremities, or, less commonly, to the abdominal wall of the groin. This is particularly true when nerve roots are involved.

Treatment of low back pain as dramatically improved over the previous decade, typically combining physical management of the injury, medications, or surgery if warranted. Conservative treatment (e.g., ice, rest, gentle activity), manipulative therapies, and therapeutic exercise interventions all have their proponents. Only rarely is surgical intervention indicated. The limited number of well-controlled, randomized studies addressing the issues related to low back pain treatment leaves this area open to continuing debate and controversy. The efficacy of each of these varies based on the injury itself and its severity.

Given the serious and pervasive nature of this musculoskeletal condition, knowledge of its causal mechanisms, and thus how to reduce risk, is essential in prescribing treatment programs and designing injury prevention strategies.

---

nucleus pulposus into the area of annular weakness. Protrusions commonly occur posteriorly, a result of more extreme forward flexion and lifting of heavy objects while flexed, often in conjunction with lateral bending or rotation. This mechanism creates tensile stresses on the posterolateral aspect of the annulus fibrosus (figure 8.28), which, when combined with a compressive load, results in disc movement. Adams and Hutton (1982) suggested that sudden disc migration occurs most often in the lower lumbar region (L4-L5 or L5-S1) and is associated with disc degeneration.

The hyperflexion mechanism is not implicated in most cases of gradual disc herniation (i.e., where there is no identifiable precipitating event). **Degeneration** of the disc, rather, is a factor of age, with 60% of people over the age of 40 showing some form of degeneration. Rates of degeneration vary, but are associated with a loss of strength in the annulus and a loss of fluid in the nucleus, which alters the mechanics of the disc as a whole.

A variety of terms are used to describe disc pathologies. Some key terms, with their recommended definitions, are presented here (Fardon and Milette 2001):

- *Bulging disc.* A disc in which the contour of the outer annulus fibrosus extends beyond the edges of the disc space in the horizontal plane, typically more than 50% of the disc circumference (180°) and less than 3 mm beyond the vertebral body edge (figure 8.29*a-b*). (Note: Disc bulging is not considered a herniation.)

- *Herniation.* Localized (i.e., less than 50% of the disc circumference, or 180°) displacement of disc material beyond the normal margins of the intervertebral disc space.

- *Protrusion.* A herniated disc in which the distance between the edges of the disc material beyond the disc space is less than the distance between the edges of the base in the same plane (figure 8.29*c*).

- *Extrusion.* A herniated disc in which any one distance between the edges of the disc material beyond the disc space is greater than the distance between the edges of the base in the same plane (figure 8.29*d*).

- *Sequestration.* An extruded disc in which part of the disc tissue is displaced beyond the outer annulus and has no connection by disc

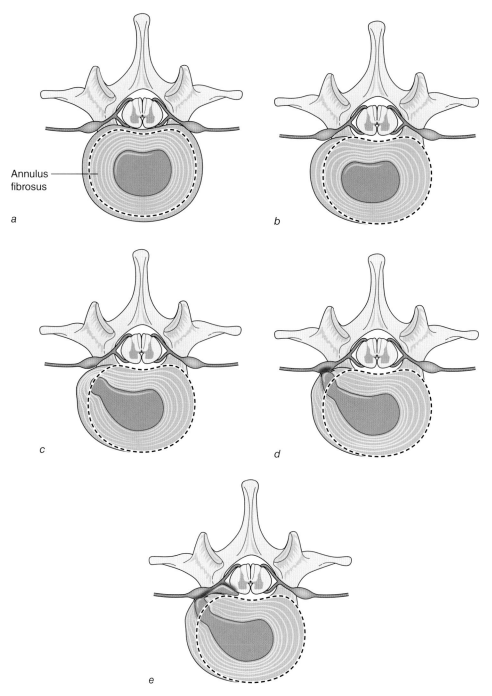

Annulus fibrosus

FIGURE 8.29 Descriptors of intervertebral disc pathology. *(a)* Symmetrical bulging disc. *(b)* Asymmetrical bulging disc. *(c)* Protrusion. *(d)* Extrusion. *(e)* Sequestration.

tissue with the original disc (i.e., a displaced fragment) (figure 8.29*e*).

Disc injury typically follows a progression from disc bulging (figure 8.29*a-b*) to sequestration. The nucleus pulposus puts such pressure on the annulus fibrosus that if there is a weak spot in the walls of the inner annular ring, that ring will rupture. In that way the nucleus pulposus can slowly make its way through successive layers of the annulus fibrosus and form a herniation, which can appear as either a protrusion (figure 8.29*c*) or extrusion (figure 8.29*d*). Eventually herniation can lead to tearing of the outer layer of the annulus fibrosus, at which point the nucleus pulposus begins to leak out of the disc altogether, which can result in sequestration (figure 8.29e).

Whatever the causal mechanism, there is a risk of the herniated disc impinging on adjacent structures. The amount of progressive herniation determines the degree of impingement. Because many disc herniation injuries occur in the posterolateral direction, the affected structure often is a nerve root. This results in mechanical, and possibly chemical or inflammatory, irritation and compression of the nerve root with resultant pain in the back, buttocks, thigh, lower leg, and possibly even the foot.

Chapter Review

Key Points

- Of all the body's regions, the head, neck, and trunk have the greatest potential for catastrophic injury. Injuries to vital structures in these regions can readily compromise essential body functions and, in all too many cases, result in paralysis or death.

- Injuries to the head and neck can be life threatening, whereas those to the trunk are typically less severe, but can be debilitating. Injury prevention is therefore paramount.

- Head injuries happen in response to the sudden application of direct or indirect forces to the head or its connected structures.

- Understanding the mechanisms responsible for head, neck, and trunk injuries can assist with their proper diagnosis, treatment, and prevention.

- The tissues of the spine are a normally balanced system of alignment and curvatures that can be disrupted acutely by excessive forces or chronically by repetitive strains.

- An improved understanding has emerged of pathologies and injury management of head, neck, and trunk injuries over the previous decade, but there is much research that remains to be done.

Questions to Consider

1. This chapter's *A Closer Look* examined concussion in detail. Select another injury presented in the chapter and write your own *A Closer Look* for that injury.

2. Explain, using specific examples, why head, neck, and trunk injuries have the greatest potential for causing catastrophic injury.

3. The sport of American football is a complex social phenomenon and the subject of controversy. Imagine that you have been selected to participate in a debate addressing the question, "Should football be banned?" Prepare a list of arguments to support the abolition of football. Prepare another list of arguments to support the retention of football.

4. Complete the same exercise addressing the pros and cons of heading in women's soccer.

5. Low back pain is a common condition that affects up to 80% of the adult population at some point in their lives. What elements would you include in a biomechanically sound program for adults to prevent low back pain?

Suggested Readings

Herman, M.J., and P.D. Pizzutillo. 2005. Spondylolysis and spondylolisthesis in the child and adolescent. *Clinical Orthopaedics and Related Research* 434: 46-54.

Kandel, E.R., J.D. Koester, S.H. Mack, and S.A. Siegelbaum. 2021. *Principles of Neural Science* (6th ed.). New York: McGraw Hill.

Kwan, O., and J. Friel. 2003. A review and methodologic critique of the literature supporting "chronic whiplash injury" Part I—research articles. *Medical Science Monitor* 9: 203-215.

McClune, T., A.K. Burton, and G. Waddell. 2002. Whiplash associated disorders: A review of the literature to guide patient information and advice. *Emergency Medicine Journal* 19: 499-506.

McGehee, D.V. 1996. Head injury in motor vehicle crashes: Human factors, effects, and prevention. In *Head Injury and Postconcussive Syndrome*, edited by M. Rizzo and D. Tranel. New York: Churchill Livingstone.

McGill, S. 2016. *Low Back Disorders: Evidence-Based Prevention and Rehabilitation* (3rd ed.). Champaign, IL: Human Kinetics.

National Center for Injury Prevention and Control. 2001. *Injury Fact Book 2001-02*. Atlanta: Centers for Disease Control and Prevention.

National Safety Council. 2004. *Injury Facts*. Itasca, IL: National Safety Council.

Nunn, K., T. Hanstock, and B. Lask. 2008. *Who's Who of the Brain*. London: Jessica Kingsley Publishers.

Petraglia, A., J. Bailes, and A. Day. 2015. *Handbook of Neurological Sports Medicine*. Champaign, IL: Human Kinetics.

Shirado, O., K. Kaneda, S. Tadano, H. Ishikawa, P.C. McAfee, and K.E. Warden. 1992. Influence of disc degeneration on mechanism of thoracolumbar burst fractures. *Spine* 17: 286-292.

Silver, J.M., T.W. McAllister, and D.B. Archiniegas, eds. 2019. *Textbook of Traumatic Brain Injury* (3rd ed.). Washington, DC: American Psychiatric Publishing.

Uscinski, R.H. 2006. Shaken baby syndrome: An odyssey. *Neurologia medico-chirurgica (Tokyo)* 46: 57-61.

abrasion—A scraping away of the superficial skin layer, usually by friction or an abnormal mechanical process.

acceleration—Measure of the time rate change in a body's velocity; change in velocity divided by change in time.

accident—Unforeseen or unplanned event or circumstance, possibly resulting from carelessness or ignorance and potentially leading to an unexpected injury.

acromioplasty—Excision of the acromion process to relieve pressure in the subacromial space.

actin—Contractile protein that forms thin myofilament in muscle fibers that acts as the binding site during muscular contraction.

action potential—Quick increase and decrease in electrical activity traveling along the membrane of a cell.

active stabilization—Contribution of muscle action to joint stability.

acute injury—Injury resulting from a single or a few overload episodes.

acute muscular strain—Overstretching a passive muscle or dynamically overloading an active muscle.

adaptation—Modification of an organism, or the parts of an organism, that makes it fit for existence within the confines of its environment.

adhesive capsulitis—Condition characterized by pain, stiffness, and limited range of motion (also known as *frozen shoulder*).

adipocytes—Cell specialized for the storage of fat, found in connective tissues.

adipose tissue—Loose connective tissue that appears as an aggregate of fat cells surrounded by areolar tissue.

aggrecan—Large aggregating proteoglycan (protein modified with carbohydrates) forming the major structural component of cartilage.

allograft—Tissue graft between two individuals of the same species.

all-or-none principle—Principle stating that all fibers within a given motor unit contract or none contract.

amenorrhea—Absence of menstrual cycles.

analytical epidemiology—Use of research strategies to reveal the determinants or underlying causes of disease and injury.

anastomoses—Connections of branches or parts (e.g., convergence of blood vessels).

anatomical position—Standard body reference position, with body erect, head facing forward, and arms hanging straight down with palms facing forward.

aneurysm—Abnormal blood-filled cavity in a blood vessel or organ.

angular acceleration—Change in angular velocity divided by the change in time.

angular displacement—Amount of rotation.

angular impulse—Product of moment × time; also torque × time.

angular momentum—Quantity of angular motion, measured by the product of mass moment of inertia × angular velocity.

angular motion—Form of movement in which a body rotates about an axis of rotation; also *rotational motion*.

angular power—Measure of angular work per unit time; also torque × angular velocity.

angular velocity—Angular displacement divided by the change in time.

angular work—Mechanical measure of torque × angular displacement.

anisotropic—Material exhibiting a direction-dependent tissue response to an applied force.

anlage—An initial clustering of embryonic cells from which a body part or organ develops; also known as the *primordium*.

annulus fibrosus—Series of fibrocartilage rings surrounding the nucleus pulposus of an intervertebral disc.

anterior drawer mechanism—Action causing anterior translation (e.g., of tibia relative to femur).

anteversion—Forward rotation or displacement relative to a reference plane.

anthropometric—Relating to the study of comparative measurements of the human body (e.g., height, weight, body composition, segment mass, and shape).

anthropometry—Study of comparative measurements of the human body (e.g., height, weight, body composition, muscle mass, and shape).

aponeuroses—Fibrous or membranous sheets connecting a muscle and the part it moves.

applied force—Muscle force; also *effort force*.

appositional growth—Growth of cells that proceeds in the cartilage layers immediately beneath the perichondrium.

arachnoid—Thin tissue membrane comprising the middle meningeal layer between the dura mater and pia mater.

Archimedes' principle—Buoyancy principle stating that the magnitude of the buoyant force is equal to the weight of the displaced liquid.

area moment of inertia—Measure of a body's resistance to bending.

areolar tissue—Weak connective tissue saturating almost all areas of the body with spaces or holes where only fluid extracellular matrix exists.

activation–resorption–formation—Series of events involved in bone remodeling.

arthritis—Joint inflammation.

arthrology—Study of joints and joint motion.

arthroplasty—Joint replacement through surgical procedures.

articular cartilage—Smooth, shiny layer of hyaline cartilage covering the joint surfaces of articulating bones.

articulation—Junction of two or more bones at their sites of contact; also *joint*.

aseptic necrosis—Cell death in the absence of infection.

atherosclerosis—Vascular disease characterized by plaque buildup in the arterial walls.

atrophy—Decrease in size.

autograft—Graft involving tissue from the same person (also *autologous graft*).

autologous graft—See *autograft*.

avascular necrosis—Cell death caused by an absent or deficient blood supply.

avulsion fracture—Fracture in which a piece of bone is pulled away at the insertion site with the osteotendinous or osteoligamentous attachment still intact.

axis of rotation—Imaginary line about which joint rotation occurs.

axis—Point about which rotation occurs; also *fulcrum* or *pivot*.

axonotmesis—Axonal nerve damage that does not completely sever the surrounding endoneurial sheath.

ballistics—(1) Study of the firing characteristics of a firearm. (2) Study of projectile motion.

Bankart lesion—Avulsion of the anteroinferior glenoid labrum at the attachment site of the inferior glenohumeral ligament complex.

Barton's fracture—Fracture of the distal radius in which the volar lip of the radial articular surface is sheared off.

basement membrane—Thin extracellular supporting layer that separates a layer of epithelial cells from the underlying layer.

basilar skull fracture—Break in a bone at the base of the skull.

beam—Structure that is relatively long and slender.

bending moment—Sum of the moments acting on a beam.

bending—Result of any force acting perpendicular to the longitudinal axis of a beam.

Bennett's fracture—Fracture subluxation of the trapeziometacarpal joint.

biaxial loading—Simultaneous loading along two axes.

biceps anchor—Attachment of the proximal tendon of the long head of the biceps brachii at the supraglenoid tubercle.

bilaminar embryonic disc—Fundamental cellular mass consisting of two cell layers (ectoderm and endoderm).

biomechanics—Area of science related to the application of mechanical principles to biology.

biotribology—Study of the friction, lubrication, and wear of diarthrodial joints.

biphasic response—Two-phase response seen in viscoelastic tissues, with an immediate first phase followed by a delayed second-phase response.

blastema—Mass of living cells capable of growth and differentiation.

blastocyst—Mass of about 64 cells arranged in a hollow ball shape.

blister—Fluid accumulation under or within the epidermis caused by heat or by chemical or mechanical means.

body mass index—Measure of body composition as a ratio of body weight to height (kg/m^2).

body—Any collection of matter.

bone mineral content (BMC)—Measure of total mineral in bone (measured in grams).

bone mineral density (BMD)—Measure of the mineral content in a volume of bone, measured either as areal BMD (g/cm^2) or volumetric BMD (g/cm^3).

boosted lubrication—Form of lubrication that incorporates elastohydrodynamic and squeeze-film types of lubrication, which in turn boost the effectiveness of the lubricating fluid film.

boundary lubrication—Form of lubrication in which a layer of molecules adheres to each of the two surfaces that are gliding past each other.

brittle—Characteristic of a material that experiences minimal deformation when a load is applied to it before failure (e.g., glass).

bucket-handle tear—Tear in the central part of a C-shaped piece of cartilage (e.g., meniscus).

buoyant force—Equal and opposite force exerted by a liquid against the weight of a body, allowing the body to float.

burst fracture—Shattering of a vertebral body attributable to a severe compressive axial loading.

butterfly fracture—Fracture with more than one fracture line.

canaliculi—Small channels or passageways found in bone.

cancellous bone—See *trabecular bone*.

cantilever bending—Type of loading in which a force offset from the longitudinal axis creates both compression and bending.

capsular ligament—Ligament seen as a thickening of a joint capsule structure.

cardiac muscle—Myocardial tissue that is striated in appearance and works involuntarily.

cardiomegaly—Enlargement of the heart.

carpal tunnel syndrome (CTS)—Overuse injury in which contents of the carpal tunnel (e.g., blood vessels, flexor tendons, and median nerve) are subjected to increased compressive forces, with symptoms including tingling, numbness, and pain.

causal association—Relation between a risk factor and a disease or injury outcome in which the risk factor has been shown to contribute to the outcome in question.

cavitation—Creation of a cavity, or space, within a tissue or body.

center of gravity—Point at which gravity has the same effect on a body in a concentrated mass as it does on the distributed mass; acts as a balance point.

center of mass—Point about which a body's mass is equally distributed.

centripetal theory—Theory suggesting that the distribution of damaging diffuse strains induced by inertial loading would decrease in magnitude from the surface to the center of brain mass.

cerebral contusion—Area of bleeding along the surface of the brain.

cerebral edema—Brain swelling caused by the accumulation of fluid in the brain as a result of trauma, tumor, hypoxia, or exposure to toxic substances.

cerebritis—Inflammation of cerebral tissue.

cerebrospinal fluid (CSF)—Liquid that circulates through the ventricles to the spaces between the meninges about the brain and spinal cord and that primarily maintains uniform pressure within the brain and spinal cord.

chemotaxis—Cellular attraction caused by chemical action.

chondral fracture—Isolated damage to articular cartilage; also *flap tear*.

chondrocyte—Mature cartilage cell.

chondromalacia—End stage of cartilage degeneration (softening), characterized by cartilage fibrillation, loss of elastic support, and disruption of collagen framework.

chondromalacia patella—Softening of the articular cartilage on the retropatellar surface.

chondron—Structural unit including a chondrocyte and its lacuna.

chronic injury—Injury caused by repeated insults that may lead progressively to degenerative conditions that set the stage for an acute injury; also *cumulative trauma disorder, overuse injury, repetitive stress syndrome*.

chronic traumatic encephalopathy (CTE)—Cumulative neurological injuries that result in decrements to neurological function after repeated head impacts (with or without concussion).

chronological age—Age determined by calendar years.

circumferential fibrocartilage—Ring of fibrocartilage that acts as a spacer in the hip and shoulder joints.

closed fracture—Fracture that remains within the body's internal environment; also known as *simple fracture*.

closure—Completion of the endochondral ossification process evidenced by disappearance of the epiphyseal growth plate.

Cobb angle—Angle between the two lines that perpendicularly bisect the lines through the surfaces of the vertebrae at each end of the curvature.

coefficient of restitution—Ratio between the relative postcollision velocity and the relative precollision velocity.

collagen—Most abundant protein in the animal world, constituting more than 30% of total protein in the human body and present in all types of connective tissue.

collagenous fibers—Containing an insoluble fibrous protein (collagen) occurring in vertebrates as the primary constituent of connective tissue fibrils and in bones.

Colles' fracture—Fracture of the distal radius with a fracture pattern showing volar (anterior) metaphyseal cortex failure in tension and varying degrees of comminution on the dorsal (posterior) surface.

collision—Forceful impact between two or more bodies.

comminuted fracture—Fracture in which the configuration consists of more than one fracture line, typically in the form of a multifragmented, shattered bone.

compact bone—Bone with high density (low porosity); also *cortical bone*.

compartment syndrome (CS)—Condition caused by the expansion of enclosed tissue within a confined anatomical space; results in increased pressure that affects blood circulation and nerve conduction.

compensatory injury—Secondary injury caused by movement compensation in response to a primary injury.

complete fracture—Bone fracture that traverses the entire bone.

complex glycoprotein—Major protein found in the extracellular matrix.

compliance—Opposite or inverse of stiffness.

compound fracture—Break in the bone that protrudes through the skin.

compression—Force that tends to push ends of a body together.

compression–flexion mechanism—Injury mechanism that combines simultaneous cervical flexion with forceful axial spinal compression; also *flexion–compression mechanism*.

compressive stress—Internal resistance to being pushed together.

concave—Arched or curved inward, or inner surface of a structure.

concavity compression—Stability created when a convex object is pressed into a concave surface.

concentric—Active muscle shortening.

concurrent force system—Force system in which all forces originate from or are focused on a common point.

concussion—A mild traumatic brain injury induced by biomechanical forces.

conductivity—Ability of a tissue to conduct an electrical impulse or signal.

congenital dislocation—Abnormal hip joint formation during development that predisposes the hip to subluxation or luxation.

connecting fibrocartilage—Fibrocartilage at joints with limited motion (e.g., intervertebral disc).

connective tissue—Classification of all tissues that are not epithelial, muscle, or nervous tissue, including blood, adipose, cartilage, ligament, bone, and fascia.

conservation of energy—No net gain or loss of energy.

conservation of momentum—No net gain or loss of momentum.

continuum mechanical model—Model that considers structures and materials as continuous matter.

contractility—Ability of a muscle to generate force and shorten.

contralateral—Situated on, appearing on, or affecting the opposite side of the body.

contrecoup lesion—Brain injury at a site opposite from impact.

contusion—Skeletal muscle injury that results from a direct compressive impact; muscle bruise, distinguished by intramuscular hemorrhage.

convex—Arched or curved outward, or outer surface of a structure.

coracoacromial arch—Superior border of the glenohumeral joint formed by the acromion process and the coracoacromial ligament.

corpus callosum—The neuronal bridge allowing for communication between the left and right cerebral hemispheres.

cortical bone—Bone with high density (low porosity); also *compact bone*.

countermoment—Moment acting in the opposite direction of an applied moment.

countertorque—Torque acting in the opposite direction of an applied torque.

coup lesion—Brain injury at the site or on the same side as impact.

coxa valga—Angle that is greater than normal between the long axis and the neck of the proximal femur.

coxa vara—Angle that is less than normal between the long axis and the neck of the proximal femur.

creep response—Additional deformation (following the initial deformation) over time when a viscoelastic tissue is exposed to a constant load.

cross-bridge—Protruding head of a myosin filament that binds to an actin filament to produce a power stroke and filament sliding during muscle contraction.

cryotherapy—Modality used to counteract the inflammatory process that includes cold compress, ice, and cooling sprays.

cumulative trauma disorder—See *chronic injury*.

curvilinear motion—Movement along a curved path.

cyclic loading—(1) Repeated force application that allows for dynamic fluid flow (with nutrients and waste products) in and out of the tissue. (2) Repeated force application above a certain threshold that can cause a material to fatigue and exhibit a decreased ability to withstand applied forces.

dampened response—Retardation of an elastic material in returning to its unloaded shape or configuration.

damping—See *dampened response*.

dashpot—Component of a rheological model that represents tissue viscous properties.

de novo—Over again, anew, or from the beginning.

debridement—Surgical removal of lacerated, dead, or contaminated tissue.

deformable-body model—Model in which segments are allowed to deform (e.g., bend).

deformation—Change in a body's shape or configuration when subjected to an external load.

deformation to failure—Amount of deformation experienced by a tissue when it reaches failure.

deformational energy—Energy stored in a tissue or body during deformation; also *strain energy*.

degeneration—Normal degradation that results in pain.

degenerative joint disease (DJD)—Noninflammatory disorder of synovial joints, particularly those with load-bearing involvement, characterized by deterioration of the hyaline articular cartilage and bone formation on joint surfaces and at the joint margins; also *osteoarthritis*.

delayed-onset muscle soreness (DOMS)—Pain resulting from connective and contractile tissue disruption 24 to 72 hours after vigorous exercise, often associated with eccentric muscle action.

dendrites—Short-branched extensions of a nerve cell, along which impulses received from other cells at synapses are transmitted to the cell body.

dense irregular connective tissue—Fibrous connective tissue with loosely and randomly interwoven fibers, such as fascia.

dense regular connective tissue—Organized fibrous tissues, such as tendons, ligaments, or aponeuroses.

density—Measure of mass concentration, determined as mass divided by volume.

depressed skull fracture—Depression of a skull fragment into the subcranial space caused by compressive force of blunt trauma.

dermatome—New layer of cells formed after the sclerotome has condensed near the notochord.

descriptive epidemiology—Systematic and ongoing collection, analysis, interpretation, and dissemination of public health information to assess public health status, define public health priorities, and evaluate programs set in place to improve the health of a community.

destabilizing component—Force component acting through a joint axis that tends to destabilize the joint.

deterministic model—Model whose output is fully determined (i.e., does not vary) for a given set of inputs.

diaphysis—Main or midsection of a long bone.

diffuse axonal injury (DAI)—Diffuse degeneration of the white matter in the brain.

diffuse injury—Tissue damage over a wide area.

diffuse traumatic axonal injury (DTAI)—See *diffuse axonal injury*.

direct injury—Fracture at the specific site of force application.

direct solution approach—See *forward solution approach*.

displaced fracture—Fracture in which the bony fragments are moved relative to their normal (prefracture) position.

displacement—Vector measure of movement from one location to another.

distance—Scalar measure of how far a body has moved along its movement path.

distraction—Action that pulls away or separates joint surfaces.

drag force—Force acting parallel to the direction of fluid flow.

ductile—Characteristic of a compliant material that undergoes considerable deformation before failure.

dura mater—Tough tissue membrane comprising the outer meningeal layer.

dynamic equilibrium—Balanced state of bodies in motion with nonzero accelerations.

dynamic friction—See *kinetic friction*.

dynamic model—Model that characterizes the nonzero acceleration of a body or system.

dyspnea—Shortness of breath.

eccentric—Active muscle lengthening.

ectoderm—Layer of cells associated with the primitive amniotic cavity that gives rise to nervous system structures.

edema—Accumulation of excessive fluid (swelling).

effort force—See *applied force*.

elastic cartilage—Flexible and extensible cartilage found in the external ear, epiglottis, portions of the larynx, and eustachian tube.

elastic deformation—Change in a structure's shape or configuration that is followed by a return to its original configuration when the force is removed.

elasticity—Ability of a material to return to its original shape when a load is removed.

elastic fibers—Slender and extensible fibers composed of elastin that can safely stretch to about 150% of their original length and return to their original length.

elastic limit—Load or stress level above which tissue becomes plastic and experiences permanent deformation.

elastic modulus—See *modulus of elasticity*.

elastic region—During mechanical loading, in this region the material (tissue) can be deformed and when released will return back to its original configuration.

elastin—Protein in connective tissue that is elastic and returns to its original shape after stretching. Composed primarily of the amino acids glycine, valine, alanine, and praline and made in a reaction that links several tropoelastin molecules catalyzed by lysyl oxidase.

elastohydrodynamic lubrication—Subtype of fluid-film lubrication in which one or both of the surfaces are deformable.

elastoplastic—Characteristic of collisions in which there is energy transfer and loss; may also be plastic deformation.

embryo (embryonic stage)—Human development from fertilization to week 8.

embryology—Study of embryos and their development.

endochondral ossification—Process of bone growth in which hyaline cartilage is replaced by bony material.

endoderm—Layer of embryonic cells that gives rise to the gastrointestinal tract.

endomysium—Layer of connective tissue, capillaries, nerves, and lymphatics that surround individual muscle fibers.

endoneurium—Delicate sheath surrounding each axon.

endotendineum—Loose connective tissue that binds tendon fascicles together.

endurance training—Form of training that enhances the ability of the cardiorespiratory and muscular systems to resist fatigue.

energy to failure—Measure of the strain energy stored by the tissue prior to failure.

energy—Capacity or ability to perform work.

epicondylitis—Inflammation or damage of an epicondyle.

epidemiology—Study of the distribution and determinants of disease and injury frequency within a given human population.

epidural hematoma—Blood accumulation between the cranial vault and the outer protective meningeal layer (dura mater).

epimysium—Connective tissue surrounding the entire muscle.

epineurium—Tough covering surrounding the nerve trunk.

epiphysis—Rounded end of a long bone filled with red marrow, which produces red blood cells.

epitendineum—Surface covering of the tendon.

epithelial tissue—Covering (lining) tissue that absorbs, secretes, transports, excretes, and protects underlying organ or tissue.

equilibrium—Balanced condition where the sum of forces and the sum of moments equals zero.

ergogenic—Intended to increase physical performance, work output, stamina, or recovery.

ergonomics—Study of how people interact with their immediate environment in a safe and productive manner.

eversion sprain—See *medial ankle sprain*.

exercise-induced muscle injury—Injury resulting from connective and contractile tissue disruption following exercise.

external ballistics—Effect of external factors (e.g., wind, velocity, drag, gravity) on projectile flight from the barrel to the target.

external mechanics—Mechanical factors that produce and control movement outside the body (e.g., gravity or ground reaction forces).

extracapsular ligament—Ligament extrinsic to the joint capsule.

extracellular bone matrix—Inorganic (mineral) and fluid component of bones.

extracellular matrix—Noncellular component of a tissue.

extrapolation—Prediction or estimation of a value beyond known or measured values.

exudate—Substances that move (exude) from blood vessels into surrounding tissues during an inflammatory response.

failure—Complete tearing or rupture.

fascia—Dense irregular fibrous tissue found in layers or sheaths around organs, blood vessels, bones, cartilage, and dermis of the skin.

fasciotomy—Surgical procedure in which fascia is cut (released) to reduce pressure or tension.

fatigue—(1) Inability to continue work. (2) Loss of strength and stiffness in materials subjected to repeated cyclic loads.

fatigue fracture—Bone fracture resulting from loss of material strength attributable to repeated loading.

female athlete triad—Pathological condition caused by the combination of disordered eating, disrupted hormone levels, and poor bone quality and quantity in young female athletes.

fetal stage—Period of human development from week 9 until birth.

fiber—Threadlike structure composed of many fibrils.

fibroblasts—Principal cells in many fibrous connective tissues that form fibers and components of the extracellular matrix.

fibrocartilage—Strong, resilient, flexible cartilage found in areas of the body where friction could pose a problem.

fibroelastic tissue—Loose, woven network of fibers that encapsulates most organs.

finite-element modeling—Form of modeling that involves assembling complex geometrical figures, or elements, to represent a structure.

first-class lever—Lever system with the axis between the resistance force and the effort force.

first-cycle effect—Mechanical response of tissue to the first loading cycle, which may differ from subsequent loading cycles.

first law of motion—Law stating that a body at rest or in uniform motion will remain at rest or in uniform motion unless acted upon by an external force.

flap tear—Isolated damage to articular cartilage; also *chondral fracture.*

flexion–compression mechanism—See *compression–flexion mechanism.*

flexural rigidity—Measure of the bending stiffness of bone.

fluid flow—Characteristics of a fluid, whether liquid or gas, that allow it to move and that govern the nature of this movement.

fluid mechanics—Branch of mechanics dealing with the properties and behaviors of gases and liquids.

fluid resistance—Opposition to flow.

fluid-film lubrication—Lubrication mechanism in which two nonparallel surfaces move past each other on a thin layer of fluid.

focal injury—Tissue damage limited to a specific location.

force couple—A pair of parallel and oppositely directed forces that tend to cause the same rotation about an axis.

force—Mechanical action or effect applied to a body that tends to produce acceleration.

force-relaxation response—Force decrease seen in a viscoelastic tissue stretched or compressed to a given length and then held at that length.

force–velocity relation—Property of skeletal muscle that shows how its force production capability depends on its contraction velocity.

forward solution approach—Problem-solving approach that uses known or measured kinetic measures (e.g., force) to calculate associated kinematic measures (e.g., acceleration); also *direct solution approach.*

four-point bending—Bending mode involving four parallel forces (two outer forces in the same direction and two remaining forces acting in the opposite direction).

fracture—Structural breakage in a hard tissue, such as bone.

free-body diagram (FBD)—Diagram depicting all the forces and moments acting in a particular system.

friction—Resistance created at the interface between two bodies that acts in the opposite direction of motion or intended motion.

fulcrum—Point about which rotation occurs; also *axis* or *pivot.*

Galeazzi fracture—Fracture of the distal third of the radius.

gastrulation—Transformation of the bilaminar embryonic disc into a three-layered disc containing the three primary germ layers—ectoderm, mesoderm, and endoderm.

general force system—Force system that is neither linear, parallel, nor concurrent.

general motion—Simultaneous linear and angular (rotational) motion.

Glasgow Coma Scale (GCS)—Scoring rubric to describe the level of consciousness following a traumatic brain injury.

glycation—Bonding of a sugar molecule to a protein or lipid molecule without the involvement of enzymes.

glycosaminoglycans—Polysaccharides that are constituents of mucoproteins, glycoproteins, and blood-group substances.

gouty arthritis—Joint inflammation caused by excess production of uric acid, with resulting uric acid (urate) crystals embedded in joint structures with attendant irritation and pain; also called *gout*.

graft—Surgically implanted living tissue.

gravitational (positional) potential energy—The energy an object or a body has due to its position in a gravitational field. A measure of the potential to perform work as a function of the height a body is elevated above a reference level.

ground reaction force (GRF)—Force exerted *by* the ground that is equal and opposite to a force applied *to* the ground by an impacting object (e.g., foot).

growth plate (physis)—Area of developing tissue (hyaline cartilage) near the end of the long bones.

Haversian canals—Small canals through which blood vessels pass, generally oriented longitudinally in bone.

hematoma—Mass of blood that forms in a tissue or body space as a result of a broken blood vessel.

hematopoiesis—Process of blood cell formation.

hemodynamics—Forces and mechanisms involved with blood circulation.

hemorrhage—Profuse bleeding.

heparin—Naturally occurring glycosaminoglycan, which acts as a blood anticoagulant.

herniation—Protrusion of the nucleus pulposus through the annulus fibrosus.

high ankle sprain—Injury to the anterior and posterior tibiofibular ligaments just above the ankle joint.

histamine—Vasodilator and organic nitrogenous compound involved in local immune responses.

homeostasis—Maintenance of a relatively stable internal physiological environment.

Hooke's law—Principle that stress and strain are linearly related; the resulting strain is proportional to the developed stress.

hoop effect—Radiating circumferential stress developed perpendicular to an applied compressive load.

hyaline cartilage—Firm, glossy appearing cartilage that lines most of the joint surfaces (articular cartilage), the anterior portions of the ribs, and areas of the respiratory system (trachea, nose, and bronchi).

hydrodynamic lubrication—Subtype of fluid-film lubrication produced by two moving surfaces that are nondeformable.

hydroxyapatite—Complex calcium–phosphate crystal that forms the primary structural element of bone.

hyperemia—Presence of excess blood in a body part or region.

hyperesthesia—Heightened or pathological sensitivity to stimulation.

hyperglycolysis—Enhanced breakdown of a carbohydrate (e.g., glucose or glycogen) by enzymatic action.

hyperplasia—Abnormal or unexpected increase in the constituents composing a part (e.g., cells in a tissue).

hypertrophy—Increase in size or bulk without an increase in number of parts (e.g., adaptive increase in muscle fiber size in response to resistance training).

hypovascular—Having a decreased or low number of blood vessels.

hypoxemia—Decrease in blood perfusion.

hypoxia—Decrease in blood (oxygen) delivery to a tissue.

hysteresis loop—Area enclosed by the loading–unloading paths on a load–deformation curve; measures energy loss during a loading–unloading cycle of a viscoelastic material.

hysteresis—Delay or retardation in a material's response when forces are changed.

idealized force vector—Single vector used to represent many vectors.

idiopathic—Of unknown origin or cause.

iliac-type luxation—Anterosuperior hip dislocation; also *pubic-type luxation.*

iliotibial band syndrome (ITBS)—Inflammatory condition caused by friction as the iliotibial band passes over the lateral femoral epicondyle during repeated flexion–extension cycles of the knee.

impact injury—Injury resulting from a direct compressive force.

impact strength—Ability of bone to resist impact loading.

impingement syndrome—Pressure increase within a confined anatomical space with deleterious effect on the enclosed tissues.

impulse—Mechanical agent that changes momentum, calculated as force × time.

impulse–momentum principle—Mechanical principle stating that the impulse equals the change in momentum.

impulsive force—Force component in an impulse.

in situ—Research approach that examines tissues in their normal place, with some elements of natural environment preserved; artificial testing.

in vitro—Research approach that examines tissues in an artificial environment that allows direct measurements.

in vivo—Research approach that examines tissues in the living body.

incidence—Number of new injuries that occur within a given population at risk over a specified time period.

incomplete fracture—Fracture that only partially traverses the bone structure.

indirect injury—Fracture that is remote from the location of force application.

inertia—Resistance to a change in a body's state of linear motion.

inflammation—Localized physiological response to injury that involves redness, heat, pain, swelling, and sometimes loss of function.

initial-cycles effect—Mechanical response of tissue to the first few loading cycles, which may differ from subsequent loading cycles.

injury—Damage to tissue caused by physical trauma.

instantaneous joint center—Axis of rotation location at an instant in time.

insufficiency fracture—Chronic fracture found in persons with no increase in physical activity but with decreased bone density.

integrins—Integral membrane proteins in the plasma membrane of cells that attach the cell to the extracellular matrix and facilitate signal transduction from the extracellular matrix to the cell.

internal ballistics—Effect of bullet and weapon design and materials on the projectile while in the barrel of the weapon.

internal impingement—Pinching where the supraspinatus tendon contacts the posterior–superior rim of the glenoid fossa.

internal mechanics—Mechanical factors that produce and control movement inside the body (e.g., forces produced by muscle action and stability provided by ligaments surrounding joints).

interpolation—Estimation of values between known or measured values.

interstitial growth—Growth occurring in young cartilage where the cells divide within the lacunae and form cell nests.

intervertebral disc—Structure between two adjacent vertebrae composed of a nucleus pulposus surrounded by the annulus fibrosus.

intra-articular fibrocartilage—Fibrocartilage that is located in a joint.

intracapsular ligament—Ligament located within a joint capsule.

intracranial pressure (ICP)—Pressure within the cranial vault (skull).

intramembranous ossification—Process of bone growth in which a membrane is replaced by bony material.

inverse dynamics—Problem-solving approach that uses known or measured kinematic measures (e.g., acceleration) to calculate associated kinetic measures (e.g., force).

inverse solution approach—See *inverse dynamics*.

inversion sprain—See *lateral ankle sprain*.

ipsilateral—Situated on, appearing on, or affecting the same side of the body.

irritability—Ability to respond to a stimulus; also known as *excitability*.

ischemia—Deficient blood supply caused by decreased flow to an area.

isotropic—Property by which a tissue's mechanical responses (e.g., strength or stiffness) to loading are not dependent on direction.

joint reaction force (JRF)—Net effect of muscle and other forces acting across a joint.

joint stability—Ability of a joint to resist dislocation and maintain an appropriate functional position throughout its range of motion.

joint—Junction of two or more bones at their sites of contact; also *articulation*.

joule—Unit of work and energy (1 J = 1 N·m).

Kelvin–Voight model—Rheological model with its spring and dashpot elements in parallel.

kinematics—Description of movement without regard to the forces involved.

kinetic energy—Energy possessed by a body by virtue of its motion.

kinetic friction—Frictional resistance created while an object is moving (e.g., sliding or rolling) along a surface; also *dynamic friction*.

kinetics—Assessment of movement with respect to the forces involved; the study of forces and their effects.

knee extensor mechanism—Functional unit that extends the knee, including the quadriceps muscle group, quadriceps tendon, patella, and patellar tendon–ligament.

kyphosis—Excessive spinal flexion (e.g., thoracic hunchback).

labrum—U-shaped ring of fibrocartilage around the rim of a joint.

laceration—Jagged tearing of the skin, as made by a knife or sharp implement.

lacunae—Small pockets or cavities.

lamellar bone—Primary bone composed of multiple thin layers (lamellae) of bone matrix and cells organized in parallel with the bone surface.

laminar flow—Flow characterized by a smooth, essentially parallel pattern of fluid movement.

lateral ankle sprain—Injury to the lateral ankle ligaments caused by violent foot and ankle supination.

length–tension relation—Property of skeletal muscle that shows how its force production capability depends on the length of the muscle's contractile and noncontractile structures.

level of dysfunction—Degree of impaired or abnormal functioning.

lever arm—See *moment arm*.

lever—Rigid structure, fixed at a single point, to which two forces are applied at two points.

lift force—Force acting perpendicular to the direction of fluid flow.

ligaments—Cords of regular dense fibrous connective tissue that connect one bone to another.

linear acceleration—Change in linear velocity divided by change in time.

linear displacement—Vector measure of the straight-line distance from starting position to the ending position.

linear force system—Force system in which all forces act along a single line.

linear fracture—Break in the bone that does not move the bone.

linear impulse—Product of force × time.

linear limit—See *proportional limit*.

linear momentum—Quantity of linear motion measured by the product of mass × linear velocity.

linear motion—Motion along a straight (rectilinear) or curved (curvilinear) line.

linear power—Measure of mechanical work per unit time; force × linear velocity.

linear region—Portion of the stress–strain (or load–deformation) curve that is in the elastic region.

linear spring—Component of a rheological model that represents tissue elastic properties.

linear velocity—Linear displacement divided by the change in time.

linear work—Mechanical measure of force × displacement.

load—Externally applied force.

load–deformation curve—Curve that shows the relation between the external force (load) and the change in shape or configuration (deformation) of a tissue.

lordosis—Excessive spinal extension (e.g., lumbar lordosis).

luxation—Complete dislocation of joint.

macrophage—Migratory cell that contains small holes or vacuoles that can assimilate foreign material, old red blood cells, and bacteria.

macrotrauma—Trauma that can be seen by the unassisted eye (e.g., tibia fracture or laceration).

magnus force—Force created by the spin of an object that creates a deviation in its normal trajectory.

mass moment of inertia—Measure of resistance to change in the state of a body's movement about a fixed axis.

mass—Quantity of matter (in SI units, measured in kilograms).

mast cells—Migratory cells that are relatively large because of their substantial amount of cytoplasm.

material discontinuity—Interruption or imperfection in the normal physical makeup of a material or structure.

material properties—Qualitative measure of a tissue's mechanical properties, usually expressed as a relative measure (e.g., stress and elastic modulus).

material strength—Ultimate stress.

material—Mechanical quality of a tissue.

maximal load—During mechanical loading of a tissue, this is the peak load at which tissue microfailures begin to develop, resulting in a loss of structural integrity and loss of load resistance.

Maxwell model—Rheological model with its spring and dashpot elements in series.

mechanical energy—Capacity or ability to perform mechanical work.

mechanics—Branch of science that deals with the effects of forces and energy on bodies.

mechanical strain—Relative measure of a change in shape or configuration of tissue when subjected to a load.

mechanical work—See *work*.

mechanism—Fundamental physical process responsible for a given action, reaction, or result.

mechanotransduction—Process by which tissue cells convert a mechanical stimulus into a biochemical response.

medial ankle sprain—Injury to the medial ankle ligaments caused by violent foot and ankle pronation.

medial tibial stress syndrome (MTSS)—Inflammatory reaction of the deep fascial tibial attachments in response to chronic loads, with pain localized to the posteromedial crest of the tibia.

medullary canal—Central canal oriented along the longitudinal axis of long bones.

megapascal (MPa)—Measure of pressure or stress (1 MPa = 1 N/mm^2, or 10^6 Pa).

meninges—Protective membrane layers surrounding the brain and spinal cord (dura mater, pia mater, and arachnoid).

meningitis—Inflammation of the meninges.

meniscus—Interposed fibrocartilage pad that acts as a shock absorber and a wedge at the joint periphery to improve the structural fit of a joint.

mesenchyme—Progenitor primitive tissue of adult connective tissue (e.g., cartilage, ligaments, fascia, tendons, blood cells, blood vessels, skin, and bone) that is loosely woven and formed from undifferentiated cells of the sclerotome.

mesoderm—Middle of the three primary germ layers of an embryo that is the source of many bodily tissues and structures (e.g., bone, muscle, connective tissue, and dermis).

metaphyseal—Deriving from the metaphysis.

metaphysis—Portion of a long bone between the epiphyses and the diaphysis.

microfibrils—Component of elastic fibers composed of microfibrillar-associated glycoproteins, fibrillin, fibulin, and the elastin receptor.

microstrain—Unit of relative deformation (με) equal to 10–^{6}.

microtrauma—Tissue injury that can only be seen under a microscope (e.g., microcracks in bone).

migratory cells—Cells that wander or move within a tissue or body system.

modeling—Formation of new or additional bone, occurring mostly during the growing years.

model—Structural or mathematical representation of one or more of an object's or system's characteristics.

modulus of elasticity—Ratio of stress to strain; slope of the linear portion of a stress–strain curve; also *elastic modulus* and *Young's modulus*.

moment—Effect of a force that tends to rotate or bend a body or segment; also *moment of force*.

moment arm—Perpendicular distance from the axis of rotation to the line of force action; also *lever arm* and *torque arm*.

moment of inertia—Resistance to a change in a body's state of angular motion or position.

momentum—Quantity of motion possessed by a moving body.

Monteggia lesion—Fracture in the proximal ulna with dislocation of the radial head.

morphology—Area of study concerned with the form and structure of plants and animals.

morula—Solid mass of cells resulting from cell division following zygote formation.

motor unit—Single motor neuron and all the muscle fibers it innervates.

multiaxial loading—Multidimensional force application to a body in either two- (biaxial) or three- (triaxial) dimensional space.

muscle—Body tissue capable of developing force in response to stimulation. There are three muscle types: skeletal, cardiac, and smooth.

musculotendinous junction—See *myotendinous junction*.

myelopathy—Disease or disorder of the spinal cord.

myofibrils—Contractile units of muscle.

myofilaments—Individual filaments (actin or myosin) that comprise a myofibril.

myosin—Thick myofilament found in muscle fibers that acts as the cross-bridge during muscular contraction.

myositis ossificans—Deposit of an ossified mass within a muscle.

myotendinous junction—Region where a muscle and tendon connect; also *musculotendinous junction*.

myotome—Developmental tissue that gives rise to the musculature.

nebulin—A protein that anchors actin to the Z discs in mammalian skeletal muscle.

negative ulnar variance—Ulnar variance with radius longer than the ulna.

neoplasm—Abnormal new or uncontrolled excessive growth in a body tissue; tumor.

nervous tissue—Body tissue responsible for communication. Develops from the ectoderm and comprises the main parts of the nervous system, including the brain, spinal cord, peripheral nerves, nerve endings, and sense organs.

net moment—Sum of all the moments acting on a body; also *net torque*.

net torque—Sum of all the torques acting on a body; also *net moment*.

neurapraxia—Injury to a nerve that disrupts conduction and causes temporary paralysis but not degeneration, followed by rapid and complete recovery.

neuron—Nerve cell.

neurotmesis—Partial or complete severance of a nerve, with axonal disruption.

neutral axis—Line (in a beam) along which neither compressive nor tensile stress exists.

Newtonian fluid—Fluid in which the stress–strain response is linear.

newton—Unit of force ($1\ N = 1\ kg \cdot m \cdot s^{-2}$).

nightstick fracture—Fracture of the ulna, named for the mechanism of blocking an overhead blow.

nonsteroidal anti-inflammatory drugs (NSAIDs)—Inflammation-reducing drugs that do not contain steroids; can produce positive or negative effects on the body's tissues and human performance, thus altering injury risk.

normal force—Force acting perpendicular to a surface.

notochord—Primitive spinal cord.

nucleus pulposus—Gelatinous mass in the interior of an intervertebral disc.

obturator-type luxation—Anteroinferior hip dislocation.

oligomenorrhea—Irregular menstrual cycles.

open fracture—Fracture that penetrates the skin and exposes bone to external environment; also known as *compound fracture*.

orthotics—Supports or braces for weak or ineffective joints.

os acromiale—Unfused acromial apophysis.

Osgood–Schlatter disease (OSD)—Traction apophysitis at the tibial tuberosity.

osteoarthritis (OA)—Noninflammatory condition that affects synovial joints, especially those involved in weight bearing, characterized by cartilage deterioration and bone outgrowth on joint surfaces and joint margins.

osteoblasts—Mononuclear bone cells that produce new bone material.

osteochondral fracture—Injury to cartilage and its underlying bone.

osteochondritis dissecans—Complete or partial detachment of a fragment of bone and cartilage at a joint.

osteochondrosis—Disease in which an ossification center, especially in the epiphyses of long bones, experiences degeneration followed by calcification.

osteoclasts—Large, multinucleated bone cells that break down, or resorb, bone.

osteocytes—Mature bone cells that are smaller and less active than an osteoblast.

osteoid—Organic portion of the extracellular matrix in bone.

osteonecrosis—Bone death caused by cessation of blood flow.

osteopenia—Mild to moderate bone loss; clinically classified as having a bone mineral density (BMD) rating 1.0 to 2.5 standard deviations below the mean BMD for young, healthy adults.

osteophyte—Bone outgrowth; also known as *bone spur*.

osteophytosis—Condition characterized by formation of osteophytes.

osteoporosis—Severe bone loss marked by increased risk of fractures, primarily of the hip, spine, and wrist; clinically identified by a bone mineral density (BMD) rating 2.5 standard deviations below the mean BMD for young, healthy adults.

osteosarcoma—Malignant bone tumor.

osteotendinous junction—Region where a bone and tendon connect.

overuse injury—Injuries resulting from repeated overloads with insufficient time for recovery; also *chronic injury*.

parallel force system—Force system in which all forces act parallel to one another.

parallel-elastic component—Component of a muscle model that accounts for muscle elasticity in parallel with the contractile component.

paresthesia—Sensation of tingling or creeping on the skin with no specific cause, usually associated with injury or irritation of a sensory nerve.

pars interarticularis—Area of the vertebral lamina between the superior and inferior articular facets.

pascal (Pa)—Unit of pressure or stress ($1\ Pa = 1\ N/m^2$).

passive joint stabilizer—Periarticular structure (e.g., ligaments or joint capsule) that stabilizes a joint.

passive stabilization—Contribution of noncontractile components (e.g., periarticular tissues) to joint stability.

patella alta—Abnormally elevated patella situated high in the intercondylar groove.

patellar ligament—Collagenous connective tissue spanning between the inferior pole of the patella and the tibial tuberosity; also *patellar tendon*.

patellar tendon—See *patellar ligament*.

patellar tracking—Sliding movement of the patella in the intercondylar groove of the femur.

peak height velocity (PHV)—Highest rate of longitudinal bone growth.

perfectly elastic collision—Collision in which bodies rebound away from each other following the collision with no energy or momentum loss.

perfectly plastic (inelastic) collision—Collision in which the bodies stick together and move together with a common velocity after impact with no loss of energy or momentum.

performance biomechanics—Study of the mechanical function of the human body across all types of movement.

perichondrium—Connective tissue membrane surrounding cartilage.

perimysium—Connective tissue that surrounds a bundle of muscle fibers (fascicle).

perineurium—Connective tissue sheath surrounding a bundle of nerve fibers.

periosteal collar—Bony ring surrounding the primary ossification center in developing bone.

peripheral neuropathy—Structural or functional disorder of the peripheral nervous system.

peritenon—Loose areolar connective tissue enveloping the tendon.

permanent set—Plastic deformation in which a tissue does not return to its preloaded shape or configuration.

pes cavus—Foot deformity characterized by a high longitudinal plantar arch.

pes planus—Foot deformity characterized by a flattened longitudinal plantar arch (flat foot).

phagocyte—Cell (e.g., white blood cell) that engulfs and consumes foreign material (e.g., microorganisms) and debris.

phagocytosis—Bodily defense process by which phagocytes engulf and destroy foreign particles and tissue debris.

physiological age—Age based on physiological quality of the tissues.

physiological range—Normal operational range for a physiological variable or measure.

pia mater—Thin tissue membrane comprising the inner meningeal layer.

pivot—Point about which rotation occurs; also *axis* or *fulcrum*.

planar model—Two-dimensional model of an object or system.

plantar fasciitis (PF)—Inflammation of the plantar fascia.

plastic deformation—Permanent change in a tissue's or body's shape or dimensions.

plastic region—When a tissue is loaded beyond its proportional limit, smaller and smaller increases in load will produce greater and greater increases in deformation and structural damage to the tissue.

pluripotent—Capable of developmental plasticity, or having multiple developmental potentials.

point mass—Concentration of a body's mass at a single point.

Poisson's effect—A body's inverse response created transversely to an axial load (e.g., a body subjected to a uniaxial compressive load increases its dimension in the axial direction and decreases its dimension in the transverse direction).

Poisson's ratio—Negative of the strain transverse to a load divided by the strain in line with an applied load.

polar moment of inertia—Resistance to torsional loading about a longitudinal axis.

positive ulnar variance—Ulnar variance with the ulna longer than the radius.

posterolateral rotatory instability (PLRI)—Elbow instability that results from combined axial compression, valgus instability, and supination.

potential energy—Energy created by virtue of a body's position (gravitational potential energy) or deformation (strain energy).

power—Rate of work production.

pressure—Total applied force divided by the area over which the force is applied ($p = F/A$).

prevalence—Number of cases (e.g., injuries) both new and old that exist in a given population at a specific point in time divided by the total population.

primary bone—Bone composed of multiple thin layers (lamellae) of bone matrix and cells organized in parallel with the bone surface, used to replace existing bone.

primary injury—Immediate injury as a consequence of trauma (e.g., skull fracture or torn medial collateral ligament).

primary ossification center—Region in developing bone where initial ossification happens (in the mid-diaphyseal region of long bones).

primary osteons—Haversian system with concentrically arranged lamellae.

primary spongiosa—Lattice of calcified cartilage.

progressive overload—Training principle that suggests the continual increase in the total workload during training sessions will stimulate muscle growth and strength gain.

pronation—Combination of ankle dorsiflexion, subtalar eversion, and external rotation of the foot.

proportional limit—Point at which a tissue's load–deformation or stress–strain response changes from linear to nonlinear; also *linear limit*.

proteoglycan—Protein to which are attached one or more specialized carbohydrate side chains, called glycosaminoglycans.

pubic-type luxation—Anterosuperior hip dislocation; also *iliac-type luxation*.

public health approach—Four-step method for gathering epidemiological information.

puncture—Wound created by a sharp implement that penetrates the skin.

Q angle—Angle measured between a line along the longitudinal midline of the thigh and a line connecting the tibial tuberosity with the centroid of the patella (Q = quadriceps).

quadriceps tendon—Tendon connecting the quadriceps muscle group with the superior pole of the patella.

quadriplegia—Paralysis in all four limbs; also *tetraplegia*.

quasi-static model—Model with negligible acceleration that mimics a static model.

range of motion (ROM)—Measure of joint mobility.

rate of elastic return—Speed at which a deformed material returns to its original shape or configuration.

reaction force—Equal and opposite force created in response to an applied force.

rectilinear motion—Linear motion in a straight line.

reduction—Replacement or realignment of a body part to its normal position following luxation or subluxation.

relative risk—Risk calculated as the injury incidence in group A divided by the injury incidence in group B.

remodeling—Adaptation of existing bone via resorption and reformation.

repetitive stress syndrome—See *chronic injury*.

resident cells—Fixed (nonmoving) cells.

resilient—Characteristic of elastic materials that quickly return to their original shapes.

resistance force—An externally applied force.

resistance training—Mode of physical conditioning designed to enhance muscular strength; also known as *strength training*.

reticular fibers—Forming or resembling a network.

reticular tissue—Connective tissue containing reticular fibers and some primitive cells; found near lymph nodes and in bone marrow, liver, and spleen.

retroversion—Rearward rotation or displacement relative to a reference plane.

rheological model—Model that characterizes the fluid-related aspects of a tissue or system.

rheology—Study of the deformation and flow of matter.

rheumatoid arthritis—Joint inflammation of autoimmune origin.

rigid-body mechanics—Approach that models each body segment as a nondeformable member.

rigid-body model—Model that treats each segment as a nondeformable member.

risk—Likelihood of injury or death associated with a particular object, task, or environment.

risk factors—Factors that may contribute to the occurrence of injury.

rotational motion—See *angular motion*.

rotatory component—Component of a force acting perpendicular to a segment that tends to cause rotation.

rupture point—Point at which a tissue reaches failure.

sarcomeres—Contractile units of the myofibril, delimited by Z bands at each end of its length.

scalar—Measure that has magnitude only.

scapulohumeral balance—Muscle action at the glenohumeral joint that maintains the net joint reaction force within the glenoid fossa.

Scheuermann's kyphosis—Spinal disorder (kyphosis) in children typically accompanied by vertebral wedging, end plate irregularities, and narrowing of the intervertebral disc spaces.

sclerotome—Group of mesenchymal cells emerging from the ventromedial part of a mesodermic somite and migrating toward the notochord.

scoliosis—Lateral (frontal plane) deviation of the spine.

screw-home mechanism—Tibiofemoral rotation during the final few degrees of knee extension.

second-class lever—Lever system with the resistance force between the axis and the effort force.

second impact syndrome (SIS)—Second head injury sustained before symptoms associated with a first head injury (most often a concussion) have fully resolved.

second law of motion—Law stating that force acting upon a body will produce an acceleration proportional to the force ($F = m \cdot a$).

secondary bone—Bone deposited only during remodeling and replacing preexisting primary bone.

secondary injury—Injury happening some time after an initial trauma or in compensation for a primary injury.

secondary ossification centers—Regions in developing bone where subsequent ossification happens (in the epiphyseal region of long bones).

secondary spongiosa—Trabecular lamellar bone formed after the resorption of the primary spongiosa.

sequelae—Aftereffects.

series-elastic component—Component of a muscle model that accounts for muscle elasticity in series with the contractile component.

serotonin—Neurotransmitter, which carries messages between nerve cells in the brain and throughout the body and affects body functions including vasoconstriction.

Sharpey's fibers—Compact bundles of perforating smaller collagen fibers that are tightly embedded in bone to reinforce attachment sites.

shear—Force that tends to produce horizontal sliding of one layer over another or angulation within a structure.

shear modulus of elasticity—Ratio of shear stress to shear strain.

shear stress—Internal resistance developed in response to a shear load.

shoulder separation—Acromioclavicular sprain.

simulation—Process of using a validated model to address questions related to a system and its operation.

skeletal muscle—Muscle tissue responsible for maintaining posture and producing movement.

SLAP lesion—Injury to the superior labrum anterior–posterior region of the glenoid labrum.

sliding filament theory—Final steps associated with excitation–contraction coupling that describe the interaction between the actin and myosin filaments needed to produce force.

Smith's fracture—Fracture of the distal radius with tensile failure on the dorsal aspect of the metaphysis and compressive comminution on the volar (palmar) aspect.

smooth muscle—Muscle tissue that facilitates substance movement through tracts in the circulatory, respiratory, digestive, urinary, and reproductive systems.

somatotype—Shape or physical classification of the human body.

somites—Cuboidal bodies that form distinct surface elevations and influence the external contours of the embryo.

spatial model—Three-dimensional model of an object or system.

speed—Scalar quantity that measures how fast a body is moving.

spinal cord injury (SCI)—Damage to the spinal cord, usually as a result of high-energy collision.

spondylolisthesis—Vertebral slippage, usually at L5-S1 or L4-L5.

spondylolysis—Fracture of the pars interarticularis.

spondylosis—Intervertebral disc deterioration.

spongy bone—See *trabecular bone*.

sprain—Ligament injury.

squeeze-film lubrication—Form of fluid-film lubrication in which two surfaces move at right angles to each other, as might happen in the knee joint at the instant of heel strike in walking, and fluid is forced out of the cartilage to produce a fluid interface between the two surfaces.

stabilizing component—Force component acting through the joint axis that tends to stabilize the joint.

static equilibrium—Balanced state where net accelerations equal zero.

static friction—Resistance created between two surfaces in the absence of movement.

static model—Model of a system that has zero net acceleration, usually motionless.

stem cells—Cells that can differentiate into a variety of cell types, such as connective tissue cells (e.g., fibroblast, chondroblast, or osteoblast) and nerve cells.

stenosis—Narrowing or constriction of a bodily passage or tract.

stiffness—Measure of the relation between stress and strain (i.e., how much a body deforms in response to a given load).

stochastic model—Model whose output varies as a function of probability algorithms within the model.

strain—Damage to a musculotendinous unit (i.e., muscle–tendon complex).

strain energy—Energy stored in a tissue during deformation; also *deformational energy*.

strain energy density—Relative measure of energy stored during deformation, as measured by the area under the stress–strain curve.

strain to failure—Measure of the mechanical strain to the point of tissue failure.

strain-rate dependent—Tissue characteristic in which its mechanical response depends on the rate at which the tissue is deformed.

stratiform fibrocartilage—Layer of fibrocartilage over bone that reduces friction where tendons act.

stress fracture—Bone fracture caused by chronic loading.

stress reaction—Area of enhanced metabolic activity in bone in response to repeated loading.

stress-relaxation response—Stress decrease seen in a viscoelastic tissue stretched or compressed to a given length and then held at that length.

stress riser—Force or stress concentration at the site of a material discontinuity.

stress—Internal resistance developed in response to an externally applied load.

stroma—Supportive tissue of an epithelial organ, consisting of connective tissues and blood vessels.

structural properties—Property based on a bone's structure, such as flexural rigidity, load behaviors, and energy.

structural strength—Absolute load a structure can withstand prior to failure.

subacromical impingement—Pinching of structures (distal tendon of the supraspinatus, proximal tendon of the biceps long head, and subacromial bursa) under the coracoacromial arch.

subarachnoid hematoma—Blood accumulation between the arachnoid and the pia mater.

subdural hematoma—Blood accumulation between the dura mater and the arachnoid.

subluxation—Partial dislocation of a joint.

supination—Combination of ankle plantar flexion, subtalar inversion, and internal rotation of the foot.

synapse—Junction where a nervous impulse is passed between a neuron and its target structure (e.g., another neuron or sarcolemma of skeletal muscle fiber).

syncytium—Multinucleated mass resulting from fusion of cells.

synovial membrane—Connective tissue that lines the cavity of a joint and produces synovial fluid.

synovitis—Inflammation of a synovial membrane.

taping—To fasten, tie, bind, cover, or support with tape, as in taping a sprained ankle.

teardrop fracture—Fracture at the anteroinferior corner of a cervical vertebral body.

tendinitis—Inflammation of a tendon.

tendon—White, collagenous flexible band that connects muscle to bone.

tensile load—Externally applied force that tends to pull ends of a body apart.

tensile stress—Internal resistance to being pulled apart.

tension—Force that tends to pull ends of a body apart.

tension–extension mechanism—Injury mechanism in which the head is forcibly hyperextended by posterior impact with forcible resistance applied to the chin, inertial forces resulting from posterior impact, or forces applied inferiorly to the posterior aspect of the head.

terminal ballistics—Projectile behavior in tissues.

tetanus—See *tetany*.

tetany—Steady skeletal muscle contraction caused by rapid arrival of signals from nerves.

third-class lever—Lever system with the effort force between the axis and the resistance force.

third law of motion—Law stating that for every action there is an equal and opposite reaction.

thoracic outlet syndrome—Compression of nerves or blood vessels between the neck and shoulders that results in neck and shoulder pain, numbness, tingling, and weakened grip.

three-point bending—Bending mode involving three parallel forces (two outer forces in the same direction with the remaining force in between acting in the opposite direction).

tide mark—Boundary between calcified and noncalcified layers of bone.

time—Measure of the duration of a particular event.

tinnitus—Ringing or whistling sounds in the ear.

tissue—Aggregation of cells and intercellular substance that together perform a specialized function.

tissue biomechanics—Study of mechanical response of tissues (e.g., bone, tendon, muscle) to external forces.

titin—Giant filamentous protein essential to the structure, development, and elasticity of muscle.

toe region—Portion of a stress–strain curve at initial loading that exhibits relatively high compliance (low stiffness) prior to the collagen fibers becoming taut and increasing tissue stiffness.

tonically recruited—Repeated recruitment of slow muscle fibers.

torque—(1) Effect of a force that tends to cause rotation or twisting about an axis. (2) Mechanical agent creating and controlling angular motion.

torque arm—See *moment arm*.

torsion—Twisting action applied to a structure.

total mechanical energy (TME)—Sum of linear kinetic energy + angular kinetic energy + positional potential energy.

toughness—Measure of a tissue's ability to absorb mechanical energy.

trabeculae—Small bars or rods of bone in the structure of spongy or cancellous bone.

trabecular bone—Bone with high porosity (low density); also *cancellous bone* and *spongy bone*.

traction apophysitis—Inflammation of the bone at a tendon or ligament insertion, caused by tensile, or pulling, force.

transfer of energy—Exchange of energy from one body to another.

transfer of momentum—Exchange of momentum from one body to another.

translational motion—See *linear motion*.

transverse tubules (T-tubules)—Invaginations of the sarcolemma that pass through the muscle fiber between the myofibrils.

traumatic axonal injury (TAI)—See *diffuse axonal injury*.

traumatic brain injury (TBI)—Term that covers numerous conditions arising from impact or acceleration–deceleration of the head.

triaxial loading—Simultaneous loading along three axes.

truss mechanism—Mechanical assemblage of two hinged segments (beams), supported at two points and arranged to transmit vertical forces to those points (e.g., longitudinal arch of the foot).

turbulent flow—Fluid flow that exhibits a chaotic pattern that contains areas of turbulence (eddies) and multidirectional movement patterns.

turf toe—Capsuloligamentous injury to the first metatarsophalangeal joint resulting from hyperflexion or hyperextension.

ulnar variance (UV)—Difference in length between the distal radius and ulna.

ultimate load—Highest load a tissue can withstand prior to failure.

undifferentiated mesenchymal stem cells—Cells that can differentiate into a variety of connective tissue cells (e.g., fibroblast, chondroblast, or osteoblast).

undisplaced fracture—Fracture in which the bony segments remain in their original (prefracture) position.

unfused tetanic contraction—Partial relaxation between muscle twitches.

unhappy triad—Knee injury caused by valgus rotation characterized by concurrent injury to the anterior cruciate ligament (ACL), medial meniscus, and medial collateral ligament.

uniaxial loading—Forces applied along a single line, typically along a primary axis of a structure.

vacuolation—Formation or development of a small cavity or space filled with air or fluid.

valgus—Medial deviation of a joint (e.g., knock-kneed).

valgus-extension overload mechanism—Mechanism of elbow injury seen in overhead throwing that involves simultaneous valgus and extension at the elbow.

varus—Lateral deviation of a joint (e.g., bowlegged).

vector—Measure that has both magnitude and direction.

velocity—Measure of the time rate (change) of displacement, calculated by displacement divided by change in time.

viscoelastic—Characteristic of tissues that can return to their original shape or configuration after a load is removed (elastic) and have strain-rate dependent response to loading (viscous effect).

viscosity—Property of a fluid that enables it to develop and maintain a resistance to flow dependent on the flow's velocity (rate of flow).

Volkmann canals—Canals containing transversely oriented blood vessels in bone.

Wallerian degeneration—Axonal degeneration distal to a site of nerve injury.

watt—Unit of mechanical power (1 W = 1 J/s).

wedge fracture—Fracture in which the front (anterior) edge of the vertebra collapses.

whiplash—Acceleration–deceleration mechanism of energy transfer to the neck.

windlass mechanism—Hyperextension of the toes to increase tension in the plantar fascia.

Wolff's law—Law that describes bone's ability to structurally adapt to the time-averaged forces applied to it.

work—Measure of a force (or torque) acting through a displacement in the direction of the force (or torque); also *mechanical work*.

wound ballistics—Study of the interaction of penetrating projectiles and living body tissues.

woven bone—Immature bone without laminar or osteonal organization.

yaw—Movement from side to side.

yellow elastic ligaments—Parallel elastic fibers that are surrounded by loose connective tissue, found in the vocal cords and the ligamenta flava of the vertebrae.

yield point—Point at which there begins a brief region of relatively large strain for little increase in stress (i.e., region of high compliance).

Young's modulus—See *modulus of elasticity*.

zone of Ranvier—Area at the cortical margins of the growth plate toward the primary ossification center.

zygote—Cell formed by the union of an egg (ovum) and sperm (spermatozoa).

References

Chapter 1

American Academy of Orthopaedic Surgeons. 2022. Hip Fractures - OrthoInfo - AAOS. https://orthoinfo.aaos.org/en/diseases--conditions/hip-fractures/

Apostolakis, E., G. Apostolaki, M. Apostolaki, and M. Chorti. 2010. The reported thoracic injuries in Homer's *Iliad*. *Journal of Cardiothoracic Surgery* 5: 114.

Bittencourt, N.F.N., W.H. Meeuwisse, L.D. Mendonca, A. Nettel-Aguirre, J.M. Ocarisno, and S.T. Fonseca. 2016. Complex systems approach for sports injuries: Moving from risk factor identification to injury pattern recognition—narrative review and new concept. *British Journal of Sports Medicine* 50: 1309-1314.

Brewer, B.W., and C.J. Redmond. 2017. *Psychology of Sport Injury*. Champaign, IL: Human Kinetics.

Caine, D.J., C.G. Caine, and K.J. Linder. 1996. *Epidemiology of Sports Injuries*. Champaign, IL: Human Kinetics.

Committee on Trauma Research. 1985. *Injury in America: A Continuing Public Health Problem*. Washington, DC: National Academy Press.

Fonseca, S.T., T.R. Souza, E. Verhagen, R. van Emmerik, N.F.N. Bittencourt, L.D.M. Mendonca, A.G.P. Andrade, R.A. Resende, and J.M. Ocariono. 2020. Sports injury forecasting and complexity: A synergetic approach. *Sports Medicine* 50(10): 1757-1770.

Fu, G., X. Xie, Q. Jia, Z. Li, P. Chen, and Y. Ge. 2020. The development history of accident causation models in the past 100 years: 24Model, a more modern accident causation model. *Process Safety and Environmental Protection* 134: 47-82.

Galanakos, S.P., A.G.J. Bot, and G.A. Macheras. 2015. Pelvic and lower extremity injuries in Homer's *Iliad*: A review of the literature. *Journal of Trauma and Acute Care Surgery* 78(1): 204-208.

Haagsma, J.A., N. Graetz, I. Bolliger, M. Naghavi, et al. 2016. The global burden of injury: Incidence, mortality, disability-adjusted life years and time trends from the Global Burden of Disease study of 2013. *Injury Prevention* 22: 3-18.

Heil, J. 1993. *Psychology of Sport Injury*. Champaign, IL: Human Kinetics.

Hulme, A., S. McLean, P.M. Salmon, J. Thompson, B.R. Lane, and R.O. Nielsen. 2019. Computational methods to model complex systems in sports injury research: Agent-based modelling (ABM) and systems dynamics (SD) modelling. *British Journal of Sports Medicine* 53(24): 1507-1510.

Hutchison, R.L., and M.A. Hirthler. 2013. Upper extremity injuries in Homer's *Iliad*. *Journal of Hand Surgery* 38(9): 1790-1793.

Ichikawa, M., W. Chadbunchachai, and E. Marui. 2003. Effect of the helmet act for motorcyclists in Thailand. *Accident Analysis and Prevention* 35: 183-189.

Ivarsson, A., U. Johnson, M.B. Andersen, U. Tranaeus, A. Stenling, and M. Lindwall. 2017. Psychosocial factors and sports injuries: Meta-analyses for prediction and prevention. *Sports Medicine* 42: 353-365.

Kanis, J. 2007. Assessment of osteoporosis at the primary health-care level. WHO Scientific Group Technical Report.

Kayhanian, S., and R.J. Machado. 2020. Head injuries in Homer's *Iliad*. *World Neurosurgery* 143: 33-37.

Keele, K.D. 1983. *Leonardo da Vinci's Elements of the Science of Man*. New York: Academic Press.

Kegler, S.R., G.T. Baldwin, R.A. Rudd, and M.F. Ballesteros. 2017. Increases in United States life expectancy through reductions in injury-related death. *Population Health Metrics* 15: 32.

Koutserimpas, C., K. Alpantaki, and G. Samonis. 2017. Trauma management in Homer's *Iliad*. *International Wound Journal* 14(4): 682-684.

LeVay, D. 1990. *The History of Orthopaedics*. Lancashire, UK: Parthenon.

Meeuwisse, W.H. 1994. Assessing causation in sport injury: A multifactorial model. *Clinical Journal of Sport Medicine* 4: 166-170.

Meeuwisse, W.H., H. Tyreman, B. Hagel, and C. Emery. 2007. A dynamic model of etiology in sport injury: The recursive nature of risk and causation. *Clinical Journal of Sport Medicine* 17(3): 215-219.

Mylonas, A.I., F.H. Tzerbos, A.C. Eftychiadis, and E.C. Papadopolou. 2008. Cranio-maxillofacial injuries in Homer's *Iliad*. *Journal of Craniomaxillofacial Surgery* 36(1): 1-7.

National Center for Health Statistics. 2022. Health, United States 2020-2021 (cdc.gov).

National Safety Council. 2022. All Injuries Overview - Injury Facts (nsc.org). https://injuryfacts.nsc.org/all-injuries/overview/

Nixon, H.L. 1992. A social network analysis of influences on athletes to play with pain and injuries. *Journal of Sport and Social Issues* 16(2): 127-135.

Philippe, P., and O. Mansi. 1998. Nonlinearity in the epidemiology of complex health and disease processes. *Theoretical Medicine and Bioethics* 19: 591-607.

Rang, M. 2000. *The Story of Orthopaedics*. Philadelphia: Saunders.

Rice, D.P., and W. Max. 1996. Annotation: The high cost of injuries in the United States. *American Journal of Public Health* 86: 14-15.

Robertson, L.S. 2018. *Injury Epidemiology* (4th ed.). Raleigh, NC: Lulu Press.

Runge, J.W. 1993. The cost of injury. *Emergency Medicine Clinics of North America* 11: 241-253.

Salari, N., H. Ghasemi, L. Moharmmadi, M.Behzadi, E. Rabieenia, S. Shohaimi, and M. Mohammadi. 2021. The global prevalence of osteoporosis in the world: a comprehensive systematic review and meta-analysis. *Journal of Orthopaedic Surgery and Research* 16:609.

Sanders, M.S., and E.J. McCormick. 1993. *Human Factors in Engineering and Design*. New York: McGraw-Hill.

Suchman, E. 1961. On accident behavior. In *Behavioural Approaches to Accident Research*, edited by E.A. Suchman. Washington, DC: Association for the Aid to Crippled Children.

Swinney, C. 2016. Helmet use and head injury in Homer's *Iliad*. *World Neurosurgery* 90: 14-19.

Vos, T., S.S. Lim, C. Abbafati, K.M. Abbas, M. Abbasi, et al. 2020. Global burden of 369 diseases and injuries in 204 countries and territories, 1990-2019: A systematic analysis for the Global Burden of Disease Study 2019. *Lancet* 396: 1204-1222.

World Health Organization (WHO). 2014. Injuries and violence: The facts. Available: https://apps.who.int/iris/handle/10665/149798

Chapter 2

Åstrand, P.-O., K. Rodahl, H.A. Dahl, and S.B. Stromme. 2003. *Textbook of Work Physiology: Physiological Bases of Exercise* (4th ed.). Champaign, IL: Human Kinetics.

Berchuck, M., T.P. Andriacchi, B.R. Bach, and B. Reider. 1990. Gait adaptations by patients who have a deficient anterior cruciate ligament. *Journal of Bone and Joint Surgery* 72A: 871-877.

Cabral, W.A., E. Makareeva, A.D. Letocha, N. Scribanu, A. Fertala, A. Steplewski, D.R. Keene, et al. 2007. Y-Position cysteine substitution in type I collagen (Alpha1(I) R888C/p.R1066C) is associated with osteogenesis imperfecta/Ehlers-Danlos Syndrome phenotype. *Human Mutation* 28(4): 396-405. doi: 10.1002/humu.20456

Carter, D.R., G.S. Beaupre, W. Wong, R.L. Smith, T.P. Andriacchi, and D.J. Schurman. 2004. The mechanobiology of articular cartilage development and degeneration. *Clinical Orthopaedics and Related Research* 427S: S69-S77.

Currey, J.D. 2002. *Bones: Structure and Mechanics*. Princeton, NJ: Princeton University Press.

Dizon, J.M.R., and J.J.B. Reyes. 2010. A systematic review on the effectiveness of external ankle supports in the prevention of inversion ankle sprains among elite and recreational players. *Journal of Science and Medicine in Sport* 13: 309-317.

Durham, M., and S.J. Dyson. 2011. Applied anatomy of the musculoskeletal system. In *Diagnosis and Management of Lameness in the Horse* (2nd ed.), edited by M.W. Ross and S.J. Dyson. St. Louis, MO: Saunders.

Eyre, D.R. 2004. Collagens and cartilage matrix homeostasis. *Clinical Orthopaedics and Related Research* 427S: S118-S122.

Fawcett, D.W., and E. Raviola. 1994. *Bloom and Fawcett: A Textbook of Histology* (12th ed.). New York: Chapman and Hall.

Garrett, W.E., and T.M. Best. 2000. Anatomy, physiology, and mechanics of skeletal muscle. In *Orthopaedic Basic Science* (2nd ed.), edited by S.R. Simon. Park Ridge, IL: American Academy of Orthopaedic Surgeons.

Hertel, J., and Corbett, R.O. 2019. An updated model of chronic ankle instability. *Journal of Athletic Training* 54(6): 572-588.

Kim, A.W., A.M. Rosen, V.A. Brander, and T.S. Buchanan. 1995. Selective muscle activation following electrical stimulation of the collateral ligaments of the human knee joint. *Archives of Physical Medicine and Rehabilitation* 76: 750-757.

Langman, J. 1969. *Medical Embryology* (2nd ed.). Baltimore: Williams & Wilkins.

Lo, I.K.Y., G. Thornton, A. Miniaci, C.B. Frank, J.B. Rattner, and R.C. Bray. 2003. Structure and function of diarthrodial joints. In *Operative Arthroscopy* (3rd ed.), edited by J.B. McGinty. Philadelphia: Lippincott Williams & Wilkins.

Martin, R.B., and D.B. Burr. 1989. *Structure, Function, and Adaptation of Compact Bone*. New York: Raven Press.

Moffatt, C.B., and O. Cohen-Fix. 2019. The multiple ways nuclei scale on a multinucleated muscle cell scale. *Developmental Cell* 49(1): 3-5.

Morel, V., A. Mercay, and T.M. Quinn. 2005. Prestrain decreases cartilage susceptibility to injury by ramp compression in vitro. *Osteoarthritis Cartilage* 13: 964-970.

Nezwek, T., and Varacallo, M. 2019. *Physiology*. Treasure Island, FL: StatsPearls Publishing. www.ncbi.nlm.nih.gov/books/NBK542226/

Ogden, J.A. 2000a. Anatomy and physiology of skeletal development. In *Skeletal Injury in the Child* (3rd ed.), edited by J.A. Ogden. New York: Springer.

Ogden, J.A. 2000b. Injury to the growth mechanisms. In *Skeletal Injury in the Child* (3rd ed.), edited by J.A. Ogden. New York: Springer.

Ogden, J.A., and D.P. Grogan. 1987. Prenatal development and growth of the musculoskeletal system. In *The Scientific Basis of Orthopaedics* (2nd ed.), edited by J.A. Albright and R.A. Brand. Norwalk, CT: Appleton-Lange.

Ogden, J.A., D.P. Grogan, and T.R. Light. 1987. In *The Scientific Basis of Orthopaedics* (2nd ed.), edited by J.A. Albright and R.A. Brand. Norwalk, CT: Appleton-Lange.

Oinas, J., A.P. Ronkainen, L. Rieppo, M.A.J. Finnila, J.T. Livarinen, P.R. van Weeren, H.J. Helminen, P.A.J. Brama, R.K. Korhonen, and S. Saarakkala. 2018. Composition, structure and tensile biomechanical properties of equine articular cartilage during growth and maturation. *Scientific Reports* 8: 11357.

Parry, D.A.D., and J.M. Squire. 2005. Fibrous proteins: coiled coils, collagen and elastomers. In *Advances in Protein Chemistry* (vol. 70), edited by D.A.D. Parry and J.M. Squire. Amsterdam: Academic Press.

Ricard-Blum, S. 2011. The collagen family. *Cold Spring Harbor Perspectives in Biology* 3(1): a004978.

Rosier, R.N, P.R. Reynolds, and R.J. O'Keefe. 2000. Molecular and cell biology in orthopaedics. In *Orthopaedic Basic Science* (2nd ed.), edited by S.R. Simon. Park Ridge, IL: American Academy of Orthopaedic Surgeons.

Sands, W.A., D.J. Caine, and J. Borms. 2003. *Scientific Aspects of Women's Gymnastics. Series: Medicine and Sport Science* (vol. 45). Basel, Switzerland: Karger.

Shaker, J., and L. Deftos. 2018. *Calcium and Phosphate Homeostasis*. South Dartmouth, MA: EndoText. www.ncbi.nlm.nih.gov/books/NBK279023/

Shim, S.S., D.H. Copp, and F.P. Patterson. 1967. An indirect method of bone blood-flow measurement based on the clearance of a circulating bone-seeking radioisotope. *Journal of Bone and Joint Surgery* 49A: 693-702.

Silver, F.H., and G. Bradica. 2002. Mechanobiology of cartilage: How do internal and external stresses affect mechanochemical transduction and elastic energy storage? *Biomechanics and Modeling in Mechanobiology* 1: 219-238.

Slater, L.V., J.M. Hart, A.R. Kelly, and C.M. Kuenze. 2017. Progressive changes in walking kinematics and kinetics after anterior cruciate ligament injury and reconstruction: A review and meta-analysis. *Journal of Athletic Training* 52(9): 847-860.

Solomonow, M. 2004. Ligaments: A source of work-related musculoskeletal disorders. *Journal of Electromyography and Kinesiology* 14: 49-60.

Surve, I., M.P. Schwellnus, T. Noakes, and C. Lombard. 1994. A fivefold reduction in the incidence of recurrent ankle sprains in soccer players using the Sport-Stirrup orthosis. *American Journal of Sports Medicine* 22: 601-606.

Tidball, J.G. 1991. Force transmission across muscle cell membranes. *Journal of Biomechanics* 24(Suppl. 1): 43-52.

Tothill, P., and J.N. MacPherson. 1986. The distribution of blood flow to the whole skeleton in dogs, rabbits and rats measured with microspheres. *Clinical Physics and Physiological Measurement* 7: 117-123.

Tskhovrebova, L., and J. Trinick. 2010. Roles of titin in the structure and elasticity of the sarcomere. *Biomedical Research International* 2010:612482. doi: 10.1155/2010/612482

Vynios, D.H. 2014. Metabolism of cartilage proteoglycans in health and disease. *Biomedical Research International* 2014:452315.

Whiting, W.C. 2019. *Dynamic Human Anatomy* (2nd ed.). Champaign, IL: Human Kinetics.

Woo, S.L.-Y., K.-N. An, C.B. Frank, G.A. Livesay, C.B. Ma, J. Zeminski, J.S. Wayne, and B.S. Myers. 2000. Anatomy, biology, and biomechanics of tendon and ligament. In *Orthopaedic Basic Science* (2nd ed.), edited by S.R. Simon. Park Ridge, IL: American Academy of Orthopaedic Surgeons.

Zelzer, E., R. Mamiuk, N. Ferrara, R.S. Johnson, E. Schipani, and B.R. Olsen. 2004. VEGFA is necessary for chondrocyte survival during bone development. *Development* 131: 2161-2171.

Chapter 3

Bergmann, G., I. Kutzner, A. Bender, J. Dymke, A. Trepczynski, G.N. Duda, D. Felsenberg, and P. Damm. 2018. Loading of the hip and knee joints during whole body vibration training. *PLoS ONE* 13(12): e0207014. doi: 10.137/journal.pone.0207014

Blemker, S.S., and S.L. Delp. 2005. Three-dimensional representation of complex muscle architectures and geometries. *Annals of Biomedical Engineering* 33: 661-673.

Burstein, A.H., and T.M. Wright. 1994. *Fundamentals of Orthopaedic Biomechanics*. Baltimore: Williams & Wilkins.

D'Lima, D.D., B.J. Fregly, and C.W. Colwell, Jr. 2013. Implantable sensor technology: Measuring bone and joint biomechanics of daily life *in vivo. Arthritis Research & Therapy* 15: 203.

Dragoo, J.L., H.J. Braun, and A.H.S. Harris. 2013. The effect of playing surface on the incidence of ACL injuries in National Collegiate Athletic Association American football. *Knee* 20(3): 191-195.

Hubbard, M. 1993. Computer simulation in sport and industry. *Journal of Biomechanics* 26(Suppl. 1): 53-61.

Kirking, B., J. Krevolin, C. Townsend, C.W. Colwell, Jr., and D.D. D'Lima. 2006. A multiaxial force-sensing implantable tibial prosthesis. *Journal of Biomechanics* 39: 1744-1751.

Robertson, L.S. 2018. *Injury Epidemiology* (4th ed.). Morrisville, NC: Lulu Press.

Rudert, M.J., B.J. Ellis, C.R. Henak, N.J. Stroud, D.R. Pederson, J.A. Weiss, and T.D. Brown. 2014. A new sensor for measurement of dynamic contact stress in the hip. *Journal of Biomechanical Engineering* 136(3). doi: 10.1115/1.4026103

Seth, A., J.L. Hicks, T.K. Uchida, A. Habib, C.L. Dambia, J.J. Dunne, et al. 2018. OpenSim: Simulating musculoskeletal dynamics and neuromuscular control to study human and animal movement. *PLoS Computational Biology* 14(7): e1006223.

Stansfield, B.W., A.C. Nicol, J.P. Paul, I.G. Kelly, F. Graichen, and G. Bergmann. 2003. Direct comparison of calculated hip joint contact forces with those measured using instrumented implants: An evaluation of a three-dimensional mathematical model of the lower limb. *Journal of Biomechanics* 36: 929-936.

Steffen, K., T.E. Andersen, and R. Bahr. 2007. Risk of injury on artificial turf and natural grass in young female football players. *British Journal of Sports Medicine* 41(Suppl 1): i33-i37.

Viidik, A. 1968. A rheological model for uncalcified parallel-fibred collagenous tissue. *Journal of Biomechanics* 1(1): 3-7.

Westerhoff, P., F. Graichen, A. Bender, A. Rohlmann, and G. Bergmann. 2009. An instrumented implant for *in vivo* measurement of contact forces and contact moment in the shoulder joint. *Medical Engineering & Physics* 31: 207-213.

Williams, J.H., E. Akogyrem, and J.R. Williams. 2013. A meta-analysis of soccer injuries on artificial turf and natural grass. *Journal of Sports Medicine*. doi: 10.1155/2013/380523

Winter, D.A. 2009. *Biomechanics and Motor Control of Human Movement* (4th ed.). New York: Wiley.

Chapter 4

Akeson, W.H., D. Amiel, M.F. Abel, S.R. Garfin, and S.L. Woo. 1987. Effects of immobilization on joints. *Clinical Orthopaedics and Related Research* 219: 28-37.

Ashizawa, N., R. Fujimura, K. Tokuyama, and M. Suzuki. 1997. A bout of resistance exercise increases urinary calcium independently of osteoblastic activation in men. *Journal of Applied Physiology* 83: 1159-1163.

Åstrand, P.-O., K. Rodahl, H.A. Dahl, and S.B. Stromme. 2003. *Textbook of Work Physiology: Physiological Bases of Exercise* (4th ed.). Champaign, IL: Human Kinetics.

Bailey, D.A., R.A. Faulkner, and H.A. McKay. 1996. Growth, physical activity, and bone mineral acquisition. *Exercise and Sport Sciences Reviews* 24: 233-266.

Baldwin, K.M., and F. Haddad. 2002. Cellular and molecular responses to altered physical activity paradigms. *American Journal of Physical Medicine and Rehabilitation* 81(Suppl.): 40-51.

Bandy, W.D., and K. Dunleavy. 1996. Adaptability of skeletal muscle: Response to increased and decreased use. In *Athletic Injuries and Rehabilitation*, edited by J.E. Zachazewski, D.J. Magee, and W.S. Quillen. Philadelphia: Saunders.

Bass, S.L., P. Eser, and R. Daly. 2005. The effect of exercise and nutrition on the mechanostat. *Journal of Musculoskeletal and Neuronal Interactions* 5: 239-254.

Benjamin, M., and B. Hillen. 2003. Mechanical influences on cells, tissues and organs—"Mechanical morphogenesis." *European Journal of Morphology* 41: 3-7.

Beveridge, W.I.B. 1957. *The art of scientific investigation* (3rd ed.). London: Heinemann.

Bilanin, J., M. Blanchard, and E. Russek-Cohen. 1989. Lower vertebral bone density in male long distance runners. *Medicine and Science in Sports and Exercise* 21: 66-70.

Bostrom, M.P.G., A. Boskey, J.J. Kaufman, and T.A. Einhorn. 2022. Form and function of bone. In *Orthopaedic Basic Science* (5th ed.), edited by R. Aaron. Park Ridge, IL: American Academy of Orthopaedic Surgeons.

Bourrin, S., A. Toromanoff, P. Ammann, J.P. Bonjour, and R. Rizzoli. 2000. Dietary protein deficiency induces osteoporosis in aged male rats. *Journal of Bone and Mineral Research* 15: 1555-1563.

Brand-Saberi, B. 2005. Genetic and epigenetic control of skeletal muscle development. *Annals of Anatomy* 187: 199-207.

Buckingham, M., L. Bajard, T. Chang, P. Daubas, J. Hadchouel, S. Meilhac, D. Montarras, D. Rocancourt, and F. Relaix. 2003. The formation of skeletal muscle: From somite to limb. *Journal of Anatomy* 202: 59-68.

Burr, D.B., C. Milgrom, D. Fyhrie, M. Forwood, M. Nyska, A. Finestone, S. Hoshaw, E. Saiag, and A. Simkin. 1996. In vivo measurement of human tibial strains during vigorous activity. *Bone* 18: 405-410.

Chakravarthy, M.V., B.S. Davis, and F.W. Booth. 2000. IGF-1 restores satellite cell proliferative potential in immobilized old skeletal muscle. *Journal of Applied Physiology* 89: 1365-1379.

Chen, C.T., M. Bhargava, P.M. Lin, and P.A. Torzilli. 2003. Time, stress, and location dependent chondrocyte death and collagen damage in cyclically loaded articular cartilage. *Journal of Orthopaedic Research* 21: 888-898.

Chen, G., L. Liu, and J. Yu, 2012. A comparative study on strength between American college male and female students in Caucasian and Asian populations. *Sport Science Review* 21: 153-165.

Couppé, C., P. Hansen, M. Kongsgaard, V. Kovanen, C. Suetta, P. Aagaard, M. Kjaer, and S.P. Magnusson, 2009. Mechanical properties and collagen cross-linking of the patellar tendon in old and young men. *Journal of Applied Physiology* 107(3): 880-886.

Croker, S.L., W. Reed, and D. Donlon. 2016. Comparative cortical bone thickness between the long bones of humans and five common non-human mammal taxa. *Forensic Science International* 260: 104.e1-104.e17.

Crowell, H.P., and I.S. Davis. 2011. Gait retraining to reduce lower extremity loading in runners. *Clinical Biomechanics* 26(1): 78-83.

Cureton, K.J., M.A. Collins, D.W. Hill, and F.M. McElhannon, Jr. 1990. Muscle hypertrophy in men and women. *Medicine and Science in Sports and Exercise* 20: 338-344.

Currey, J.D. 1979. Mechanical properties of bone tissues with greatly differing functions. *Journal of Biomechanics* 12: 313-319.

Currey, J.D. 1988. The effect of porosity and mineral content on the Young's modulus of elasticity of compact bone. *Journal of Biomechanics* 21: 131-139.

Currey, J.D. 2002. *Bones: Structure and Mechanics*. Princeton, NJ: Princeton University Press.

Currey, J.D. 2003a. How well are bones designed to resist fracture? *Journal of Bone and Mineral Research* 18: 591-598.

Currey, J.D. 2003b. The many adaptations of bone. *Journal of Biomechanics* 36: 1487-1495.

Currey, J.D. 2005. Bone architecture and fracture. *Current Osteoporosis Reports* 3: 52-56.

Currey, J.D., and R.M. Alexander. 1985. The thickness of walls of tubular bones. *Journal of Zoology* 206: 453-468.

Darling, A.L., D.L. Millward, D.J. Torgerson, C.E. Hewitt, and S.A. Lanham-New. 2009. Dietary protein and bone health: A systematic review and meta-analysis. *The American Journal of Clinical Nutrition* 90(6): 1674-1692.

Dean, J.C., J.M. Clair-Auger, O. Lagerquist, and D.F. Collins. 2014. Asynchronous recruitment of low-threshold motor units during repetitive, low-current stimulation of the human tibial nerve. *Frontiers in Human Neuroscience* 8: 1002.

Deprez, X., and P. Fardellone. 2003. Nonpharmacological prevention of osteoporotic fractures. *Joint Bone Spine* 70: 448-457.

Doschak, M.R., and R.F. Zernicke. 2005. Structure, function and adaptation of bone-tendon and bone-ligament complexes. *Journal of Musculoskeletal and Neuronal Interactions* 5: 35-40.

Doty, S.B. 2004. Space flight and bone formation. *Materwiss Werksttech* 35: 951-961.

Ehrhardt, J., and J. Morgan. 2005. Regenerative capacity of skeletal muscle. *Current Opinion in Neurology* 18: 548-553.

Engelke, K., W. Kemmler, D. Lauber, C. Beeskow, R. Pintag, and W.A. Kalender. 2006. Exercise maintains bone density at spine and hip EFOPS: A 3-year longitudinal study in early post-menopausal women. *Osteoporosis International* 17: 133-142.

Englemark, V.E. 1961. Functionally induced changes in articular cartilage. In *Biomechanical Studies of the Musculoskeletal System*, edited by F.G. Evans. Springfield, IL: Charles C Thomas.

Flanagan, S., C. Dunn-Lewis, D. Hatfield, L. Distefanso, M. Fragala, M. Shoap, M. Gotwald, J. Trail, A. Gomez, J. Voler, C. Cortis, B. Comstock, D. Hooper, T. Szivak, D. Looney, W. DuPont, D. McDermott, M. Gaudiose, and W. Kraemer. 2015. Developmental differences between boys and girls result in sex-specific physical fitness changes from fourth to fifth grade. *Journal of Strength and Conditioning Research* 29: 175-180.

Frank, C.B. 1996. Ligament injuries: Pathophysiology and healing. In *Athletic Injuries and Rehabilitation*, edited by J.E. Zachazewski, D.J. Magee, and W.S. Quillen. Philadelphia: Saunders.

Galloway, M.T., A.L. Lalley, and J.T. Shearn. 2013. The role of mechanical loading in tendon development, maintenance, injury, and repair. *The Journal of Bone and Joint Surgery* 95(17): 1620-1628. doi: 10.2106/JBJS.L.01004

Garrett, W.E., Jr., and T.M. Best. 2022. Anatomy, physiology, and mechanics of skeletal muscle. In *Orthopaedic Basic Science* (5th ed.), edited by R. Aaron. Park Ridge, IL: American Academy of Orthopaedic Surgeons.

Gentil, P., J. Steele, M.C. Pereira, R.P. Castanheira, A. Paoli, and M. Bottaro. 2016. Comparison of upper body strength gains between men and women after 10 weeks of resistance training. *PeerJ* 4: e1627.

Giannini, S., M. Nobile, S. Sella, and L. Dalle Carbonare. 2005. Bone disease in primary hypercalciuria. *Critical Reviews in Clinical Laboratory Science* 42: 229-248.

Gregor, R.J., P.V. Komi, R.C. Browning, and M. Jarvinen. 1991. A comparison of the triceps surae and residual muscle moments at the ankle during cycling. *Journal of Biomechanics* 24: 287-297.

Haizlip, K.M., B.C. Harrison, and L.A. Leinwand. 2015. Sex-based differences in skeletal muscle kinetics and fiber-type composition. *Physiology* 30(1): 30-39.

Hakkinen, K. 2002. *Strength Training for Sport*. Malden, MA: Blackwell.

Harwood, F.L., and D. Amiel. 1992. Differential metabolic responses of periarticular ligaments and tendon to joint immobilization. *Journal of Applied Physiology* 72: 1687-1691.

Hengsberger, S., P. Ammann, B. Legros, R. Rizzoli, and P. Zysset. 2005. Intrinsic bone tissue properties in adult rat vertebrae: Modulation by dietary protein. *Bone* 36: 134-141.

Hetland, M.L., J. Haarbo, and C. Christiansen. 1993. Low bone mass and high bone turnover in male long distance runners. *Journal of Clinical Endocrinology and Metabolism* 77(3): 770-775. doi: 10.1210/jcem.77.3.8370698

Hiney, K.M., B.D. Nielsen, D. Rosenstein, M.W. Orth, and B.P. Marks. 2004. High-density exercise of short duration alters bovine bone density and shape. *Journal of Animal Science* 82: 1612-1620.

Ikai, M., and T. Fukunaga. 1968. Calculation of muscle strength per unit cross-sectional area of human muscle by means of ultrasonic measurements. *Internationale Zeitschrift Fur Angewandte Physiologie* 6: 174-177.

Iwamoto, J., C. Shimamura, T. Takeda, H. Abe, S. Ichimura, Y. Sato, and Y. Toyama. 2004. Effects of treadmill exercise on bone mass, bone metabolism, and calcitrophic hormones in young growing rats. *Journal of Bone and Mineral Research* 22: 26-31.

Jin, M., E.H. Frank, T.M. Quinn, E.B. Hunziker, and A.J. Grodzinsky. 2001. Tissue shear deformation stimulates proteoglycan and protein biosynthesis in bovine cartilage explants. *Archives of Biochemistry and Biophysics* 395: 41-48.

Kadi, F., N. Charifi, C. Denis, J. Lexell, J.L. Andersen, P. Schjerling, S. Olsen, and M. Kjaer. 2005. The behaviour of satellite cells in response to exercise: What have we learned from human studies? *Pflugers Archives* 451: 319-327.

Kaplan, F.S., W.C. Hayes, T.M. Keaveny, A. Boskey, T.A. Einhorn, and J.P. Iannotti. 1994. Form and function of bone. In *Orthopaedic Basic Science*, edited by S.R. Simon. Park Ridge, IL: American Academy of Orthopaedic Surgeons.

Kasashima, Y., R.K. Smith, H.L. Birch, T. Takahashi, K. Kusano, and A.E. Goodship. 2002. Exercise-induced tendon hypertrophy: Cross-sectional area changes during growth are influenced by exercise. *Equine Veterinary Journal* 34(Suppl.): 264-268.

Kjaer, M. 2004. Role of extracellular matrix in adaptation of tendon and skeletal muscle to mechanical loading. *Physiological Reviews* 84: 649-698.

Komi, P.V. 2003. *Strength and Power in Sport*. Oxford, UK: Blackwell Scientific.

Kopiczko, A. 2014. Assessment of intake of calcium and vitamin D and sun exposure in the context of osteoporosis risk in a study conducted on perimenopausal women. *Menopause Review (Przeglad menopauzalny)* 13(2): 79-83. doi: 10.5114/pm.2014.42707

Korpelainen, R., S. Keinanen-Kiukaanniemi, J. Heikkinen, K. Vaananen, and L. Korpelainen. 2006. Effect of impact exercise on bone mineral density in elderly women with low bone mineral density: A population-based randomized controlled 30-month intervention. *Osteoporosis International* 21: 772-779.

Lanyon, L.E. 1987. Functional strain in bone tissue as an objective and controlling stimulus for adaptive bone remodeling. *Journal of Biomechanics* 20: 1083-1093.

Lee, J.H. 2019. The effect of long-distance running on bone strength and bone biochemical markers. *Journal of Exercise Rehabilitation* 15(1): 26-30.

Li, F., E. Eckstrom, P. Harmer, K. Fitzgerald, J. Voit, and K.A. Cameron. 2016. Exercise and fall prevention: Narrowing the research-to-practice gap and enhancing integration of clinical and community practice. *Journal of the American Geriatric Society* 64(2): 425-431.

Lieberman, D.E., O.M. Pearson, J.D. Polk, B. Demes, and A.W. Crompton. 2003. Optimization of bone growth and remodeling in response to loading in tapered mammalian limbs. *Journal of Experimental Biology* 206: 3125-3138.

Linnamo, V., A. Pakarinen, P.V. Komi, W.J. Kraemer, and K. Hakkinen. 2005. Acute hormonal responses to submaximal and maximal heavy resistance and explosive exercises in men and women. *Journal of Strength Conditioning Research* 19: 566-571.

Liu, D., H.P. Veit, and D.M. Denbow. 2004. Effects of long-term dietary lipids on mature bone mineral content, collagen, crosslinks, and prostaglandin E2 production in Japanese quail. *Poultry Science* 83: 1876-1883.

Lo, I.K.Y., G. Thornton, A. Miniaci, C.B. Frank, J.B. Rattner, and R.C. Bray. 2012. Structure and function of diarthrodial joints. In *Operative Arthroscopy* (4th ed.), edited by M.D. Johnson et al. Philadelphia: Lippincott Williams & Wilkins.

Loitz, B.J., and R.F. Zernicke. 1992. Strenuous exercise-induced remodeling of mature bone: Relationships between in vivo strains and bone mechanics. *Journal of Experimental Biology* 170: 1-18.

Loitz-Ramage, B.J., and R.F. Zernicke. 1996. Bone biology and mechanics. In *Athletic Injuries and Rehabilitation*, edited by J.E. Zachazewski, D.J. Magee, and W.S. Quillen. Philadelphia: Saunders.

Lorentzon, M., D. Mellstrom, and C. Ohlsson. 2005. Association of amount of physical activity with cortical bone size and trabecular volumetric BMD in young adult men: The GOOD study. *Journal of Bone and Mineral Research* 20: 1936-1943.

Lorenz, D.S., Reiman, M.P., and Walker, J.C. 2010. Periodization: Current review and suggested implementation for athletic rehabilitation. *Sports Health* 2(6): 509-518.

Macaluso, A., and G. De Vito. 2004. Muscle strength, power, and resistance training in older people. *European Journal of Applied Physiology* 91: 450-472.

MacDougall, J., C. Webber, J. Martin, S. Ormerod, A. Chesley, E. Younglai, C. Gordon, and C. Blimkie. 1992. Relationship among running mileage, bone density, and serum testosterone in male runners. *Journal of Applied Physiology* 73: 1165-1170.

MacDougall, J.D. 2003. Hypertrophy or hyperplasia? In *Strength and Power in Sport: The Encyclopedia of Sports Medicine* (2nd ed.), edited by P. Komi. Oxford, UK: Blackwell.

Maddalozzo, G.G., J.J. Widrick, B.J. Cardinal, K.M. Winters-Stone, M.A. Hoffman, and C.M. Snow. 2007. The effects of hormone replacement therapy and resistance training on spine bone mineral density in early postmenopausal women. *Bone* 40: 1244-1251.

Mankin, H.J., V.C. Mow, J.A. Buckwalter, J.P. Iannotti, and A. Ratcliffe. 2022. Articular cartilage structure, composition and function. In *Orthopaedic Basic Science* (5th ed.), edited by R. Aaron. Park Ridge, IL: American Academy of Orthopaedic Surgeons.

Marcus, R., C. Cann, P. Madvig, J. Minkoff, M. Goddard, M. Bayer, M. Martin, W. Haskell, and H. Genant. 1985. Menstrual function and bone mass in elite women distance runners. Endocrine and metabolic features. *Annals of Internal Medicine* 102: 158-163.

Martin, R.B., D.B. Burr, and N.A. Sharkey. 2015. *Skeletal Tissue Mechanics* (2nd ed.). New York: Springer.

Matsuda, J.J., R.F. Zernicke, A.C. Vailas, A. Pedrini-Mille, and J.A. Maynard. 1986. Morphological and mechanical adaptation of immature bone to strenuous exercise. *Journal of Applied Physiology: Respiratory, Environmental, and Exercise Physiology* 60: 2028-2034.

McArdle, W.D., F.I. Katch, and V.L. Katch. 2001. *Exercise Physiology*. Philadelphia: Lippincott Williams & Wilkins.

McCall, G.E., W.C. Byrnes, and S.J. Fleck. 1999. Acute and chronic hormonal responses to resistance training designed to promote muscle hypertrophy. *Canadian Journal of Applied Physiology* 24: 96-107.

McCormack, S., D. Cousminer, A. Chesi, J. Mitchell, S. Roy, H. Kalkwarf, J. Lappe, V. Gilsanz, S. Obefield, J. Shepherd, K. Winer, A. Kelly, S. Grant, and B. Zermei. 2017. Association between linear growth and bone accrual in a diverse cohort of children and adolescents. *JAMA Pediatrics* 171(9): e171769.

Mehta, J., J. Kling, and J. Manson. 2021. Risks, benefits, and treatment modalities of menopausal hormone therapy: Current concepts. *Frontiers in Endocrinology*. 26 March. doi: 10.3389/fendo.2021.564781

Merriam-Webster. 2003. *Merriam-Webster's Collegiate Dictionary* (11th ed.). Springfield, MA: Merriam-Webster.

Mow, V.C., A. Ratcliffe, and A.R. Poole. 1992. Cartilage and diarthrodial joints as paradigms for hierarchical materials and structures. *Biomaterials* 1: 67-97.

Mullner, T., O. Kwasny, R. Reihsner, V. Lohnert, and R. Schabus. 2000. Mechanical properties of a rat patellar tendon stress-shielded in situ. *Archives of Orthopaedic and Trauma Surgery* 120: 70-74.

Musumeci, G. 2016. The effect of mechanical loading on articular cartilage. *The Journal of Functional Morphology and Kinesiology* 1(2): 154-161.

Nickien M., A. Heuijerjans, K. Ito, and C.C. van Donkelaar. 2018. Comparison between in vitro and in vivo cartilage overloading studies based on a systematic literature review. *Journal of Orthopedic Research* 36(8): 2076-2086.

North American Hormone Therapy Position Statement Advisory Panel (NHTPSAP). 2017. The 2017 hormone therapy position statement of The North American Menopause Society. *Menopause* 24(7): 728-753. doi: 10.1097/GME.0000000000000921

O'Brien, M. 2001. Exercise and osteoporosis. *Irish Journal of Medical Science* 170: 58-62.

Oftadeh, R., M. Perez-Viloria, J.C. Villa-Camacho, A. Vaziri, and A. Nazarian. 2015. Biomechanics and mechanobiology of trabecular bone: A review. *Journal of Biomechanical Engineering* 137(1): 0108021-01080215. doi: 10.1115/1.4029176

Oganov, V.S. 2004. Modern analysis of bone loss mechanisms in microgravity. *Journal of Gravitational Physiology* 11: P143-P146.

Ormerod, S., J. MacDougall, and C. Webber. 1988. The effects of different forms of exercise on bone mineral content. *Canadian Journal of Sport Science* 13: 74P.

Palmes, D., H.U. Spiegel, T.O. Schneider, M. Langer, U. Stratmann, T. Budny, and A. Probst. 2002. Achilles tendon healing: Long-term biomechanical effects of postoperative mobilization and immobilization in a new mouse model. *Journal of Orthopaedic Research* 20: 939-946.

Parfitt, A.M. 1984. The cellular basis of bone remodeling: The quantum concept reexamined in light of recent advances in the cell biology of bone. *Calcified Tissue International* 36: S38.

Parry, H.A., M.D. Roberts, and A.N. Kavazis. 2020. Human skeletal muscle mitochondrial adaptations following resistance exercise training. *International Journal of Sports Medicine* 41(6): 349-359. doi: 10.1055/a-1121-7851

Pimentel Neto, J., L.C. Rocha, G.K. Barbosa, C. dos Santos Jacob, W.K. Neto, L. Watanabe, and A.P. Ciena. 2020. Myotendinous junction adaptations to ladder-based resistance training: Identification of a new telocyte niche. *Scientific Reports* 10: 14124. doi: 10.1038/s41598-020-70971-6

Platt, M.A. 2005. Tendon repair and healing. *Clinics in Podiatric Medicine and Surgery* 22: 553-560.

Robinson, T., C. Snow-Harter, D. Taafe, D. Gillis, J. Shaw, and R. Marcus. 1995. Gymnasts exhibit higher bone mass than runners despite prevalence of amenorrhea and oligomenorrhea. *Journal of Bone and Mineral Research* 19: 26-35.

Ross, A.C., C.L. Taylor, A.L. Yaktine et al., eds. 2011. *Dietary Reference Intakes for Calcium and Vitamin D.* Washington, DC: National Academies Press. Available from: www.ncbi.nlm.nih.gov/books/NBK56060/

Rubin, C.T., and L.E. Lanyon. 1985. Regulation of bone mass by mechanical strain magnitude. *Calcified Tissue International* 37: 411-417.

Schoenfeld, B.J., B. Contreras, J. Krieger, J. Grgic, K. Delcastillo, R. Belliard, and A. Alto. 2019. Resistance training volume enhances muscle hypertrophy but not strength in trained men. *Medicine and Science in Sports and Exercise* 51(1): 94-103. doi: 10.1249/MSS.0000000000001764

Senderovich, H., and A. Kosmopoulos. 2018. An insight into the effect of exercises on the prevention of osteoporosis and associated fractures in high-risk individuals. *Rambam Maimonides Medical Journal* 9(1): e0005. doi: 10.5041/RMMJ.10325

Siddiqui, J.A., and N.C. Partridge. 2016. Physiological bone remodeling: Systemic regulation and growth factor involvement. *Physiology* 31(3): 233-245. doi: 10.1152/physiol.00061.2014

Singh, K., K. Masuda, E.J. Thonar, H.S. An, and G. Cs-Szabo. 2009. Age-related changes in the extracellular matrix of nucleus pulposus and annulus fibrosus of human intervertebral disc. *Spine* 34(1): 10-16. doi: 10.1097/BRS.0b013e31818e5ddd

Snow-Harter, C., and R. Marcus. 1991. Exercise, bone mineral density, and osteoporosis. *Exercise and Sport Sciences Reviews* 19: 351-388.

Sorrenti, S.J. 2006. Achilles tendon rupture: Effect of early mobilization in rehabilitation after surgical repair. *Foot Ankle International* 27: 407-410.

Specker, B., T. Binkley, and N. Fahrenwald. 2004. Increased periosteal circumference remains present 12 months after an exercise intervention in preschool children. *Bone* 35: 1383-1388.

Staud, R. 2005. Vitamin D: More than just affecting calcium and bone. *Current Rheumatology Reports* 7: 356-364.

Suva, L.J., D. Gaddy, D.S. Perrien, R.L. Thomas, and D.M. Findlay. 2005. Regulation of bone mass by mechanical loading: Microarchitecture and genetics. *Current Osteoporosis Report* 3: 46-51.

Tajbakhsh, S. 2003. Stem cells to tissue: Molecular, cellular and anatomical heterogeneity in skeletal muscle. *Current Opinion in Genetics and Development* 13: 413-422.

Taylor, A.H., N.T. Cable, G. Faulkner, M. Hillsdon, M. Narici, and A.K. Van Der Bij. 2004. Physical activity and older adults: A review of health benefits and the effectiveness of interventions. *Journal of Sports Science* 22: 703-725.

Tidball, J.G. 1983. The geometry of actin filament-membrane associations can modify adhesive strength of the myotendinous junction. *Cell Motility and the Cytoskeleton* 3: 439-447.

Tipton, C.M., R.D. Matthes, J.A. Maynard, and R.A. Carey. 1975. The influence of physical activity on ligaments and tendons. *Medicine and Science in Sports* 7: 165-175.

Tuukkanen, J., B. Wallmark, P. Jalovaara, T. Takala, S. Sjogren, and K. Vaananen. 1991. Changes induced in growing rat bone by immobilization and remobilization. *Bone* 12: 113-118.

Vaitkeviciute, D., E. Lätt, J. Mäestu, T. Jürimäe, M. Saar, P. Purge, K. Maasalu, and J. Jürimäe. 2014. Physical activity and bone mineral accrual in boys with different body mass parameters during puberty: A longitudinal study. *PLoS One* 9(10): e107759. doi: 10.1371/journal.pone.0107759

Wackerhage, H., B.J. Schoenfeld, D.L. Hamilton, M. Lehti, and J.J. Hulmi. 2019. Stimuli and sensors that initiate skeletal muscle hypertrophy following resistance exercise. *The Journal of Applied Physiology* 126: 30-43. doi: 10.1152/japplphysiol.00685.2018

Walker, J.M. 1996. Cartilage of human joints and related structures. In *Athletic Injuries and Rehabilitation*, edited by J.E. Zachazewski, D.J. Magee, and W.S. Quillen. Philadelphia: Saunders.

Weinkamer, R., C. Eberl, and P. Fratzl. 2019. Mechanoregulation of bone remodeling and healing as inspiration for self-repair in materials. *Biomimetics (Basel, Switzerland)* 4(3): 46. doi: 10.3390/biomimetics4030046

Williams, P.E., and G. Goldspink. 1981. Longitudinal growth of striated muscle. *Journal of Cell Science* 9: 751-767.

Wilmore, J.H. 1979. The application of science to sport: Physiological profiles of male and female athletes. *Canadian Journal of Applied Sport Science* 4: 102-115.

Woo, S.L.-Y., K.-N. An, C.B. Frank, G.A. Livesay, C.B. Ma, J. Zeminski, J.S. Wayne, and B.S. Myers. 2022. Anatomy, biology, and biomechanics of tendon and ligament. In *Orthopaedic Basic Science* (5th ed.), edited by R. Aaron. Park Ridge, IL: American Academy of Orthopaedic Surgeons.

Woo, S.L.-Y., M.A. Gomez, T.J. Sites, P.O. Newton, C.A. Orlando, and W.H. Akeson. 1987. The biomechanical and morphological changes in the medial collateral ligament of the rabbit after immobilization and remobilization. *Journal of Bone and Joint Surgery* 69A: 1200-1211.

Woo, S.L., M. Thomas, and S.S. Chan Saw. 2004. Contribution of biomechanics, orthopaedics and rehabilitation: The past, present and future. *Surgeon* 2: 125-136.

Wren, T.A.L., G.S. Beaupre, and D.R. Carter. 2000. Tendon and ligament adaptation to exercise, immobilization, and remobilization. *Journal of Rehabilitation Research and Development* 37: 217-224.

Yamada, H. 1973. *Strength of Biological Materials*. Huntington, NY: Krieger.

Yin, H., F. Price, and M.A. Rudnicki. 2013. Satellite cells and the muscle stem cell niche. *Physiological Reviews* 93(1): 23-67. doi: 10.1152/physrev.00043.2011

Zernicke, R.F., J.J. Garhammer, and F.W. Jobe. 1977. Human patellar tendon rupture: A kinetic analysis. *Journal of Bone and Joint Surgery* 59A: 179-183.

Zernicke, R.F., J. McNitt-Gray, C. Otis, B. Loitz, G. Salem, and G. Finerman. 1994. Stress fracture risk assessment among elite collegiate women runners. *Journal of Biomechanics* 27: 978-986.

Zioupos, P., and J.D. Currey. 1994. The extent of microcracking and the morphology of microcracks in damaged bone. *Journal of Materials Science* 29: 978-986.

Chapter 5

American Academy of Orthopaedic Surgeons (AAOS). 2020. *The Seventh Annual Report of the AJRR on Hip and Knee Arthroplasty*. Rosemont, IL: AAOS.

Andarawis-Puri, N., E.L. Flatow, and L.J. Soslowsky. 2015. Tendon basic science: Development, repair, regeneration, and healing. *Journal of Orthopaedic Research* 33(6): 780-784.

Anderson, R.N., A.M. Minino, L.A. Fingerhut, M. Warner, and M.A. Heinen. 2004. Deaths: Injuries, 2001. *National Vital Statistics Reports* 52: 1-86.

Brandt, K.D. 1992. The pathogenesis of osteoarthritis. *EULAR Bulletin* 3: 75-81.

Bray, R.C., P.T. Salo, I.K. Lo, P. Ackermann, J.B. Rattner, and D.A. Hart. 2005. Normal ligament structure, physiology and function. *Sports Medicine and Arthroscopy Review* 13: 127-135.

Bunn, T.L., S. Slavova, T.W. Struttmann, and S.R. Browning. 2005. Sleepiness/fatigue and distraction/inattention as factors for fatal versus nonfatal commercial motor vehicle driver injuries. *Accident Analysis and Prevention* 37: 862-869.

Cai, Y., S. Li, S. Chen, Y. Hua, and J. Shan. 2017. An ultrasound classification of anterior talofibular ligament (ATFL) injury. *Open Orthopaedics Journal* 11 (Suppl-4, M2): 610-616.

Cavaillon, J.-M., and M. Singer, eds. 2018. *Inflammation: From Molecular and Cellular Mechanisms to the Clinic*. New York: Wiley.

Chartered Institute for Ergonomics and Human Factors. 2022. Aims and Scope. *Ergonomics*. Available: tandfonline.com/journals/terg20

Chikritzhs, T., and M. Livingston. 2021. Alcohol and the risk of injury. *Nutrients* 13(8): 2777.

Close, G.L., T. Ashton, A. McArdle, and D.P.M. MacLaren. 2005. The emerging role of free radicals in delayed onset muscle soreness and contraction-induced muscle injury. *Comparative Biochemistry and Physiology, Part A* 142: 257-266.

Collins, K.H., W. Herzog, G.Z. MacDonald, R.A. Reimer, J.L. Rios, I.C. Smith, R.F. Zernicke, and D.A. Hart. 2018. Obesity, metabolic syndrome, and musculoskeletal disease: Common inflammatory pathways suggest a central role for loss of muscle integrity. *Frontiers in Physiology* 9: 1-25. doi: 10.3389/fphys.2018.00112

Committee on Trauma Research. 1985. *Injury in America: A Continuing Public Health Problem*. Washington, DC: National Academy Press.

Croft, P., C. Cooper, C. Wickham, and D. Coggon. 1992. Osteoarthritis of the hip and occupational activity. *Scandinavian Journal of Work and Environmental Health* 18: 59-63.

Day, S.M., R.F. Ostrum, E.Y.S. Chao, C.T. Rubin, H.T. Aro, and T.A. Einhorn. 1994. Bone injury, regeneration, and repair. In *Orthopaedic Basic Science*, edited by J.A. Buckwalter, T.A. Einhorn, and S.R. Simon. Park Ridge, IL: American Academy of Orthopaedic Surgeons.

Ellender, L., and M.M. Linder. 2005. Sports pharmacology and ergogenic aids. *Primary Care: Clinics in Office Practice* 32: 277-292.

Farnaghi, S., I. Prasadam, G. Cai, T. Friis, Z. Du, R. Crawford, et al. 2017. Protective effects of mitochondria-targeted antioxidant and statin on cholesterol-induced osteoarthritis. *FASEB Journal* 31: 356-367.

Felson, D.T., J.J. Anderson, A. Naimark, A.M. Walker, and R.F. Meenan. 1988. Obesity and knee osteoarthritis: The Framingham study. *Annals of Internal Medicine* 109(1): 18-24.

Frank, C.B. 1996. Ligament injuries: Pathophysiology and healing. In *Athletic Injuries and Rehabilitation* (2nd ed.), edited by J.E. Zachazewski, D.J. Magee, and W.S. Quillen. Philadelphia: Saunders.

Frank, C.B. 2004. Ligament structure, physiology and function. *Journal of Musculoskeletal and Neuronal Interactions*. 4(2): 199-201

Friel, N.A., and C.R. Chu. 2013. The role of ACL injury in the development of posttraumatic knee osteoarthritis. *Clinics in Sports Medicine* 32(1): 1-12.

Fulkerson, J.P., C.C. Edwards, and O.D. Chrisman. 1987. Articular cartilage. In *The Scientific Basis of Orthopaedics* (2nd ed.), edited by J.A. Albright and R.A. Brand. Norwalk, CT: Appleton-Lange.

Garrett, W.E., Jr., P.K. Nikolaou, B.M. Ribbeck, R.R. Glisson, and A.V. Seaber. 1988. The effect of muscle architecture on the biomechanical failure properties of skeletal muscle under passive conditions. *American Journal of Sports Medicine* 16: 7-12.

Garrett, W.E., Jr., M.R. Safran, A.V. Seaber, R.R. Glisson, and B.M. Ribbeck. 1987. Biomechanical comparison of stimulated and nonstimulated skeletal muscle pulled to failure. *American Journal of Sports Medicine* 15: 448-454.

Gorbaty, J.D., J.E. Hsu, and A.O. Gee. 2017. Classifications in brief: Rockwood classification of acromioclavicular joints separations. *Clinical Orthopaedics & Related Research* 475: 283-287.

Harris, W.H. 1986. Etiology of osteoarthritis of the hip. *Clinical Orthopaedics and Related Research* 213: 20-33.

Hartgens, F., and H. Kuipers. 2004. Effects of androgenic-anabolic steroids in athletes. *Sports Medicine* 34(8): 513-554.

Hauser, R.A., and E.E. Dolan. 2011. Ligament injury and healing: An overview of current clinical concepts. *Journal of Prolotherapy* 3(4): 836-846.

Henriksen, K., and M.A. Karsdal. 2019. Type I collagen. In *Biochemistry of Collagens, Laminins and Elastin* (2nd ed.), edited by M.A. Karsdal. Waltham, MA: Academic Press.

Hipp, J.A., and W.C. Hayes. 2003. Biomechanics of fractures. In *Skeletal Trauma: Basic Science, Management, and Reconstruction* (2nd ed.), edited by B.D. Browner, J.B. Jupiter, A.M. Levine, and P.G. Trafton. Philadelphia: Saunders.

Horton, W.E., R. Yagi, D. Laverty, and S. Weiner. 2005. Overview of studies comparing human normal cartilage with minimal and advanced osteoarthritic cartilage. *Clinical and Experimental Rheumatology* 23: 103-112.

Hotfiel, T., J. Freiwald, M.W. Hoppe, C. Lutter, R. Forst, C. Grim, W. Bloch, M. Hüttel, and R. Heiss. 2018. Advances in delayed-onset muscle soreness (DOMS): Part I: Pathogenesis and diagnostics. *Sportverletz Sportschaden* 32(4): 243-250.

Houston, C.S., and L.E. Swischuk. 1980. Varus and valgus—no wonder they are confused. *New England Journal of Medicine* 302: 471-472.

Hoy, D., J.A. Geere, F. Davatchi, B. Meggitt, and L.H. Barrero. 2014. A time for action: Opportunities for preventing the growing burden and disability from musculoskeletal conditions in low- and middle-income countries. *Best Practice & Research: Clinical Rheumatology* 28: 377-393.

Jacofsky, D.J., and M. Allen. 2016. Robotics in arthroplasty: A comprehensive review. *The Journal of Arthroplasty* 31: 2353-2363.

Jones, I.A., R. Togashi, G.F.R Hatch, III, A.E. Weber, and C.T. Vangsness, Jr. 2018. Anabolic steroids and tendons: A review of their mechanical, structural, and biologic effects. *Journal of Orthopaedic Research* 36: 2830-2841.

Kannus, P. 2000. Structure of the tendon connective tissue. *Scandinavian Journal of Medicine & Science in Sports* 10(6): 312-320.

Kanis, J.A. O. Johnell, A. Oden, H. Johansson, and E. McCloskey. 2008. FRAX™ and the assessment of fracture probability in men and women from the UK. *Osteoporosis International* 19: 385-397.

Kannus, P., and L. Józsa. 1991. Histopathological changes preceding spontaneous rupture of a tendon. A controlled study of 891 patients. *Journal of Bone and Joint Surgery* 73(10): 1507-1525.

Karsdal, M.A. 2019. *Biochemistry of Collagens, Laminins and Elastin* (2nd ed.). Waltham, MA: Academic Press.

Lawrence, R.C., M.C. Hochberg, J.L. Kelsey, F.C. McDuffie, T.A. Medsger, Jr., W.R. Felts, and L.E. Shulman. 1989. Estimates of the prevalence of selected arthritic and musculoskeletal diseases in the United States. *Journal of Rheumatology* 16(4): 427-441.

Leadbetter, W.B. 2001. Soft tissue athletic injury. In *Sports Injuries: Mechanisms, Prevention, Treatment* (2nd ed.), edited by F.H. Fu and D.A. Stone. Philadelphia: Lippincott Williams & Wilkins.

Lee, S., T.-N. Kim, and S.-H. Kim. 2012. Sarcopenic obesity is more closely associated with knee osteoarthritis than is nonsarcopenic obesity: A cross-sectional study. *Arthritis & Rheumatology*, 64: 3947-3954.

Leong, N.L., J.L. Kator, T.L. Clemens, A. James, M. Enomoto-Iwamoto, and J. Jie. 2020. Tendon and ligament healing and current approaches to tendon and ligament regeneration. *Journal of Orthopaedic Research* 38(1): 7-12.

Longo, U.G., F. Franceschi, L. Ruzzini, C. Rabitti, S. Morini, N. Maffulli, F. Forriol, and V. Denaro. 2007. Light microscopic histology of supraspinatus tendon ruptures. *Knee Surgery, Sports Traumatology, Arthroscopy* 15(11): 1390-1394.

Makhmalbaf, H., and O. Shahpari. 2018. Medial collateral ligament injury; a new classification based on MRI and clinical findings. A guide for patient selection and early surgical intervention. *Archives of Bone and Joint Surgery* 6(1): 3-7.

Mankin, H.J., V.C. Mow, J.A. Buckwalter, J.P. Iannotti, and A. Ratcliffe. 1994. Articular cartilage structure, composition and function. In *Orthopaedic Basic Science*, edited by S.R. Simon. Park Ridge, IL: American Academy of Orthopaedic Surgeons.

McMaster, P.E. 1933. Tendon and muscle ruptures. *Journal of Bone and Joint Surgery* 15: 705-722.

Merola, M., and S. Affatato. 2019. Materials for hip prostheses: A review of wear and loading considerations. *Materials* 12(3): 495.

Miller, T.R., D.C. Lestina, and G.S. Smith. 2001. Injury risk among medically identified alcohol and drug abusers. *Alcoholism: Clinical and Experimental Research* 25: 54-59.

Mueller-Wohlfahrt, H-W., L. Haensel, K. Mithoefer, J. Ekstrand, B. English, S. McNally, J. Orchard, C.N. van Dijk, G.M. Kerkhoffs, P. Schamasch, D. Blottner, L. Swaerd, E. Goedhart, and P. Ueblacker. 2013. Terminology and classification of muscle injuries in sport: The Munich consensus statement. *British Journal of Sports Medicine* 47:342-350.

National Safety Council. 2019. *Injury Facts.* Itasca, IL: National Safety Council.

Pouresmaeili, F., B. Kamalidehghan, M. Kamarehei, and Y.M. Goh. 2018. A comprehensive overview on osteoporosis and its risk factors. *Therapeutics and Clinical Risk Management* 14: 2029-2049.

Reginster, J.-Y., E. Abadie, P. Delmas, R. Rizzoli, W. Dere, P. van der Auwere, B. Avouac, M.-L. Brandi, A. Daifotis, A. Diez-Perez, G. Calvo, O. Johnell, J.-M. Kaufman, G. Kreutz, A. Laslop, F. Lekkerkerker, B. Mitlak, P. Nilsson, J. Orloff, M. Smillie, A. Taylor, Y. Tsouderos, D. Ethgen, and B. Flamion. 2006. Recommendations for an update of the current (2001) regulatory requirements for registration of drugs to be used in the treatment of osteoporosis in postmenopausal women and in men. *Osteoporosis International* 17: 1-7.

Salter, R.B. 1999. *Textbook of Disorders and Injuries of the Musculoskeletal System.* Baltimore: Williams & Wilkins.

Si, L., T.M. Winzenberg, Q. Jiang, M. Chen, and A.J. Palmer. 2015. Projection of osteoporosis-related fractures and costs in China: 2010-2050. *Osteoporosis International* 26(7): 1929-1937.

Smith, E.U.R., D.G. Hoy, M.J. Cross, L. Sanchez-Riera, F. Blyth, R. Buchbinder, R., et al. 2014. Burden of disability due to musculoskeletal (MSK) disorders. *Best Practice & Research: Clinical Rheumatology* 28: 353-366.

Sunderland, S. 1990. The anatomy and physiology of nerve injury. *Muscle Nerve* 13: 771-784.

Tanzer, M., and N. Noiseux. 2004. Osseous abnormalities and early osteoarthritis: The role of hip impingement. *Clinical Orthopaedics and Related Research* 429: 170-77.

Taylor, B., H.M. Irving, F. Kanteres, R. Room, G. Borges, C. Cherpitel, T. Greenfield, and J. Rehm. 2010. The more you drink, the harder you fall: a systematic review and meta-analysis of how acute alcohol consumption and injury or collision risk increase together. *Drug and Alcohol Dependence* 110(1-2): 108-116.

Tidball, J.G., and M. Chan. 1989. Adhesive strength of single muscle cells to basement membrane at myotendinous junction. *Journal of Applied Physiology* 67: 1063-1069.

Tidball, J.G., G. Salem, and R.F. Zernicke. 1993. Site and mechanical conditions for failure of skeletal muscle in experimental strain injuries. *Journal of Applied Physiology* 74: 1280-1286.

Viguet-Carrin, S., P. Garnero, and P.D. Delmas. 2006. The role of collagen in bone strength. *Osteoporosis International* 17(3): 319-336.

Weissmann, G. 1992. Inflammation: Historical perspective. In *Inflammation: Basic Principles and Clinical Correlates* (2nd ed.), edited by J.I. Gallin, I.M. Goldstein, and R. Snyderman. New York: Raven Press.

Woo, S.L.-Y., S.D. Abramowitch, R. Kilger, and R. Liang. 2006. Biomechanics of knee ligaments: Injury, healing, and repair. *Journal of Biomechanics* 39(1): 1-20.

Woo, S.L.-Y., K.-N. An, S.P. Arnoczky, J.S. Wayne, D.C. Fithian, and B.S. Myers. 1994. Anatomy, biology, and biomechanics of tendon, ligament, and meniscus. In *Orthopaedic Basic Science*, edited by J.A. Buckwalter, T.A. Einhorn, and S.R. Simon. Park Ridge, IL: American Academy of Orthopaedic Surgeons.

Chapter 6

Agel, J., R. Rockwood, and D. Klossner. 2016. Collegiate ACL injury rates across 15 sports: National Collegiate Athletic Association Injury Surveillance System data update (2004-2005 through 2012-2013). *Clinical Journal of Sports Medicine* 26(6): 518-523.

Agel, J., E. Arendt, and B. Bershadsky. 2005. Anterior cruciate ligament injury in National Collegiate Athletic Association basketball and soccer. *American Journal of Sports Medicine* 33: 524-531.

Ahmed, A.M., and D.L. Burke. 1983. In-vitro measurement of static pressure distribution in synovial joints: Part I. Tibial surface of the knee. *Journal of Biomechanical Engineering* 105: 216-225.

Ahmed, A.M., D.L. Burke, and A. Hyder. 1987. Force analysis of the patellar mechanism. *Journal of Orthopaedic Research* 5: 69-85.

Ahmed, A.M., D.L. Burke, and A. Yu. 1983. In-vitro measurement of static pressure distribution in synovial joints: Part II. Retropatellar surface. *Journal of Biomechanical Engineering* 105: 226-236.

Ahmed, I.M., M. Lagopoulos, P. McConnell, R.W. Soames, and G.K. Sefton. 1998. Blood supply of the Achilles tendon. *Journal of Orthopaedic Research* 16: 591-596.

Allen, C.R., G.A. Livesay, E.K. Wong, and S.L.-Y. Woo. 1999. Injury and reconstruction of the anterior cruciate ligament and knee osteoarthritis. *Osteoarthritis and Cartilage* 7: 110-121.

Allen, L.R., D. Flemming, and T.G. Sanders. 2004. Turf toe: Ligamentous injury of the first metatarsophalangeal joint. *Military Medicine* 169: xix-xxiv.

Almeida, S.A., K.M. Williams, R.A. Shaffer, and S.K. Brodine. 1999. Epidemiological patterns of musculoskeletal injuries and physical training. *Medicine and Science in Sports and Exercise* 31: 1176-1182.

Anderson, C.J., C.G. Ziegler, C.A. Wijdicks, L. Engebretsen, and R.F. LaPrade. 2012. Arthroscopically pertinent anatomy of the anterolateral and posteromedial bundles of the posterior cruciate ligament. *Journal of Bone & Joint Surgery (American)* 94: 1936-1945.

Andrews, J.R., J.C. Edwards, and Y.E. Satterwhite. 1994. Isolated posterior cruciate ligament injuries. *Clinics in Sports Medicine* 13: 519-530.

Andrews, K., A. Lu, L. Mckean, and N. Ebraheim. 2017. Review: Medial collateral ligament injuries. *Journal of Orthopaedics* 14: 550-554.

Arendt, E., B. Bershadsky, and J. Agel. 2002. Periodicity of noncontact anterior cruciate ligament injuries during the menstrual cycle. *Journal of Gender-Specific Medicine* 5: 19-26.

Arendt, E., and R. Dick. 1995. Knee injury patterns among men and women in collegiate basketball and soccer. NCAA data and review of literature. *American Journal of Sports Medicine* 23: 694-701.

Arndt, A.N., P.V. Komi, G.-P. Bruggemann, and J. Lukkariniemi. 1998. Individual muscle contributions to the in vivo Achilles tendon force. *Clinical Biomechanics* 13(7): 532-541.

Arnason, A., T.E. Andersen, I. Holme, L. Engebretsen, and R. Bahr. 2008. Prevention of hamstring strains in elite soccer: An intervention study. *Scandinavian Journal of Medicine & Science in Sports* 18(1): 40-48.

Arthur, J.R., J.M. Haglin, J.L. Makovicka, and A. Chhabra. 2020. Anatomy and biomechanics of the posterior cruciate ligament and their surgical implications. *Sports Medicine and Arthroscopy Review* 28(1): e1-e10.

Askling, C., J. Karlsson, and A. Thorstensson. 2003. Hamstring injury occurrence in elite soccer players after preseason training with eccentric overload. *Scandinavian Journal of Medicine and Science in Sports* 13: 244-250.

Bakalakos, R., I.S. Benetos, M. Rozis, J. Vlamis, and S. Pneumaticos. 2019. Posterior hip dislocation in a nonprofessional football player: A case report and review of the literature. *European Journal of Orthopaedic Surgery & Traumatology* 29: 231-234.

Baker, S.P. 1985. Fall injuries in the elderly. *Clinics in Geriatric Medicine* 1: 501-511.

Barbour, K.E., C.G. Helmick, M. Boring, and T.J. Brady. 2017. Vital signs: Prevalence of doctor-diagnosed arthritis and arthritis-attributable activity limitation—United States, 2013-2015. *Morbidity and Mortality Weekly Report* 66(9): 246-253.

Batt, M.E. 1995. Shin splints—a review of terminology. *Clinical Journal of Sports Medicine* 5: 53-57.

Beck, B.R. 1998. Tibial stress injuries. An aetiological review for the purposes of guiding management. *Sports Medicine* 26: 265-279.

Behnke, R.S., and Plant, J.L. 2022. *Kinetic Anatomy* (4th ed.). Champaign, IL: Human Kinetics.

Beiner, J.M., and P. Jokl. 2001. Muscle contusion injuries: Current treatment options. *Journal of the American Academy of Orthopaedic Surgeons* 9: 227-237.

Beiner, J.M., and P.J. Jokl. 2002. Muscle contusion injury and myositis ossificans traumatica. *Clinical Orthopaedics and Related Research* 403S: S110-S119.

Besier, T.F., C.E. Draper, G.E. Gold, G.S. Beaupré, and S.L. Delp. 2005. Patellofemoral joint contact area increases with knee flexion and weight-bearing. *Journal of Orthopaedic Research* 23: 345-350.

Bjordal, J., F. Arnly, B. Hannestad, and T. Strand. 1997. Epidemiology of anterior cruciate ligament injuries in soccer. *American Journal of Sports Medicine* 25: 341-345.

Boden, B., G. Dean, J. Feagin, and W. Garrett. 2000. Mechanisms of anterior cruciate ligament injury. *Orthopedics* 23: 573-578.

Bogey, R.A., J. Perry, and A.J. Gitter. 2005. An EMG-to-force processing approach for determining ankle muscle forces during normal human gait. *IEEE Transactions of Neural Systems and Rehabilitation Engineering* 13: 302-310.

Bradley, J., J. Klimkiewicz, M. Rytel, and J. Powell. 2002. Anterior cruciate ligament injuries in the National Football League: Epidemiology and current treatment trends among team physicians. *Arthroscopy* 18: 502-509.

Brechter, J.H., and C.M. Powers. 2002. Patellofemoral stress during walking in persons with and without patellofemoral pain. *Medicine and Science in Sports and Exercise* 34: 1582-1593.

Brechter, J.H., C.M. Powers, M.R. Terk, S.R. Ward, and T.Q. Lee. 2003. Quantification of patellofemoral joint contact area using magnetic resonance imaging. *Magnetic Resonance Imaging* 21: 955-959.

Breiul, V., C.H. Roux, and G.F. Carle. 2016. Pelvic fractures: Epidemiology, consequences, and medical management. *Current Opinion in Rheumatology* 28(4): 442-447.

Brien, W.W., S.H. Kuschner, E.W. Brien, and D.A. Wiss. 1995. The management of gunshot wounds to the femur. *Orthopedic Clinics of North America* 26: 133-138.

Brockett, C.L., D.L. Morgan, and U. Proske. 2004. Predicting hamstring strain injury in elite athletes. *Medicine and Science in Sports and Exercise* 36: 379-387.

Buerba, R.A., N.F. Fretes, S.K. Davana, and J.J. Beck. 2019. Chronic exertional compartment syndrome: Current management strategies. *Open Access Journal of Sports Medicine* 10: 71-79.

Burdett, R.G. 1982. Forces predicted at the ankle during running. *Medicine and Science in Sports and Exercise* 14: 308-316.

Butler, D.L., Y. Guan, M.D. Kay, J.F. Cummings, S.M. Feder, and M.S. Levy. 1992. Location-dependent variations in the material properties of the anterior cruciate ligament. *Journal of Biomechanics* 25: 511-518.

Carr, J.B. 2003. Malleolar fractures and soft tissue injuries of the ankle. In *Skeletal Trauma: Basic Science, Management, and Reconstruction* (3rd ed.), edited by B.D. Browner, J.B. Jupiter, A.M. Levine, and P.T. Trafton. Philadelphia: Saunders.

Cascio, B., L. Culp, and A. Cosgarea. 2004. Return to play after anterior cruciate ligament reconstruction. *Clinics in Sports Medicine* 23: 395-408.

Casparian, J.M., M. Luchi, R.E. Moffat, and D. Hinthorn. 2000. Quinolones and tendon ruptures. *Southern Medical Journal* 93: 488-491.

Centers for Disease Control and Prevention (CDC). 2022. Fact sheet risk factors for falls. Available: https://www.cdc.gov/steadi/pdf/steadi-factsheet-riskfactors-508.pdf

Chudik, S.C., A.A. Allen, V.B.S. Lopez, and R.F. Warren. 2002. Hip dislocations in athletes. *Sports Medicine and Arthroscopy Review* 10(2): 123-133.

Church, J.S., and W.J.P. Radford. 2001. Isolated compartment syndrome of the tibialis anterior muscle. *Injury, International Journal of the Care of the Injured* 32: 170-171.

Ciullo, J.V., and J.D. Shapiro. 1994. Track and field. In *Sports Injuries: Mechanisms, Prevention, Treatment*, edited by F.H. Fu and D.A. Stone. Baltimore: Williams & Wilkins.

Clark, D., J.M. Stevens, D. Tortonese, M.R. Whitehouse, D. Simpson, and J. Eldridge. 2019. Mapping the contact area of the patellofemoral joint: The relationship between stability and joint congruence. *The Bone & Joint Journal* 101-B: 552-558.

Coccolini, F., P.F. Stahel, G. Montori, W. Biffl, T.M. Horer, F. Catena, et al. 2017. Pelvic trauma: WSES classification and guidelines. *World Journal of Emergency Surgery* 12: 5.

Cooper, C., H. Inskip, P. Croft, L. Campbell, G. Smith, M. McLaren, and D. Coggon. 1998. Individual risk factors for hip osteoarthritis: Obesity, hip injury, and physical activity. *American Journal of Epidemiology* 147: 516-522.

Cooper, J., J. Tilan, A.D. Rounds, S. Rosario, K. Inaba, and G.S. Marecek. 2018. Hip dislocations and concurrent injuries in motor vehicle collisions. *Injury* 49(7): 1297-1301.

Court-Brown, C., and J. McBirnie. 1995. The epidemiology of tibial fractures. *Journal of Bone and Joint Surgery* 77B: 417-421.

Crisco, J.J., P. Jokl, G.T. Heinen, M.D. Connell, and M.M. Panjabi. 1994. A muscle contusion injury model: Biomechanics, physiology, and histology. *American Journal of Sports Medicine* 22: 702-710.

Croisier, J.L., B. Forthomme, M.H. Namurois, M. Vanderthommen, and J.M. Crielaard. 2002. Hamstring muscle strain recurrence and strength performance disorders. *American Journal of Sports Medicine* 30: 199-203.

Crossley, K.M., M. van Middelkoop, C.J. Barton, and A.G. Culvenor. 2019. Rethinking patellofemoral pain. Prevention, management and long-term consequences. *Best Practice & Research Clinical Rheumatology* 33: 48-65.

Cummings, S.R., and L.J. Melton, III. 2002. Epidemiology and outcomes of osteoporotic fractures. *The Lancet* 359: 1761-1767.

Curtis, E.M., R.J. Moon, N.C. Harvey, and C. Cooper. 2017. The impact of fragility fracture and approaches to osteoporosis risk assessment worldwide. *Bone* 104: 29-38.

Dandy, D.J. 2002. General observations on surgery of the anterior cruciate ligament. In *Oxford Textbook of Orthopedics and Trauma*, edited by C. Bulstrode, J. Buckwalter, A. Carr, L. Marsh, J. Fairbank, J. Wilson-MacDonald, and G. Bowden. Oxford, UK: Oxford University Press.

Davidson, C.W., M.J. Meriles, T.J. Wilkinson, J.S. McKie, and N.L. Gilchrist. 2001. Hip fracture mortality and morbidity—Can we do better? *New Zealand Medical Journal* 114: 329-332.

Dayton, P.D., and R.T. Bouche. 1994. Compartment syndromes. In *Musculoskeletal Disorders of the Lower Extremities*, edited by L.M. Oloff. Philadelphia: Saunders.

DeCoster, T.A., and D.R. Swenson. 2002. Femur shaft fractures. In *Oxford Textbook of Orthopedics and Trauma*, edited by C. Bulstrode, J. Buckwalter, A. Carr, L. Marsh, J. Fairbank, J. Wilson-MacDonald, and G. Bowden. Oxford, UK: Oxford University Press.

Demirag, B., C. Ozturk, Z. Yazici, and B. Sarisozen. 2004. The pathophysiology of Osgood-Schlatter disease: A magnetic resonance investigation. *Journal of Pediatric Orthopaedics B* 13: 379-382.

Diaz, J.A., D.A. Fischer, A.C. Rettig, T.J. Davis, and K.D. Shelbourne. 2003. Severe quadriceps muscle contusions in athletes. *American Journal of Sports Medicine* 31: 289-293.

Diaz, A.R., and P.Z. Navas. 2018. Risk factors for trochanteric and femoral neck fracture. *Revista Española de Cirugía Ortopédica y Traumatología* (English Edition) 62(2): 134-141.

Dictionary.com. 2022. Shin splints. https://www.dictionary.com/browse/shin-splints

Dienst, M., R.T. Burks, and P.E. Greis. 2002. Anatomy and biomechanics of the anterior cruciate ligament. *Orthopedic Clinics of North America* 33: 605-620.

Divani, K., P. Subramanian, K. Tsitskaris, D. Crone, and M. Lamba. 2013. Bilateral patellar tendon rupture. *JRSM Short Reports*. doi: 10.1177/2042533313499557

Dodwell, E.R., L.E. LaMont, D.W. Green, T.J. Pan, R.G. Marx, and S. Lyman. 2014. 20 years of pediatric anterior cruciate ligament reconstruction in New York State. *The American Journal of Sports Medicine* 42(3): 675-680.

Doherty, C., E. Delahunt, B. Caulfield, J. Hertel, J. Ryan, and C. Bleakley. 2014. The incidence and prevalence of ankle sprain injury: A systematic review and meta-analysis of prospective epidemiological studies. *Sports Medicine* 44: 123-140.

Dragoo, J.L., R.S. Lee, P. Benhaim, G.A. Finerman, and S.L. Hame. 2003. Relaxin receptors in the human female anterior cruciate ligament. *American Journal of Sports Medicine* 31: 577-584.

Duethman, N.C., R.K. Martin, A.J. Krych, M.J. Stuart, and B.A. Levy. 2020. Surgical treatment of combined ACL PCL medial side injuries. *Sports Medicine and Arthroscopy Review* 28(3): e18-e24.

Dye, S.F. 2004. Reflections on patellofemoral disorders. In *Patellofemoral Disorders: Diagnosis and Treatment*, edited by R.M. Biedert. West Sussex, UK: Wiley.

Eriksen, H.A., A. Pajala, J. Leppilahti, and J. Risteli. 2002. Increased content of type III collagen at the rupture site of human Achilles tendon. *Journal of Orthopaedic Research* 20: 1352-1357.

Etheridge, B.S., D.P. Beason, R.R. Lopez, J.E. Alonso, G. McGwin, and A.W. Eberhardt. 2005. Effects of trochanteric soft tissues and bone density on fracture of the female pelvis in experimental side impacts. *Annals of Biomedical Engineering* 33: 248-254.

Evangelidis, P.E., G.J. Massey, R.A. Ferguson, P.C. Wheeler, M.T.G. Pain, and J.P Folland. 2017. The functional significance of hamstrings composition: Is it really a "fast" muscle group? *Scandinavian Journal of Medicine & Science in Sports* 27(11): 1181-1189.

Fairclough, J., K. Hayashi, H. Toumi, K. Lyons, G. Bydder, N. Phillips, T.M. Best, and M. Benjamin. 2006. The functional anatomy of the iliotibial band during flexion and extension of the knee: Implications for understanding iliotibial band syndrome. *Journal of Anatomy* 208: 309-316.

Fanelli, G.C., and C.J. Edson. 1995. Posterior cruciate ligament injuries in trauma patients: Part II. *Arthroscopy* 11: 526-529.

Fanelli, G.C., and C.J. Edson. 2020. Combined ACL-PC-medial and lateral side injuries. *Sports Medicine and Arthroscopy Review* 28(3): 100-109.

Farrell, K.C., K.D. Reisinger, and M.D. Tillman. 2003. Force and repetition in cycling: Possible implications for iliotibial band friction syndrome. *The Knee* 10: 103-109.

Filbay, S.R., and H. Grindem. 2019. Evidence-based recommendations for the management of anterior cruciate ligament (ACL) rupture. *Best Practice & Research Clinical Rheumatology* 33: 33-47.

Foley, J., R. Elhelali, and D. Moiloa. 2019. Spontaneous simultaneous bilateral patellar tendon rupture. *British Medical Journal Case Reports* 12: e227931.

Fox, K.M., S.R. Cummings, E. Williams, and K. Stone. 2000. Femoral neck and intertrochanteric fractures have different risk factors: a prospective study. *Osteoporosis International* 11: 1018-1023.

Fredericson, M., A.G. Bergman, K.L. Hoffman, and M.S. Dillingham. 1995. Tibial stress reaction in runners: Correlation of clinical symptoms and scintigraphy with a new magnetic resonance imaging grading system. *American Journal of Sports Medicine* 23: 472-481.

Freedman, B.R., F.T. Sheehan, and A.L. Lerner. 2015. MRI-based analysis of patellofemoral cartilage contact, thickness, and alignment in extension, and during moderate and deep flexion. *Knee* 22(5): 405-410.

Fukashiro, S., P.V. Komi, M. Jarvinen, and M. Miyashita. 1995. In vivo Achilles tendon loading during jumping in humans. *European Journal of Applied Physiology and Occupational Physiology* 71: 453-458.

Funsten, R.V., P. Kinser, and C.J. Frankel. 1938. Dashboard dislocation of the hip: A report of 20 cases of traumatic dislocations. *Journal of Bone and Joint Surgery* 20A: 124-132.

Garneti, N., C. Holton, and A. Shenolikar. 2005. Bilateral Achilles tendon rupture: A case report. *Accident and Emergency Nursing* 13: 220-223.

Garrett, W.E. 1995. Basic science of musculotendinous injuries. In *The Lower Extremity and Spine in Sports Medicine*, edited by J.A. Nicholas and E.B. Hershman. St. Louis: Mosby-Year Book.

Garrett, W.E., F.R. Rich, P.K. Nikolaou, and J.B. Vogler. 1989. Computed tomography of hamstring muscle strains. *Medicine and Science in Sports and Exercise* 21: 506-514.

Garrett, W.E., Jr., M.R. Safran, A.V. Seaber, R.R. Glisson, and B.M. Ribbeck. 1987. Biomechanical comparison of stimulated and nonstimulated skeletal muscle pulled to failure. *American Journal of Sports Medicine* 15: 448-454.

Gheidi, N., T.W. Keernozek, J.D. Willson, A. Revak, and K. Diers. 2018. Achilles tendon loading during weight bearing exercises. *Physical Therapy in Sport* 32: 260-268.

Giddings, V.L., G.S. Beaupre, R.T. Whalen, and D.R. Carter. 2000. Calcaneal loading during walking and running. *Medicine and Science in Sports and Exercise* 32: 627-634.

Gindele, A., D. Schwamborn, K. Tsironis, and G. Benz-Bohm. 2000. Myositis ossificans traumatica in young children: Report of three cases and review of the literature. *Pediatric Radiology* 30: 451-459.

Goff, J.D., and R. Crawford. 2011. Diagnosis and treatment of plantar fasciitis. *American Family Physician* 84(6): 676-682.

Gokcen, E.C., A.R. Burgess, J.H. Siegel, S. Mason-Gonzalez, P.C. Dischinger, and S.M. Ho. 1994. Pelvic fracture mechanism of injury in vehicular trauma patients. *Journal of Trauma* 36: 789-796.

Goldblatt, J., S. Fitzsimmons, E. Balk, and J. Richmond. 2005. Reconstruction of the anterior cruciate ligament: Meta-analysis of patellar tendon versus hamstring tendon autograft. *Arthroscopy* 21: 791-803.

Gornitzky, A.L., A. Lott, J.L. Yellin, P.D. Fabricant, J.T. Lawrence, and T.J. Ganley. 2015. Sport-specific yearly risk and incidence of anterior cruciate ligament tears in high school athletes: A systematic review and meta-analysis. *The American Journal of Sports Medicine* 44(10): 2716-2723.

Grabiner, M.D., M.J. Pavol, and T.M. Owings. 2002. Can fall-related hip fractures be prevented by characterizing the biomechanical mechanisms of failed recovery? *Endocrine* 17: 15-20.

Griffin, L.Y., J. Agel, M.J. Albohm, E.A. Arendt, R.W. Dick, W.E. Garrett, J.G. Garrick, T.E. Hewett, L. Huston, M.L. Ireland, R.J. Johnson, W.B. Kibler, S. Lephart, J.L. Lewis, T.N. Lindenfeld, B.R. Mandelbaum, P. Marchak, C.C. Teitz, and E.M. Wojtys. 2000. Noncontact anterior cruciate ligament injuries: Risk factors and prevention strategies. *Journal of the American Academy of Orthopaedic Surgeons* 8: 141-150.

Grood, E.S., F.R. Noyes, D.L. Butler, and W.J. Suntary. 1981. Ligamentous and capsular restraints preventing straight medial and lateral laxity in intact human cadaver knees. *Journal of Bone and Joint Surgery* 63A: 1257-1269.

Gulli, B., and D. Templeman. 1994. Compartment syndrome of the lower extremity. *Orthopedic Clinics of North America* 25: 677-684.

Hallén, L.G., and O. Lindahl. 1965. Rotation in the knee-joint in experimental injury to the ligaments. *Acta Orthopaedica Scandinavica* 36(4): 400-407.

Hallén, L.G., and O. Lindahl. 1966. The "screw-home" movement in the knee-joint. *Acta Orthopaedica Scandinavica* 37(1): 97-106.

Hammad, Y.N., A. Johnson, and A. Norrish. 2018. Chronic osteomyelitis of the tibia in a runner; catastrophic consequences of shin splints. *British Medical Journal Case Reports.* doi: 10.1136/bcr-2017-223186

Hayes, W.C., E.G. Myers, J.N. Morris, T.N. Gerhart, H.S. Yett, and L.A. Lipsitz. 1993. Impact near the hip dominates fracture risk in elderly nursing home residents who fall. *Calcified Tissue International* 52: 192-198.

Herzog, M.M., Z.Y. Kerr, S.W. Marshall, and E.A. Wikstrom. 2019. Epidemiology of ankle sprains and chronic ankle instability. *Journal of Athletic Training* 54(6): 603-610.

Hewett, T., G. Myer, and K. Ford. 2005. Reducing knee and anterior cruciate ligament injuries among female athletes: A systematic review of neuromuscular training interventions. *Journal of Knee Surgery* 18: 82-88.

Hicks, J.H. 1954. The mechanics of the foot. II. The plantar aponeurosis and the arch. *Journal of Anatomy* 88: 25-30.

Hierton, C. 1983. Regional blood flow in experimental myositis ossificans. *Acta Orthopaedica Scandinavica* 54: 58-63.

Hirano, A., T. Fukubayashi, T. Ishii, and N. Ochiai. 2002. Magnetic resonance imaging of Osgood-Schlatter disease: The course of the disease. *Skeletal Radiology* 31: 334-342.

Hubbell, J.D., and E. Schwartz. 2005. Anterior cruciate ligament injury. Available: www.emedicine.com/sports /topic9.htm.

Huberti, H.H., and W.C. Hayes. 1984. Patellofemoral contact pressures: The influence of q-angle and tendofemoral contact. *Journal of Bone and Joint Surgery* 66A: 715-724.

Huberti, H.H., W.C. Hayes, J.L. Stone, and G.T. Shybut. 1984. Force ratios in the quadriceps tendon and ligamentum patellae. *Journal of Orthopaedic Research* 2: 49-54.

Hull, M.L., and C.D. Mote. 1980. Leg loading in snow skiing: Computer analyses. *Journal of Biomechanics* 13: 481-491.

Hungerford, D.S., and M. Barry. 1979. Biomechanics of the patellofemoral joint. *Clinical Orthopaedics and Related Research* 144: 9-15.

Hunt, K.J., P. Phisitkul, J. Pirolo, and A. Amendola. 2015. High ankle sprains and syndesmotic injuries in athletes. *Journal of the American Academy of Orthopaedic Surgeons* 23: 661-673.

Hurschler, C., R. Vanderby, Jr., D.A. Martinez, A.C. Vailas, and W.D. Turnipseed. 1994. Mechanical and biochemical analyses of tibial compartment fascia in chronic compartment syndrome. *Annals of Biomedical Engineering* 22: 272-279.

Inman, V.T. 1976. *The Joints of the Ankle*. Baltimore: Williams & Wilkins.

Inoue, M., E. McGurk-Burleson, J.M. Hollis, and S.L.-Y. Woo. 1987. Treatment of the medial collateral ligament injury. *American Journal of Sports Medicine* 15: 15-21.

Ireland, M.L. 2002. The female ACL: Why is it more prone to injury? *Orthopedic Clinics of North America* 33: 637-651.

Ireland, M.L., and S.M. Ott. 2001. Special concerns of the female athlete. In *Sports Injuries: Mechanisms, Prevention, Treatment*, edited by F.H. Fu and D.A. Stone. Philadelphia: Lippincott Williams & Wilkins.

Jarvholm, B., R. Lundstrom, H. Malchau, B. Rehn, and E. Vingard. 2004. Osteoarthritis in the hip and whole-body vibration in heavy vehicles. *International Archives of Occupational and Environmental Health* 77: 424-426.

Järvinen, T.A., P. Kannus, M. Paavola, T.L. Järvinen, L. Józsa, and M. Järvinen. 2001. Achilles tendon injuries. *Current Opinions in Rheumatology* 13: 150-155.

Joglekar, S.B., and S. Rehman. 2009. Delayed onset thigh compartment syndrome secondary to contusion. *Orthopedics* 32(8): doi: 10.3928/01477447-20090624-09

Johnell, O., and J.A. Kanis. 2004. An estimate of the world-wide prevalence, mortality and disability associated with hip fracture. *Osteoporosis International* 15: 897-902.

Johnell, O., A. Rausing, B. Wendeberg, and N. Westlin. 1982. Morphological bone changes in shin splints. *Clinical Orthopaedics and Related Research* 167: 180-184.

Józsa, L., J.B. Balint, P. Kannus, A. Reffy, and M. Barzo. 1989. Distribution of blood groups in patients with tendon rupture. *Journal of Bone and Joint Surgery* 71B: 272-274.

Kaeding, C.C., B. Léger-St-Jean, and R.A. Magnussen. 2016. Epidemiology and diagnosis of anterior cruciate ligament injuries. *Clinics in Sports Medicine.* doi: 10.1016/j. csm.2016.08.001

Kanis, J.A., A. Odén, E.V. McCloskey, H. Johansson, D.A. Wahl, and C. Cooper. 2012. A systematic review of hip fracture incidence and probability of fracture worldwide. *Osteoporosis International* 23: 2239-2256.

Kannus, P., J. Bergfeld, M. Järvinen, R.J. Johnson, M. Pope, P. Renström, and K. Yasuda. 1991. Injuries to the posterior cruciate ligament of the knee. *Sports Medicine* 12: 110-131.

Kellersmann, R., T.R. Blattert, and A. Weckbach. 2005. Bilateral patellar tendon rupture without predisposing systemic disease or steroid use: A case report and review of the literature. *Archives of Orthopaedic Trauma and Surgery* 125: 127-133.

Khaund, R., and S.H. Flynn. 2005. Iliotibial band syndrome: A common source of knee pain. *American Family Physician* 71: 1545-1550.

Kibler, W.B., and T.J. Chandler. 1994. Racquet sports. In *Sports Injuries: Mechanisms, Prevention, Treatment*, edited by F.H. Fu and D.A. Stone. Baltimore: Williams & Wilkins.

Kibler, W.B., C. Goldberg, and T.J. Chandler. 1991. Functional biomechanical deficits in running athletes with plantar fasciitis. *American Journal of Sports Medicine* 19: 66-71.

King, J.B. 1998. Post-traumatic ectopic calcification in the muscles of athletes: A review. *British Journal of Sports Medicine* 32: 287-290.

Kirk, K.L., T. Kuklo, and W. Klemme. 2000. Iliotibial band friction syndrome. *Orthopedics* 23: 1209-1214.

Komi, P.V., S. Fukashiro, and M. Järvinen. 1992. Biomechanical loading of Achilles tendon during normal locomotion. *Clinics in Sports Medicine* 11: 521-531.

Koulouris, G., and D. Connell. 2003. Evaluation of the hamstring muscle complex following acute injury. *Skeletal Radiology* 32: 582-589.

Kransdorf, M.J., J.M. Meis, and J.S. Jelinek. 1991. Myositis ossificans: MR appearance with radiologic-pathologic correlation. *American Journal of Roentgenology* 157: 1243-1248.

Kujala, U.M., M. Järvinen, A. Natri, M. Lehto, O. Nelimarkka, M. Hurme, L. Virta, and J. Finne. 1992. ABO blood groups and musculoskeletal injuries. *Injury* 23: 131-133.

Kumar, G., and R.W. Parkinson. 2002. Is the mechanism of traumatic posterior dislocation of the hip a brake pedal injury rather than a dashboard injury? *Injury* 33(6): 548.

Kvist, M. 1994. Achilles tendon injuries in athletes. *Sports Medicine* 18: 173-201.

Lam, F., J. Walczak, and A. Franklin. 2001. Traumatic asymmetrical bilateral hip dislocation in an adult. *Emergency Medicine Journal* 18: 506-507.

Ladenhauf, H.N., G. Seitliner, and D.W. Green. 2020. Osgood-Schlatter disease: A 2020 update of a common knee condition in children. *Current Opinion in Pediatrics* 32(1): 107-112.

Lange, T., E. Taghizadeh, B.R. Knowles, N.P Südkamp, M. Zaitsev, H. Meine, and K. Izadpanah. 2019. Quantification of patellofemoral cartilage deformation and contact area changes in response to static loading via high-resolution MRI with prospective motion correction. *Journal of Magnetic Resonance Imaging* 50(5): 1561-1570.

La Porta, G.A., and P.C. La Fata. 2005. Pathologic conditions of the plantar fascia. *Clinics in Podiatric Medicine and Surgery* 22(1): 1-9.

LaPrade, C.M., D.M. Civitarese, M.T. Rasmussen, and R.F. LaPrade. 2015. Emerging updates on the posterior cruciate ligament: A review of the current literature. *American Journal of Sports Medicine* 43(12): 3077-3092.

Lau, S., M. Bozin, and T. Thillainadesan. 2017. Lisfranc fracture dislocation: A review of a commonly missed injury of the midfoot. *Emergency Medicine Journal* 34: 52-56.

Lauritzen, J.B. 1997. Hip fractures. Epidemiology, risk factors, falls, energy absorption, hip protectors, and prevention. *Danish Medical Bulletin* 44: 155-168.

Leadbetter, W.B. 2001. Soft tissue athletic injury. In *Sports Injuries: Mechanisms, Prevention, Treatment*, edited by F.H. Fu and D.A. Stone. Philadelphia: Lippincott Williams & Wilkins.

LeBlanc, K.E., H.L. Muncie, Jr., and L.L. LeBlanc. 2014. Hip fracture: Diagnosis, treatment, and secondary prevention. *American Family Physician* 89(12): 945-951.

Lee, H.L. 2019. Causal association between smoking behavior and the decreased risk of

osteoarthritis: A Mendelian randomization. Zeitschrift für Rheumatologie 78(5): 461-466.

Levin, P.E., and B.D. Browner. 1991. Dislocations and fracture-dislocations of the hip. In *The Hip and Its Disorders*, edited by M.E. Steinberg. Philadelphia: Saunders.

Levy, A.S., J. Bromberg, and D. Jasper. 1994. Tibia fractures produced from the impact of a baseball bat. *Journal of Orthopaedic Trauma* 8: 154-158.

Lewiecki, E.M., N.C. Wright, J.R. Curtis, E. Siris, R.F. Gagel, K.G. Saag, A.J. Singer, P.M. Steven, and R.A. Adler. 2018. Hip fracture trends in the United States, 2022 to 2015. *Osteoporosis International* 29: 717-722.

Lieber, R.L., and J. Friden. 2002. Mechanisms of muscle injury gleaned from animal models. *American Journal of Physical Medicine and Rehabilitation* 81(11 Suppl.): S70-S79.

Lievense, A.M., S.M.A. Bierma-Zeinstra, A.P. Verhagen, M.E. van Baar, J.A.N. Verhaar, and B.W. Koes. 2002. Influence of obesity on the development of osteoarthritis of the hip: A systematic review. *Rheumatology* 41: 1155-1162.

Linko, E., A. Harilainen, A. Malmivaara, and S. Seitsalo. 2005. Surgical versus conservative interventions for anterior cruciate ligament ruptures in adults. *The Cochrane Database of Systematic Reviews* 2: CD001356.

Lofman, O., K. Berglund, L. Larsson, and G. Toss. 2002. Changes in hip fracture epidemiology: Redistribution between ages, genders and fracture types. *Osteoporosis International* 13: 18-25.

Long, W.T., W. Chang, and E.W. Brien. 2003. Grading system for gunshot injuries to the femoral diaphysis in civilians. *Clinical Orthopedics* 408: 92-100.

Louw, M., and C. Deary. 2014. The biomechanical variables involved in the aetiology of iliotibial band syndrome in distance runners—A systematic review of the literature. *Physical Therapy in Sport* 15(1): 64-75.

Maffulli, N., J.A. Reaper, S.W. Waterston, and T. Ahya. 2000. ABO blood groups and Achilles tendon rupture in the Grampian Region of Scotland. *Clinical Journal of Sports Medicine* 10: 269-271.

Maffulli, N., and J. Wong. 2003. Rupture of the Achilles and patellar tendons. *Clinics in Sports Medicine* 22: 761-776.

Magnusson, H.I., N.E. Westlin, F. Nyqvist, P. Gärdsell, E. Seeman, and M.K. Karlsson. 2001. Abnormally decreased regional bone density in athletes with medial tibial stress syndrome. *American Journal of Sports Medicine* 29: 712-715.

Mahan, K.T., and S.R. Carter. 1992. Multiple ruptures of the tendo Achillis. *Journal of Foot Surgery* 31: 548-559.

Mandelbaum, B.R., H.J. Silvers, D.S. Watanabe, J.F. Knarr, S.D. Thomas, L.Y. Griffin, D.T. Kirkendall, and W. Garrett. 2005. Effectiveness of a neuromuscular and proprioceptive training program in preventing anterior cruciate ligament injuries in female athletes: 2-year follow-up. *American Journal of Sports Medicine* 33: 1003-1010.

Markolf, K.L., D.M. Burchfield, M.M. Shapiro, M.F. Shepard, G.A. Finerman, and J.L. Slauterbeck. 1995. Combined knee loading states that generate high anterior cruciate ligament forces. *Journal of Orthopaedic Research* 13: 930-935.

Markolf, K.L., J.R. Slauterbeck, K.L. Armstrong, M.S. Shapiro, and G.A. Finerman. 1996. Effects of combined knee loadings on posterior cruciate ligament force generation. *Journal of Orthopaedic Research* 14: 633-638.

Markolf, K.L., J.R. Slauterbeck, K.L. Armstrong, M.S. Shapiro, and G.A. Finerman. 1997. A biomechanical study of replacement of the posterior cruciate ligament with a graft. Part II: Forces in the graft compared with forces in the intact ligament. *Journal of Bone and Joint Surgery* 79A: 381-386.

Marks, R., J.P. Allegrante, C.R. MacKenzie, and J.M. Lane. 2003. Hip fractures among the elderly: Causes, consequences and control. *Ageing Research Reviews* 2: 57-93.

Matsumoto, K., H. Sumi, Y. Sumi, and K. Shimizu. 2003. An analysis of hip dislocations among snowboarders and skiers: A 10-year prospective study from 1992 to 2002. *Journal of Trauma* 55: 946-948.

Mauntel, T.C., E.A. Wikstrom, K.G. Roos, A. Djoko, T.P. Dompier, and Z.Y. Kerr. 2017. The epidemiology of high ankle sprains in National Collegiate Athletic Association sports. *The American Journal of Sports Medicine* 45(9): 2156-2163.

McLean, S., X. Huang, A. Su, A. Van den Bogert. 2004. Sagittal plane biomechanics cannot injure the ACL during sidestep cutting. *Clinical Biomechanics* 19: 828-838.

McLean, S., X. Huang, A. Su, A. Van den Bogert. 2005. Association between lower extremity posture at contact and peak knee valgus moment during sidestepping: Implications for ACL injury. *Clinical Biomechanics* 20: 863-870.

McNulty, A.L., and F. Guilak. 2015. Mechanobiology of the meniscus. *Journal of Biomechanics* 48(8): 1469-1478.

Medici, D., and B.R. Olsen. 2012. The role of endothelial-mesenchymal transition in heterotopic ossification. *Journal of Bone & Mineral Research*, 27(8): 1619-1622.

Merriam-Webster. 2005. *Merriam-Webster's Medical Desk Dictionary*. Springfield, MA: Merriam-Webster.

Michelson, J.D., A. Myers, R. Jinnah, Q. Cox, and M. Van Natta. 1995. Epidemiology of hip fractures among the elderly. Risk factors for fracture type. *Clinical Orthopaedics and Related Research* 311: 129-135.

Miyasaka, K.C., D.M. Daniel, M.L. Stone, and P. Hirshman. 1991. The incidence of knee ligament injuries in the general population. *American Journal of Knee Surgery* 4: 3-8.

Moen, M.H., J.L. Tol, A. Weir, M. Steunebrink, and T.C. De Winter. 2009. Medial tibial stress syndrome: A critical review. *Sports Medicine* 39(7): 523-546.

Monma, H., and T. Sugita. 2001. Is the mechanism of traumatic posterior dislocation of the hip a brake pedal injury rather than a dashboard injury? *Injury, International Journal for Care of the Injured* 32: 221-222.

Montalvo, A.M., D.K. Schneider, K.E. Webster, L. Yut, M.T. Galloway, R.S. Heidt, Jr., C.C. Kaeding, T.E. Kremcheck, R.A. Magnussen, S.N. Parikh, D.T. Stanfield, E.J. Wall, and G.D. Myer. 2019. Anterior cruciate ligament injury risk in sport: A systematic review and meta-analysis of injury incidence by sex and sport classification. *Journal of Athletic Training* 54(5): 472-482.

Moorman, C.T., III, R.F. Warren, E.B. Hershman, J.F. Crowe, H.G. Potter, R. Barnes, S.J. O'Brien, and J.H. Guettler. 2003. Traumatic posterior hip subluxation in American football. *Journal of Bone and Joint Surgery* 85A: 1190-1196.

Morse, K.W., A. Premkumar, A. Zhu, R. Morgenstern, and E.P. Su. 2021. Return to sport after hip resurfacing arthroplasty. *Orthopaedic Journal of Sports Medicine* 9(5): 1-8.

Mubarak, S.J. 1981. *Compartment Syndromes and Volkmann's Contracture*. Philadelphia: W.B. Saunders.

Mulvad, B., R.O. Nielsen, M. Lind, and D. Ramskov. 2018. Diagnoses and time to recovery among injured recreational runners in the RUN CLEVER trial. *PLoS ONE* 13(10): e0204742.

Myer, G., K. Ford, and T. Hewett. 2005. The effects of gender on quadriceps muscle activation strategies during a maneuver that mimics a high ACL injury risk position. *Journal of Electromyographical Kinesiology* 115: 181-189.

Myer, G.D., D. Sugimoto, S. Thomas, and T.E. Hewett. 2013. The influence of age on the M effectiveness of neuromuscular training to reduce anterior cruciate ligament injury in female athletes: A meta-analysis. *American Journal of Sports Medicine* 41(1): 203-215.

Myklebust, G., L. Engebretsen, I. Braekken, A. Skjolberg, O. Olsen, and R. Bahr. 2003. Prevention of anterior cruciate ligament injuries in female team handball players: A prospective intervention study over three seasons. *Clinical Journal of Sports Medicine* 13: 71-78.

Noonan, T.J., and W.E. Garrett. 1992. Injuries at the myotendinous junction. *Clinics in Sports Medicine* 11: 783-806.

Norman, A., and H.D. Dorfman. 1970. Juxtacortical circumscribed myositis ossificans: Evolution and radiographic features. *Radiology* 96: 304-306.

Nowinski, R.J., and C.T. Mehlman. 1998. Hyphenated history: Osgood-Schlatter disease. *American Journal of Orthopaedics* 27: 584-585.

Noyes, F.R., and S. Barber-Westin, eds. 2018. *ACL Injuries in the Female Athlete: Causes, Impacts, and Conditioning Programs* (2nd ed.). New York: Springer.

O'Donoghue, D.H. 1984. *Treatment of Injuries to Athletes* (4th ed.). Philadelphia: Saunders.

Opar, D.A., M.D. Williams, and A.J. Shield. 2012. Hamstring strain injuries: Factors that lead to injury and re-injury. *Sports Medicine* 42(3): 209-226.

Orava, S., J.-J. Siinikumpu, J. Sarimo, L. Lempainen, G. Mann, and I. Hetsroni. 2017. Surgical excision of symptomatic mature posttraumatic myositis ossificans: Characteristics and outcomes in 32 athletes. *Knee Surgery, Sports Traumatology, Arthroscopy* 25(12): 3961-3968.

Orchard, J.W. 2001. Intrinsic and extrinsic risk factors for muscle strains in Australian football. *American Journal of Sports Medicine* 29: 300-303.

Owings, T.M., M.J. Pavol, and M.D. Grabiner. 2001. Mechanisms of failed recovery following postural perturbations on a motorized treadmill mimic those associated with an actual forward trip. *Clinical Biomechanics* 16: 813-819.

Pajala, A., J. Melkko, J. Leppilahti, P. Ohtonen, Y. Soini, and J. Risteli. 2009. Tenascin-C and type I and III collagen expression in total Achilles tendon rupture. An immunohistochemical study. *Histology and Histopathology* 24(10): 1207-1211.

Papadimitropoulos, E.A., P.C. Coyte, R.G. Josse, and C.E. Greenwood. 1997. Current and projected rates of hip fracture in Canada. *Canadian Medical Association Journal* 157: 1357-1363.

Paul, J., K. Spindler, J. Andrish, R. Parker, M. Secic, and J. Bergfeld. 2003. Jumping versus nonjumping anterior cruciate ligament injuries: A comparison of pathology. *Clinical Journal of Sports Medicine* 13: 1-5.

Pavol, M.J., T.M. Owings, K.T. Foley, and M.D. Grabiner. 1999. Gait characteristics as risk factors for falling from trips induced in older adults. *The Journals of Gerontology Series A Biological Sciences and Medical Sciences* 54: M583-M590.

Pavol, M.J., T.M. Owings, K.T. Foley, and M.D. Grabiner. 2001. Mechanisms leading to a fall from an induced trip in healthy older adults. *The Journals of Gerontology Series A Biological Sciences and Medical Sciences* 56: M428-M437.

Petersen, W., C. Braun, W. Bock, K. Schmidt, A. Weimann, W. Drescher, E. Eiling, R. Stange, T. Fuchs, J. Hedderich, and T. Zantop. 2005. A controlled prospective case control study of a prevention training program in female team handball players: The German experience. *Archives of Orthopaedic Trauma and Surgery* 125: 614-621.

Peterson, L., and P. Renström. 2001. *Sports Injuries: Their Prevention and Treatment.* Champaign, IL: Human Kinetics.

Peterson, L., and P. Renström. 2017. *Sports Injuries: Prevention, Treatment and Rehabilitation* (4th ed.). Champaign, IL: Human Kinetics.

Petushek, E.J., D. Sugimoto, M. Stoolmiller, G. Smith, and G.D. Myer. 2019. Evidence-based best-practice guidelines for preventing anterior cruciate ligament injuries in young female athletes: A systematic review and meta-analysis. *American Journal of Sports Medicine* 47(7): 1744-1753.

Piziali, R.L., J. Rastegar, D.A. Nagel, and D.J. Schurman. 1980. The contribution of the cruciate ligaments to the load-displacement characteristics of the human knee joint. *Journal of Biomechanical Engineering* 102: 277-283.

Poppe, T., D. Reinhardt, A. Tarakemeh, B.G. Vopat, and M.K. Mulcahey. 2019. Turf toe: Presentation, diagnosis, and management. *Journal of Bone and Joint Surgery Reviews* 7(8): e7. doi: 10.2106/JBJS.RVW.18.00188

Pourcelot, P., M. Defontaine, B. Ravary, M. Lemâtre, and N. Crevier-Denoix. 2005. A non-invasive method of tendon force measurement. *Journal of Biomechanics* 38: 2124-2129.

Powers, C.M. 2003. The influence of altered lower-extremity kinematics on patellofemoral joint dysfunction: A theoretical approach. *Journal of Orthopaedic and Sports Physical Therapy* 33: 639-646.

Powers, C.M., Y.-J. Chen, I.S. Scher, and T.Q. Lee. 2010. Multiplane loading of the extensor mechanism alters the patellar ligament force/quadriceps force ratio. *Journal of Biomechanical Engineering* 132(2): 024503. doi: 10.1115/1.4000852

Powers, C.M., J.C. Lilley, and T.Q. Lee. 1998. The effects of axial and multi-plane loading of the extensor mechanism on the patellofemoral joint. *Clinical Biomechanics* 13: 616-624.

Powers, C.M., E. Witvrouw, I.S. Davis, and K.M. Crossley. 2017. Evidence-based framework for a pathomechanical model of patellofemoral pain: 2017 patellofemoral pain consensus statement from the 4th International Patellofemoral Pain Research Retreat, Manchester, UK: part 3. *British Journal of Sports Medicine* 51: 1713-1723.

Proske, U., D.L. Morgan, C.L. Brockett, and P. Percival. 2004. Identifying athletes at risk of hamstring strains and how

to protect them. *Clinical Experiments in Pharmacology and Physiology* 31: 546-550.

Quarles, J.D., and R.G. Hosey. 2004. Medial and lateral collateral injuries: Prognosis and treatment. *Primary Care* 31: 957-975.

Quintana, J.M., I. Arostegui, A. Escobar, J. Azkarate, J.I. Goenaga, and I. Lafuente. 2008. Prevalence of knee and hip osteoarthritis and the appropriateness of joint replacement in an older population. *Archives of Internal Medicine* 168(14): 1576-1584.

Ramirez, R.N., K. Baldwin, and C.C.D. Franklin. 2014. Prevention of anterior cruciate ligament rupture in female athletes. *JBJS Reviews* 2(9): e3.

Reeves, N.D., and G. Cooper. 2017. Is human Achilles tendon deformation greater in regions where cross-sectional area is smaller? *Journal of Experimental Biology* 220: 1634-1642.

Ren, Y., J. Hu, B. Lu, W. Zhou, and B. Tan. 2019. Prevalence and risk factors of hip fracture in a middle-aged and older Chinese population. *Bone* 122: 143-149.

Revak, A., K. Diers, T.W. Kernozek, N. Gheidi, and C. Olbrantz. 2017. Achilles tendon loading during heel-raising and -lowering exercises. *Journal of Athletic Training* 52(2): 89-96.

Ribbans, W.J., and M. Collins. 2013. Pathology of the tendo Achillis: Do our genes contribute? *The Bone and Joint Journal* 95-B: 306-313.

Robinovitch, S.N., T.A. McMahon, and W.C. Hayes. 1995. Force attenuation in trochanteric soft tissues during impact from a fall. *Journal of Orthopaedic Research* 13: 956-962.

Rose, P.S., and F.J. Frassica. 2001. Atraumatic bilateral patellar tendon rupture, a case report and review of the literature. *Journal of Bone and Joint Surgery* 83: 1382-1386.

Ross, M.D., and D. Villard. 2003. Disability levels of college-aged men with a history of Osgood-Schlatter disease. *Journal of Strength and Conditioning Research* 17: 659-663.

Rossettini, G., D. Ristori, and M. Testa. 2018. Myositis ossificans: Delayed complications of severe muscle contusion. *Journal of Orthopaedic & Sports Physical Therapy* 48(5): 420.

Rothwell, A.G. 1982. Quadriceps hematoma: A prospective clinical study. *Clinical Orthopaedics and Related Research* 171: 97-103.

Roux, C.H., J. Coste, C. Roger, E. Fontas, A.-C. Rat, and F. Guillemin. 2021. Impact of smoking on femorotibial and hip osteoarthritis progression: 3-year follow-up data from the KHOALA cohort. *Joint Bone Spine* 88(2). doi: 10.1016/j.jbspin.2020.09.009

Safran, M.R., R.S. Benedetti, A.R. Bartolozzi, III, and B.R. Mandelbaum. 1999. Lateral ankle sprains: A comprehensive review. Part 1: Etiology, pathoanatomy, histopathogenesis, and diagnosis. *Medicine and Science in Sports and Exercise* 31: S429-S437.

Salem, G.J., and C.M. Powers. 2001. Patellofemoral joint kinetics during squatting in collegiate women athletes. *Clinical Biomechanics* 16: 424-430.

Salsich, G.B., S.R. Ward, M.R. Terk, and C.M. Powers. 2003. In vivo assessment of patellofemoral joint contact area in individuals who are pain free. *Clinical Orthopaedics and Related Research* 417: 277-284.

Schepsis, A.A., M. Fitzgerald, and R. Nicoletta. 2005. Revision surgery for exertional anterior compartment syndrome of the lower leg. *American Journal of Sports Medicine* 33: 1040-1047.

Schepsis, A.A., H. Jones, and A.L. Haas. 2002. Achilles tendon disorders in athletes. *American Journal of Sports Medicine* 30: 287-305.

Schmidt, A.H. 2017. Acute compartment syndrome. *Injury* 48S: S22-S25.

Schneider, H.P., J.M. Baca, B.B. Carpenter, P.D. Dayton, A.E. Fleischer, and B.D. Sachs. 2018. American College of Foot and Ankle Surgeons clinical consensus statement: Diagnosis and treatment of adult acquired infracalcaneal heel pain. *The Journal of Foot & Ankle Surgery* 57: 370-381.

Scott, S.H., and D.A. Winter. 1990. Internal forces at chronic running injury sites. *Medicine and Science in Sports and Exercise* 22: 357-369.

Seedhom, B.B., and V. Wright. 1974. Functions of the menisci: A preliminary study. *Journal of Bone and Joint Surgery* 56B: 381-382.

Seering, W.P., R.L. Piziali, D.A. Nagel, and D.J. Schurman. 1980. The function of the primary ligaments of the knee in varus-valgus and axial rotation. *Journal of Biomechanics* 13: 785-794.

Seow, D., T.N.B.T. Yusof, Y. Yasui, Y. Shimozono, and J.G. Kennedy. 2020. Treatment options for turf toe: A systematic review. *The Journal of Foot & Ankle Surgery* S9: 112-116.

Sibley, T., D.A. Algren, and S. Ellison. 2012. Bilateral patellar tendon ruptures without predisposing systemic disease or steroid use: A case report and review of the literature. *American Journal of Emergency Medicine* 30(1):261.e3-5. doi: 10.1016/j.ajem.2010.11.011

Siegler, S., J. Block, and C.D. Schneck. 1988. The mechanical characteristics of the collateral ligaments of the human ankle joint. *Foot and Ankle* 8: 234-242.

Siliski, J.M. 2003. Dislocations and soft tissue injuries of the knee. In *Skeletal Trauma: Basic Science, Management, and Reconstruction*, edited by B.D. Browner, J.B. Jupiter, A.M. Levine, and P.T. Trafton. Philadelphia: Saunders.

Singh, N. 2018. International epidemiology of anterior cruciate ligament injuries. *Orthopedic Research Online Journal* 1(5): 94-96.

Speer, K.P., C.E. Spritzer, F.H. Bassett, J.A. Feagin, and W.E. Garrett. 1992. Osseous injury associated with acute tears of the anterior cruciate ligament. *American Journal of Sports Medicine* 20: 382-389.

Speer, K.P., R.F. Warren, T.L. Wickiewicz, L. Horowitz, and L. Henderson. 1995. Observations on the injury mechanism of anterior cruciate ligament tears in skiers. *American Journal of Sports Medicine* 23: 77-81.

Spilker, R.L., P.S. Donzelli, and V.C. Mow. 1992. A transversely isotropic biphasic finite element model of the meniscus. *Journal of Biomechanics* 25: 1027-1045.

Stanitski, C.L. 2002. Sports injuries in children and adolescents. In *Oxford Textbook of Orthopedics and Trauma*, edited by C. Bulstrode, J. Buckwalter, A. Carr, L. Marsh, J. Fairbank, J. Wilson-MacDonald, and G. Bowden. Oxford, UK: Oxford University Press.

Stannard, J.P., J.T. Stannard, and J.L. Cook. 2020. Surgical treatment of combined ACL, PCL, and lateral side injuries. *Sports Medicine and Arthroscopy Review* 28(3): 94-99.

Staubli, H.U., U. Durrenmatt, B. Porcellini, and W. Rauschning. 1999. Anatomy and surface geometry of the patellofemoral joint in the axial plane. *Journal of Bone and Joint Surgery* 81B: 452-458.

Stedman's Medical Dictionary for the Health Professions and Nursing (5th ed.). 2005. Philadelphia: Lippincott Williams & Wilkins.

Sterett, W.I., and W.B. Krissoff. 1994. Femur fractures in alpine skiing: Classification and mechanisms of injury in 85 cases. *Journal of Orthopaedic Trauma* 8: 310-314.

Stevenson, H., J. Webster, R. Johnson, and B. Beynnon. 1998. Gender differences in knee injury epidemiology among competitive alpine ski racers. *Iowa Orthopaedic Journal* 18: 64-66.

Stødle, A.H., K.H. Hvaal, M. Enger, H. Brøgger, J.E. Madsen, and E.E. Husebye. 2020. Lisfranc injuries: Incidence, mechanisms of injury and predictors of instability. *Foot and Ankle Surgery* 26: 535-540.

St-Onge, N., Y. Chevalier, N. Hagemeister, M. Van De Putte, and J. De Guise. 2004. Effect of ski binding parameters on knee biomechanics: A three-dimensional computational study. *Medicine and Science in Sports and Exercise* 36: 1218-1225.

Swenson, T.M., and C.D. Harner. 1995. Knee ligament and meniscal injuries: Current concepts. *Orthopaedic Clinics of North America* 26: 529-546.

Tarazi, N., P. O'loughlin, A. Amin, and P. Keogh. 2016. A rare case of bilateral tendon ruptures: A case report and literature review. *Case Reports in Orthopedics.* doi: 10.1155/2016/6912968

Tearse, D., J.A. Buckwalter, J.L. Marsh, and E.A. Brandser. 2002. Stress fractures. In *Oxford Textbook of Orthopedics and Trauma*, edited by C. Bulstrode, J. Buckwalter, A. Carr, L. Marsh, J. Fairbank, J. Wilson-MacDonald, and G. Bowden. Oxford, UK: Oxford University Press.

Thelen, D.G., E.S. Chumanov, D.M. Hoerth, T.M. Best, S.C. Swanson, L. Li, M. Young, and B.C. Heiderscheit. 2005. Hamstring muscle kinematics during treadmill sprinting. *Medicine and Science in Sports and Exercise* 37: 108-114.

Thomas, J.L., J.C. Christensen, S.R. Kravitz, R.W. Mendicino, J.M. Schuberth, J.V. Vanore, L.S. Weil Sr., H.J. Zlotoff, R. Bouché, and J. Baker. 2010. The diagnosis and treatment of heel pain: A clinical practice. *The Journal of Foot & Ankle Surgery* 49 (Suppl. 3): S1-S19.

Thomeé, R., P. Renström, J. Karlsson, and G. Grimby. 1995. Patellofemoral pain syndrome in young women. I. A clinical analysis of alignment, pain parameters, common symptoms and functional activity level. *Scandinavian Journal of Medicine and Science in Sports* 5: 237-244.

Trojian, T., and A.K. Tucker. 2019. Plantar fasciitis. *American Academy of Family Physicians* 99(12): 744-750.

Upadhyay, S.S., A. Moulton, and R.G. Burwell. 1985. Biological factors predisposing to traumatic posterior dislocation of the hip. *Journal of Bone and Joint Surgery* 67B: 232-236.

Urabe, Y., M. Ochi, K. Onari, and Y. Ikuta. 2002. Anterior cruciate ligament injury in recreational alpine skiers: Analysis of mechanisms and strategy for prevention. *Journal of Orthopaedic Science* 7: 1-5.

van den Bogert, A.J., M.J. Pavol, and M.D. Grabiner. 2002. Response time is more important than walking speed for the ability of older adults to avoid a fall after a trip. *Journal of Biomechanics* 35: 199-205.

van den Kroonenberg, A.J., W.C. Hayes, and T.A. McMahon. 1995. Dynamic models for sideways falls from standing height. *Journal of Biomechanical Engineering* 117: 309-318.

van der Worp, M.P., N. van der Horst, A. de Wijer, F.J.G. Backx, and M.W.G. Nijhuis-van der Sanden. 2012. Iliotibial band syndrome in runners: A systematic review. *Sports Medicine* 42(11): 969-992.

Vanek, D., A. Saxena, and J.M. Boggs. 2003. Fluoroquinolone therapy and Achilles tendon rupture. *Journal of the American Podiatric Medical Association* 93: 333-335.

van Kuijk, K.S.R., V. Eggerding, M. Reijman, B.L. van Meer, S.M.A. Bierma-Zeinstra, E. van Arkel, J.H. Waarsing, and D.E. Meuffels. 2021. Differences in knee shape between ACL injured and non-injured: A matched case-control study of 168 patients. *Journal of Clinical Medicine* 10: 968.

van Kuijk, K.S.R., M. Reijman, S.M.A. Bierma-Zeinstra, J.H. Waarsing, and D.E. Meuffels. 2019. Posterior cruciate ligament injury is influenced by intercondylar shape and size of tibial eminence. *The Bone & Joint Journal* 101-B(9): 1058-1062.

Vavken, P., and M.M. Murray. 2013. ACL injury epidemiology. In *The ACL Handbook*, edited by M. Murray, P. Vavken, and B. Fleming. New York: Springer.

Venes, D., ed. 2005. *Taber's Cyclopedic Medical Dictionary.* Philadelphia: Davis.

Veronese, N., and S. Maggi. 2018. Epidemiology and social costs of hip fracture. *Injury* 49(8): 1458-1460.

Verrall, G.M., J.P. Slavotinek, and P.G. Barnes. 2005. The effect of sports specific training on reducing the incidence of hamstring injuries in professional Australian Rules football players. *British Journal of Sports Medicine* 39: 363-368.

Verrall, G.M., J.P. Slavotinek, P.G. Barnes, and G.T. Fon. 2003. Diagnostic and prognostic value of clinical findings in 83 athletes with posterior thigh injury: Comparison of clinical findings with magnetic resonance imaging documentation of hamstring muscle strain. *American Journal of Sports Medicine* 31: 969-973.

Verzijl, N., R.A. Bank, J.M. TeKoppele, and J. DeGroot. 2003. Ageing and osteoarthritis: A different perspective. *Current Opinions in Rheumatology* 15: 616-622.

Verzijl, N., J. DeGroot, Z.C. Ben, O. Brau-Benjamin, A. Maroudas, R.A. Bank, J. Mizrahi, C.G. Schalkwijk, S.R. Thorpe, J.W. Baynes, J.W. Bijlsma, F.P. Lafeber, and J.M. TeKoppele. 2002. Crosslinking by advanced glycation end products increases the stiffness of the collagen network in human articular cartilage: A possible mechanism through which age is a risk factor for osteoarthritis. *Arthritis and Rheumatology* 46: 114-123.

Vuori, J.-P., and H.T. Aro. 1993. Lisfranc joint injuries: Trauma mechanisms and associated injuries. *Journal of Trauma* 35: 40-45.

Walczak, B.E., C.N. Johnson, and B.M. Howe. 2015. Myositis ossificans. *Journal of the American Academy of Orthopaedic Surgeons* 23: 612-622.

Walker, P., and M. Erkman. 1975. The role of the menisci in force transmission across the knee. *Clinical Orthopaedics* 109: 184-192.

Ward, S.R., and C.M. Powers. 2004. The influence of patella alta on patellofemoral joint stress during normal and fast walking. *Clinical Biomechanics* 19: 1040-1047.

Ward, S.R., M.R. Terk, and C.M. Powers. 2007. Patella alta: Association with patellofemoral alignment and changes in contact area during weight-bearing. *Journal of Bone & Joint Surgery* 89(8): 1749-1755.

Watson, J.T. 2002. Tibial shaft fractures. In *Oxford Textbook of Orthopedics and Trauma* (vol. 3), edited by C. Bulstrode, J. Buckwalter, A. Carr, L. Marsh, J. Fairbank, J. Wilson-MacDonald, and G. Bowden. Oxford, UK: Oxford University Press.

Weiss, R.J., S.M. Montgomery, Z. Al Dabbagh, and K.A. Jansson. 2009. National data of 6409 Swedish inpatients with femoral shaft fractures: stable incidence between 1998 and 2004. *Injury* 40(3): 304-308.

Wind, W.M., Jr., J.A. Bergfeld, and R.D. Parker. 2004. Evaluation and treatment of posterior cruciate ligament injuries: Revisited. *American Journal of Sports Medicine* 32: 1765-1775.

Winquist, R.A., and S.T. Hansen, Jr. 1980. Comminuted fractures of the femoral shaft treated by intramedullary nailing. *Orthopedic Clinics of North America* 11: 633-648.

Winquist, R.A., S.T. Hansen, Jr., and D.K. Clawson. 1984. Closed intramedullary nailing of femoral fractures: A report of five hundred and twenty cases. *Journal of Bone and Joint Surgery* 66A: 529-539.

Winters, M. 2020. The diagnosis and management of medial tibial stress syndrome. *Der Unfallchirurg* 123 (Suppl. 1): S15-S19.

Wiss, D.A., W.W. Brien, and V. Becker, Jr. 1991. Interlocking nailing for the treatment of femoral fractures due to gunshot wounds. *Journal of Bone and Joint Surgery* 73A: 598-606.

Wojtys, E.M., L.J. Huston, M.D. Boynton, K.P. Spindler, and T.N. Lindenfeld. 2002. The effect of the menstrual cycle on anterior cruciate ligament injuries in women as determined by hormone levels. *American Journal of Sports Medicine* 30: 182-188.

Woo, S.L., J.M. Hollis, D.J. Adams, R.M. Lyon, and S. Takai. 1991. Tensile properties of the human femur-anterior cruciate ligament-tibia complex. The effects of specimen age and orientation. *American Journal of Sports Medicine* 19: 217-225.

Woo, S. L.-Y., M.A. Knaub, and M. Apreleva. 2001. Biomechanics of ligaments in sports medicine. In *Sports Injuries: Mechanisms, Prevention, Treatment*, edited by F.H. Fu and D.A. Stone. Philadelphia: Lippincott Williams & Wilkins.

Worrell, T.W. 1994. Factors associated with hamstring injuries: An approach to treatment and preventative measures. *Sports Medicine* 17: 338-345.

Yates, B., M.J. Allen, and M.R. Barnes. 2003. Outcome of surgical treatment of medial tibial stress syndrome. *Journal of Bone and Joint Surgery* 85A: 1974-1980.

Yates, B., and S. White. 2004. The incidence and risk factors in the development of medial tibial stress syndrome among naval recruits. *American Journal of Sports Medicine* 32: 772-780.

Yinger, K., B.R. Mandelbaum, and L.C. Almekinders. 2002. Achilles rupture in the athlete: Current science and treatment. *Clinics in Podiatric Medicine and Surgery* 19: 231-250.

Yu, B., and W.E. Garrett. 2007. Mechanisms of non-contact ACL injuries. *British Journal of Sports Medicine* 41(Suppl. 1): i47-i51.

Zantop, T., B. Tillmann, and W. Petersen. 2003. Quantitative assessment of blood vessels of the human Achilles tendon: An immunohistochemical cadaver study. *Archives of Orthopaedic Trauma Surgery* 123: 501-504.

Zernicke, R.F. 1981. Biomechanical evaluation of bilateral tibial spiral fractures during skiing: A case study. *Medicine and Science in Sports and Exercise* 13: 243-245.

Zernicke, R.F., J. Garhammer, and F.W. Jobe. 1977. Human patellar-tendon rupture: A kinetic analysis. *Journal of Bone and Joint Surgery* 59A: 179-183.

Zhang, K., L. Li, L. Yang, J. Shi, L. Zhu, H. Liang, X. Wang, X. Yang, and Q. Jiang. 2019. The biomechanical changes of load distribution with longitudinal tears of meniscal horns on knee joint: A finite element analysis. *Journal of Orthopaedic Surgery and Research* 14.

Chapter 7

Abrams, G.D., P.A. Renstrom, and M.R. Safran. 2012. Epidemiology of musculoskeletal injury in the tennis player. *British Journal of Sports Medicine*. doi: 10.1136/bjsports-2012-091164

Agrahari, Y., M.J.L. Agrahari, and S.K. Kunwor. 2020. Simultaneous bilateral anterior glenohumeral joint dislocation: A case report. *Journal of Nepal Medical Association* 58(277): 512-514.

Ahmad, C.S., and N.S. ElAttrache. 2004. Valgus extension overload syndrome and stress injury of the olecranon. *Clinics in Sports Medicine* 23: 665-676.

Alashkham, A., A. Alraddadi, P. Felts, and R. Soames. 2017. Blood supply and vascularity of the glenoid labrum: Its clinical implications. *Journal of Orthopaedic Surgery (Hong Kong)* 25(3): 2309499017731632.

Allman, F.L., Jr. 1967. Fractures and ligamentous injuries of the clavicle and its articulation. *Journal of Bone and Joint Surgery* 49A: 774-784.

Anakwenze, O.A., V.K. Kancherla, J. Iyengar, C.S. Ahmad, and W.N. Levine. 2014. Posterolateral rotatory instability of the elbow. *American Journal of Sports Medicine* 42(2): 485-491.

Andrews, J.R., W.G. Carson, Jr., and W.D. McLeod. 1985. Glenoid labrum tears related to the long head of the biceps. *American Journal of Sports Medicine* 13: 337-341.

Atroshi, I., C. Gummesson, R. Johnsson, E. Ornstein, J. Manstam, and I. Rosén. 1999. Prevalence of carpal tunnel syndrome in a general population. *Journal of the American Medical Association* 282(2): 153-158.

Bado, J.L. 1967. The Monteggia lesion. *Clinical Orthopaedics and Related Research* 50: 71-86.

Balke, M., C. Schmidt, N. Dedy, M. Banerjee, B. Bouillon, and D. Liem. 2013. Correlation of acromial morphology with impingement syndrome and rotator cuff tears. *Acta Orthopaedica* 84(2): 178-183.

Banas, M.P., R.J. Miller, and S. Totterman. 1995. Relationship between the lateral acromion angle and rotator cuff disease. *Journal of Shoulder and Elbow Surgery* 4: 454-461.

Bankart, A.S.B. 1923. Recurrent or habitual dislocation of the shoulder joint. *British Medical Journal* 2: 1132-1133.

Barco, R., and S.A. Antuña. 2017. Medial elbow pain. *EFORT Open Reviews* 2(8): 362-371.

Bartolozzi, A., D. Andreychik, and S. Ahmad. 1994. Determinants of outcome in the treatment of rotator cuff disease. *Clinical Orthopaedics and Related Research* 308: 90-97.

Bigliani, L.U., and W.N. Levine. 1997. Subacromial impingement syndrome. *Journal of Bone and Joint Surgery* 79A: 1854-1868.

Bigliani, L.U., D.S. Morrison, and E.W. April. 1986. The morphology of the acromion and its relationship to rotator cuff tears. *Orthopaedic Transactions* 10: 228.

Blevins, F.T. 1997. Rotator cuff pathology in athletes. *Sports Medicine* 24: 205-220.

Bonza, J.E., S.K. Fields, E.E. Yard, and R.D. Comstock. 2009. Shoulder injuries among United States high school athletes during the 2005-2006 and 2006-2007 school years. *Journal of Athletic Training* 44(1): 76-83.

Botte, M.J., and R.H. Gelberman. 1987. Fractures of the carpus, excluding the scaphoid. *Hand Clinics of North America* 3: 149-161.

Branch, T., C. Partin, P. Chamberland, E. Emeterio, and M. Sabetelle. 1992. Spontaneous fractures of the humerus during pitching: A series of 12 cases. *American Journal of Sports Medicine* 20: 468-470.

Bright, A.S., B. Torpey, D. Magid, T. Codd, and E.G. McFarland. 1997. Reliability of radiographic evaluation for acromial morphology. *Skeletal Radiology* 26: 718-721.

Budoff, J.E., R.P. Nirschl, O.A. Ilahi, and D.M. Rodin. 2003. Internal impingement in the etiology of rotator cuff tendinosis revisited. *Arthroscopy* 19: 810-814.

Buess, E., K.U. Steuber, and B. Waibl. 2005. Open versus arthroscopic rotator cuff repair: A comparative view of 96 cases. *Arthroscopy* 21: 597-604.

Burkhart, S.S. 1993. Arthroscopic debridement and decompression for selected rotator cuff tears. Clinical results, pathomechanics, and patient selection based on biomechanical parameters. *Orthopedic Clinics of North America* 24: 111-123.

Burkhart, S.S. 2000. A stepwise approach to arthroscopic rotator cuff repair based on biomechanical principles. *Arthroscopy* 16: 82-90.

Burkhart, S.S., and C.D. Morgan. 1998. The peel-back mechanism: Its role in producing and extending posterior type II SLAP lesions and its effect on SLAP repair rehabilitation. *Arthroscopy* 14: 637-640.

Burkhart, S.S., and C. Morgan. 2001. SLAP lesions in the overhead athlete. *Orthopedic Clinics of North America* 32: 431-441.

Burkhart, S.S., C.D. Morgan, and W.B. Kibler. 2000. Shoulder injuries in overhead athletes: The "dead arm" revisited. *Clinics in Sports Medicine* 19: 125-158.

Burnham, R.S., L. May, E. Nelson, R. Steadward, and D.C. Reid. 1993. Shoulder pain in wheelchair athletes: The role of muscle imbalance. *American Journal of Sports Medicine* 21: 238-242.

Burnier, M., B.T. Elhassan, and J. Sanchez-Sotelo. 2019. Surgical management of irreparable rotator cuff tears. *Journal of Bone and Joint Surgery* 101A(17): 1603-1612.

Buss, D.D., and J.D. Watts. 2003. Acromioclavicular injuries in the throwing athlete. *Clinics in Sports Medicine* 22: 327-341.

Caine, D., W. Howe, W. Ross, and G. Bergman. 1997. Does repetitive physical loading inhibit radial growth in female gymnasts? *Clinical Journal of Sport Medicine* 7: 302-308.

Callaghan, E.B., D.L. Bennett, G.Y. El-Khoury, and K. Ohashi. 2004. Ball-thrower's fracture of the humerus. *Skeletal Radiology* 33: 355-358.

Chalmers, P.N., L. Beck, M. Miller, J. Kawakami, A.G. Dukas, R.T. Burks, P.E. Greis, and R.Z. Tashjian. 2020. Acromial morphology is not associated with rotator cuff tearing or repair healing. *Journal of Shoulder and Elbow Surgery* 29(11): 2229-2239.

Chan, H.B.Y., P.Y. Pua, and C.H. How. 2017. Physical therapy in the management of frozen shoulder. *Singapore Medical Journal* 58(12): 685-689.

Chen, C.H., K.Y. Hsu, W.J. Chen, and C.H. Shih. 2005. Incidence and severity of biceps long head tendon lesion in patients with complete rotator cuff tears. *Journal of Trauma* 58: 1189-1193.

Cho, C.-H., K.-C. Bae, and D.-H. Kim. 2019. Treatment strategy for frozen shoulder. *Clinics in Orthopedic Surgery* 11(3): 249-257.

Ciccotti, M.G., and W.P.H. Charlton. 2001. Epicondylitis in the athlete. *Clinics in Sports Medicine* 20: 77-93.

Clasper, J. 2002. Frozen shoulder. In *Oxford Textbook of Orthopedics and Trauma*, edited by C. Bulstrode, J. Buckwalter, A. Carr, L. Marsh, J. Fairbank, J. Wilson-MacDonald, and G. Bowden. Oxford, UK: Oxford University Press.

Codman, E.A. 1911. Complete rupture of the supraspinatus tendon: Operative treatment with report of two successful cases. *Boston Medical and Surgical Journal* 164: 708-710.

Codman, E.A. 1934. Tendinitis of the short rotators. In *Ruptures of the Supraspinatus Tendon and Other Lesions on or About the Subacromial Bursa*, edited by E.A. Codman. Boston: Thomas Todd.

Cohen, M.S. 2004. Fractures of the coronoid process. *Hand Clinics* 20: 443-453.

Conway, J.E., F.W. Jobe, R.E. Glousman, and M. Pink. 1992. Medial instability of the elbow in throwing athletes: Treatment by repair or reconstruction of the ulnar collateral ligament. *Journal of Bone and Joint Surgery* 74A: 67-83.

Cooper, D.E., S.P. Arnoczky, S.J. O'Brien, R.F. Warren, E. DeCarlo, and A.A. Allen. 1992. Anatomy, histology, and vascularity of the glenoid labrum: An anatomical study. *Journal of Bone and Joint Surgery* 74A: 46-52.

Corpus, K.T., C.L. Camp, D.M. Dines, D.W. Altchek, and J.S. Dines. 2016. Evaluation and treatment of internal impingement of the shoulder in overhead athletes. *World Journal of Orthopaedics* 7(12): 776-784.

Court-Brown, C.M., and B. Caesar. 2006. Epidemiology of adult fractures: A review. *Injury—International Journal of the Care of the Injured* 37: 691-697.

Cresswell, T.R., and R.B. Smith. 1998. Bilateral anterior shoulder dislocations in bench pressing: An unusual cause. *British Journal of Sports Medicine* 32: 71-72.

Cunningham, G., and A. Lädermann. 2018. Redefining anterior shoulder impingement: A literature review. *International Orthopaedics* 42: 359-366.

Després-Tremblay, G., A. Chevrier, M. Snow, M.B. Hurtig, S. Rodeo, and M.D. Buschmann. 2016. Rotator cuff repair: A review of surgical techniques, animal models, and new technologies under development. *Journal of Shoulder and Elbow Surgery* 25: 2078-2085.

De Smet, L. 1994. Ulnar variance: Facts and fiction. Review article. *Acta Orthopaedica Belgica* 60: 1-9.

De Smet, L., A. Clasessens, J. Lefevre, and G. Beunen. 1994. Gymnast wrist: An epidemiologic survey of ulnar variance and stress changes of the radial physis in elite female gymnasts. *American Journal of Sports Medicine* 22: 846-850.

Dias, J. 2002. Scaphoid fractures. In *Oxford Textbook of Orthopedics and Trauma*, edited by C. Bulstrode, J. Buckwalter, A.

Carr, L. Marsh, J. Fairbank, J. Wilson-MacDonald, and G. Bowden. Oxford, UK: Oxford University Press.

Dias, R., S. Cutts, and S. Massoud. 2005. Frozen shoulder. *British Medical Journal* 331: 1453-1456.

DiFiori, J.P., J.C. Puffer, B. Aish, and F. Dorey. 2002. Wrist pain, distal radial physeal injury, and ulnar variance in young gymnasts: Does a relationship exist? *American Journal of Sports Medicine* 30: 879-885.

DiFiori, J.P., J.C. Puffer, B.R. Mandelbaum, and F. Dorey. 1997. Distal radial growth plate injury and positive ulnar variance in nonelite gymnasts. *American Journal of Sports Medicine* 25: 763-768.

DiFiori, J.P., J.C. Puffer, B.R. Mandelbaum, and S. Mar. 1996. Factors associated with wrist pain in the young gymnast. *American Journal of Sports Medicine* 24: 9-14.

Doehrmann, R., and T.J. Frush. 2021. *Posterior Shoulder Instability*. Treasure Island, FL: StatPearls. NBK557648.

Duplay, E.S. 1872. De la periarthritis scapulohumerale et des raiderus de l'epaule qui en son la consequence. *Archives of General Medicine* 20: 513-542.

Edelson, G., and C. Teitz. 2000. Internal impingement in the shoulder. *Journal of Shoulder and Elbow Surgery* 9: 308-315.

Edgar, C. 2019. Acromioclavicular and sternoclavicular joint injuries. In *Rockwood and Green's Fractures in Adults* (9th ed.), edited by P. Tornetta, III, W. Ricci, C.M. Court-Brown, M.M. McQueen, and M. McKee. Philadelphia: Wolters Kluwer.

Ekholm, R., J. Adami, J. Tidermark, K. Hansson, H. Törnkvist, and S. Ponzer. 2006. Fractures of the shaft of the humerus: An epidemiological study of 401 fractures. *Journal of Bone and Joint Surgery* 88B(11): 1469-1473.

Emond, M., N. Le Sage, A. Lavoie, and L. Rochette. 2004. Clinical factors predicting fractures associated with an anterior shoulder dislocation. *Academy of Emergency Medicine* 11: 853-858.

Enger, M., S.A. Skjaker, L. Nordsletten, A.H. Pripp, K. Melhuus, S. Moosmayer, and J.I. Brox. 2019. Sports-related acute shoulder injuries in an urban population. *BMJ Open Sport & Exercise Medicine* 5:e000551. doi: 10.1136/bmjsem-2019-000551

Evans, M. 1949. Pronation injuries of the forearm. *Journal of Bone and Joint Surgery* 31B: 578-588.

Farley, T.E., C.H. Neumann, L.S. Steinbach, and S.A. Petersen. 1994. The coracoacromial arch: MR evaluation and correlation with rotator cuff pathology. *Skeletal Radiology* 23: 641-645.

Fernandez, D.L., and J.B. Jupiter. 1996. *Fractures of the Distal Radius*. New York: Springer-Verlag.

Fleisig, G.S., J.R. Andrews, C.J. Dillman, and R.F. Escamilla. 1995. Kinetics of baseball pitching with implications about injury mechanisms. *American Journal of Sports Medicine* 23: 233-239.

Foulk, D.A., M.P. Darmelio, A.C. Rettig, and G. Misamore. 2002. Full-thickness rotator-cuff tears in professional football players. *American Journal of Orthopedics* 31: 622-624.

Fowler, J.R., and T.B. Hughes. 2015. Scaphoid fractures. *Clinics in Sports Medicine* 34(1): 37-50.

Fu, F.H., and D.A. Stone. 2001. *Sports Injuries: Mechanisms, Prevention, Treatment* (2nd ed.). Philadelphia: Lippincott Williams & Wilkins.

Funakoshi, T., T. Majima, N. Suenaga, N. Iwasaki, S. Yamane, and A. Minami. 2006. Rotator cuff regeneration using chitin fabric as an acellular matrix. *Journal of Shoulder and Elbow Surgery* 15(1): 112-118.

Funakoshi, T., T. Majima, N. Iwasaki, N. Suenaga, N. Sawaguchi, K. Shimode, A. Minami, K. Harada, and S. Nishimura. 2005. Application of tissue engineering techniques for rotator cuff regeneration using a chitosan-based hyaluronan hybrid fiber scaffold. *American Journal of Sports Medicine* 33: 1193-1201.

Galeazzi, R. 1934. Uber ein besonderes syndrom bei verltzunger im bereich der unterarmknochen. *Archiv Fur Orthopadische und Unfall-Chirurgie* 35: 557-562.

Giangarra, C.E., B. Conroy, F.W. Jobe, M. Pink, and J. Perry. 1993. Electromyographic and cinematographic analysis of elbow function in tennis players using single- and double-handed backhand strokes. *American Journal of Sports Medicine* 21: 394-399.

Giaroli, E.L., N.M. Major, and L.D. Higgins. 2005. MRI of internal impingement of the shoulder. *American Journal of Roentgenology* 185: 925-929.

Goldberg, B.A., R.J. Nowinski, and F.A. Matsen, III. 2001. Outcome of nonoperative management of full-thickness rotator cuff tears. *Clinical Orthopaedics and Related Research* 382: 99-107.

Grana, W. 2001. Medial epicondylitis and cubital tunnel syndrome in the throwing athlete. *Clinics in Sports Medicine* 20: 541-548.

Guntern, D.V., C.W. Pfirrmann, M.R. Schmid, M. Zanetti, C.A. Binkert, A.G. Schneeberger, and J. Hodler. 2003. Articular cartilage lesions of the glenohumeral joint: Diagnostic effectiveness of MR arthrography and prevalence in patients with subacromial impingement syndrome. *Radiology* 226: 165-170.

Haahr, J.P., and J.H. Anderson. 2003. Physical and psychosocial risk factors for lateral epicondylitis: A population based case-referent study. *Occupational & Environmental Medicine* 60(5): 322-329.

Hafner, R.A., K. Poznanski, and J.M. Donovan. 1989. Ulnar variance in children—standard measurements for evaluation of ulnar shortening in juvenile rheumatoid arthritis, hereditary multiple exostosis and other bone or joint disorders in childhood. *Skeletal Radiology* 18: 513-516.

Halder, A.M., K.D. Zhao, S.W. O'Driscoll, B.F. Morrey, and K.N. An. 2001. Dynamic contributions to superior shoulder stability. *Journal of Orthopedic Research* 19: 206-212.

Handelberg, F., S. Willems, M. Shahabpour, J.-P. Huskin, and J. Kuta. 1998. SLAP lesions: A retrospective multicenter study. *Arthroscopy* 14: 856-862.

Harryman, D.T., II, J.A. Sidles, J.M. Clark, K.J. McQuade, T.D. Gibb, and F.A. Matsen, III. 1990. Translation of the humeral head on the glenoid with passive glenohumeral motion. *Journal of Bone and Joint Surgery* 72A: 1334-1343.

Hatta, T., H. Sano, J. Zuo, N. Yamamoto, and E. Itoi. 2013. Localization of degenerative changes of the acromioclavicular joint: A cadaveric study. *Surgical and Radiologic Anatomy* 35: 89-94.

Hawkins, R.H., and R. Dunlop. 1995. Nonoperative treatment of rotator cuff tears. *Clinical Orthopedics* 321: 178-188.

Haygood, T.M., C.P. Langlotz, J.B. Kneeland, J.P. Iannotti, G.R. Williams, Jr., and M.K. Dalinka. 1994. Categorization of acromial shape: Interobserver variability with MR imaging and conventional radiography. *American Journal of Roentgenology* 162: 1377-1382.

Healey, J.H., S. Barton, P. Noble, U.W. Kohi 3rd, and O.A. Ilahi. 2001. Biomechanical evaluation of the origin of the long head of the biceps tendon. *Arthroscopy* 17(4): 378-382.

Hey, H.W.D., and A.K.S. Chong. 2011. Prevalence of carpal fracture in Singapore. *Journal of Hand Surgery (Am.)* 36(2): 278-283. Hong, J., M. Yeo, G.H. Yang, and G. Kim. 2019. Cell-electrospinning and its application for tissue engineering. *International Journal of Molecular Sciences* 20: 6208.

Horii, E., R. Nakamura, K. Watanabe, and K. Tsunoda. 1994. Scaphoid fracture as a "puncher's" fracture. *Journal of Orthopaedic Trauma* 8: 107-110.

Horvath, F., and L. Kery. 1984. Degenerative deformations of the acromioclavicular joint in elderly. *Archives of Gerontology and Geriatrics* 3: 259-265.

Hotchkiss, R.N. 1996. Fractures and dislocations of the elbow. In *Rockwood and Green's Fractures in Adults,* edited by C.A. Rockwood, D.P. Green, R.W. Bucholz, and J.D. Heckman. Philadelphia: Lippincott-Raven.

Hotchkiss, R.N. 2000. Epicondylitis—lateral and medial. *Hand Clinics* 16: 505-508.

Hutchinson, M.R., and M.A. Veenstra. 1993. Arthroscopic decompression of shoulder impingement secondary to os acromiale. *Arthroscopy* 9: 28-32.

Itoi, E., and S. Tabata. 1992. Conservative treatment of rotator cuff tears. *Clinical Orthopaedics and Related Research* 275: 165-173.

Jacobson, S.R., K.P. Speer, J.T. Moor, D.H. Janda, S.R. Saddemi, P.B. MacDonald, and W.J. Mallon. 1995. Reliability of radiographic assessment of acromial morphology. *Journal of Shoulder and Elbow Surgery* 4: 449-453.

Jobe, C.M. 1995. Posterior superior glenoid impingement: expanded spectrum. *Arthroscopy* 11: 530-536.

Jobe, C.M. 1997. Superior glenoid impingement. *Orthopedic Clinics of North America* 28: 137-143.

Jobe, F.W., and M. Pink. 1993. Classification and treatment of shoulder dysfunction in the overhead athlete. *Journal of Orthopaedic and Sports Physical Therapy* 18: 427-432.

Jobe, F.W., H. Stark, and S.J. Lombardo. 1986. Reconstruction of the ulnar collateral ligament in athletes. *Journal of Bone and Joint Surgery* 68A: 1158-1163.

Jupiter, J.B., and J.F. Kellam. 2003. Diaphyseal fractures of the forearm. In *Skeletal Trauma* (3rd ed.), edited by B.D. Browner, J.B. Jupiter, A.M. Levine, and P.G. Trafton. Philadelphia: Saunders.

Jupiter, J.B., S.J. Leibovic, W. Ribbans, and R.M. Wilk. 1991. Posterior Monteggia lesion. *Journal of Orthopaedic Trauma* 5: 395-402.

Kannus, P., and L. Józsa. 1991. Histopathological changes preceding spontaneous rupture of a tendon. A controlled study of 891 patients. *Journal of Bone and Joint Surgery* 73(10): 1517-1525.

Kany, J. 2020. Tendon transfers in rotator-cuff surgery. *Orthopaedics & Traumatology: Surgery & Research* 106(1S): S43-S51.

Kaplan, H., A. Kiral, M. Kuskucu, M.O. Arpacioglu, A. Sarioslu, and O. Rodop. 1998. Report of eight cases of humeral fracture following the throwing of hand grenades. *Archives of Orthopaedic Trauma and Surgery* 117: 50-52.

Karakoc, Y., and Ï.B. Atalay. 2020. Comparison of mini-open versus all-arthroscopic rotator cuff repair: Retrospective analysis of a single center. *Pan African Medical Journal* 37: 132.

Kaur, R., A. Dahuja, S. Garg, K. Bansal, R.S. Garg, and P. Singh. 2019. Correlation of acromial morphology in association with rotator cuff tear: a retrospective study. *Polish Journal of Radiology* 84: e459-e463.

Keener, J.D., L.M. Galatz, S.A. Teefey, W.D. Middleton, K. Steger-May, G. Stobbs-Cucchi, R. Patton, and K. Yamaguchi. 2015. A prospective evaluation of survivorship of asymptomatic degenerative rotator cuff tears. *Journal of Bone & Joint Surgery* 97(2): 89-98.

Keener, J.D., B.M. Patterson, N. Orveets, and A.M. Chamberlain. 2019. Degenerative rotator cuff tears: Refining surgical indications based on natural history data. *Journal of the American Academy of Orthopaedic Surgeons* 27(5): 156-165.

Kelly, B.C., D.S. Constantinescu, and A.R. Vap. 2019. Arthroscopic and open or mini-open rotator cuff repair trends and complication rates among American Board of Orthopaedic Surgeons part II examinees (2007-2017). *Arthroscopy* 35(11): 3019-3024.

Khedr, H., A. Al-Zahrani, A. Al-Zahrani, and M.M. Al-Qattan. 2017. Bilateral irreducible inferior shoulder dislocation: A case report. *International Journal of Surgery Case Reports* 31: 124-127.

Kibler, W.B. 1995. Pathophysiology of overload injuries around the elbow. *Clinics in Sports Medicine* 14: 447-457.

Kim, J.M., and D.A. London. 2020. Complex Monteggia fractures in the adult cohort: Injury and management. *Journal of the American Academy of Orthopaedic Surgeons* 28(19): e839-e848.

Kim, S.H., R.M. Szabo, and R.A. Marder. 2012. Epidemiology of humerus fractures in the United States: Nationwide emergency department sample, 2008. *Arthritis Care & Research* 64(3): 407-414.

Kim, T.K., W.S. Queale, A.J. Cosgarea, and E.G. McFarland. 2003. Clinical features of the different types of SLAP lesions. *Journal of Bone and Joint Surgery* 85A: 66-71.

Klemt, C., J.A. Prinold, S. Morgans, S.H.L. Smith, D. Nolte, P. Reilly, and A.M.J. Bull. 2018. Analysis of shoulder compressive and shear forces during functional activities of daily life. *Clinical Biomechanics* 54: 34-41.

Koh, T.J., M.D. Grabiner, and G.G. Weiker. 1992. Technique and ground reaction forces in the back handspring. *American Journal of Sports Medicine* 20: 61-66.

Kraushaar, B.S., and R.P. Nirschl. 1999. Tendinosis of the elbow (tennis elbow). Clinical features and findings of histological, immunohistochemical, and electron microscopy studies. *Journal of Bone and Joint Surgery* 81A: 259-278.

Kristensen, S.S., E. Thomassen, and F. Christensen. 1986. Ulnar variance determination. *Journal of Hand Surgery* 11B: 255-257.

Kukkonen, J., A. Joukainen, J. Lehtinen, K.T. Mattila, E.K.J. Tuominen, T. Kauko, and V. Äärimaa. 2014. Treatment of non-traumatic rotator cuff tears: A randomized controlled trial with one-year clinical results. *Bone & Joint Journal* 96-B(1): 75-81.

Kukkonen, J., A. Joukainen, J. Lehtinen, K.T. Mattila, E.K.J. Tuominen, T. Kauko, and V. Äärimaa. 2015. Treatment of nontraumatic rotator cuff tears: A randomized controlled trial with two years of clinical and imaging follow-up. *Journal of Bone and Joint Surgery (Am)* 97(21): 1729-1737.

Labriola, J.E., T.Q. Lee, R.E. Debski, and P.J. McMahon. 2005. Stability and instability of the glenohumeral joint: The role of shoulder muscles. *Journal of Shoulder and Elbow Surgery* 14(Suppl.): 32S-38S.

Lädermann, A., P.J. Denard, and P. Collin. 2015. Massive rotator cuff tears: Definition and treatment. *International Orthopaedics* 39(12): 2403-2014.

Lambers Heerspink, F.O., J.J.A.M. van Raay, R.C.T. Koorevaar, P.J.M. van Eerden, R.E. Westerbeek, E. van 't Riet, I. van den Akker-Scheek, and R.L. Diercks. 2015. Comparing surgical repair with conservative treatment for degenerative rotator cuff tears: A randomized controlled trial. *Journal of Shoulder and Elbow Surgery* 24(8): 1274-1281.

Lambert, S.M., and R. Hertel. 2002. Dislocations about the shoulder girdle, scapular fractures, and clavicle fractures. In *Oxford Textbook of Orthopedics and Trauma*, edited by C. Bulstrode, J. Buckwalter, A. Carr, L. Marsh, J. Fairbank, J. Wilson-MacDonald, and G. Bowden. Oxford, UK: Oxford University Press.

Lawrence, R.L., V. Moutzouros, and M.J. Bey. 2019. Asymptomatic rotator cuff tears. *JBJS Reviews* 7(6): e9.

Leach, R.E., and J.K. Miller. 1987. Lateral and medial epicondylitis of the elbow. *Clinics in Sports Medicine* 6: 259-272.

Lehman, C., F. Cuomo, F.J. Kummer, and J.D. Zuckerman. 1995. The incidence of full thickness rotator cuff tears in a large cadaveric population. *Bulletin of the Hospital for Joint Diseases* 54: 30-31.

Lin, D.J., T.T. Wong, and J.K. Kazam. 2018. Shoulder injuries in the overhead-throwing athlete: Epidemiology, mechanisms of injury, and imaging findings. *Radiology* 286(2): 370-387.

Lippitt, S., and F. Matsen. 1993. Mechanisms of glenohumeral joint stability. *Clinical Orthopaedics and Related Research* 291: 20-28.

Liu, J., L. Fan, Y. Zhu, H. Yu, T. Xu, and G. Li. 2017. Comparison of clinical outcomes in all-arthroscopic versus mini-open repair of rotator cuff tears: A randomized clinical trial. *Medicine* 96(11): e6322.

Lo, S.L., K. Raskin, H. Lester, and B. Lester. 2002. Carpal tunnel syndrome: a historical perspective. *Hand Clinics* 18(2): 211-217.

Maffet, M.W., G.M. Gartsman, and B. Moseley. 1995. Superior labrum-biceps tendon complex lesions of the shoulder. *American Journal of Sports Medicine* 23: 93-98.

Malcarney, H.L., and G.A.C. Murrell. 2003. The rotator cuff: Biological adaptations to its environment. *Sports Medicine* 33: 993-1002.

Markolf, K.L., M.S. Shapiro, B.R. Mandelbaum, and L. Teurlings. 1990. Wrist loading patterns during pommel horse exercises. *Journal of Biomechanics* 23: 1001-1011.

McFarland, E.G., C.Y. Hsu, C. Neira, and O. O'Neil. 1999. Internal impingement of the shoulder: A clinical and arthroscopic analysis. *Journal of Shoulder and Elbow Surgery* 8: 458-460.

McLean, A., and F. Taylor. 2019. Classifications in brief: Bigliani classification of acromial morphology. *Clinical Orthopaedics and Related Research* 477: 1958-1961.

Meeuwisse, W.H. 1994. Assessing causation in sport injury: A multifactorial model. *Clinical Journal of Sports Medicine* 4: 166-170.

Mengiardi, B., C.W.A. Pfirrmann, C. Gerber, J. Hodler, and M. Zanetti. 2004. Frozen shoulder: MR arthrographic findings. *Radiology* 233: 486-492.

Michener, L.A., P.W. McClure, and A.R. Karduna. 2003. Anatomical and biomechanical mechanisms of subacromial impingement syndrome. *Clinical Biomechanics* 18: 369-379.

Milgrom, C., M. Schaffler, S. Gilbert, and M. van Holsbeeck. 1995. Rotator-cuff changes in asymptomatic adults. The effect of age, hand dominance and gender. *Journal of Bone and Joint Surgery* 77B: 296-298.

Millstein, E.S., and S.J. Snyder. 2003. Arthroscopic management of partial, full-thickness, and complex rotator cuff tears: Indications, techniques, and complications. *Arthroscopy* 19: 189-199.

Minagawa, H. N. Yamamoto, H. Abe, M. Fukuda, N. Seki, K. Kikuchi, H. Kijima, and E. Itoi. 2013. Prevalence of symptomatic and asymptomatic rotator cuff tears in the general population: From mass-screening in one village. *Journal of Orthopaedics* 10(1): 8-12.

Moosmayer, S., G. Lund, U.S. Seljom, B. Haldorsen, I.C. Svege, T. Hennig, A.H. Pripp, and H.-J. Smith. 2019. At a 10-year follow-up, tendon repair is superior to physiotherapy in the treatment of small and medium-sized rotator cuff tears. *Journal of Bone and Joint Surgery (Am.)* 101(12): 1050-1060.

Morgan, C.D., S.S. Burkhart, M. Palmeri, and M. Gillespie. 1998. Type II SLAP lesions: Three subtypes and their relationships to superior instability and rotator cuff tears. *Arthroscopy* 14: 553-565.

Morris, M., F.W. Jobe, J. Perry, M. Pink, and B.S. Healy. 1989. Electromyographic analysis of elbow function in tennis players. *American Journal of Sports Medicine* 17: 241-247.

Mozingo, J.D., M. Akbari-Shandiz, N.S. Murthy, M.G. Van Straaten, B.A. Schueler, D.R. Holmes, III, C.H. McCollough, and K.D. Zhao. 2020. Shoulder mechanical impingement risk associated with manual wheelchair tasks in individuals with spinal cord injury. *Clinical Biomechanics* 71: 221-229.

Nakamura, R., Y. Tanaka, T. Imaeda, and T. Miura. 1991. The influence of age and sex on ulnar variance. *Journal of Hand Surgery* 16B: 84-88.

Nam, E.K., and S.J. Snyder. 2003. The diagnosis and treatment of superior labrum, anterior and posterior (SLAP) lesions. *American Journal of Sports Medicine* 31: 798-810.

Nazari, G., J.C. MacDermid, D. Bryant, N. Dewan, and G.S. Athwal. 2019. Effects of arthroscopic vs. mini-open rotator cuff repair on function, pain & range of motion. A systematic review and meta-analysis. *PLoS ONE.* doi: 10.1371/journal.pone.0222953

Neer, C.S., II. 1972. Anterior acromioplasty for the chronic impingement syndrome in the shoulder: A preliminary report. *Journal of Bone and Joint Surgery* 54A: 41-50.

Neer, C.S., II. 1990. *Shoulder Reconstruction.* Philadelphia: Saunders.

Nestor, B.J., S.W. O'Driscoll, and B.F. Morrey. 1992. Ligamentous reconstruction for posterolateral instability of the elbow. *Journal of Bone and Joint Surgery* 74A: 1235-1241.

Neviaser, J.S. 1945. Adhesive capsulitis of the shoulder. *Journal of Bone and Joint Surgery* 27A: 211-212.

Nirschl, R.P. 1988. Prevention and treatment of elbow and shoulder injuries in the tennis player. *Clinics in Sports Medicine* 7: 289-308.

Nirschl, R.P., and E.S. Ashman. 2003. Elbow tendinopathy: Tennis elbow. *Clinics in Sports Medicine* 22: 813-836.

Nirschl, R., and F. Pettrone. 1979. Tennis elbow: The surgical treatment of lateral epicondylitis. *Journal of Bone and Joint Surgery* 61A: 832-841.

Nordt, W.E., III, R.B. Garretson, III, and E. Plotkin. 1999. The measurement of subacromial contact pressure in patients with impingement syndrome. *Arthroscopy* 15: 121-125.

O'Driscoll, S.W. 2000. Classification and evaluation of recurrent instability of the elbow. *Clinical Orthopaedics and Related Research* 370: 34-43.

O'Driscoll, S.W., D.F. Bell, and B.F. Morrey. 1991. Posterolateral rotatory instability of the elbow. *Journal of Bone and Joint Surgery* 73A: 440-446.

O'Driscoll, S.W., B.F. Morrey, S. Korinek, and K.N. An. 1992. Elbow subluxation and dislocation: A spectrum of instability. *Clinical Orthopaedics* 280: 186-197.

Ogata, S., and H.K. Uhthoff. 1990. Acromial enthesopathy and rotator cuff tear. A radiologic and histologic postmortem investigation of the coracoacromial arch. *Clinical Orthopaedics and Related Research* 254: 39-48.

Padua, L., D. Coraci, C. Erra, C. Pazzaglia, I. Paolasso, C. Loreti, P. Caliandro, and L.D. Hobson-Webb. 2016. Carpal tunnel syndrome: Clinical features, diagnosis, and management. *Lancet Neurology* 15: 1273-1284.

Paley, K.J., F.W. Jobe, M.M. Pink, R.S. Kvitne, and N.S. ElAttrache. 2000. Arthroscopic findings in the overhand throwing athlete: Evidence for posterior internal impingement of the rotator cuff. *Arthroscopy* 16: 35-40.

Penrose, J.H. 1951. The Monteggia fracture with posterior dislocation of the radial head. *Journal of Bone and Joint Surgery* 33B: 65-73.

Perry, J.J., and L.D. Higgins. 2001. Shoulder injuries. In *Sports Injuries: Mechanisms, Prevention, Treatment*, edited by F.H. Fu and D.A. Stone. Philadelphia: Lippincott Williams & Wilkins.

Peterson, L., and P. Renström. 2001. *Sports Injuries: Their Prevention and Treatment.* Champaign, IL: Human Kinetics.

Phalen, G.S. 1966. The carpal-tunnel syndrome. *Journal of Bone and Joint Surgery* 48A: 211-218.

Piper, C.C., A.J. Hughes, Y. Ma, H. Wang, and A.S. Neviaser. 2018. Operative versus nonoperative treatment for the management of full-thickness rotator cuff tears: A systematic review and meta-analysis. *Journal of Shoulder and Elbow Surgery* 27(3): 572-576.

Praemer, A., S. Furner, and D.P. Rice. 1999. *Musculoskeletal Conditions in the United States.* Park Ridge, IL: American Academy of Orthopaedic Surgeons.

Prato, N., D. Peloso, A. Franconeri, G. Tegaldo, G.B. Ravera, E. Silvestri, and L.E. Derchi. 1998. The anterior tilt of the acromion: Radiographic evaluation and correlation with shoulder diseases. *European Journal of Radiology* 8: 1639-1646.

Priest, J.D., J. Braden, and S.G. Gerberich. 1980. The elbow and tennis. *The Physician and Sportsmedicine* 8: 80-85.

Ptasznik, R., and O. Hennessy. 1995. Abnormalities of the biceps tendon of the shoulder: Sonographic findings. *American Journal of Roentgenology* 164: 409-414.

Rasool, M.N. 2004. Dislocations of the elbow in children. *Journal of Bone and Joint Surgery* 86B: 1050-1058.

Rebuzzi, E., N. Coletti, S. Schiavetti, and F. Giusto. 2005. Arthroscopic rotator cuff repair in patients older than 60 years. *Arthroscopy* 21: 48-54.

Reddy, A.S., K.J. Mohr, M.M. Pink, and F.W. Jobe. 2000. Electromyographic analysis of the deltoid and rotator cuff muscles in persons with subacromial impingement. *Journal of Shoulder and Elbow Surgery* 9: 519-523.

Rettig, A.C. 2002. Traumatic elbow injuries in the athlete. *Orthopedic Clinics of North America* 33: 509-522.

Rettig, M.E., and K.B. Raskin. 2000. Acute fractures of the distal radius. *Hand Clinics* 16: 405-415.

Robinson, C.M., K.T.M. Seah, Y.H. Chee, P. Hindle, and I.R. Murray. 2012. Frozen shoulder. *Journal of Bone and Joint Surgery* 94(1): 1-9.

Ruby, L.K., and C. Cassidy. 2003. Fractures and dislocations of the carpus. In *Skeletal Trauma* (3rd ed.), edited by B.D. Browner, J.B. Jupiter, A.M. Levine, and P.G. Trafton. Philadelphia: Saunders.

Rudy, B.S., and W.L. Hennrikus. 2017. Bilateral anterior shoulder dislocation. *JAAPA* 30(7): 25-27.

Ruotolo, C., and W.M. Nottage. 2002. Surgical and non-surgical management of rotator cuff tears. *Arthroscopy* 18: 527-531.

Sabbah, M.D., M. Morsy, and S.L. Moran. 2019. Diagnosis and management of acute schaphoid fractures. *Hand Clinics* 35(3): 259-269.

Safran, M.R. 2004. Ulnar collateral ligament injury in the overhead athlete: Diagnosis and treatment. *Clinics in Sports Medicine* 23: 643-663.

Samilson, R.L., and V. Prieto. 1983. Posterior dislocation of the shoulder in athletes. *Clinics in Sports Medicine* 2: 369-378.

Sauerbrey, A.M., C.L. Getz, M. Piancastelli, J.P. Iannotti, M.L. Ramsey, and G.R. Williams, Jr. 2005. Arthroscopic versus mini-open rotator cuff repair: A comparison of clinical outcome. *Arthroscopy* 21: 1415-1420.

Sayit, E., A.T. Sayit, M. Bagir, and Y. Terzi. 2018. Ulnar variance according to gender and side during aging: An analysis of 600 wrists. *Orthopaedics & Traumatology: Surgery & Research* 104: 865-869.

Schemitsch, C., J. Chahal, M. Vicente, L. Nowak, P-H Flurin, F. Lambers Heerspink, P. Henry, and A. Nauth. 2019. Surgical repair versus conservative treatment and subacromial decompression for the treatment of rotator cuff tears: a meta-analysis of randomized trials. *Bone & Joint Journal* 101-B(9): 1100-1106.

Sher, J.S., J.W. Uribe, A. Posada, B.J. Murphy, and M.B. Zlatkin. 1995. Abnormal findings on magnetic resonance images of asymptomatic shoulders. *Journal of Bone and Joint Surgery* 77B: 10-15.

Shiri, R., E. Viikari-Juntura, H. Varonen, and M. Heliövaara. 2006. Prevalence and determinants of lateral and medial epicondylitis: A population study. *American Journal of Epidemiology* 164(11): 1065-1074.

Silva, L.P., C.V. Sousa, E. Rodrigues, B. Alpoim, and M. Leal. 2015. Bilateral anterior glenohumeral dislocation: Clinical case. *Revista Brasileira de Ortopedia* 46(3): 318-320.

Silverstein, B.A., L.J. Fine, and T.J. Armstrong. 1987. Occupational factors and carpal tunnel syndrome. *American Journal of Industrial Medicine* 11: 343-358.

Smith, F.M. 1947. Monteggia fractures: An analysis of 25 consecutive fresh injuries. *Surgery, Gynecology and Obstetrics* 85: 630-640.

Snijders, C.J., A.C.W. Volkers, K. Mechelse, and A. Vleeming. 1987. Provocation of epicondylalgia lateralis (tennis elbow) by power grip or pinching. *Medicine and Science in Sports and Exercise* 19: 518-523.

Snyder, S.J., M.P. Banas, and R.P. Karzel. 1995. An analysis of 140 injuries to the superior glenoid labrum. *Journal of Shoulder and Elbow Surgery* 4: 243-248.

Snyder, S.J., R.P. Karzel, W. Del Pizzo, R.D. Ferkel, and M.J. Friedman. 1990. SLAP lesions of the shoulder. *Arthroscopy* 6: 274-279.

Soslowsky, L.J., C.H. An, C.M. DeBano, and J.E. Carpenter. 1996. Coracoacromial ligament: In situ load and viscoelastic properties in rotator cuff disease. *Clinical Orthopaedics and Related Research* 330: 40-44.

Speed, J.S., and H.B. Boyd. 1940. Treatment of fractures of ulna with dislocation of head of radius. *Journal of the American Medical Association* 125: 1699-1704.

Speer, K.P. 1995. Anatomy and pathomechanics of shoulder instability. *Clinics in Sports Medicine* 14: 751-760.

Stoll, L.E., and J.L. Codding. 2019. Lower trapezius tendon transfer for massive irreparable rotator cuff tears. *Orthopedic Clinics of North America* 50(3): 375-382.

Suh, N., E.T. Ek, and S.W. Wolfe. 2014. Carpal fractures. *Journal of Hand Surgery (American)* 39(4): 785-791.

Taneja, A.K., L.P. Neto, and A. Skaf. 2013. Bilateral anterior glenohumeral dislocation and coracoid processes fracture after seizure: Acute MRI findings of this rare condition. *Clinical Imaging* 37(6): 1131-1134.

Tashjian, R.Z. 2012. Epidemiology, natural history, and indications for treatment of rotator cuff tears. *Clinics in Sports Medicine* 31(4): 589-604.

Templehof, S., S. Rupp, and R. Seil. 1999. Age-related prevalence of rotator cuff tears in asymptomatic shoulders. *Journal of Shoulder and Elbow Surgery* 8: 296-299.

Thigpin, C.A., M.A. Shaffer, B.W. Gaunt, B.G. Leggin, G.R. Williams, and R.B. Wilcox, III. 2016. The American Society of Shoulder and Elbow Therapists' consensus statement of rehabilitation following arthroscopic rotator cuff repair. *Journal of Shoulder and Elbow Surgery* 25: 521-535.

Thorsness, R., and A. Romeo. 2016. Massive rotator cuff tears: Trends in surgical management. *Orthopedics* 39(3): 145-151.

Toivonen, D.A., M.J. Tuite, and J.F. Orwin. 1995. Acromial structure and tears of the rotator cuff. *Journal of Shoulder and Elbow Surgery* 4: 376-383.

Tompkins, D.G. 1971. The anterior Monteggia fracture. *Journal of Bone and Joint Surgery* 53A: 1109-1114.

Tossy, J.D., N.C. Mead, and H.M. Sigmond. 1963. Acromioclavicular separations: useful and practical classification for treatment. *Clinical Orthopaedics and Related Research* 28: 111-119.

Tosti, R., J. Jennings, and J.M. Sewards. 2013. Lateral epicondylitis of the elbow. *American Journal of Medicine* 126(4):357.e1-6.

Tuite, M.J., D.A. Toivonen, J.F. Orwin, and D.H. Wright. 1995. Acromial angle on radiographs of the shoulder: Correlation with the impingement syndrome and rotator cuff tears. *American Journal of Roentgenology* 165: 609-613.

Turhan, E., and M. Demirel. 2008. Bilateral anterior gleno-humeral dislocation in a horse rider: A case report and a review of the literature. *Archives of Orthopaedic Trauma and Surgery* 128(1): 79-82.

Tytherleigh-Strong, G., N. Walls, and M.M. McQueen. 1998. The epidemiology of humeral shaft fractures. *Journal of Bone and Joint Surgery* 80B: 249-253.

Updegrove, G.F., W. Mourad, and J.A. Abboud. 2018. Humeral shaft fractures. *Journal of Shoulder and Elbow Surgery* 27: e87-e97.

Varacallo, M., D.C. Tapscott, and S.D. Mair. 2021. Superior labrum anterior posterior lesions. *National Library of Medicine* NBK538284.

van Rijn, R.M., B.M.A. Huisstede, B.W. Koes, and A. Burdorf. 2009. Associations between work-related factors and specific disorders at the elbow: A systematic literature review. *Rheumatology* 48: 528-536.

Vaz, S., J. Soyer, P. Pries, and J.P. Clarac. 2000. Subacromial impingement: Influence of coracoacromial arch geometry on shoulder function. *Joint Bone Spine* 67: 305-309.

Viikari-Juntura, E., and B. Silverstein. 1999. Role of physical load factors in carpal tunnel syndrome. *Scandinavian Journal of Work and Environmental Health* 25: 163-185.

Walch, G., P. Boileau, E. Noel, and S.T. Donell. 1992. Impingement of the deep surface of the supraspinatus tendon on the posterior glenoid rim: An arthroscopic study. *Journal of Shoulder and Elbow Surgery* 1: 238-245.

Wang, J.C., and M.S. Shapiro. 1997. Changes in acromial morphology with age. *Journal of Shoulder and Elbow Surgery* 6: 55-59.

Warner, J.J., and I.M. Parsons, IV. 2001. Latissimus dorsi tendon transfer: A comparative analysis of primary and salvage reconstruction of massive, irreparable rotator cuff tears. *Journal of Shoulder and Elbow Surgery* 10: 514-521.

Warner, J.J., P. Tetreault, J. Lehtinen, and D. Zurakowski. 2005. Arthroscopic versus mini-open rotator cuff repair: A cohort comparison study. *Arthroscopy* 21: 328-332.

Weber, E.R., and E.Y. Chao. 1978. An experimental approach to the mechanism of scaphoid wrist fractures. *Journal of Hand Surgery* 3: 142-148.

Werner, R.A., and M. Andary. 2002. Carpal tunnel syndrome: Pathophysiology and clinical neurophysiology. *Clinical Neurophysiology* 113: 1373-1381.

Werner, S.L., G.S. Fleisig, C.J. Dillman, and J. Andrews. 1993. Biomechanics of the elbow during baseball pitching. *Journal of Orthopaedic and Sports Physical Therapy* 17: 274-278.

Whaley, A.L., and C.L. Baker. 2004. Lateral epicondylitis. *Clinics in Sports Medicine* 23: 677-691.

Wilkins, K.E. 2002. Changes in the management of Monteggia fractures. *Journal of Pediatric Orthopaedics* 22: 548-554.

Wilkinson, G.T. 1895. Complete transverse fracture of the humerus by muscular action. *Lancet* 2: 733.

Williams, G.R., V.D. Nguyen, and C.A. Rockwood, Jr. 1989. Classification and radiographic analysis of acromioclavicular dislocations. *Applied Radiology* 18: 29-34.

Williams, G.R., C.A. Rockwood, Jr., L.U. Bigliani, J.P. Iannotti, and W. Stanwood. 2004. Rotator cuff tears: Why do we repair them? *Journal of Bone and Joint Surgery* 86A: 2764-2776.

Wilson, F.D., J.R. Andrews, T.A. Blackburn, and G. McCluskey. 1983. Valgus extension overload in the pitching elbow. *American Journal of Sports Medicine* 11: 83-88.

Wirth, M.A., and C.A. Rockwood, Jr. 1997. Operative treatment of irreparable rupture of the subscapularis. *Journal of Bone and Joint Surgery* 79A: 722-731.

Wittenberg, R.H., F. Rubenthaler, T. Wolk, J. Ludwig, R.E. Willburger, and R. Steffen. 2001. Surgical or conservative treatment for chronic rotator cuff calcifying tendinitis—a matched-pair analysis of 100 patients. *Archives of Orthopaedic and Trauma Surgery* 121: 56-59.

Worland, R.L., D. Lee, C.G. Orozco, F. SozaRex, and J. Keenan. 2003. Correlation of age, acromial morphology, and rotator cuff tear pathology diagnosed by ultrasound in asymptomatic patients. *Journal of the Southern Orthopedic Association* 12: 23-26.

Wright, P.R. 1963. Greenstick fracture of the upper end of the ulna with dislocation of the radio-humeral joint or displacement of the superior radial epiphysis. *Journal of Bone and Joint Surgery* 45B: 727-731.

Yamaguchi, K., J.S. Sher, W.K. Anderson, R. Garretson, J.W. Uribe, K. Hechtman, and R.J. Neviaser. 2000. Glenohumeral motion in patients with rotator cuff tears: A comparison of asymptomatic and symptomatic shoulders. *Journal of Shoulder and Elbow Surgery* 9: 6-11.

Youm, T., D.H. Murray, E.N. Kubiak, A.S. Rokito, and J.D. Zuckerman. 2005. Arthroscopic versus mini-open rotator cuff repair: a comparison of clinical outcomes and patient satisfaction. *Journal of Shoulder and Elbow Surgery* 14: 455-459.

Zuckerman, J.D., F.J. Kummer, F. Cuomo, and M. Greller. 1997. Interobserver reliability of acromial morphology classification: An anatomic study. *Journal of Shoulder and Elbow Surgery* 6: 286-287.

Chapter 8

Adams, J.H., D. Doyle, I. Ford, T.A. Gennarelli, D.I. Graham, and D.R. McLellan. 1989. Diffuse axonal injury in head injury: Definition, diagnosis and grading. *Histopathology* 15: 49-59.

Adams, M.A., and W.C. Hutton. 1982. Prolapsed intervertebral disc. A hyperflexion injury. *Spine* 7: 184-191.

Adebayo, E.T., O.S. Ajike, and E.O. Adekeye. 2003. Analysis of the pattern of maxillofacial fractures in Kaduna, Nigeria. *British Journal of Oral and Maxillofacial Surgery* 41: 396-400.

Agarwal, Y., P. Gulati, B. Sureka, and N. Kumar. 2015. Radiologic imaging in spinal trauma. In *ISCoS Textbook of Comprehensive Management of Spinal Cord Injuries*, edited by H.S. Chhabra. New Delhi: Wolters Kluwer-India.

Allsop, D., and K. Kennett. 2001. Skull and facial bone trauma. In *Accidental Injury*, edited by A.M. Nahum and J.W. Melvin. New York: Springer.

Alvi, A., T. Doherty, and G. Lewen. 2003. Facial fractures and concomitant injuries in trauma patients. *Laryngoscope* 113: 102-106.

American Psychiatric Association. 2013. *Diagnostic and Statistical Manual of Mental Disorders* (5th ed.). Washington, DC: Author.

Amonoo-Kuofi, H.S. 1992. Changes in the lumbosacral angle, sacral inclination and the curvature of the lumbar spine during aging. *Acta Anatomica* 145: 373-377.

Bailes, J.E., and R.C. Cantu. 2001. Head injury in athletes. *Neurosurgery* 48: 26-46.

Barnsley, L., S. Lord, and N. Bogduk. 1994. Whiplash injury. *Pain* 58: 283-307.

Bartlett, C.S. 2003. Clinical update: Gunshot wound ballistics. *Clinical Orthopaedics and Related Research* 408: 28-57.

Bartynski, W.S., M.T. Heller, S.Z. Grahovac, W.E. Rothfus, and M. Kurs-Lasky. 2005. Severe thoracic kyphosis in the older patient in the absence of vertebral fracture: Association of extreme curve with age. *American Journal of Neuroradiology* 26(8): 2077-2085.

Bazarian, J.J., J. McClung, M.N. Shah, Y.T. Cheng, W. Flesher, and J. Kraus. 2005. Mild traumatic brain injury in the United States, 1998-2000. *Brain Injury* 19: 85-91.

Beutler, W.J., B.E. Fredrickson, A. Murtland, C.A. Sweeney, W.D. Grant, and D. Baker. 2003. The natural history of spondylolysis and spondylolisthesis: 45-year follow-up evaluation. *Spine* 28: 1027-1035.

Bogduk, N., and N. Yoganandan. 2001. Biomechanics of the cervical spine. Part 3: Minor injuries. *Clinical Biomechanics* 16: 267-275.

Boos, N., and M. Aebi. 2008. *Spinal Disorders: Fundamentals of Diagnosis and Treatment.* Bern, Switzerland: Springer Science & Business Media.

Bradford, D.S. 1995. Kyphosis in the elderly. In *Moe's Textbook of Scoliosis and Other Spinal Deformities*, edited by J.E. Lonstein, D.S. Bradford, R.B. Winter, and J.W. Ogilvie. Philadelphia: Saunders.

Brasileiro, B.F., and L.A. Passeri. 2006. Epidemiological analysis of maxillofacial fractures in Brazil: A 5-year prospective study. *Oral Surgery, Oral Medicine, Oral Pathology, Oral Radiology and Endodontics* 102: 28-34.

Broglio, S.P., R.C. Cantu, G.A. Gioia, K.M. Guskiewicz, J. Kutcher, M. Palm, et al. 2014. National Athletic Trainers' Association position statement: Management of sport concussion. *Journal of Athletic Training* 49(2): 245-265. doi: 10.4085/1062-6050-49.1.07

Broglio, S.P., B. Schnebel, J.J. Sosnoff, S. Shin, X. Fend, X. He, and J. Zimmerman, J. 2010. Biomechanical properties of concussions in high school football. *Medicine and Science in Sports and Exercise* 42(11): 2064-2071. doi: 10.1249/MSS.0b013e3181dd9156

Broglio, S.P., R.M. Williams, K.L. O'Connor, and J. Goldstick. 2016. Football players' head-impact exposure after limiting of full-contact practices. *Journal of Athletic Training* 51(7): 511-518. doi: 10.4085/1062-6050-51.7.04

Bryden, D.W., J.I. Tilghman, and S.R. Hinds, II. 2019. Blast-related traumatic brain injury: Current concepts and research considerations. *Journal of Experimental Neuroscience* 13, 1179069519872213. doi: 10.1177/1179069519872213

Cantu, R.C. 1998. Second-impact syndrome. *Clinics in Sports Medicine* 17: 37-44.

Cantu, R.C. 2001. Posttraumatic retrograde and anterograde amnesia: Pathophysiology and implications in grading and safe return to play. *Journal of Athletic Training* 36(3): 244-248.

Case, M.E., M.A. Graham, T.C. Handy, J.M. Jentzen, and J.A. Monteleone. 2001. Position paper on fatal abusive head injuries in infants and young children. *American Journal of Forensic Medicine and Pathology* 22: 112-122.

Cassidy, J.D., J. Duranceau, M.H. Liang, L.R. Salmi, M.L. Skovon, and W.O. Spitzer. 1995. Scientific monograph of the Quebec Task Force on whiplash associated disorders. *Spine* 20: S8-S58.

Centers for Disease Control and Prevention (CDC). 2019. Surveillance report of traumatic brain injury-related emergency department visits, hospitalizations, and deaths—United States, 2014. Available: https://www.cdc.gov/traumaticbraininjury/pdf/TBI-Surveillance-Report-FINAL_508.pdf

Chisholm, D.A., A.M. Black, L. Palacios-Derflingher, P.H. Eliason, K.J. Schneider, C.A. Emery, and B.E. Hagel. 2020. Mouthguard use in youth ice hockey and the risk of concussion: Nested case-control study of 315 cases. *British Journal of Sports Medicine* 54(14): 866-870. doi: 10.1136/bjsports-2019-101011

Cobb, S., and B. Battin. 2004. Second-impact syndrome. *Journal of School Nursing* 20: 262-267.

Cormier, J., Manoogian, S., Bisplinghoff, J., Rowson, S., Santago, A., McNally, C., Duma, S., and Bolte Iv, J. 2010. The tolerance of the nasal bone to blunt impact. *Annals of advances in automotive medicine. Association for the Advancement of Automotive Medicine. Annual Scientific Conference*, 54, 3-14.

Cusick, J.F., and N. Yoganandan. 2002. Biomechanics of the cervical spine 4: Major injuries. *Clinical Biomechanics* 17: 1-20.

Cutler, W.B., E. Friedmann, and E. Genovese-Stone. 1993. Prevalence of kyphosis in a healthy sample of pre- and postmenopausal women. *American Journal of Physical Medicine and Rehabilitation* 72: 219-225.

Damasio, A.R. 1994. *Descartes' Error: Emotion, Reason, and the Human Brain.* New York: Grosset/Putnam.

Damasio, H., T. Grabowski, R. Frank, A.M. Galaburda, and A.R. Damasio. 1994. The return of Phineas Gage: Clues about the brain from the skull of a famous patient. *Science* 264: 1102-1105.

Davis, C.G. 2000. Injury threshold: Whiplash-associated disorders. *Journal of Manipulative and Physiological Therapeutics* 23: 420-427.

Denny-Brown, D., and W.R. Russell. 1941. Experimental cerebral concussion. *Brain* 64: 93-164.

Duhaime, A.C., C.W. Christian, L.B. Rorke, and R.A. Zimmerman. 1998. Non-accidental head injury in infants—the "shaken-baby syndrome." *New England Journal of Medicine* 338: 1822-1829.

Eck, J.C., S.D. Hodges, and S.C. Humphreys. 2001. Whiplash: A review of a commonly misunderstood injury. *American Journal of Medicine* 110: 651-656.

Fackler, M.L. 1996. Gunshot wound review. *Annals of Emergency Medicine* 28: 194-203.

Fackler, M.L. 1998. Civilian gunshot wounds and ballistics: Dispelling the myths. *Emergency Medicine Clinics of North America* 16: 17-28.

Fardon, D.F., and P.C. Milette. 2001. Nomenclature and classification of lumbar disc pathology. *Spine* 26: E93-E113.

Gardner, B. 2002. Rehabilitation of spinal cord injuries. In *Oxford Textbook of Orthopedics and Trauma*, edited by C. Bulstrode, J. Buckwalter, A. Carr, L. Marsh, J. Fairbank, J. Wilson-MacDonald, and G. Bowden. Oxford, UK: Oxford University Press.

Gennarelli, T.A., and D.I. Graham. 2005. Neuropathology. In *Textbook of Traumatic Brain Injury*, edited by J.M. Silver, T.W. McAllister, and S.C. Yudofsky. Washington, DC: American Psychiatric Publishing.

Gennarelli, T.A., L.E. Thibault, J.H. Adams, D.I. Graham, C.J. Thompson, and R.P. Marcincin. 1982. Diffuse axonal injury and traumatic coma in the primate. *Annals of Neurology* 12: 564-574.

Giza, C.C., and D.A. Hovda. 2014. The new neurometabolic cascade of concussion. *Neurosurgery* 75(Suppl. 4): S24-33. doi: 10.1227/NEU.0000000000000505

Giza, C.C., J.S. Kutcher, S., Ashwal, J. Barth, T.S. Getchius, G.A. Gioia, et al. 2013. Summary of evidence-based guideline update: Evaluation and management of concussion in sports: Report of the Guideline Development Subcommittee of the American Academy of Neurology. *Neurology* 80(24): 2250-2257. doi: 10.1212/WNL.0b013e31828d57dd

Goldsmith, W., and J. Plunkett. 2004. A biomechanical analysis of the causes of traumatic brain injury in infants and children. *American Journal of Forensic Medicine and Pathology* 25: 89-100.

Grauer, J.N., M.M. Panjabi, J. Cholewicki, K. Nibu, and J. Dvorak. 1997. Whiplash produces an S-shaped curvature of the neck with hyperextension at lower levels. *Spine* 22: 2489-2494.

Grobler, L.J., P.A. Robertson, J.E. Novotny, and M.H. Pope. 1993. Assessment of the role played by lumbar facet joint morphology. *Spine* 18: 80-91.

Gross, A.G. 1958. Impact thresholds of brain concussion. *Journal of Aviation Medicine* 29: 725-732.

Gurdjian, E.S., and J.E. Webster. 1946. Deformation of the skull in head injury studied by stresscoat technique. *Surgery, Gynecology & Obstetrics* 83: 219-233.

Gurdjian, E.S., J.E. Webster, and H.R. Lissner. 1947. The mechanism of production of linear skull fractures. *American Journal of Surgery* 85: 195-210.

Gurdjian, E.S., J.E. Webster, and H.R. Lissner. 1949. Studies on skull fracture with particular reference to engineering factors. *American Journal of Surgery* 87: 736-742.

Gurdjian, E.S., J.E. Webster, and H.R. Lissner. 1953. Observations on prediction of fracture site in head injury. *Radiology* 60: 226-235.

Gurdjian, E.S., J.E. Webster, and H.R. Lissner. 1955. Observations on the mechanism of brain concussion, contusion, and laceration. *Surgery, Gynecology & Obstetrics* 101: 680-690.

Guskiewicz, K.M., J.P. Mihalik, V. Shankar, S.W. Marshall, D.H. Crowell, S.M. Oliaro, et al. 2007. Measurement of head impacts in collegiate football players: Relationship between head impact biomechanics and acute clinical outcome after concussion. *Neurosurgery* 61(6): 1244-1252. doi: 10.1227/01.neu.0000306103.68635.1a

Hampson, D. 1995. Facial injury: A review of biomechanical studies and test procedures for facial injury assessment. *Journal of Biomechanics* 28: 1-7.

Harmon, K.G., J.R. Clugston, K. Dec, B. Hainline, S. Herring, S.F. Kane, et al. 2019. American Medical Society for Sports Medicine position statement on concussion in sport. *British Journal of Sports Medicine* 53(4): 213-225. doi: 10.1136/bjsports-2018-100338

Hart, C., and E. Williams. 1994. Epidemiology of spinal cord injuries: A reflection of changes in South African society. *Paraplegia* 32: 709-714.

Haug, R.H., J.M. Adams, P.J. Conforti, and M.J. Likavec. 1994. Cranial fractures associated with facial fractures: A review of mechanism, type, and severity of injury. *Journal of Oral and Maxillofacial Surgery* 52: 729-733.

Hawes, M.C. 2003. The use of exercises in the treatment of scoliosis: An evidence-based critical review of the literature. *Pediatric Rehabilitation* 6: 171-182.

Hodgson, V.R. 1967. Tolerance of the facial bones to impact. *American Journal of Anatomy* 120: 113-122.

Hodgson, V.R., and L.M. Thomas. 1971. *Breaking Strength of the Human Skull vs. Impact Surface Curvature* (HS-800-583). Springfield, VA: U.S. Department of Transportation.

Hodgson, V.R., and L.M. Thomas. 1972. Effect of long-duration impact on head. In *Proceedings of the 16th Stapp Car Crash Conference*, Warrendale, PA: Society of Automotive Engineers.

Hodgson, V.R., and L.M. Thomas. 1973. *Breaking Strength of the Human Skull vs. Impact Surface Curvature* (HS-801-002). Springfield, VA: U.S. Department of Transportation.

Hogg, N.J., T.C. Stewart, J.E. Armstrong, and M.J. Girotti. 2000. Epidemiology of maxillofacial injuries at trauma hospitals in Ontario, Canada, between 1992 and 1997. *Journal of Trauma* 49: 425-432.

Holbourn, A.H.S. 1943. Mechanics of head injuries. *Lancet* 2: 438-441.

Holdsworth, F.W. 1970. Fractures, dislocations, and fracture-dislocations of the spine. *Journal of Bone and Joint Surgery* 52A: 1534-1541.

Hopper, R.H., J.H. McElhaney, and B.S. Myers. 1994. Mandibular and basilar skull fracture tolerance (SAE 942213). In *Proceedings of the 38th Stapp Car Crash Conference*, Warrendale, PA: Society of Automotive Engineers.

Ikata, T., R. Miyake, S. Katoh, T. Morita, and M. Murase. 1996. Pathogenesis of sports-related spondylolisthesis in adolescents. *American Journal of Sports Medicine* 24: 94-98.

Ito, S., P.C. Ivancic, M.M. Panjabi, and B.W. Cunningham. 2004. Soft tissue injury threshold during simulated whiplash. *Spine* 29: 979-987.

Karacan, I., H. Koyuncu, O. Pekel, G. Sumbuloglu, M. Kirnap, H. Dursun, A. Kalkan, A. Cengiz, A. Yalinkilic, H.I. Unalan, K. Nas, S. Orkun, and I. Tekeoglu. 2000. Traumatic spinal cord injuries in Turkey: A nation-wide epidemiological study. *Spinal Cord* 38: 697-701.

Kristman, V.L., J. Borg, A.K. Godbolt, L.R. Salmi, C. Cancelliere, L.J. Carroll, et al. 2014. Methodological issues and research recommendations for prognosis after mild traumatic brain injury: Results of the International Collaboration on Mild Traumatic Brain Injury Prognosis. *Archives of Physical Medicine and Rehabilitation* 95(Suppl. 3): S265-277. doi: 10.1016/j.apmr.2013.04.026

Kucera, K.L., D. Klossner, B. Colgate, and R.C. Cantu. 2020. Annual survey of football injury research 1931-2019. Available: https://nccsir.unc.edu/files/2020/09/Annual-Football-2019-Fatalities-FINAL-updated-20200618.pdf.

Kühne, C.A., C. Krueger, M. Homann, C. Mohr, and S. Ruchholtz. 2007. Epidemiology and management in emergency room patients with maxillofacial fractures. *Mund Kiefer und Gesichtschirurgie* 11: 201-208.

Kumar, S., R. Ferrari, and Y. Narayan. 2005. Kinematic and electromyographic response to whiplash loading in low-velocity whiplash impacts—a review. *Clinical Biomechanics* 20: 343-356.

Langlois, J.A., W. Rutland-Brown, and M.M. Wald. 2006. The epidemiology and impact of traumatic brain injury: A brief overview. *Journal of Head Trauma Rehabilitation* 21(5): 375-378. doi: 10.1097/00001199-200609000-00001

Langlois, J.A., W. Rutland-Brown, and K.E. Thomas. 2004. *Traumatic Brain Injury in the United States: Emergency Department Visits, Hospitalizations, and Deaths*. Atlanta: Centers for Disease Control and Prevention, National Center for Injury Prevention and Control.

Lestini, W.F., and S.W. Wiesel. 1989. The pathogenesis of cervical spondylosis. *Clinical Orthopaedics and Related Research* 239: 69-93.

Lim, L.H., L.K. Lam, M.H. Moore, J.A. Trott, and D.J. David. 1993. Associated injuries in facial fractures: Review of 839 patients. *British Journal of Plastic Surgery* 46: 635-638.

Lindh, M. 1989. Biomechanics of the lumbar spine. In *Basic Biomechanics of the Musculoskeletal System* (2nd ed.), edited by M. Nordin and V.H. Frankel. Philadelphia: Lea & Febiger.

Lowe, T.G., M. Edgar, J.Y. Margulies, N.H. Miller, V.J. Raso, K.A. Reinker, and C.-H. Rivard. 2000. Etiology of idiopathic scoliosis: Current trends in research. *Journal of Bone and Joint Surgery* 82A: 1157-1168.

Luan, F., K.H. Yang, B. Deng, P.C. Begeman, S. Tashman, and A.I. King. 2000. Qualitative analysis of neck kinematics during low-speed rear-end impact. *Clinical Biomechanics* 15: 649-657.

Martland, H.S. 1928. Punch drunk. *Journal of the American Medical Association* 91(15): 1103-1107. doi: 10.1001/jama.1928.02700150029009

Maxwell, W.L., C. Watt, D.I. Graham, and T.A. Gennarelli. 1993. Ultrastructural evidence of axonal shearing as a result of lateral acceleration of the head in non-human primates. *Acta Neuropathologica* 86: 136-144.

McCormack, B.M., and P.R. Weinstein. 1996. Cervical spondylosis: An update. *Western Journal of Medicine* 165: 43-51.

McCrea, M., K. Guskiewicz, C. Randolph, W.B. Barr, T.A. Hammeke, S.W. Marshall, et al. 2013. Incidence, clinical course, and predictors of prolonged recovery time following sport-related concussion in high school and college athletes. *Journal of the International Neuropsychological Society* 19(1): 22-33. doi: 10.1017/S1355617712000872

McCrea, M., T. Hammeke, G. Olsen, P. Leo, and K. Guskiewicz. 2004. Unreported concussion in high school football players: Implications for prevention. *Clinical Journal of Sport Medicine* 14(1): 13-17. doi: 10.1097/00042752-200401000-00003

McCrory, P. 2001. Does second impact syndrome exist? *Clinical Journal of Sport Medicine* 11: 144-149.

McCrory, P.R., and S.F. Berkovic. 2001. Concussion: The history of clinical and pathophysiological concepts and misconceptions. *Neurology* 57(12): 2283-2289. doi: 10.1212/wnl.57.12.2283

McCrory, P., K. Johnston, W. Meeuwisse, M. Aubry, R. Cantu, J. Dvorak, T. Graf-Baumann, J. Kelly, M. Lovell, and P. Schamasch. 2005. Summary and agreement statement of the 2nd International Conference on Concussion in Sport, Prague 2004. *Clinical Journal of Sports Medicine* 15: 48-55.

McCrory, P., W. Meeuwisse, J. Dvorak, M. Aubry, J. Bailes, S. Broglio, et al. 2017. Consensus statement on concussion in sport—the 5th International Conference on Concussion in Sport held in Berlin, October 2016. *British Journal of Sports Medicine* 51(11): 838-847. doi: 10.1136/bjsports-2017-097699

McElhaney, J.H., R.W. Nightingale, B.A. Winkelstein, V.C. Chancey, and B.S. Myers. 2001. Biomechanical aspects of cervical trauma. In *Accidental Injury*, edited by A.M. Nahum and J.W. Melvin. New York: Springer.

Melton, L.J., III. 1997. Epidemiology of spinal osteoporosis. *Spine* 22(Suppl. 24): 2S-11S.

Meythaler, J.M., J.D. Peduzzi, E. Eleftheriou, and T.A. Novack. 2001. Current concepts: Diffuse axonal injury—associated traumatic brain injury. *Archives of Physical Medicine and Rehabilitation* 82: 1461-1471.

Mihalik, J.P., M.A. McCaffrey, E.M. Rivera, J.E. Pardini, K.M. Guskiewicz, M.W. Collins, and M.E. Lovell. 2007. Effectiveness of mouthguards in reducing neurocognitive deficits following sports-related cerebral concussion. *Dental Traumatology* 23(1): 14-20. doi: 10.1111/j.1600-9657.2006.00488.x

Miller, J.D. 1993. Traumatic brain swelling and edema. In *Head Injury* (3rd ed.), edited by P.R. Cooper. Baltimore: Williams & Wilkins.

Miller, N.H. 2000. Genetics of familial idiopathic scoliosis. *Spine* 25: 2416-2418.

Murata, Y., K. Takahashi, M. Yamagata, E. Hanaoka, and H. Moriya. 2003. The knee-spine syndrome. *Journal of Bone and Joint Surgery* 85B: 95-99.

Murrie, V.L., A.K. Dixon, W. Hollingworth, H. Wilson, and T.A.C. Doyle. 2003. Lumbar lordosis: Study of patients with and without low back pain. *Clinical Anatomy* 16: 144-147.

Nachemson, A. 1975. Towards a better understanding of low-back pain: A review of the mechanics of the lumbar disc. *Rheumatology and Rehabilitation* 14: 129-143.

Nahum, A.M., J.D. Gatts, C.W. Gadd, and J.P. Danforth. 1968. Impact tolerance of the skull and face (680785). In *Proceedings of the 12th Stapp Car Crash Conference*, Warrendale, PA: Society of Automotive Engineers.

Natarajan, R.N., R.B. Garretson, III, A. Biyani, T.H. Lim, G.B. Andersson, and H.S. An. 2003. Effects of slip severity and loading directions on the stability of isthmic spondylolisthesis: A finite element model study. *Spine* 28: 1103-1112.

Neuman, M., and E. Eriksson. 2006. Facial trauma. In *Textbook of Pediatric Emergency Medicine*, edited by G.R. Fleisher, S. Ludwig, and F.M. Henretig. Hagerstown, MD: Lippincott Williams & Wilkins.

Offierski, C.M., and I. MacNab. 1983. Hip-spine syndrome. *Spine* 8: 316-321.

Old, J.L., and M. Calvert. 2004. Vertebral compression fractures in the elderly. *American Family Physician* 69: 111-116.

Omalu, B.I., S.T. DeKosky, R.L. Minster, M.I. Kamboh, R.L. Hamilton, and C.H. Wecht. 2005. Chronic traumatic encephalopathy in a National Football League player. *Neurosurgery* 57(1): 128-134. doi: 10.1227/01.neu.0000163407.92769.ed

Ommaya, A.K. 1995. Head injury mechanisms and the concept of preventive management: A review and critical synthesis. *Journal of Neurotrauma* 12: 527-546.

Ommaya, A.K., and T.A. Gennarelli. 1974. Cerebral concussion and traumatic unconsciousness: Correlations and experimental and clinical observations on blunt head injuries. *Brain* 97: 633-654.

Ommaya, A.K., R.L. Grubb, Jr., and R.A. Naumann. 1971. Coup and contre-coup injury: Observations on the mechanics of visible brain injuries in the rhesus monkey. *Journal of Neurosurgery* 35: 503-516.

Ommaya, A.K., W. Goldsmith, and L. Thibault. 2002. Biomechanics and neuropathology of adult and paediatric head injury. *British Journal of Neurosurgery* 16: 220-242.

Padman, R. 1995. Scoliosis and spine deformities. *Delaware Medical Journal* 67: 528-533.

Panjabi, M.M., A.M. Pearson, S. Ito, P.C. Ivancic, and J.-L. Wang. 2004. Cervical spine curvature during simulated whiplash. *Clinical Biomechanics* 19: 1-9.

Panjabi, M.M., S. Ito, A.M. Pearson, and P.C. Ivancic. 2004. Injury mechanisms of the cervical intervertebral disc during simulated whiplash. *Spine* 29: 1217-1225.

Panjabi, M.M., T.R. Oxland, R.-M. Lin, and T.W. McGowen. 1994. Thoracolumbar burst fracture: A biomechanical investigation of its multidirectional flexibility. *Spine* 19: 578-585.

Pappachan, B., and Alexander, M. 2012. Biomechanics of cranio-maxillofacial trauma. *Journal of maxillofacial and oral surgery* 11(2), 224-230. doi: 10.1007/s12663-011-0289-7

Parent, S., P.O. Newton, and D.R. Wenger. 2005. Adolescent idiopathic scoliosis: Etiology, anatomy, natural history, and bracing. *Instructional Course Lectures* 54: 529-536.

Pastakia, K., and S. Kumar. 2011. Acute whiplash associated disorders (WAD). *Open Access Emergency Medicine* 3, 29-32. doi: 10.2147/OAEM.S17853

Pearson, A.M., P.C. Ivancic, S. Ito, and M.M. Panjabi. 2004. Facet joint kinematics and injury mechanisms during simulated whiplash. *Spine* 29: 390-397.

Pellman, E.J., D.C. Viano, A.M. Tucker, I.R. Casson, and J.F. Waeckerle. 2003. Concussion in professional football: Reconstruction of game impacts and injuries. *Neurosurgery* 53(4): 799-812. doi: 10.1093/neurosurgery/53.3.799

Pintar, F.A., N. Yoganandan, L.M. Voo, J.F. Cusick, D.J. Maiman, and A. Sances, Jr. 1995. Dynamic characteristics of the human cervical spine. *SAE Transactions* 104: 3087-3094.

Powell, J.W., and K.D. Barber-Foss. 1999. Traumatic brain injury in high school athletes. *Journal of the American Medical Association* 282: 958-963.

Radanov, B.P., M. Sturzenegger, and G. Di Stefano. 1995. Long-term outcome after whiplash injury: A 2-year follow-up considering features of injury mechanism and somatic, radiologic, and psychosocial findings. *Medicine* 74: 281-297.

Rhee, J.S., L. Posey, N. Yoganandan, and F. Pintar. 2001. Experimental trauma to the malar eminence: Fracture biomechanics and injury patterns. *Otolaryngology Head and Neck Surgery* 125: 351-355.

Rowson, S., S.M. Duma, R.M. Greenwald, J.G. Beckwith, J.J. Chu, K.M. Guskiewicz, et al. 2014. Can helmet design reduce the risk of concussion in football? *Journal of Neurosurgery* 120(4): 919-922. doi: 10.3171/2014.1.JNS13916

Rydevik, B., M. Szpalski, M. Aebi, et al. 2008. Whiplash injuries and associated disorders: New insights into an old problem. *European Spine Journal* 17, 359-416. doi: 10.1007/s00586-007-0484-x

Sahuquillo, J., and M.A. Poca. 2002. Diffuse axonal injury after head trauma. A review. *Advances and Technical Standards in Neurosurgery* 27: 23-86.

Sano, K., N. Nakamura, K. Hirakawa, H. Masuzawa, and K. Hashizume. 1967. Mechanism and dynamics of closed head injuries (preliminary report). *Neurologia medico-chirurgica (Tokyo)* 9: 21-33.

Santucci, R.A., and Y.-J. Chang. 2004. Ballistics for physicians: Myths about wound ballistics and gunshot injuries. *Journal of Urology* 171: 1408-1414.

Schneider, D.C., and A.M. Nahum. 1972. Impact studies of facial bones and skull (SAE 720965). In *Proceedings of the 16th Stapp Car Crash Conference*, Warrendale, PA: Society of Automotive Engineers.

Schroeder, G.D., A.R. Vaccaro, C.K. Kepler, J.D. Koerner, F.C. Oner, M.F. Dvorak, et al. 2015. Establishing the injury severity of thoracolumbar trauma: Confirmation of the hierarchical structure of the AOSpine Thoracolumbar Spine Injury Classification System. *Spine (Phila Pa 1976)* 40(8): E498-503. doi: 10.1097/BRS.0000000000000824

Severy, D.M., J.H. Mathewson, and C.O. Bechtol. 1955. Controlled automobile rearend collisions, an investigation of related engineering and medical phenomena. *Canadian Services Medical Journal* 11: 727-759.

Sokolove, P.E., N. Kuppermann, and J.F. Holmes. 2005. Association between the "seat belt sign" and intra-abdominal injury in children with blunt torso trauma. *Academy of Emergency Medicine* 12: 808-813.

Stehbens, W.E. 2003. Pathogenesis of idiopathic scoliosis revisited. *Experimental and Molecular Pathology* 74: 49-60.

Stinson, J.T. 1993. Spondylolysis and spondylolisthesis in the athlete. *Clinics in Sports Medicine* 12: 517-528.

Swartz, E.E., R.T. Floyd, and M. Cendoma. 2005. Cervical spine functional anatomy and the biomechanics of injury due to compressive loading. *Journal of Athletic Training* 40(3): 155-161.

Teasdale, G., and B. Jennett. 1974. Assessment of coma and impaired consciousness. A practical scale. *Lancet* 2(7872): 81-84.

Tegner, Y., and R. Lorentzon. 1996. Concussion among Swedish elite ice hockey players. *British Journal of Sports Medicine* 30: 251-255.

Tierney, R.T., M.R. Sitler, C.B. Swanik, K.A. Swanik, M. Higgins, and J. Torg, 2005. Gender differences in head-neck segment dynamic stabilization during head acceleration. *Medicine and Science in Sports and Exercise* 37(2): 272-279. doi: 10.1249/01.mss.0000152734.47516.aa

Torg, J.S., J.J. Vegso, M.J. O'Neill, and B. Sennett. 1990. The epidemiologic, pathologic, biomechanical, and cinematographic analysis of football-induced cervical spine trauma. *American Journal of Sports Medicine* 18: 50-57.

Tran, N.T., N.A. Watson, A.F. Tencer, R.P. Ching, and P.A. Anderson. 1995. Mechanism of the burst fracture in the thoracolumbar spine: The effect of loading rate. *Spine* 20: 1984-1988.

Tuzun, C., I. Yorulmaz, A. Cindas, and S. Vatan. 1999. Low back pain and posture. *Clinical Rheumatology* 18: 308-312.

Valsamis, M.P. 1994. Pathology of trauma. *Neurosurgery Clinics of North America* 5: 175-183.

Van Pelt, K L., T. Puetz, J. Swallow, A.P. Lapointe, and S.P. Broglio. 2021. Data-driven risk classification of concussion rates: A systematic review and meta-analysis. *Sports Medicine* 51(6): 1227-1244.

Volgas, D.A., J.P. Stannard, and J.E. Alonso. 2005. Ballistics: A primer for the surgeon. *Injury* 36: 373-379.

Watkins, R.G., and W.G. Watkins, IV. 2001. Cervical spine and spinal cord injuries. In *Sports Injuries: Mechanisms, Prevention, Treatment*, edited by F.H. Fu and D.A. Stone. Philadelphia: Lippincott Williams & Wilkins.

Watkins, R.G., and L.A. Williams. 2001. Lumbar spine injuries. In *Sports Injuries: Mechanisms, Prevention, Treatment*, edited by F.H. Fu and D.A. Stone. Philadelphia: Lippincott Williams & Wilkins.

Wegner, D.R., and S.L. Frick. 1999. Scheuermann kyphosis. *Spine* 24: 2630-2639.

White, A.A., and M.M. Panjabi. 1990. *Clinical Biomechanics of the Spine* (2nd ed.). Philadelphia: Lippincott.

Wiebe, D.J., B.A. D'Alonzo, R. Harris, M. Putukian, and C. Campbell-McGovern. 2018. Association between the experimental kickoff rule and concussion rates in Ivy League football. *Journal of the American Medical Association* 320(19): 2035-2036. doi: 10.1001/jama.2018.14165

Weisenbach, C.A., Gomez, J., Daniel, R.W., and Brozoski, F.T. 2020. Summary of available craniomaxiollofacial injury criteria for use with the FOCUS headform. United States Army Aeromedical Research Laboratory: Fort Rucker, AL.

Wiltse, L.L., P.H. Newman, and I. MacNab. 1976. Classification of spondylolysis and spondylolisthesis. *Clinical Orthopaedics and Related Research* 117: 23-29.

Wotherspoon, S., K. Chu, and A.F. Brown. 2001. Abdominal injury and the seat-belt sign. *Emergency Medicine (Fremantle)* 13: 61-65.

Wunderle, K., K.M. Hoeger, E. Wasserman, and J.J. Bazarian. 2014. Menstrual phase as predictor of outcome after mild traumatic brain injury in women. *The Journal of Head Trauma Rehabilitation* 29(5): E1-E8. doi: 10.1097/HTR.0000000000000006

Yoganandan, N., N.M. Haffner, D.J. Maiman, H. Nichols, F.A. Pintar, J. Jentzen, S.S. Weinshel, S.J. Larson, and A. Sances, Jr. 1989. Epidemiology and injury biomechanics of motor vehicle related trauma to the human spine. In *Proceedings of the 3rd Stapp Car Crash Conference* (SAE 892438), Warrendale, PA: Society of Automotive Engineers.

Yoganandan, N., and F.A. Pintar. 2004. Biomechanics of temporo-parietal skull fracture. *Clinical Biomechanics* 19: 225-239.

Yoganadan, N., F.A. Pintar, A. Sances, Jr., P.R. Walsh, C.L. Ewing, D.J. Thomas, and R.G. Snyder. 1995. Biomechanics of skull fracture. *Journal of Neurotrauma* 12: 659-668.

Yoganandan, N., F. Pintar, J. Reinartz, and A.J. Sances. 1993. Human facial tolerance to steering wheel impact: A biomechanical study. *Journal of Safety Research* 24: 77-85.

Zemper, E.D. 2003. Two-year prospective study of relative risk of a second cerebral concussion. *American Journal of Physical Medicine & Rehabilitation* 82: 653-659.

Zhang, L., K.H. Yang, and A.I. King. 2001. Biomechanics of neurotrauma. *Neurological Research* 23: 144-156.

Note: The italicized *f* and *t* following page numbers refer to figures and tables, respectively.

A

acceleration
  angular 54*f*, 55, 62, 64, 261
  average vs. instantaneous 54*f*
  linear 54*f*, 55, 55*f*, 64, 257, 259-260
  in rear-end collisions 273
  rotational 248, 257, 259-260
  second law of motion and 62, 62*f*, 63
  as vector measurement 53
acceleration injuries 248, 250
accident-liability theory 13
accident-proneness theory 13
accidents, defined 5
Achilles tendon
  compressive and tensile loading in 111, 113, 201
  injuries to 115-116, 122, 200-203, 202*f*
acromioclavicular (AC) joint 207, 210-213, 211*f*, 212*f*
acromion 207, 210-211, 216-221, 218*f*
acromioplasty 217, 221, 222
action potentials 41, 44
active stabilization 214
acute muscular strain 143
acute vs. chronic injuries 122, 124, 125
adaptations
  of articular cartilage 112-113
  of bone 105-111
  defined 99
  factors affecting 99-100
  of skeletal muscle 117-119
  of tendons and ligaments 114-116
adhesive capsulitis 213
adipocytes 24
adipose tissue 23-24
adjustment-to-stress theory 13
age, chronological vs. physiological 125
aggrecan 34, 34*f*, 111
all-or-none principle 44
anabolic steroids 126
analytical epidemiology 10
anastomoses 30-32
anatomical drawings 7, 7*f*
anatomical position 58*f*, 71, 71*f*, 236
aneurysms 251
angular acceleration 54*f*, 55, 62, 64, 261

angular displacement 53, 54*f*, 75, 75*f*
angular impulse 67
angular kinetics 58-61
angular momentum 67
angular motion 52-53, 52*f*, 58, 61-62, 67
angular power 64, 65
angular velocity 53-54, 54*f*, 61, 62, 64-67, 75, 75*f*
angular work 64
ankle and foot injuries 193-205
  Achilles tendon pathologies 115, 122, 200-203, 202*f*
  anatomy of 188*t*, 193-196, 193*f*, 194*f*, 195*f*, 196*f*
  plantar fasciitis 203, 204*f*
  sprains 38, 196-200, 197*f*, 198*f*, 199*f*, 200*f*
  taping and bracing for prevention of 38, 39
  toe injuries 204-205, 204*f*, 205*f*
annulus fibrosus 279-283, 280*f*
anterior cruciate ligament (ACL) injuries
  anatomy of 168, 168*f*, 173
  artificial turf and 69
  conservative treatment of 175
  epidemiology of 172-173
  injury mechanisms 173-175, 174*f*
  neuromotor control patterns following 38-39
  osteoarthritis following 39, 136, 175
  prevention of 176-177
  rehabilitation of 176, 177*t*
  surgical repair of 175-176, 176*f*
  tissue mechanics and 173
anterior drawer mechanism 175
anterior talofibular ligament (ATFL) 193, 197, 199*f*
anthropometry and anthropometrics 69, 90, 127, 201
aponeuroses 37, 196, 204*f*, 235*f*
appositional growth 33
arachnoid mater 247, 251
Archimedes' principle 71
area moment of inertia 83-85, 84*f*, 102
areolar tissue 23, 36
arm injuries 225-227, 226*f*. *See also* forearm injuries

arousal–alertness theory 13
arthritis. *See also* osteoarthritis
  causes of 34
  in early humans 5
  inflammatory response and 127
  pathology of 144-145
  spondylolisthesis and 277
arthrology 45-48, 45*t*, 46*t*, 47*t*. *See also* joints
arthroplasty 8, 135, 138, 160, 161, 222
arthroscopy 8, 218, 222-223
articular cartilage
  adaptive capabilities 112-113
  biomechanics of 111-112
  cellular organization of 33-34, 33*f*, 135
  development and maturation of 112-113
  durability of 71
  healing of 137
  injuries to 135-137
  loading of 34, 34*f*, 111-112, 111*f*
  lubrication mechanisms 112
  use vs. disuse effects on 113
articulations. *See* joints
artificial turf 69
atherosclerosis 70, 126
atrophy 113-119, 126, 136, 139, 218, 223, 227
auditory ossicles 245
automobile collisions. *See* vehicle collisions
avascular necrosis 131, 157, 160
average velocity 54, 54*f*
avulsion fracture 113, 114, 133-134, 231, 238, 270*f*
axis of rotation 52, 52*f*, 58, 60-61, 73, 76, 167
axonotmesis 148
axons 22, 44, 44*f*, 146, 148

B

ballistics 164, 253-254
Bankart lesions 224, 224*f*
Barton's fractures 239, 239*f*
baseball pitching, kinetics of 231, 232*f*
basement membrane 21
basilar skull fractures 250
bending
  bone 101-104, 101*f*, 102*f*, 103*t*
  cantilever 63, 85-86, 86*f*

bending *(continued)*
    four-point 85, 85*f*
    material stresses in response to 83-85, 84*f*, 85*f*
    three-point 85, 85*f*, 101*f*, 104
Bennett's fracture 243
biaxial loading 81-82, 82*f*, 83*f*
biceps tendon injuries 227
bilaminar embryonic discs 20-21
biomechanics. *See also* kinematics; kinetics; tissue biomechanics
    bending modes in 85
    defined 4
    models and simulations in 89-93
    nutrition considerations 125
    performance 69
    research needs on 16-17
    of skull fractures 250
    terminology issues 122
biotribology 69
bipennate muscles 43-44, 43*f*
blastemas 48
blastocysts 20, 20*f*, 21*t*
blast-related injuries 248, 253
body mass index (BMI) 157, 161, 276
bone. *See also* cortical bone; trabecular bone; *specific bones*
    adaptive capabilities 105-111
    biomechanics of 100-105
    comparative properties of 105
    deformities of 29, 29*f*
    development and maturation of 26-29, 26*f*, 27*f*, 106-107, 107*f*
    female athlete triad and 108-109
    injuries to 130-135
    mass of 102, 104, 106-110, 107*f*, 131-132, 156
    modeling and remodeling of 26, 26*f*, 30, 32, 106-109, 106*t*, 135
    nutrition considerations 107-108
    structure of 32, 32*t*, 124
    tissue components 29-32
    use vs. disuse effects on 109-111
bone mineral content (BMC) 106-109, 117, 252
bone mineral density (BMD) 26, 107-110, 131-132, 131*f*, 156, 160, 189
bone-on-bone force 76, 77*f*
bone–patellar tendon–bone (BPTB) grafts 175-176, 176*f*
bracing
    of ankles 38, 39
    for ligament injuries 123
    for scoliosis 275, 276*f*
brain stem 246-247, 247*f*, 260, 262
bruises. *See* contusions
bucket-handle tears 179, 179*f*
buoyant forces 71
bursitis 127, 203, 219, 229

burst fractures 274
butterfly fractures 133

C
calcaneal tendon. *See* Achilles tendon
calcaneofibular ligament (CFL) 193, 197, 199*f*
canaliculi 27, 30, 31*f*
cancellous bone. *See* trabecular bone
cantilever bending 63, 85-86, 86*f*
capability–demand theory 13
car crashes. *See* vehicle collisions
cardiac muscle 39-40
carpal fractures 242, 242*f*
carpal tunnel syndrome (CTS) 125, 130, 148, 241-242
cartilage. *See* fibrocartilage; hyaline cartilage
cavitation 164, 254, 254*f*, 260
center of gravity 57, 58*f*, 60
center of mass 57, 58*f*, 62*f*, 64, 66-67, 76-77, 248, 249*f*
Centers for Disease Control and Prevention (CDC) 4, 12, 157-158, 255
centripetal theory 262
cerebellum 246, 247*f*
cerebral contusions 250, 256-258, 257*f*
cerebral edema 130, 258, 261
cerebrospinal fluid (CSF) 247-248, 250, 258
cerebrum 246, 247, 247*f*
cervical spondylosis 270-271
cervical trauma 265-268, 266*f*, 266*t*, 267*f*, 268*f*
chondral fractures 135-136
chondroblasts 21, 24, 33
chondrocytes 24-25, 27-28, 33-35, 34*f*, 112-113, 135
chondromalacia 136, 183-184, 231
chronic compartment syndrome (CCS) 188-189
chronic traumatic encephalopathy (CTE) 255
chronic vs. acute injuries 122, 124, 125
chronological age 125
cigarette smoking 132, 161
circumferential fibrocartilage 35
closed fractures 133
closure of epiphyseal plates 28
Cobb angle 275*f*, 276
coefficient of restitution 68
collagen
    Achilles tendon ruptures and 203
    in bone 30, 32, 103, 124
    in cartilage 33-35, 33*f*, 34*f*, 111, 111*f*, 112
    in connective tissue 22-23
    in extracellular matrix 24, 30
    in ligaments 37, 113-115, 124

mass of 115
structure of 25, 25*f*
in tendons 35, 36*f*, 114-116, 124, 216
collateral ligament injuries 171, 172*f*, 179-180, 180*f*
Colles' fractures 238-239, 239*f*
collisions. *See also* vehicle collisions
    bodily 243, 251
    continuum of 68
    defined 67
    facial fractures from 251
    SLAP lesions from 225
columnar epithelium 21-22, 23*f*
comminuted fractures 133
compact bone. *See* cortical bone
compartment syndromes 130, 146, 161, 186, 188-189, 189*f*, 191
compensatory injuries 124
complete fractures 133
complex glycoproteins 25
compound fractures 250
compression–flexion mechanism 265-266
compressive stress 28, 78, 82*f*, 83, 84*f*, 103
concavity compression 214
concurrent force systems 56, 57*f*
concussions 255, 256, 258-261
congenital hip dislocations 159-160
connecting fibrocartilage 35
connective tissue 22-37. *See also specific types of connective tissue*
    bone 26-32
    cartilage 33-35
    constituents of 24-26
    defined 22
    dense 25, 36-37
    fascia 37
    loose 22-25, 36
    organization of 22*f*
    tendons and ligaments 35-37
conservation of energy 66
conservation of momentum 67
continuum mechanical models 91
contrecoup lesions 256-258, 257*f*
contusions
    cerebral 250, 256-258, 257*f*
    compartment syndromes and 188
    from impact injuries 143, 145
    quadriceps 161-162
coronoid fractures 234, 235*f*
corpus callosum 246, 247*f*, 261
cortical bone
    arterial supply of 30*f*, 31
    biomechanics of 101-104, 101*f*, 102*f*, 103*t*
    endochondral ossification of 27*f*
    fatigue and failure in 103-105

injuries to 131, 133
structure of 26, 31*f*, 32, 32*t*, 100
countertorque (countermoment) 61
coup lesions 256-258, 257*f*
coxa vara/coxa valga 63
cramps 143
cranial bones 245, 246*f*
cranial nerves 247, 248*t*, 250
crash-test dummies 89, 90, 158
creep response 34, 88, 88*f*, 103, 111, 113
cross-bridge cycles 41-42, 42*f*, 45, 116
cryotherapy 127, 175
cuboidal epithelium 21-22, 23*f*
curvilinear motion 52, 52*f*
cyclic loading 103-105, 112, 113, 139

D
deformable-body models 91
deformation. *See also* load–deformation curve
elastic 67
to failure 80
plastic 67, 80, 80*f*, 101
spinal 6, 9, 274-277, 275*f*, 276*f*, 277*f*
of tissue 76, 88, 122, 249
degenerative joint disease. *See* osteoarthritis
delayed-onset muscle soreness (DOMS) 143
dendrites 22, 44*f*
de novo deposition of woven bone 32
dense irregular connective tissue 37
dense regular connective tissue 25, 36-37
density. *See also* bone mineral density
compartment syndromes and 130
of connective tissue 22, 24
fluid mechanics and 69
material mechanics and 77
of muscle fibers 42-43
strain energy and 80
depressed skull fractures 249*f*, 250
dermatome 21
descriptive epidemiology 9-10
destabilizing component of force 60, 60*f*
deterministic models 91
diabetes 52, 126, 148, 161, 213
diaphyses 27*f*, 28, 30, 30*f*, 101-102
diarthrodial joints 45, 48, 69, 71, 112
diet. *See* nutrition
diffuse axonal injuries (DAIs) 260-262
direct injuries 132, 226, 248
dislocations
biceps tendon 227
elbow 234, 234*f*
hip 158-160, 159*f*
joint 72, 131, 144, 144*f*, 148
metacarpal and phalangeal 243

shoulder 9, 211, 213-216, 216*f*, 224
vertebral 265-266
displacement
angular 53, 54*f*, 75, 75*f*
of bone fragments 133
linear 53, 54*f*, 75, 76
of medial meniscus 178
posterior vertebral 266
of radial head 237, 238
of tarsometatarsal joints 204
as vector measurement 53
distal radius fractures 238-239, 238*f*, 239*f*
distance 53, 55*f*, 64, 65*f*
drag forces 71
drug use 126, 130, 156, 159
dura mater 247, 250, 251
dynamic equilibrium 64
dynamic models 91

E
ectoderm 20-22, 21*f*
edema
cerebral 130, 258, 261
muscle strains and 143
in Osgood–Schlatter disease 184
pressure and 111, 127, 129, 148
quadriceps contusions and 161
skin injuries and 145
tissue fluid and 26, 129
eggs (oocytes) 20
elastic cartilage 34-35
elastic deformation 67
elastic fibers 22, 23, 25, 33, 35, 37
elasticity 67, 79, 86-88, 92, 279
elastic modulus. *See* modulus of elasticity
elastin 24, 25
elbow injuries 227-234
anatomy of 227-229, 228*f*, 229*t*
dislocations 234, 234*f*
epicondylitis 230-231
fractures 234, 235*f*
sport-specific 229, 229*t*
valgus-extension loading 231-232, 232*f*, 234
embryonic stage of development 20-21, 20*f*, 21*f*, 21*t*
endochondral ossification 27, 27*f*, 28, 32, 48
endoderm 20-21, 21*f*
endomysium 40*f*, 41, 44
endoneurium 146-148, 147*f*
endotendineum 35
endurance training 115, 117, 118
energy
conservation of 66
defined 65
to failure 80

kinetic 65-66, 164, 254, 260
mechanical 16, 45, 65-66, 103
potential 65-66, 103
strain 28, 66, 173
transfer of 66, 254-255, 269, 273
entrapment conditions. *See* compartment syndromes
epicondylitis 230-231
epidemiology
of ACL injuries 172-173
analytical 10
of concussions 259
data collection issues 11-12
defined 8
descriptive 9-10
of injuries 8-12, 65
of osteoarthritis 137
relative risk and 11, 13
epidural hematomas 250
epimysium 40, 40*f*
epineurium 146-148, 147*f*
epiphyses 27-32, 27*f*, 30*f*
epitendineum 35
epithelial tissue 21-22, 22*f*, 23*f*
equilibrium 63-64, 83*f*, 99, 111, 231, 246
ergogenic aids 126
ergonomics 128
estrogen 29, 108, 110, 132
eversion sprains 198
exercise-induced muscle injuries 143
external mechanics 53, 76
extracellular matrix 22-30, 33-35, 33*f*, 34*f*, 37, 111, 116, 130-131

F
facial bones 245, 246*f*, 252, 252*f*
facial fractures 251-252, 251*f*
falls
AC injuries from 211
dislocations from 158, 215, 227
fractures from 154, 156-158, 164, 192, 225, 227, 234
as impact injuries 67, 68
labral injuries from 224
prevention strategies 117
spinal cord injuries from 268
thumb injuries from 242-243
traumatic brain injuries from 255, 259
fascia 37, 130, 185-186, 188, 189
fatigue fractures 190
female athlete triad 108-109
femoral fractures 163-164, 163*f*
fetal stage of development 20
fibroblasts 21, 23-24, 33, 35, 37, 115, 135
fibrocartilage
of acetabular labrum 153-154

fibrocartilage (*continued*)
　development of 35
　of glenohumeral labrum 223
　injuries to 137
　of menisci 35, 137, 170, 177, 178*f*
　of osteotendinous junction 36*f*
　in vertebral column 264
fibrocytes 24
fibroelastic tissue 23
fibular fractures 192-193, 193*f*
finite-element modeling 91, 93, 93*f*
first-class lever systems 73, 74*f*
first law of motion 62-63, 62*f*, 68
flattened tendons. *See* aponeuroses
flexural rigidity 101, 101*f*
fluid flow 70, 112
fluid mechanics 69-71
fluid resistance 70-71
football
　ACL injuries in 69, 173
　ankle sprains in 200
　concussions in 255, 259
　contusions in 161
　energy transfer in 66
　hip injuries in 159, 160
　macrotrauma in 220
　spinal cord injuries in 268
　strain injuries in 164
foot injuries. *See* ankle and foot injuries
force. *See also* torque
　bone-on-bone 76, 77*f*
　components of 60, 60*f*
　defined 55
　fluid resistance and 71
　ground reaction 62*f*, 63, 77*f*, 90, 178
　impulsive 67, 258
　joint reaction 76, 77*f*, 171*f*, 182, 183, 214, 215*f*
　lever systems and 72-73, 74*f*
　linear power and 64-65
　linear work and 64, 65*f*
　in second law of motion 62, 62*f*, 63
force couple 56, 57*f*
force systems 56, 57*f*
force–velocity relation curve 44, 44*f*
forearm injuries 235-240
　anatomy of 235-236, 235*f*, 236*t*
　diaphyseal fractures of radius and ulna 236-238, 237*f*
　distal radius fractures 238-239, 238*f*, 239*f*
　ulnar variance 240
four-point bending 85, 85*f*
fractures. *See also* stress fractures
　avulsion 113, 114, 133-134, 231, 238, 270*f*
　carpal fractures 242, 242*f*
　cervical 265, 266, 268*f*

classification of 133-134, 133*f*
complications of 133-134
elbow 234, 235*f*
facial 251-252, 251*f*
femoral 163-164, 163*f*
forearm 236-239, 237*f*, 238*f*, 239*f*
growth disturbances and 29
healing 134-135, 134*f*
hip 10, 63, 132, 154, 156-158, 156*f*
humeral 225-226, 226*f*, 234, 235*f*
metacarpal and phalangeal 243
nightstick 5, 236
pathology of 132-133
pelvic 156
shoulder dislocations and 215
skull 249*f*, 250-251
tibial and fibular 192-193, 193*f*
vertebral 271, 274
free-body diagrams (FBDs) 56, 57*f*
friction
　defined 68
　in joints 35, 69, 71, 112
　kinetic 68-69, 68*f*, 71
　in rheological models 92
　skin injuries and 145
　static 68, 68*f*, 71
frozen shoulder 213
funny bone 231
fusiform muscles 43, 43*f*
G
Galeazzi fractures 236
gastrulation 20, 21
general force systems 56, 57*f*
general motion 52
genetics 117, 125, 137, 160, 203, 240, 275
Glasgow Coma Scale (GCS) 256, 256*t*
glenohumeral (GH) joint
　impingement syndrome 130, 217-221, 217*f*
　instability and dislocation of 213-216, 216*f*
　joint reaction force and 214, 215*f*
　loads during activities of daily living 214, 215*t*
　musculature of 209, 209*f*, 210*t*
　structure of 207-209, 208*f*
glycosaminoglycans 25, 26
goals–freedom–alertness theory 13
gravitational potential energy 66
gravity, center of 57, 58*f*, 60
ground reaction force (GRF) 62*f*, 63, 77*f*, 90, 178
ground substance of connective tissue 25
growth plates. *See* physes
H
hamstring strains 164-166, 165*f*

hamstring tendon (HT) grafts 175-176
hand injuries. *See* wrist and hand injuries
head injuries 245-262
　anatomy of 245-248, 246*f*, 247*f*, 248*t*
　cerebral contusions 250, 256-258, 257*f*
　cerebral edema 130, 258, 261
　concussions 255, 256, 258-261
　diffuse axonal injuries 260-262
　facial fractures 251-252, 251*f*
　injury mechanisms 248-250, 249*f*
　penetrating 249, 252-255
　skull fractures 249*f*, 250-251
　traumatic brain injuries 255-262
health education programs 14
hematomas 134, 161, 250-251
hematopoiesis 26, 130
hemodynamics 69, 89
hemorrhage 130, 143, 145, 161, 186, 250-251, 260-261
herniated discs 137, 276, 280-283, 282*f*
high ankle sprains 200, 200*f*
hip injuries 153-161
　anatomy of 153-154, 154*f*, 155*f*, 155*t*
　dislocations 158-160, 159*f*
　fractures 10, 63, 132, 154, 156-158, 156*f*
　osteoarthritis 160-161
homeostasis 32, 99, 125, 259
Hooke's law 79, 101
hoop effect 178
human error 5, 13, 125
humeral fractures 225-226, 226*f*, 234, 235*f*
hyaline cartilage 27*f*, 33-34, 33*f*, 111, 137, 279. *See also* articular cartilage
hydroxyapatite 30, 32, 106
hypertrophy 27, 113, 116-119, 270
hysteresis 87*f*, 88, 99, 103, 113
I
idealized force vectors 55, 56
iliotibial band syndrome (ITBS) 185, 185*f*
impingement syndromes 130, 217-221, 217*f*
impulse–momentum principle 67
impulsive force 67, 258
incidence, defined 10
incomplete fractures 133
indirect injuries 133, 164, 226, 248
inertia
　area moment of 83-85, 84*f*, 102
　defined 55
　first law of motion and 62-63, 62*f*
　mass moment of 61, 62*f*, 66, 67

polar moment of 86, 86*f*

inflammation. *See also specific conditions*

of Achilles tendon 122

as injury response 38, 116, 126, 127, 129-130, 129*f*

migratory cells and 24

in Osgood–Schlatter disease 184

quadriceps contusions and 161

initial-cycles effect 88-89, 89*f*

injuries. *See also* head injuries; injury mechanisms; lower-extremity injuries; neck injuries; rehabilitation; trunk injuries; upper-extremity injuries; *specific names and types of injuries*

to articular cartilage 135-137

to bone 130-135

contributory factors 124-127

definitions of 4, 122

economic perspective on 12

epidemiological perspective on 8-12, 65

ergonomics and 128

fatalities resulting from 3-4, 4*f*, 11-12

to fibrocartilage 137

health professional perspective on 12

historical perspective on 5-8, 6*f*, 7*f*, 8*f*

inflammatory response to 38, 116, 126, 127, 129-130, 129*f*

to joints 144-145

to ligaments 123, 139-140

to nervous tissue 145-148, 147*f*

prevention strategies 10, 12, 14-15, 166, 281

psychosocial perspective on 12-14, 14*t*, 125

safety professional perspective on 14-16

scientific perspective on 16-17

severity classification 123, 123*f*

to skeletal muscle 140-143

to skin 145, 146*f*

to tendons 137-139

terminology issues 122-123

tissue structure and 124

types of 122-125

unintentional 3-5, 12, 125

injury control programs 14

Injury in America (Committee on Trauma Research) 12, 16

injury mechanisms

for Achilles tendon ruptures 201, 202*f*

for ACL injuries 173-175, 174*f*

for ankle injuries 196, 198, 199*f*

bending modes and 85, 85*f*

for carpal fractures 242, 242*f*

categorization of 122

for cervical trauma 265-268, 267*f*

for femoral fractures 164

for hamstring strains 165

for head injuries 248-250, 249*f*, 260, 261

identification of 121-122

meniscal 178

for metacarpal and phalangeal conditions 243

models in discovery of 89

for Osgood–Schlatter disease 184

for osteoarthritis 137

for quadriceps contusions 161

for radius and ulna fractures 236, 238*f*

research needs on 16, 17

for skin injuries 145

for spinal cord injuries 268-269

for tendon ruptures 184

for thumb injuries 243

tissue deformation and 76

for toe injuries 204

in whiplash 62-63, 62*f*, 269

in situ research approach 99, 100, 105, 173

instantaneous joint center 76

instantaneous velocity 54-55, 54*f*

insufficiency fractures 190

internal impingement 217-218

internal mechanics 53, 76

interstitial growth 33

intervertebral discs

aging process and 270

degeneration of 125, 280, 281

herniated 137, 276, 280-283, 282*f*

structure of 35, 137, 264, 279, 280*f*

intra-articular fibrocartilage 35

intracranial hemorrhage 250, 251

intracranial pressure (ICP) 251, 258, 261

intramembranous ossification 26, 26*f*, 28

inversion sprains 38, 197-198

in vitro research approach 99, 100

in vivo research approach 76, 99, 100

ischemia 124, 188-189, 191, 242, 258, 271

J

joint reaction force (JRF) 76, 77*f*, 171*f*, 182, 183, 214, 215*f*

joint replacement. *See* arthroplasty

joints. *See also specific joints*

arthrology 45-48, 45*t*, 46*t*, 47*t*

diarthrodial 45, 48, 69, 71, 112

friction in 35, 69, 71, 112

injuries to 144-145

as lever systems 72-75, 74*f*, 75*f*

mobility and stability of 72, 73*t*

primary movement planes 71, 71*f*, 72*t*

as shock absorbers 7

stiffness of 16

torque and motion of 75-76, 75*f*, 76*f*

K

Kelvin–Voight models 92

kilogram, history of 56

kinematics

Achilles tendon loading and 201

defined 53

models for prediction of 91

patellar 183

rotator cuff lesions and 220

subacromial impingement and 218

variables related to 53-55, 54*f*

kinetics

angular 58-61

of baseball pitching 231, 232*f*

collisions and 67-68

defined 53

energy and 65-66, 164, 254, 260

equilibrium and 63-64, 83*f*

friction and 68-69, 68*f*, 71

laws of motion and 62-63, 62*f*, 65, 68

linear 55-58

models for prediction of 91

momentum and 66-68

power and 64-65

work and 64-65, 65*f*

knee injuries 166-186. *See also* anterior cruciate ligament injuries

anatomy of 166-167*f*, 166-171, 168*t*, 170*f*, 181*f*

collateral ligament injuries 171, 172*f*, 179-180, 180*f*

extensor disorders 180-184

iliotibial band syndrome 185, 185*f*

meniscus injuries 137, 177-179, 179*f*

Osgood–Schlatter disease 184, 184*f*

patellofemoral pain 180-184, 182*f*

quadriceps and patellar tendon ruptures 184, 186

knee joint 45, 48*f*

kyphosis 6, 274, 275*f*, 276

L

labral pathologies 223-225, 224*f*, 225*t*

lamellar bone 32, 32*t*

laminar flow 70

lateral ankle sprains 197

lateral collateral ligament (LCL) 168, 170, 180, 180*f*

lateral epicondylitis 230-231

laws of motion 62-63, 62*f*, 65, 68, 278

leg injuries. *See* lower-leg injuries; thigh injuries
length–tension relation curve 44, 44*f*
level of dysfunction 123
lever arm. *See* torque arm
lever systems 72-75, 74*f*, 75*f*
ligaments. *See also specific ligaments*
 adaptive capabilities 114-115
 biomechanics of 113-114, 114*f*
 development and maturation of 114
 healing of 140
 injuries to 123, 139-140
 structure of 37, 135
 use vs. disuse effects on 114-115, 115*f*
linear acceleration 54*f*, 55, 55*f*, 64, 257, 259-260
linear displacement 53, 54*f*, 75, 76
linear force systems 56, 57*f*
linear fractures 250
linear impulse 67
linear kinetics 55-58
linear momentum 67
linear motion 52-53, 52*f*, 55, 58, 61-62, 257, 277
linear power 64-65
linear velocity 53-54, 54*f*, 55*f*, 64-67, 75, 75*f*, 254
linear work 64, 65*f*
Lisfranc fracture–dislocations 204, 204*f*
load–deformation (L–d) curve
 bone bending test and 101, 101*f*
 stress–strain curve compared to 80, 81*f*
 tissue response to loading and 77, 78*f*
 viscoelasticity and 87*f*, 88
longitudinal muscles 43, 43*f*
loose connective tissue 22-25, 36
lordosis 6, 265, 274-277, 275*f*, 277*f*
low back pain 137, 277, 281
lower-extremity injuries 153-205
 ankle and foot 193-205
 hip 153-161
 knee 166-186
 lower-leg 185-193
 overview 153
 thigh 161-166
lower-leg injuries 185-193. *See also* knee injuries
 anatomy of 185-186, 187*f*, 188*t*
 compartment syndrome 186, 188-189, 189*f*, 191
 medial tibial stress syndrome 189-191
 tibial stress reaction and stress fracture 190-191, 190*f*

traumatic fractures of tibia and fibula 192-193, 193*f*
lubrication mechanisms 112

M

macrophages 23, 24, 129*f*, 135
macrotrauma vs. microtrauma 124
magnus forces 71
mass. *See also* center of mass
 body mass index 157, 161, 276
 of bone 102, 104, 106-110, 107*f*, 131-132, 156
 of collagen 115
 defined 55
 momentum and 67
 of muscle 117, 118, 127, 186
 point mass 57, 61, 62*f*
 velocity and 162, 254
 volume and 130, 188
massive rotator cuff tears (MRCT) 222
mass moment of inertia 61, 62*f*, 66, 67
mast cells 24
material mechanics 76-89
 fatigue and failure in 88-89, 89*f*
 loading types and 77, 79-87
 tissue response to loading and 77-79
 viscoelasticity and 87-88, 87*f*, 88*f*
Maxwell models 92
mechanical energy 16, 45, 65-66, 103
mechanical loading
 axial 79-83, 82*f*, 83*f*
 bending and 83-86, 84*f*, 85*f*, 86*f*
 bone response to 26, 106
 deformation and stiffness in 77, 78*f*
 loading types 77, 79-87
 of proximal femur 63
 stress and strain of 77-79
 tissue response to 71, 77-79
 torsion and 86-87, 86*f*, 87*f*
mechanical strain 78-79, 164
mechanical work 64, 65*f*, 103
mechanics. *See also* biomechanics
 defined 4
 external 53, 76
 fluid 69-71
 internal 53, 76
 joint 71-76
 material 76-89
 of muscle 40, 45
 Newtonian (classical) 62
 rigid-body 76
mechanisms. *See also* injury mechanisms
 defined 4, 121, 122
 of energy transfer 66
 of lubrication 112
 of momentum transfer 67
 protective 108

mechanotransduction 24
medial ankle sprains 198
medial collateral ligament (MCL) 168, 170, 175, 178-180, 180*f*
medial epicondylitis 231
medial tibial stress syndrome (MTSS) 189-191
medullary canals 31, 31*f*
meninges 247, 250
menisci
 blastema and 48
 fibrocartilage of 35, 137, 170, 177, 178*f*
 injuries to 137, 177-179, 179*f*
 shape of 170, 170*f*
menopause 107-110, 132, 271
menstrual dysfunction 108-109
mesenchyme 21, 33, 48
mesoderm 20-22, 26, 39, 117
metacarpal injuries 243
metaphyses 27*f*, 28, 30-32
microcracks 104, 105, 124
microfibrils 25, 35, 36*f*
microtears 116, 124, 203, 219
microtrauma vs. macrotrauma 124
migratory cells 24
mild traumatic brain injuries (MTBIs) 258
modeling
 in biomechanics 89-93
 of bone 26*f*, 106, 106*t*
 mathematical 273
modulus of elasticity 79, 79*f*, 87, 92, 101-105, 113-114, 114*f*
moment arm. *See* torque arm
moment of force. *See* torque
momentum 66-68, 260, 273
Monteggia lesions 236-238, 237*f*
morulas 20
motion, laws of 62-63, 62*f*, 65, 68, 278
motor units 44-45, 44*f*
motor vehicle collisions. *See* vehicle collisions
multiaxial loading 81-83, 82*f*, 83*f*
multifactorial model of causation 10, 11*f*
multipennate muscles 43-44, 43*f*
muscle tissue. *See also* skeletal muscle
 cardiac 39-40
 mass of 117, 118, 127, 186
 necrosis of 164
 organization of 22*f*
 smooth 39
myofibrils 40*f*, 41, 45, 117
myofilaments 40*f*, 41
myositis ossificans (MO) 143, 162-163, 162*f*
myotendinous junction 36-37, 117, 138-143, 139*f*, 161, 165-166, 165*f*

myotome 21

N

National Safety Council 3, 11, 12
neck injuries 262-271
    anatomy of 262, 262-263*f*
    cervical spondylosis 270-271
    cervical trauma 265-268, 266*f*, 266*t*, 267*f*, 268*f*
    spinal cord injuries 219, 264, 268-269
    whiplash 62-63, 62*f*, 269-270, 269*f*, 270*f*, 271*t*
nervous tissue 22, 22*f*, 145-148, 147*f*, 252
net torque (moment) 60, 61, 61*f*, 64
neurapraxia 148, 264-265
neurons 22, 148
neurotmesis 148
nightstick fractures 5, 236
notochord 20, 21, 21*t*
nucleus pulposus 279-283, 280*f*
nutrition
    in bone growth and remodeling 107-108
    as contributory factor to injury 125
    hip osteoarthritis and 160
    muscle endurance capacity and 119

O

obesity 107, 127, 136-137, 157, 161
oocytes (eggs) 20
open fractures 133
orthotics 38
Osgood–Schlatter disease (OSD) 184, 184*f*
ossification 26-28, 26*f*, 27*f*, 32, 48
osteoarthritis (OA)
    ACL injuries and 39, 136, 175
    femoral fracture and 164
    in hip 160-161
    pathology of 33, 113, 136-137, 136*f*
osteoblasts 21, 24, 26, 26*f*, 28-30, 106, 135
osteochondral fractures 135
osteoclasts 26*f*, 28, 30, 32, 106, 110, 115, 135
osteocytes 24, 27, 29-32, 31*f*, 36, 130
osteoid 26*f*, 28, 29
osteonecrosis 131
osteons 31*f*, 32, 32*t*, 100, 104
osteopenia 26, 108, 131, 131*f*
osteophytes 136, 136*f*, 161, 220, 223, 231, 270
osteoporosis
    bone mineral density in 131, 131*f*
    definitions of 131
    exercise and 110
    female athlete triad and 108
    kyphosis and 276

    pathology of 132
    prevalence of 10, 131-132, 131*f*
    sex-specific differences in 125
    vertebral fractures and 271
osteosarcoma 126
osteotendinous junction 36, 36*f*, 134, 137, 139-140
overuse injuries 115-116, 122, 126, 218, 230

P

pain
    in frozen shoulder 213
    in inflammatory response 127
    in low back 137, 277, 281
    in medial tibial stress syndrome 189
    in neck 270
    patellofemoral 180-184, 182*f*
    protective function of 7
    in quadriceps contusions 161
    in spinal cord injuries 268
    in sprains 38
    tolerance to 14
    in vertebral fractures 274
palmar aponeurosis 37, 235*f*
parallel-elastic components 45
parallel force systems 56, 57*f*
pars interarticularis 277, 277*f*
passive stabilization 214
patellar tendon 113, 116, 170, 184, 186
patellar tracking 181
patellofemoral joint (PFJ) 171, 171*f*
patellofemoral pain (PFP) 180-184, 182*f*
pelvic fractures 156
penetrating head injuries 249, 252-255
pennate muscles 43-44, 43*f*
perfectly elastic/inelastic collisions 68
performance biomechanics 69
perichondrium 33, 33*f*, 34
perimysium 40, 40*f*
perineurium 146-148, 147*f*
periosteum 30, 30*f*, 31*f*, 37, 134-135
peripheral neuropathies 126, 148
peritenon 36
phagocytes 24, 129*f*, 130
phalangeal injuries 243
physes 27-32, 27*f*, 30*f*, 117
physiological age 125
pia mater 247, 251
planar kinematics 53, 54*f*
planar models 91
plantar aponeurosis 196, 204*f*
plantar fasciitis (PF) 203, 204*f*
plastic deformation 67, 80, 80*f*, 101
point mass 57, 61, 62*f*
Poisson's effect 81, 82, 82*f*
Poisson's ratio 81, 103
polar moment of inertia 86, 86*f*

position, as kinematic variable 53, 54*f*
positional potential energy 66
posterior cruciate ligament (PCL) 168, 170-173, 170*f*, 172*f*
posterior talofibular ligament (PTFL) 193, 197, 199*f*
posterolateral rotatory instability (PLRI) 234
potential energy 65-66, 103
power 64-65
pressure
    compartment syndromes and 130
    defined 58, 78
    intracranial 251, 258
    swelling and 111, 127, 129, 148
prevalence, defined 10
primary bone 32, 32*t*
primary injuries 123-124
primary ossification centers 28
primary osteons 32
progression of injuries 123
progressive overload principle 116
pronation 185, 198, 198*f*, 203, 229, 235*f*, 236-237
proteoglycans 25-26, 34, 34*f*, 37, 111-113, 136, 279
puberty 108, 118
public health approach 10

Q

Q angle 181-182, 182*f*
quadriceps-avoidance gait 39
quadriceps contusions 161-162
quadriceps tendon ruptures 184
quadriplegia 269
quasi-static models 91

R

radial collateral ligament (RCL) 228*f*, 229, 234
radial head fractures 234-238, 235*f*, 237*f*
radiate muscles 43*f*
range of motion (ROM)
    ACL injuries and 175, 176
    in delayed-onset muscle soreness 143
    joint mechanics and 72, 73*t*
    preventing loss of 115
    rotator cuff pathologies and 221-223
    whiplash injuries and 270
rear-end collisions 269, 273
rectilinear motion 52, 52*f*
rehabilitation
    of ACL injuries 176, 177*t*
    of concussions 260
    factors for success 126, 127
    psychosocial perspective on 12-13
    of rotator cuff pathologies 222-223

relative risk 11, 13
remodeling of bone 26, 26f, 30, 32, 106-109, 106t, 135
resident cells 24
resistance (strength) training 116-118
reticular fibers 22, 23, 37
reticular tissue 23
rheological models 91-92, 92f, 93f
rigid-body mechanics 76
rigid-body models 91
risk
    culture of 14
    defined 13
    relative 11, 13
risk factors, defined 10
rotational acceleration 248, 257, 259-260
rotational motion. *See* angular motion
rotator cuff pathologies 216-223
    age-related considerations 223
    glenohumeral impingement 130, 217-221, 217f
    postoperative care and rehabilitation 222-223
    prevention strategies 223
    rotator cuff rupture 219-220, 219f
    tissue structure and function in 216-217, 217t
    treatment strategies 220-223
rotatory component of force 60, 60f

S

safety education programs 14
sarcomeres 41, 41f, 43-44, 116, 117, 164, 165
scalar measurements 53, 54, 64
scapulohumeral balance 214
Scheuermann's kyphosis 276
sclerotome 21
scoliosis 6, 274-276, 275f, 276f
screw-home mechanism 167
secondary bone 32, 32t
secondary injuries 123-124
secondary ossification centers 28
second-class lever systems 73, 74f
second impact syndrome (SIS) 261
second law of motion 62, 62f, 63, 278
series-elastic components 45
Sharpey's fibers 36, 37
shear stress 37, 78, 82-83, 83f, 85-87, 85f, 86f, 260
shin splints 191
shoulder injuries 207-225
    AC sprains 210-213, 211f, 212f
    anatomy of 207-209, 208f, 209f, 210t
    dislocations 9, 211, 213-216, 216f, 224

    glenohumeral instability and 213-216
    labral pathologies 223-225, 224f, 225t
    rotator cuff pathologies 216-223
    sport-specific 209-210, 210t
simple epithelium 21-22, 23f
skeletal muscle
    adaptive capabilities 117-119
    biomechanics of 116-117
    development and maturation of 117
    fiber types in 42-44, 43f, 43t, 117
    injuries to 140-143
    motor units and 44-45, 44f
    rotator cuff 216, 217f
    sex-related effects on 118
    stiffness of 37, 40, 45
    stimulated vs. passive 140-142, 141f, 142f, 143f
    structure of 40-41, 40f, 41f
    of trunk 271, 272-273f
    use vs. disuse effects on 118-119
skin injuries 145, 146f
skull fractures 249f, 250-251
SLAP lesions 224-225, 224f, 225t
sliding filament theory 41
Smith's fractures 239, 239f
smoking 132, 161
smooth muscle 39
somites 21, 21t, 48
spatial kinematics 53
spatial models 91
speed, as scalar measurement 54
sperm cells (spermatozoa) 20
spinal cord injuries (SCIs) 219, 264, 268-269
spinal deformities 6, 9, 274-277, 275f, 276f, 277f
spinal stenosis 270-271
spine. *See* vertebral column
spiral fractures 192
spondylolysis and spondylolisthesis 277-279, 277f, 279f, 279t
spongy bone. *See* trabecular bone
sprains
    acromioclavicular 210-213, 211f, 212f
    ankle 38, 196-200, 197f, 198f, 199f, 200f
    pathology of 140
    thumb 242-243
squamous epithelium 21-22, 23f
stabilizing component of force 60, 60f
static equilibrium 64
static friction 68, 68f, 71
static models 91
stem cells 21, 24, 132, 222
steroids, anabolic 126
stiffness

    of bone 30, 32, 103
    of cartilage 34
    in frozen shoulder 213
    of joints 16
    of ligaments 114, 115
    mechanical loading and 77, 78f
    of muscles 37, 40, 45
    of neck 270
    of tendons 113
stochastic models 91
strain. *See also* stress–strain curve
    to failure 80
    in fractures 135
    hamstring 164-166, 165f
    mechanical 78-79, 164
    musculotendinous 138-139, 142-143
strain energy 28, 66, 80, 173
stratified epithelium 21-22, 23f
stratiform fibrocartilage 35
strength (resistance) training 116-118
stress
    compressive 28, 78, 82f, 83, 84f, 103
    shear 37, 78, 82-83, 83f, 85-87, 85f, 86f, 260
    tensile 78, 82f, 83, 83f, 84f, 103-104, 113-114, 279-281
stress fractures
    cortical bone and 104
    differential diagnoses and 189
    female athlete triad and 108
    pathology of 132
    of proximal femur 277
    spondylolysis and 277
    tibial 190-191
stress reactions 189, 190, 190f
stress-relaxation response 88, 88f, 99, 113
stress risers 89, 165, 220
stress–strain curve 78-80, 79f, 80f, 81f, 87, 113
striated muscle. *See* skeletal muscle
subacromial impingement 217, 217f, 218, 220-221
subarachnoid hematomas 251
subarachnoid space 247
subdural hematomas 251
supination 197, 198f, 229, 230, 234-236, 235f
swelling. *See* edema

T

taping of ankles 38, 39
teardrop fractures 266, 268f
tendinitis
    bicipital 209, 219
    differential diagnoses and 189, 203
    inflammatory response and 69, 127, 139

patellar 184
shin splints and 191
tendon ruptures
Achilles 115, 122
anabolic steroid use and 126
genetic influences on 125
injury mechanisms for 184
as macrotrauma 124
patellar 184, 186
quadriceps 184
spontaneous 139
tendons. *See also specific tendons*
adaptive capabilities 114-115
biomechanics of 113-114
development and maturation of 114
healing of 139
injuries to 137-139
structure of 35-36, 36*f*, 135
use vs. disuse effects on 114-116
tendon transplantation surgery 233
tensile stress 78, 82*f*, 83, 83*f*, 84*f*, 103-104, 113-114, 279-281
tension–extension mechanism 266, 267*f*
testosterone 29, 118, 126
thigh injuries 161-166
femoral fractures 163-164, 163*f*
hamstring strains 164-166, 165*f*
myositis ossificans 143, 162-163, 162*f*
quadriceps contusions 161-162
third-class lever systems 73, 74*f*
third law of motion 62, 62*f*, 63
three-point bending 85, 85*f*, 101*f*, 104
thumb injuries 242-243, 243*f*
tibial fractures 192-193, 193*f*
tide mark 33*f*
time, as kinematic variable 53, 54*f*
tissue. *See also* connective tissue; muscle tissue; tissue biomechanics
adaptive capabilities 99-100, 105-119
defined 19
deformation of 76, 88, 122, 249
elasticity of 67
embryology of 20-21, 20*f*, 21*f*, 21*t*
epithelial 21-22, 22*f*, 23*f*
injuries and structure of 124
models of 91-93, 92*f*, 93*f*
nervous 22, 22*f*, 145-148, 147*f*, 252
response to loading 71, 77-79
structural strength of 23, 79, 114-115, 168
tissue biomechanics
articular cartilage 111-112
bone 100-105
defined 69
methodology for study of 99, 100

skeletal muscle 116-117
tendons and ligaments 113-114, 114*f*
tissue fluid 22, 24-26, 33, 34, 34*f*, 258
toe injuries 204-205, 204*f*, 205*f*
Tommy John surgery 233
torque. *See also* force
angular power and 65
angular work and 64
applied 59, 59*f*, 86-87, 86*f*, 87*f*
countertorque 61
defined 58, 278
joint motion and 75-76, 75*f*, 76*f*
net 60, 61, 61*f*, 64
in second law of motion 62
torque arm 58-60, 59*f*, 63, 73, 278
torsion, mechanical loading and 86-87, 86*f*, 87*f*
total mechanical energy (TME) 66
trabecular bone
biomechanics of 104-105
female athlete triad and 108
injuries to 131
structure of 26, 32, 32*t*, 100-101
use vs. disuse effects on 109
traction apophysitis 184
transfer of energy 66, 254-255, 269, 273
transfer of momentum 67
translational motion. *See* linear motion
transverse tubules (T-tubules) 41
traumatic brain injuries (TBIs) 255-262
triaxial loading 82-83, 83*f*
trunk injuries 271-283
anatomy of 271, 272-273*f*
intervertebral disc pathologies 279-283, 282*f*
spinal deformities 6, 9, 274-277, 275*f*, 276*f*, 277*f*
spondylolysis and spondylolisthesis 277-279, 277*f*, 279*f*, 279*t*
vertebral fractures 271, 274
truss mechanism 203, 204*f*
turbulent flow 70
turf toe 204-205, 205*f*

U
ulnar collateral ligament (UCL) 228*f*, 229, 231-234, 242, 243*f*
ulnar fractures 234-238, 235*f*, 237*f*
ulnar variance 240
undifferentiated mesenchymal stem cells 24
unhappy triad 175
uniaxial loading 79-81
unintentional injuries 3-5, 12, 125
unipennate muscles 43-44, 43*f*
upper-extremity injuries 207-243

elbow 227-234
forearm 235-240
overview 207
shoulder 207-225
upper-arm 225-227
wrist and hand 240-243

V
valgus, use of term 169
valgus-extension loading injuries 231-232, 232*f*, 234
varus, use of term 169
vector measurements 53-55, 54*f*
vehicle collisions
drug use and 126
facial fractures from 251-252, 251*f*
fatigue-related 125
femoral fractures from 163
head injuries from 255, 259, 261
hip and pelvic injuries from 154, 156-159, 159*f*
knee injuries from 171
neck injuries from 266, 268
rear-end 269, 273
terminology issues 5
whiplash from 269
velocity
angular 53-54, 54*f*, 61, 62, 64-67, 75, 75*f*
average vs. instantaneous 54-55, 54*f*
force–velocity relation curve 44, 44*f*
linear 53-54, 54*f*, 55*f*, 64-67, 75, 75*f*, 254
mass and 162, 254
momentum and 67
as vector measurement 53
vertebral column 264, 264*f*, 265*f*
vertebral fractures 271, 274
viscoelasticity 87-88, 87*f*, 88*f*, 103-105, 113, 132, 134, 279
viscosity 71, 87, 112, 114

W
Wallerian degeneration 148, 261
warning signs 16
wedge fractures 265
weightlifting 62*f*, 63, 64, 65*f*, 186, 278
whiplash 62-63, 62*f*, 269-270, 269*f*, 270*f*, 271*t*
windlass mechanism 203, 204*f*
Wolff's law 105-106, 190
work 64-65, 65*f*, 103
World Health Organization (WHO) 3, 10-12, 131, 132
wound ballistics 164, 253-254
woven bone 32, 32*t*
wrist and hand injuries 240-243
anatomy of 240-241, 240*f*, 241*f*

carpal fractures 242, 242*f*
carpal tunnel syndrome 125, 130, 148, 241-242
metacarpal and phalangeal 243
thumb injuries 242-243, 243*f*

Y
yellow elastic ligaments 37
Young's modulus. *See* modulus of elasticity

Z
zone of Ranvier 28
zygotes 20, 20*f*

Name Index

Note: The italicized *f* and *t* following page numbers refer to figures and tables, respectively.

A

Abrams, G.D. 230
Achilles (warrior) 200
Adams, J.H. 261
Adams, M.A. 281
Adebayo, E.T. 251
Aebi, M. 276
Affatato, S. 138
Agarwal, Y. 266*t*
Agel, J. 173, 176
Agrahari, Y. 215
Ahmad, C.S. 231
Ahmed, A.M. 178, 180
Ahmed, I.M. 201
Akeson, W.H. 115
Alashkham, A. 223
Alexander, M. 252*f*
Alexander, R.M. 102, 104
Allen, C.R. 173
Allen, L.R. 205
Allen, M. 138
Allman, F.L., Jr. 211
Allsop, D. 252
Almeida, S.A. 185
Alvi, A. 251
Amiel, D. 115
Amonoo-Kuofi, H.S. 276-277
Anakwenze, O.A. 234
Andarawis-Puri, N. 139
Andary, M. 242
Andersen, J.H. 230
Anderson, C.J. 168
Anderson, R.N. 125
Andrews, J.R. 171, 225
Andrews, K. 179
Antuña, S.A. 231
Apostolakis, E. 6
Arendt, E. 177
Arnason, A. 166
Arndt, A.N. 201
Aro, H.T. 204
Arthur, J.R. 171
Ashizawa, N. 108
Ashman, E.S. 230
Askling, C. 166
Åstrand, P.-O. 45, 118
Atalay, İ.B. 222
Atroshi, I. 241
Avicenna (Inb Sina) 7

B

Bado, J.L. 236
Bailes, J.E. 260
Bailey, D.A. 108, 109
Bakalakos, R. 159
Baker, C.L. 230
Baker, S.P. 158
Baldwin, K.M. 117
Banas, M.P. 220
Bandy, W.D. 117, 118
Bankart, A. 224

Barber-Foss, K.D. 261
Barber-Westin, S. 177
Barbour, K.E. 161
Barco, R. 231
Barnsley, L. 270, 273
Barry, M. 182
Bartlett, C.S. 254
Bartolozzi, A. 221
Bartynski, W.S. 276
Bass, S.L. 109
Batt, M.E. 191
Battin, B. 261
Bazarian, J.J. 259
Beck, B.R. 189
Beiner, J.M. 161, 162
Benjamin, M. 115
Berchuck, M. 38-39
Bergmann, G. 76
Berkovic, S.F. 258
Besier, T.F. 183
Best, T.M. 42, 43*t*, 117, 118
Beutler, W.J. 278
Beveridge, W.I.B. 100
Bigliani, L.U. 218, 220
Bilanin, J. 110
Biles, S. 153
Bircher, E. 8
Bittencourt, N.F.N. 11
Bjordal, J. 173
Blemker, S.S. 93
Blevins, F.T. 220
Boden, B. 173
Bogduk, N. 269, 273
Bogey, R.A. 201
Bonza, J.E. 210*t*
Boos, N. 276
Bostrom, M.P.G. 107-108
Botte, M.J. 242
Bouche, R.T. 189
Bourrin, S. 108
Boyd, H.B. 237
Boyd, S. 93*f*
Bradford, D.S. 276-278
Bradica, G. 25, 34
Bradley, J. 173
Branch, T. 227
Brand-Saberi, B. 117
Brandt, K.D. 136
Brasileiro, B.F. 251
Brechter, J.H. 182, 183
Breuil, V. 156
Brewer, B.W. 12
Brien, W.W. 164
Bright, A.S. 220
Brockett, C.L. 166
Broglio, S.P. 259, 260
Browner, B.D. 158, 159, 226*f*
Bryden, D.W. 248
Buckingham, M. 117
Budoff, J.E. 218
Buerba, R.A. 188

Buess, E. 222
Bunn, T.L. 125
Burdett, R.G. 201
Burke, D.L. 178
Burkhart, S.S. 220, 221, 225
Burnham, R.S. 219
Burnier, M. 222
Burr, D.B. 32*t*, 100
Burstein, A.H. 72
Buss, D.D. 211
Butler, D.L. 173

C

Cabral, W.A. 30
Caesar, B. 225
Cai, Y. 123
Caine, D.J. 5, 240
Callaghan, E.B. 227
Calvert, M. 271
Cantu, R.C. 258, 260, 261
Carr, J.B. 196, 197
Carter, D.R. 28-29
Carter, S.R. 201
Cascio, B. 176
Case, M.E. 261
Casparian, J.M. 201
Cassidy, C. 242
Cassidy, J.D. 269
Cavaillon, J.-M. 130
Celsus, A.C. 127
Chakravarthy, M.V. 116
Chalmers, P.N. 220
Chan, H.B.Y. 213
Chan, M. 140
Chandler, T.J. 191
Chang, Y.-J. 254
Chao, E.Y. 242
Charlton, W.P.H. 230
Chen, C.H. 222
Chen, C.T. 113
Chen, G. 118
Chhabra, H.S. 266*t*
Chikritzhs, T. 126
Chisholm, D.A. 260
Cho, C.-H. 213
Chong, A.K.S. 242
Chu, C.R. 136
Chudik, S.C. 159
Church, J.S. 188
Ciccotti, M.G. 230
Ciullo, J.V. 191
Clark, D. 183
Clasper, J. 213
Close, G.L. 143
Cobb, S. 261
Coccolini, F. 156
Codding, J.L. 222
Codman, E.A. 213, 221
Cohen, M.S. 234
Cohen-Fix, O. 40
Collins, K.H. 136, 137

Collins, M. 203
Connell, D. 165
Conway, J.E. 233
Cooper, C. 161
Cooper, D.E. 223
Cooper, G. 202
Cooper, J. 158
Corbett, R.O. 38
Cormier, J. 252*f*
Corpus, K.T. 218
Couppé, C. 114
Court-Brown, C.M. 192, 225
Crabb, W.A. 169
Crawford, R. 203
Cresswell, T.R. 215
Crisco, J.J. 161-162
Croft, P. 137
Croisier, J.L. 165, 166
Croker, S.L. 102-103
Crossley, K.M. 183
Crowell, H.P. 104
Cummings, S.R. 156
Cunningham, G. 218
Cureton, K.J. 118
Curie, M. 3
Currey, J.D. 30, 102-105
Curtis, E.M. 156
Cusick, J.F. 265, 268
Cutler, W.B. 276

D

Damasio, A.R. 253
Dandy, D.J. 172
Darling, A.L. 108
da Vinci, L. 7-8, 51
Davis, C.G. 270
Davis, I.S. 104
Day, S.M. 131
Dayton, P.D. 189
Dean, D. 124
Dean, J.C. 116
Deary, L. 185
DeCoster, T.A. 163
Deftos, L. 32
Delp, S.L. 93
Demirag, B. 184
Demirel, M. 215
Denny-Brown, D. 258
Deprés-Tremblay, G. 222
Deprez, X. 108
De Smet, L. 240
De Vito, G. 116
Dias, J. 242
Dias, R. 213
Diaz, A.R. 157
Diaz, J.A. 161
Dick, R. 177
Dienst, M. 173
DiFiori, J.P. 240
Divani, K. 184

Dizon, J.M.R. 38
D'Lima, D.D. 76
Dodwell, E.R. 175
Doehrmann, R. 215
Doherty, C. 197
Donlon, D. 102-103
Dorfman, H.D. 162
Doschak, M.R. 115
Doty, S.B. 109
Dragoo, J.L. 69, 177
Duethman, N.C. 171
Duhaime, A.C. 261
Dunleavy, K. 117, 118
Dunlop, R. 221
Duplay, E.S. 213
Durham, M. 35
Dye, S.F. 183
Dyson, S.J. 35

E
Eck, J.C. 270
Edelson, G. 217
Edgar, C. 211
Edson, C.J. 171
Ehrhardt, J. 116
Ekholm, R. 225
ElAttrache, N.S. 231
Ellender, L. 126
Emond, M. 215
Engelke, K. 109
Enger, M. 210
Englemark, V.E. 113
Eriksen, H.A. 203
Eriksson, E. 251
Erkman, M. 178
Etheridge, B.S. 156
Evangelidis, P.E. 165
Evans, M. 237
Eyre, D.R. 25

F
Fackler, M.L. 253, 254
Fairclough, J. 185
Fanelli, G.C. 171
Fardellone, P. 108
Fardon, D.F. 281
Farley, T.E. 218-220
Farnaghi, S. 136
Farrell, K.C. 185
Fawcett, D.W. 24, 25
Felson, D.T. 137
Fernandez, D.L. 238
Filbay, S.R. 176, 177t
Flanagan, S. 118
Fleisig, G.S. 231, 232f
Flynn, S.H. 185
Foley, J. 184
Fonseca, S.T. 11
Foulk, D.A. 220
Fowler, J.R. 242
Fox, K.M. 157
Frank, C.B. 114, 115, 140
Frassica, F.J. 184
Fredericson, M. 190f
Freedman, B.R. 183
Frick, S.L. 276
Friden, J. 164
Friel, N.A. 136
Frush, T.J. 215
Fu, G. 15
Fukashiro, S. 201
Fukunaga, T. 118

Fulkerson, J.P. 136
Funakoshi, T. 222
Funsten, R.V. 158

G
Gage, P. 253
Galanakos, S.P. 6
Galeazzi, R. 236
Galen (physician) 6, 127
Galloway, M.T. 114-116
Gardner, B. 269
Garhammer, J. 186
Garneti, N. 201
Garrett, W.E., Jr. 42, 43t, 117,
    118, 140-141, 164-166, 173, 188
Gelberman, R.H. 242
Gennarelli, T.A. 251, 260-262
Gentil, P. 118
Gheidi, N. 201
Giangarra, C.E. 230
Giannini, S. 108
Giaroli, E.L. 217
Giddings, V.L. 201
Gindele, A. 162
Giza, C.C. 255, 259
Goff, J.D. 203
Gokcen, E.C. 156
Goldberg, B.A. 219
Goldblatt, J. 176
Goldsmith, W. 260
Goldspink, G. 117
Gorbaty, J.D. 123
Gornitzky, A.L. 172
Grabiner, M.D. 158
Graham, D.I. 251, 261
Grana, W. 231
Grauer, J.N. 269
Gregor, R.J. 100
Griffin, L.Y. 172, 173
Grindem, H. 176, 177t
Grobler, L.J. 277
Grogan, D.P. 28
Grood, E.S. 179
Gross, A.G. 260
Guilak, F. 178
Gulati, P. 266t
Gulli, B. 189
Guntern, D.V. 217
Gurdjian, E.S. 250, 260
Guskiewicz, K.M. 259
Gusmer, P.G. 144f

H
Haagsma, J.A. 3
Haahr, J.P. 230
Haddad, F. 117
Hafner, R.A. 240
Haizlip, K.M. 118
Hakkinen, K. 118
Halder, A.M. 218
Hallén, L.G. 167
Hammad, Y.N. 191
Hampson, D. 252, 252f
Handelberg, F. 225
Hansen, S.T. 163
Harmon, K.G. 259, 260
Harner, C.D. 179
Harris, W.H. 137
Harryman, D.T. 214
Hart, C. 268
Hartgens, F. 126
Harwood, F.L. 115

Hatta, T. 210
Haug, R.H. 251
Hawes, M.C. 275
Hawkins, R.H. 221
Hayes, W.C. 132, 157, 182, 183
Haygood, T.M. 220
Healey, J.H. 227
Heil, J. 13, 14, 14t
Hengsberger, S. 108
Hennessy, O. 227
Hennrikus, W.L. 215
Herman, M.J. 277
Hertel, J. 38
Hertel, R. 211
Herzog, M.M. 200
Hetland, M.L. 110
Hewett, T. 177
Hey, H.W.D. 242
Hicks, J.H. 204f
Hierton, C. 162
Higgins, L.D. 209
Hillen, B. 115
Hiney, K.M. 109
Hipp, J.A. 132
Hirano, A. 184
Hirthler, M.A. 6
Hodgson, V.R. 250, 252
Hogg, N.J. 251
Holbourn, A.H.S. 256-257, 260
Holdsworth, F.W. 274
Homer (poet) 6
Hopper, R.H. 252
Horii, E. 242
Horton, W.E. 136
Horvath, F. 210
Hosey, R.G. 179
Hotchkiss, R.N. 230, 234
Hotfiel, T. 143
Houston, C.S. 169
Hovda, D.A. 259
Howe, T.E. 109
Hoy, D. 136
Hubbard, M. 91
Hubbell, J.D. 172
Huberti, H.H. 180, 182, 183
Hughes, T.B. 242
Hull, M.L. 192
Hulme, A. 11
Hungerford, D.S. 182
Hunt, K.J. 200
Hurschler, C. 188
Hutchinson, M.R. 219
Hutchison, R.L. 6
Hutton, W.C. 281

I
Ichikawa, M. 15
Ikai, M. 118
Ikata, T. 277
Inman, V.T. 197
Inoue, M. 180
Ireland, M.L. 176, 177
Ito, S. 270
Itoi, E. 221
Ivarsson, A. 13
Iwamoto, J. 109

J
Jackson, B. 160
Jacobson, S.R. 220

Jacofsky, D.J. 138
Jarvholm, B. 160
Järvinen, T.A. 201
Jin, M. 113
Jobe, C.M. 223, 225
Jobe, F. 218, 233
Joglekar, S.B. 161
John, T. 233
Johnell, O. 156, 189
Jokl, P.J. 161, 162
Jones, I.A. 126
Jove, F.W. 186
Józsa, L. 139, 202, 230
Julian, M.J. 144f
Jupiter, J.B. 236-238

K
Kadi, F. 116
Kaeding, C.C. 172
Kanis, J. 10, 132, 156
Kannus, P. 139, 171, 230
Kany, J. 222
Kaplan, F.S. 107f
Kaplan, H. 227
Karacan, I. 268
Karakoc, Y. 222
Kasashima, Y. 115
Kaur, R. 219
Kayhanian, S. 6
Keele, K.D. 8
Keener, J.D. 218, 223
Kegler, S.R. 4
Kellam, J.F. 236
Kellersmann, R. 184
Kelly, B.C. 222
Kennett, K. 252
Kery, L. 210
Khaund, R. 185
Khedr, H. 215
Kibler, W.B. 191, 203, 232
Kim, A.W. 238
Kim, J.M. 238
Kim, S.H. 225-227
Kim, T.K. 225
King, J.B. 162
Kirk, K.L. 185
Kirking, B. 76
Kjaer, M. 115
Klemt, C. 214, 215t
Koh, T.J. 240
Komi, P.V. 118, 201
Kon, K. 165f
Kopiczko, A. 108
Korpelainen, R. 109
Kosmopoulos, A. 109
Koulouris, G. 165
Koutserimpas, C. 6
Kransdorf, M.J. 162
Kraushaar, B.S. 230
Krissoff, W.B. 164
Kristensen, S.S. 240
Kristman, V.L. 258
Kucera, K.L. 255
Kühne, C.A. 251
Kuipers, H. 126
Kujala, U.M. 202
Kukkonen, J. 221
Kumar, G. 158-159
Kumar, N. 266t, 273
Kumar, S. 270
Kvist, M. 201

L

Labriola, J.E. 214
Ladenhauf, H.N. 184
Lädermann, A. 218, 222
La Fata, P.C. 203
Lam, F. 159
Lambers Heerspink, F.O. 221
Lambert, S.M. 211
Lange, T. 183
Langlois, J.A. 255, 259
Lanyon, L.E. 106
La Porta, G.A. 203
LaPrade, C.M. 171
Lau, S. 204
Lauritzen, J.B. 157
Lawrence, R.C. 137
Lawrence, R.L. 223
Leach, R.E. 231
Leadbetter, W.B. 122, 123, 162
LeBlanc, K.E. 157
Lee, H.L. 161
Lee, J.H. 109
Lee, S. 136
Lehman, C. 223
Leong, N.L. 140
Lestini, W.F. 270
LeVay, D. 7, 9
Levin, P.E. 158, 159
Levine, R. 267f
Levine, W.N. 220
Levy, A.S. 192
Lewiecki, E.M. 156
Li, F. 117
Lieber, R.L. 164
Lieberman, D.E. 109
Lievense, A.M. 161
Lim, L.H. 251
Lin, D.J. 218
Lindahl, O. 167
Linder, M.M. 126
Linko, E. 175
Linnamo, V. 118
Lippitt, S. 214
Lisfranc, J. 204
Liu, D. 108
Liu, J. 222
Livingston, M. 126
Lo, I.K.Y. 25, 34, 37, 48, 112
Lo, S.L. 241
Lofman, O. 156
Loitz-Ramage, B.J. 104, 109, 111
London, D.A. 238
Long, W.T. 164
Longo, U.G. 139
Lord, S. 273
Lorentzon, M. 109
Lorentzon, R. 261
Lorenz, D.S. 116
Louw, M. 185
Lowe, T.G. 275
Luan, F. 273
Lyman, S. 175

M

Macaluso, A. 116
MacDougall, J. 110, 116
Machado, R.J. 6
MacNab, I. 277
MacPherson, J.N. 30
Maddalozzo, G.G. 110
Maffet, M.W. 225

Maffulli, N. 201, 203
Maggi, S. 156
Magnusson, H.I. 189
Mahan, K.T. 201
Makhmalbaf, H. 123
Malcarney, H.L. 216
Mandelbaum, B.R. 177
Mankin, H.J. 113, 136
Mansi, O. 11
Marazzi, P. 162f
Marcus, R. 108, 110
Markolf, K.L. 171, 173, 240
Marks, R. 156
Martin, R.B. 32, 32t, 103-106
Martland, H.S. 255
Mathews, M. 144f
Matsen, F. 214
Matsuda, J.J. 104
Matsumoto, K. 159
Mauntel, T.C. 200
Max, W. 12
Maxwell, W.L. 261
McArdle, W.D. 116
McBirnie, J. 192
McCall, G.E. 116
McCormack, S. 107, 270
McCormick, E.J. 13
McCrea, M. 259
McCrory, P. 255, 258-261
McElhaney, J.H. 265, 266
McFarland, E.G. 217
McKee, A. 245
McLean, A. 219
McLean, S. 173, 177
McMaster, P.E. 140
McNulty, A.L. 178
Medici, D. 163
Meeuwisse, W.H. 10, 11f, 231-232
Mehlman, C.T. 184
Mehta, J. 110
Mellion, M.B. 144f
Melton, L.J., III 156, 271
Mengiardi, B. 213
Merola, M. 138
Meythaler, J.M. 261
Michelson, J.D. 157
Michener, L.A. 221
Mihalik, J.P. 260
Milette, P.C. 281
Milgrom, C. 223
Miller, J.D. 258
Miller, J.K. 231
Miller, N.H. 275
Miller, T.R. 126
Millstein, E.S. 222
Milne, A.A. 5
Minagawa, H. 223
Miyasaka, K.C. 172
Moen, M.H. 189
Moffatt, C.B. 40
Monma, H. 158
Montalvo, A.M. 173
Monteggia, G. 236-238
Moorman, C.T., III 159
Moosmayer, S. 221
Morel, V. 34
Morgan, C.D. 225
Morgan, J. 116
Morris, M. 230
Morse, K.W. 160
Mote, C.D. 192

Mow, V.C. 111, 112
Mozingo, J.D. 219
Mubarak, S.J. 189f
Mueller-Wohlfahrt, H.-W. 142
Mullner, T. 115
Mulvad, B. 189
Murata, Y. 277
Murray, M.M. 172
Murrell, G.A.C. 216
Murrie, V.L. 276-277
Musumeci, G. 113
Myer, G. 173, 177
Myklebust, G. 177
Mylonas, A.I. 6

N

Nachemson, A. 280
Nahum, A.M. 252
Nakamura, R. 240
Nam, E.K. 223
Natarajan, R.N. 277
Navas, P.Z. 157
Nazari, G. 222
Needell, S. 200f
Neer, C. 221
Nestor, B.J. 234
Neuman, M. 251
Neviaser, J.S. 213
Newton, I. 62-63, 65, 68, 269, 278
Nezwek, T. 22
Nickien, M. 100
Nicolle, C.J.H. 100
Nightingale, F. 8, 8f
Nirschl, R.P. 230
Nixon, H.L. 14
Noiseux, N. 137
Noonan, T.J. 165-166
Nordt, W.E., III 217
Norman, A. 162
Nottage, W.M. 221
Nowinski, R.J. 184
Noyes, F.R. 177

O

O'Brien, M. 110
O'Donoghue, D.H. 122, 175, 191
O'Driscoll, S.W. 234
Offierski, C.M. 277
Oftadeh, R. 101
Oganov, V.S. 109
Ogata, S. 219
Ogden, J.A. 27-29
Oinas, J. 34
Old, J.L. 271
Olsen, B.R. 163
Omalu, B. 255
Ommaya, A.K. 257-258, 260, 262
Opar, D.A. 165
Orava, S. 163
Orchard, J.W. 164
Ormerod, S. 110
Osgood, R.B. 184
Ott, S.M. 177
Owings, T.M. 158

P

Padman, R. 274, 275
Padua, L. 241
Pajala, A. 203
Paley, K.J. 218
Palmes, D. 115
Panjabi, M.M. 269, 270, 274

Papadimitropoulos, E.A. 156
Pappachan, B. 252f
Parent, S. 275
Parker, L. 216f
Parkinson, R.W. 158-159
Parry, D.A.D. 25
Parry, H.A. 117
Parsons, I.M. 222
Partridge, N.C. 106
Passeri, L.A. 251
Pastakia, K. 270
Paul, J. 174
Pavol, M.J. 158
Pearson, A.M. 269, 270
Pellman, E.J. 259
Penrose, J.H. 237
Perry, J.J. 209
Petersen, W. 177
Peterson, L. 164, 168, 173, 179, 180, 184, 185, 203, 211
Pettrone, F. 230
Petushek, E.J. 177
Phalen, G.S. 241
Philippe, P. 11
Pimentel Neto, J. 117
Pink, M. 218
Pintar, F.A. 250, 265
Piper, C.C. 221
Piziali, R.L. 179
Platt, M.A. 117
Plunkett, J. 260
Poca, M.A. 262
Poppe, T. 205
Poroy, D. 211f
Potter, H.G. 144f
Pourcelot, P. 201
Pouresmaeili, F. 132
Powell, J.W. 261
Powers, C.M. 180-181, 183
Praemer, A. 225, 234, 241
Prato, N. 219
Priest, J.D. 230
Prieto, V. 215
Proske, U. 166
Ptasznik, R. 227

Q

Quarles, J.D. 179
Quintana, J.M. 160

R

Radanov, B.P. 273
Radford, W.J.P. 188
Ramirez, R.N. 177
Rang, M. 6
Raskin, K.B. 238
Rasool, M.N. 234
Raviola, E. 24, 25
Rebuzzi, E. 222
Reddy, A.S. 218
Redmond, C.J. 12
Reed, W. 102-103
Reeves, N.D. 202
Reginster, J.-Y. 132
Rehman, S. 161
Ren, Y. 156
Renström, P. 164, 168, 173, 179, 180, 184, 185, 203, 211
Rettig, A.C. 234
Rettig, M.E. 238
Revak, A. 201
Reyes, J.J.B. 38

Rhee, J.S. 251
Ribbans, W.J. 203
Ricard-Blum, S. 25
Rice, D.P. 12
Robertson, L.S. 5, 65
Robinovitch, S.N. 157
Robinson, C.M. 213
Robinson, T. 109
Rockwood, C.A., Jr. 222
Romeo, A. 222
Rose, P.S. 184
Rosier, R.N. 30
Ross, A.C. 108
Ross, M.D. 184
Rossettini, G. 162
Rothwell, A.G. 162
Roux, C.H. 161
Rowson, S. 255, 260
Rubin, C.T. 106
Ruby, L.K. 242
Rudert, M.J. 76
Rudy, B.S. 215
Runge, J.W. 12
Ruotolo, C. 221
Russell, W.R. 258
Rydevik, B. 271t

S

Sabbagh, M.D. 242
Safran, M.R. 196, 231
Sahuquillo, J. 262
Salem, G. 141f, 142f, 143f, 183
Salsich, G.B. 182
Salter, R.B. 29, 133, 169
Samilson, R.L. 215
Sanders, M.S. 13
Sands, W.A. 29
Sano, K. 257f
Santucci, R.A. 254
Sarafrazi, N. 131f
Sauerbrey, A.M. 222
Saunders, W.B. 189f
Sayit, E. 240
Schemitsch, C. 221
Schepsis, A.A. 188, 200, 201
Schlatter, C. 184
Schmidt, A.H. 188
Schneider, D.C. 252
Schneider, H.P. 203
Schoenfeld, B.J. 116
Schroeder, G.D. 274
Schwartz, E. 172
Scott, S.H. 203
Seedhom, B.B. 178
Seering, W.P. 179
Seinfeld, J. 51
Senderovich, H. 109
Seow, D. 205
Seth, A. 93
Severy, D.M. 273
Shahpari, O. 123
Shaker, J. 32
Shapiro, J.D. 191
Shapiro, M.S. 219
Shepherd, J.A. 131f
Sher, J.S. 223
Shim, S.S. 30
Shiri, R. 231
Si, L. 132
Sibley, T. 178, 184
Siddiqui, J.A. 106

Siegler, S. 197
Siliski, J.M. 178
Silva, L.P. 215
Silver, F.H. 25, 34
Silverstein, B. 242
Simon, S.R. 43t, 107f
Singer, M. 130
Singh, K. 113
Singh, N. 172
Slater, L.V. 39
Smith, E.U.R. 136
Smith, F.M. 237
Smith, R.B. 215
Snijders, C.J. 231
Snow-Harter, C. 110
Snyder, S.J. 222-225
Sokolove, P.E. 252
Solomonow, M. 37
Sorrenti, S.J. 115
Soslowsky, L.J. 219
Specker, B. 109
Speed, J.S. 237
Speer, K.P. 174-175, 214
Spilker, R.L. 178
Squire, J.M. 25
Stanitski, C.L. 178
Stannard, J.P. 171
Stansfield, B.W. 76
Staubli, H.U. 181
Staud, R. 108
Steffen, K. 69
Stehbens, W.E. 275
Sterett, W.I. 164
Stevenson, H. 176
Stinson, J.T. 278
Stødle, A.H. 204
Stoll, L.E. 222
St-Onge, N. 175
Suchman, E. 5
Sugita, T. 158
Suh, N. 242
Sullivan, L.H. 19
Sunderland, S. 146
Sureka, B. 266t
Surve, I. 38
Sushruta (surgeon) 5
Suva, L.J. 106, 107, 109
Swartz, E.E. 260
Swenson, D.R. 163
Swenson, T.M. 179
Swinney, C. 6
Swischuk, L.E. 169

T

Tabata, S. 221
Tajbakhsh, S. 117
Taneja, A.K. 215
Tanzer, M. 137
Tarazi, N. 184
Tashjian, R.Z. 223
Taylor, A.H. 114
Taylor, B. 126
Taylor, F. 219
Tearse, D. 190
Tegner, Y. 261
Teitz, C. 217
Templehof, S. 223
Templeman, D. 189
Thackeray, W.M. 121
Thelen, D.G. 165
Thigpen, C.A. 222-223

Thomas, J.L. 203
Thomas, L.M. 250
Thomeé, R. 183
Thompson, D. 99
Thorsness, R. 222
Tidball, J.G. 37, 117, 140, 141, 141f, 142f, 143f
Tierney, R.T. 259
Tipton, C.M. 115
Toivonen, D.A. 220
Tompkins, D.G. 237
Tossy, J.D. 211
Tosti, R. 230
Tothill, P. 30
Tran, N.T. 274
Trinick, J. 41
Trojian, T. 203
Tshovrebova, L. 41
Tucker, A.K. 203
Tuite, M.J. 219
Tuukkanen, J. 109
Tuzun, C. 276
Tytherleigh-Strong, G. 227

U

Uhthoff, H.K. 219
Ulreich, R. 216f
Upadhyay, S.S. 159
Updegrove, G.F. 225
Urabe, Y. 177

V

Vaitkeviciute, D. 107
Valsamis, M.P. 256
van den Bogert, A.J. 158
van den Kroonenberg, A.J. 157
van der Worp, M.P. 185
Vanek, D. 201
van Kuijk, K.S.R. 171, 177
Van Pelt, K.L. 255, 259
van Rijn, R.M. 230
Varacallo, M. 22, 225
Vavken, P. 172
Vaz, S. 219
Veenstra, M.A. 219
Venes, D. 191
Veronese, N. 156
Verrall, G.M. 165, 166
Verzijl, N. 160
Vesalius, A. 7, 7f
Viidik, A. 92
Viikari-Juntura, E. 242
Villard, D. 184
Volgas, D.A. 253-254
Vos, T. 3
Vuori, J.-P. 204
Vynios, D.H. 34

W

Wackerhage, H. 116
Walch, G. 217, 225
Walczak, B.E. 163
Walker, J.M. 113
Walker, P. 178
Wambogo, E.A. 131f
Wang, J.C. 219
Ward, S.R. 183
Warner, J.J. 222
Watkins, R.G. 268, 269, 279
Watkins, W.G. 268, 269
Watson, J.T. 192

Watts, J.D. 211
Weber, E.R. 242
Webster, J.E. 250
Webster, M. 255
Wegner, D.R. 276
Weinkamer, R. 106
Weinstein, P.R. 270
Weisenbach, C.A. 252f
Weiss, R.J. 163
Weissmann, G. 130
Werner, R.A. 242
Werner, S.L. 231
Westerhoff, P. 76
Whaley, A.L. 230
White, S. 189
Whiting, W.C. 31f, 45t, 46t, 47t, 58f, 59f, 61f, 65f, 74f, 75f, 196f, 275f
Wiebe, D.J. 255, 260
Wiesel, S.W. 270
Wilkins, K.E. 236
Wilkinson, G.T. 226
Williams, E. 268
Williams, G.R. 211, 221, 222
Williams, J.H. 69
Williams, L.A. 279
Williams, P.E. 117
Wilmore, J.H. 118
Wilson, F.D. 231
Wind, W.M. 171
Winquist, R.A. 163
Winter, D.A. 76, 203
Winters, M. 189
Wirth, M.A. 222
Wiss, D.A. 164
Wittenberg, R.H. 221
Wojtys, E.M. 177
Wong, J. 201
Woo, S.L.-Y. 35, 37, 114, 115f, 139, 140, 173, 175
Worland, R.L. 223
Worrell, T.W. 165
Wotherspoon, S. 252
Wren, T.A.L. 115f
Wright, P.R. 238
Wright, T.M. 72
Wright, V. 178
Wunderle, K. 259

Y

Yamada, H. 103
Yamaguchi, K. 218
Yates, B. 189-190
Yin, H. 116, 117
Yinger, K. 201, 203
Yoganandan, N. 250, 252, 265, 266, 268, 269, 273
Youm, T. 222
Yu, B. 173

Z

Zantop, T. 202
Zelzer, E. 28
Zernicke, R.F. 93f, 104, 108, 109, 111, 113, 115f, 141f, 142f, 143f, 186, 192
Zhang, K. 178
Zhang, L. 260
Zioupos, P. 105
Zuckerman, J.D. 220

About the Authors

Ronald F. Zernicke, PhD, DSc, is a professor at the University of Michigan's medical center (department of orthopedic surgery), school of kinesiology, and department of biomedical engineering. He is also the director of the University of Michigan Exercise & Sport Science Initiative.

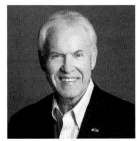

Courtesy of Kathleen Zernicke

Before moving to Ann Arbor in 2007, Zernicke was a professor and the chair of the department of kinesiology at the University of California, Los Angeles (UCLA). At the University of Calgary he was a professor for joint injury research (department of surgery, Cumming School of Medicine), the dean of kinesiology (1998-2005), and a professor of engineering. Zernicke was the executive director of the Alberta Bone and Joint Health Institute and served as director of the Alberta Provincial CIHR training program in bone and joint health, a combined graduate program of the University of Calgary and University of Alberta.

Zernicke has taught courses in biomechanics and injury mechanisms at the university level for more than 45 years. He received the UCLA Distinguished Teaching Award as well as the City of Calgary Community Achievement Award in Education. He has authored more than 545 peer-reviewed research publications and two books, including the first two editions of this book, which received the Preeminent Scholarly Publication Award from California State University at Northridge (CSUN) in 2002.

Steven P. Broglio, PhD, is a professor of kinesiology and adjunct professor of neurology and of physical medicine and rehabilitation at the University of Michigan in Ann Arbor. Broglio completed his training at the University

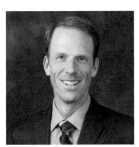

Courtesy of the University of Michigan

of Georgia, took his first faculty position at the University of Illinois at Urbana-Champaign, and has been at the University of Michigan since 2011.

At Michigan, Broglio is the director of the Michigan Concussion Center and the NeuroTrauma Research Laboratory, where he oversees clinical care, educational outreach, and multidisciplinary research aimed at fundamental questions on concussion prevention, identification, diagnosis, management, and outcomes. His research has been supported by the National Athletic Trainers' Association Research and Education Foundation, the National Institutes of Health, the National Collegiate Athletic Association, and the Department of Defense. Broglio was awarded the Early Career Investigator Award by the International Brain Injury Association as well as the Early Career and Outstanding Research awards by the National Athletic Trainers' Association. He was awarded fellowship in the American College of Sports Medicine, National Athletic Trainers' Association, and National Academy of Kinesiology.

William C. Whiting, PhD, is a professor and codirector of the biomechanics laboratory in the department of kinesiology at California State University at Northridge (CSUN) and an adjunct professor in the department of physiological science at the University of California, Los Angeles (UCLA). He has taught undergraduate and graduate courses in biomechanics and human anatomy for more than 40 years. As an author and researcher, Whiting has written more than 60 research articles, abstracts, and book chapters as well as the book Dynamic Human Anatomy, Second Edition.

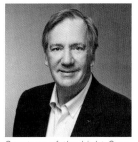

Courtesy of the Light Committee

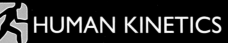

HUMAN KINETICS

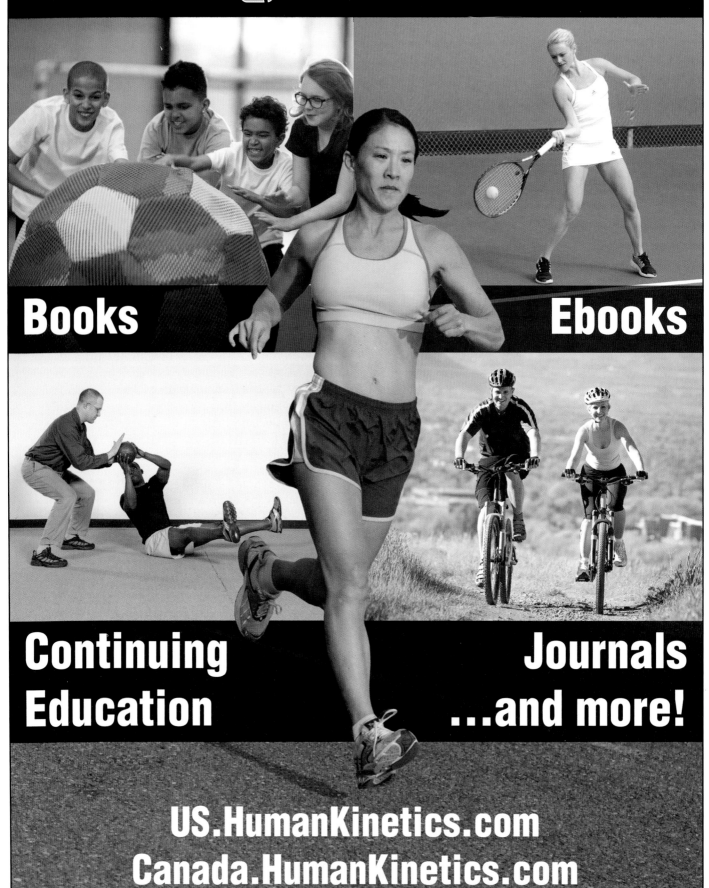

Books

Ebooks

Continuing Education

Journals ...and more!

US.HumanKinetics.com
Canada.HumanKinetics.com